SURFACTANT THERAPY FOR LUNG DISEASE

LUNG BIOLOGY IN HEALTH AND DISEASE

Executive Editor

Claude Lenfant
Director, National Heart, Lung and Blood Institute
National Institutes of Health
Bethesda, Maryland

1. Immunologic and Infectious Reactions in the Lung, *edited by Charles H. Kirkpatrick and Herbert Y. Reynolds*
2. The Biochemical Basis of Pulmonary Function, *edited by Ronald G. Crystal*
3. Bioengineering Aspects of the Lung, *edited by John B. West*
4. Metabolic Functions of the Lung, *edited by Y. S. Bakhle and John R. Vane*
5. Respiratory Defense Mechanisms (in two parts), *edited by Joseph D. Brain, Donald F. Proctor, and Lynne M. Reid*
6. Development of the Lung, *edited by W. Alan Hodson*
7. Lung Water and Solute Exchange, *edited by Norman C. Staub*
8. Extrapulmonary Manifestations of Respiratory Disease, *edited by Eugene Debs Robin*
9. Chronic Obstructive Pulmonary Disease, *edited by Thomas L. Petty*
10. Pathogenesis and Therapy of Lung Cancer, *edited by Curtis C. Harris*
11. Genetic Determinants of Pulmonary Disease, *edited by Stephen D. Litwin*
12. The Lung in the Transition Between Health and Disease, *edited by Peter T. Macklem and Solbert Permutt*
13. Evolution of Respiratory Processes: A Comparative Approach, *edited by Stephen C. Wood and Claude Lenfant*
14. Pulmonary Vascular Diseases, *edited by Kenneth M. Moser*
15. Physiology and Pharmacology of the Airways, *edited by Jay A. Nadel*
16. Diagnostic Techniques in Pulmonary Disease (in two parts), *edited by Marvin A. Sackner*
17. Regulation of Breathing (in two parts), *edited by Thomas F. Hornbein*
18. Occupational Lung Diseases: Research Approaches and Methods, *edited by Hans Weill and Margaret Turner-Warwick*
19. Immunopharmacology of the Lung, *edited by Harold H. Newball*
20. Sarcoidosis and Other Granulomatous Diseases of the Lung, *edited by Barry L. Fanburg*
21. Sleep and Breathing, *edited by Nicholas A. Saunders and Colin E. Sullivan*
22. *Pneumocystis carinii* Pneumonia: Pathogenesis, Diagnosis, and Treatment, *edited by Lowell S. Young*

23. Pulmonary Nuclear Medicine: Techniques in Diagnosis of Lung Disease, *edited by Harold L. Atkins*
24. Acute Respiratory Failure, *edited by Warren M. Zapol and Konrad J. Falke*
25. Gas Mixing and Distribution in the Lung, *edited by Ludwig A. Engel and Manuel Paiva*
26. High-Frequency Ventilation in Intensive Care and During Surgery, *edited by Graziano Carlon and William S. Howland*
27. Pulmonary Development: Transition from Intrauterine to Extrauterine Life, *edited by George H. Nelson*
28. Chronic Obstructive Pulmonary Disease: Second Edition, Revised and Expanded, *edited by Thomas L. Petty*
29. The Thorax (in two parts), *edited by Charis Roussos and Peter T. Macklem*
30. The Pleura in Health and Disease, *edited by Jacques Chrétien, Jean Bignon, and Albert Hirsch*
31. Drug Therapy for Asthma: Research and Clinical Practice, *edited by John W. Jenne and Shirley Murphy*
32. Pulmonary Endothelium in Health and Disease, *edited by Una S. Ryan*
33. The Airways: Neural Control in Health and Disease, *edited by Michael A. Kaliner and Peter J. Barnes*
34. Pathophysiology and Treatment of Inhalation Injuries, *edited by Jacob Loke*
35. Respiratory Function of the Upper Airway, *edited by Oommen P. Mathew and Giuseppe Sant'Ambrogio*
36. Chronic Obstructive Pulmonary Disease: A Behavioral Perspective, *edited by A. John McSweeny and Igor Grant*
37. Biology of Lung Cancer: Diagnosis and Treatment, *edited by Steven T. Rosen, James L. Mulshine, Frank Cuttitta, and Paul G. Abrams*
38. Pulmonary Vascular Physiology and Pathophysiology, *edited by E. Kenneth Weir and John T. Reeves*
39. Comparative Pulmonary Physiology: Current Concepts, *edited by Stephen C. Wood*
40. Respiratory Physiology: An Analytical Approach, *edited by H. K. Chang and Manuel Paiva*
41. Lung Cell Biology, *edited by Donald Massaro*
42. Heart–Lung Interactions in Health and Disease, *edited by Steven M. Scharf and Sharon S. Cassidy*
43. Clinical Epidemiology of Chronic Obstructive Pulmonary Disease, *edited by Michael J. Hensley and Nicholas A. Saunders*
44. Surgical Pathology of Lung Neoplasms, *edited by Alberto M. Marchevsky*
45. The Lung in Rheumatic Diseases, *edited by Grant W. Cannon and Guy A. Zimmerman*
46. Diagnostic Imaging of the Lung, *edited by Charles E. Putman*
47. Models of Lung Disease: Microscopy and Structural Methods, *edited by Joan Gil*

48. Electron Microscopy of the Lung, *edited by Dean E. Schraufnagel*
49. Asthma: Its Pathology and Treatment, *edited by Michael A. Kaliner, Peter J. Barnes, and Carl G. A. Persson*
50. Acute Respiratory Failure: Second Edition, *edited by Warren M. Zapol and Francois Lemaire*
51. Lung Disease in the Tropics, *edited by Om P. Sharma*
52. Exercise: Pulmonary Physiology and Pathophysiology, *edited by Brian J. Whipp and Karlman Wasserman*
53. Developmental Neurobiology of Breathing, *edited by Gabriel G. Haddad and Jay P. Farber*
54. Mediators of Pulmonary Inflammation, *edited by Michael A. Bray and Wayne H. Anderson*
55. The Airway Epithelium, *edited by Stephen G. Farmer and Douglas Hay*
56. Physiological Adaptations in Vertebrates: Respiration, Circulation, and Metabolism, *edited by Stephen C. Wood, Roy E. Weber, Alan R. Hargens, and Ronald W. Millard*
57. The Bronchial Circulation, *edited by John Butler*
58. Lung Cancer Differentiation: Implications for Diagnosis and Treatment, *edited by Samuel D. Bernal and Paul J. Hesketh*
59. Pulmonary Complications of Systemic Disease, *edited by John F. Murray*
60. Lung Vascular Injury: Molecular and Cellular Response, *edited by Arnold Johnson and Thomas J. Ferro*
61. Cytokines of the Lung, *edited by Jason Kelley*
62. The Mast Cell in Health and Disease, *edited by Michael A. Kaliner and Dean D. Metcalfe*
63. Pulmonary Disease in the Elderly Patient, *edited by Donald A. Mahler*
64. Cystic Fibrosis, *edited by Pamela B. Davis*
65. Signal Transduction in Lung Cells, *edited by Jerome S. Brody, David M. Center, and Vsevolod A. Tkachuk*
66. Tuberculosis: A Comprehensive International Approach, *edited by Lee B. Reichman and Earl S. Hershfield*
67. Pharmacology of the Respiratory Tract: Experimental and Clinical Research, *edited by K. Fan Chung and Peter J. Barnes*
68. Prevention of Respiratory Diseases, *edited by Albert Hirsch, Marcel Goldberg, Jean-Pierre Martin, and Roland Masse*
69. *Pneumocystis carinii* Pneumonia: Second Edition, Revised and Expanded, *edited by Peter D. Walzer*
70. Fluid and Solute Transport in the Airspaces of the Lungs, *edited by Richard M. Effros and H. K. Chang*
71. Sleep and Breathing: Second Edition, Revised and Expanded, *edited by Nicholas A. Saunders and Colin E. Sullivan*
72. Airway Secretion: Physiological Bases for the Control of Mucous Hypersecretion, *edited by Tamotsu Takishima and Sanae Shimura*
73. Sarcoidosis and Other Granulomatous Disorders, *edited by D. Geraint James*
74. Epidemiology of Lung Cancer, *edited by Jonathan M. Samet*

75. Pulmonary Embolism, *edited by Mario Morpurgo*
76. Sports and Exercise Medicine, *edited by Stephen C. Wood and Robert C. Roach*
77. Endotoxin and the Lungs, *edited by Kenneth L. Brigham*
78. The Mesothelial Cell and Mesothelioma, *edited by Marie-Claude Jaurand and Jean Bignon*
79. Regulation of Breathing: Second Edition, Revised and Expanded, *edited by Jerome A. Dempsey and Allan I. Pack*
80. Pulmonary Fibrosis, *edited by Sem Hin Phan and Roger S. Thrall*
81. Long-Term Oxygen Therapy: Scientific Basis and Clinical Application, *edited by Walter J. O'Donohue, Jr.*
82. Ventral Brainstem Mechanisms and Control of Respiration and Blood Pressure, *edited by C. Ovid Trouth, Richard M. Millis, Heidrun F. Kiwull-Schöne, and Marianne E. Schläfke*
83. A History of Breathing Physiology, *edited by Donald F. Proctor*
84. Surfactant Therapy for Lung Disease, *edited by Bengt Robertson and H. William Taeusch*

ADDITIONAL VOLUMES IN PREPARATION

The Thorax: Second Edition, Revised and Expanded (in three parts), *edited by Charis Roussos*

Severe Asthma: Pathogenesis and Clinical Management, *edited by Stanley Szefler and Donald Y. M. Leung*

Respiratory Sensation, *edited by Lewis Adams and Abraham Guz*

Mycobacterium avium–Complex Infection: Progress in Research and Treatment, *edited by Joyce A. Korvick and Constance A. Benson*

Alpha 1–Antitrypsin Deficiency: Biology · Pathogenesis · Clinical Manifestations · Therapy, *edited by Ronald G. Crystal*

Adhesion Molecules and the Lung, *edited by Peter A. Ward and Joseph C. Fantone*

Acute Respiratory Failure in Chronic Obstructive Pulmonary Disease, *edited by Jean-Phillippe Derenne, W. A. Whitelaw, and Thomas Similowski*

Pulmonary Rehabilitation, *edited by Alfred P. Fishman*

SURFACTANT THERAPY FOR LUNG DISEASE

Edited by

Bengt Robertson
Karolinska Institute
Stockholm, Sweden

H. William Taeusch
University of California, San Francisco, and
San Francisco General Hospital
San Francisco, California

Marcel Dekker, Inc. **New York • Basel • Hong Kong**

Library of Congress Cataloging-in-Publication Data

Surfactant therapy for lung disease / edited by Bengt Robertson, H. William Taeusch.
p. cm. — (Lung biology in health and disease ; v.84)
Includes bibliographical references and indexes.
ISBN 0-8247-9502-4 (hardcover : alk. paper)
1. Respiratory distress syndrome—Chemotherapy. 2. Pulmonary surfactant—Therapeutic use. I. Robertson, Bengt. II. Taeusch, H. William. III. Series.
[DNLM: 1. Pulmonary Surfactants—therapeutic use. 2. Pulmonary Surfactants—physiology. 3. Respiratory Distress Syndrome—therapy. 4. Respiratory Distress Syndrome—physiopathology. 5. Lung Diseases—therapy. W1 LU62 v. 84 1995 / WF 600 S9625 1995]
RC776.R38S88 1995
616.2'4—dc20
DNLM/DLC
for Library of Congress 95-22122
CIP

The publisher offers discounts on this book when ordered in bulk quantities. For more information, write to Special Sales/Professional Marketing at the address below.

This book is printed on acid-free paper.

Marcel Dekker, Inc.
270 Madison Avenue, New York, New York 10016

Current printing (last digit):
10 9 8 7 6 5 4 3 2 1

PRINTED IN THE UNITED STATES OF AMERICA

INTRODUCTION

> An almost perfect model of an interdisciplinary approach to determining the cause and learning how to diagnose, prevent and treat a serious disease, has been the virtually total understanding of the respiratory distress syndrome.
>
> —Julius H. Comroe,
> in *Advances in American Medicine: Essays at the Bicentennial*, 1976

Indeed, indeed!!

This book, *Surfactant Therapy for Lung Disease*, is almost the last chapter of a wonderful story that has spanned several decades. The exceptional value of this story stems from two very important facts. First, as implied by Comroe's statement, it illustrates how an almost Cartesian approach from very basic to applied research led to the understanding of a disease that constituted a major public health problem worldwide. Second, it shows how research conducted with foresight and perseverance gave us considerable mastery over a public health problem.

Although most of the scientific advances that led to our understanding of the pathogenesis of the neonatal respiratory distress syndrome were made in the second half of this century, none of them would have occurred without the description of the Theory of Capillary Action by Pierre Simon de Laplace in France at the beginning of the 19th century. Subsequently, the application of Laplaces's theorem by K. von Neergaard to his work on respiratory mechanics in the 1920s opened the door to a succession of major discoveries that were a tribute to interdisciplinary research. A model, indeed!

Premature birth, lung prematurity, and the resultant neonatal respiratory distress syndrome have for generations been the major cause of infant mortality in many countries, including the United States. But brilliant research led to the development of exogenous surfactant, and good medicine led to surfactant therapy. Granted, the death rate for neonatal respiratory distress syndrome began to decline with the use of ventilatory support, especially CPAP, and improvements in ancillary treatments. But, undoubtedly, the death rate reduction has accelerated with the use of exogenous surfactant therapy. As a result of decades of research, the number of deaths in the United States from this disease has declined by an order of magnitude, from more than 50,000 to less than 5000 per year.

This book ends with a postscript titled "Perspectives for the Future." The last year or so has revealed new insights on surfactant composition and determinants. It is safe to predict that the next chapter of this wonderful story will be in the domain of molecular medicine and gene therapy. But we must not fail to recognize that no matter how good that chapter will be, it would not be possible without the successes reported in this volume.

Drs. Robertson and Taeusch have assembled a roster of distinguished researchers and clinicians; in one way or another, they have been the architects of our understanding of neonatal respiratory distress syndrome. Since its beginning, this series of monographs Lung Biology in Health and Disease has included several volumes on this disease or on related aspects. However, the series would be incomplete without this volume. I am grateful to the editors and to the authors for giving me the opportunity to add the wonderful story of a "perfect model" to the series.

Claude Lenfant, M.D.
Bethesda, Maryland

FOREWORD

The late 1940s marked the increasing concern of pediatricians and pathologists with the most common cause of death in premature infants, respiratory distress; death followed within a few days after birth. The syndrome was called hyaline membrane disease after the most conspicuous histological finding, but it was soon realized that the sine qua non of the diagnosis was atelectasis, and the reaction to injury (hyaline membranes) depended on air breathing; that is, the findings were not seen in the first hour or so after birth, but worsened in the subsequent few days. Those infants who recovered usually did so within several days of birth, and recovery was usually complete by a week or so of age.

The subsequent decades have borne witness to the basic science that illuminated the role of the alveolar lining layer (pulmonary surfactant) in the pathogenesis of the disorder. Surfactant treatment for lung disease has its roots in the musings of alchemists, in the careful experiments of laboratory scientists, and in the brave, farsighted innovations of clinical pioneers. First one had to understand something of the physics of surfaces and of how chemicals modify them. Then one had to be curious about the bizarre stress-strain characteristics of the lung and how these are compatible with the sponge-like nature of the organ. Next there had to be a rapprochement of physics and chemistry and pulmonary physiology and the consequent discovery of intrinsic surface-active material, followed by the appreciation and demonstration that lack of the material might cause hyaline membrane disease.

Prenatal diagnosis of lung immaturity with respect to surfactant production made possible the use of hormonal stimulation by glucocorticoids in selected preterm infants. Knowledge that atelectasis was the consequence of deficient surfactant led to application of continuous distending airway pressure and appropriately designed ventilators. Deaths from hyaline membrane disease, synonymous with respiratory distress syndrome, were reduced by more than 75% by these interventions.

Further reduction in mortality and morbidity was made possible by continued elucidation of the physical and chemical properties of pulmonary surfactant. In 1980, Fujiwara and co-workers reported the first successful administration of bovine lung surfactant given as a liquid, instilled into the trachea of preterm infants with respiratory distress. Today, hyaline membrane disease is no longer the leading cause of neonatal deaths, and the subsequent morbidities of chronic lung disease and intraventricular hemorrhage are much reduced.

Now that this success is clear to all but the most committed therapeutic nihilists, there is a new flurry of activity, and new questions demand attention. Why do some babies fail to respond to surfactant treatment? Are better surfactants really needed? Will surfactant administration help patients with other lung diseases that cause atelectasis or small airway obstruction? Can surfactant metabolism be manipulated to the patient's advantage? Does surfactant have other important, but as yet unproved, actions? Are there feasible methods to prevent the pulmonary calamities that are presently being treated with surfactant before they occur? All these and many other issues discussed in this volume can profitably engage present-day surfactophiles.

The story of lung surfactant has not yet arrived at its last chapter. We compliment the authors of this volume for recognizing this fact and clearly pointing the way for future investigators.

Mary Ellen Avery, M.D.
Thomas Morgan Rotch Professor of Pediatrics
Department of Pediatrics
Harvard Medical School
Boston, Massachusetts

John A. Clements, M.D.
Julius H. Comroe Professor of Pulmonary Medicine
Professor of Pediatrics
Department of Pediatrics
University of California, San Francisco
San Francisco, California

PREFACE

The idea that lung disease might be amenable to treatment with exogenous surfactant was expressed as early as 1947 by the American pathologist Peter Gruenwald, who on the basis of postmortem lung pressure-volume recordings and histological observations postulated that ". . . the addition of surface active substances to the air or oxygen which is being spontaneously breathed in or introduced by a respirator might aid in relieving the initial atelectasis of newborn infants." Gruenwald's imaginative thinking did not get proper attention at that time and was not tested in experimental models or clinical practice until much later, when the basic biochemical, biophysical, and physiological properties of the pulmonary surfactant system were better understood. The scenario changed dramatically when the first successful clinical pilot studies of surfactant replacement were reported from Japan about 15 years ago, as a logical extension of experimental studies showing beneficial effects of this treatment in immature newborn animals. Since then, several thousand babies with respiratory distress syndrome have received various exogenous surfactants in controlled trials. The efficacy of this treatment has been confirmed, and surfactant therapy is now part of routine management of babies with immature lungs all over the world. Surfactant replacement is regarded by many as one of the major advances in neonatology in our time.

This rapid, recent clinical development has been paralleled by growing insight into the functional role of various surfactant components and the mechanisms by which exogenous surfactant exerts its therapeutic effect. Of particular interest in this context are the specific surfactant-associated hydrophilic and hydrophobic proteins. These proteins control important phases in the normal life cycle of endogenous surfactant, by regulating secretion, surface adsorption, and recycling of material desorbed from the air-liquid interface. At least the hydrophobic proteins seem to be essential components of exogenous surfactant preparations isolated from mammalian lungs. The hydrophilic surfactant proteins also serve in the pulmonary defense system, stimulating the phagocytosis of bacteria and viruses by alveolar macrophages.

Indications for surfactant substitution have widened in recent years, and promising results have been obtained with this therapy in babies with meconium aspiration and pneumonia. Controlled trials of surfactant therapy for adult respiratory distress syndrome are in progress. In these forms of respiratory failure, not caused by primary surfactant deficiency, the disturbance of surfactant function is probably caused by increased alveolar permeability with a vascular-to-alveolar leakage of plasma proteins interfering with surfactant function. The efficacy of surfactant treatment then depends on whether the exogenous material can resist inactivation by the plasma constituents. The sensitivity to inactivation apparently depends on the composition of the surfactant, especially on its content of the specific proteins referred to above. In infectious lung disease, possible interactions between the exogenous surfactant, alveolar macrophages, and invading bacteria may determine the result of surfactant therapy. These examples illustrate the complexity of the surfactant system and of the number of problems that need to be addressed in the development of surfactant substitutes and in the exploration of clinical targets for surfactant therapy.

This book opens with a section dealing with basic surfactant biophysics, physiology, and biochemistry. The background provided in these chapters is necessary for proper understanding of pathophysiological mechanisms interfering with surfactant function in various forms of lung disease. The major part of the book addresses clinical problems related to surfactant deficiency in immature babies and surfactant inactivation in various forms of inflammatory lung disease, and to the use of exogenous surfactant to compensate for these defects. Controlled clinical trials of surfactant replacement are reviewed in detail, and special chapters are devoted to techniques for administering surfactant, and to the combination of antenatal hormone and postnatal surfactant treatment for prevention of the respiratory distress syndrome. Dosage and timing of therapy and ventilator strategies for patients receiving surfactant are other important issues dealt with in separate chapters. Particular attention is paid also to lung mechanics, metabolic responses of the lung, and radiological, cardiovascular, and cerebral effects of surfactant replacement. Cost-benefit aspects of this new and, in many clinical situations, lifesaving therapy are analyzed in depth in another chapter.

The full potential of surfactant therapy remains to be established. We undertook the assignment to edit this volume in an optimistic mood because we believe there is still a lot to gain with growing experience in the field, and that this learning process can be accelerated by bringing together the ideas of leading experts representing basic science as well as clinical practice. This volume represents the joint work of no fewer than 57 authors. We are pleased that so many leaders in the field agreed to collaborate, and we thank all the contributing authors for their efforts to make this volume as complete and up to date as possible. Total concordance of ideas cannot be expected in a multiauthor volume of this format, but we hope that the diverging opinions will catalyze the creative thinking of the reader. We also wish to thank Christina Ingvarsson, Stockholm, and Cathy Duran, San Francisco, for excellent secretarial assistance throughout the editing of this book.

Bengt Robertson
H. Willliam Taeusch

CONTRIBUTORS

Gad Alpan, M.D. Associate Professor, Department of Neonatology, Johns Hopkins Bayview Medical Center, and Department of Pediatrics, Johns Hopkins University School of Medicine, Baltimore, Maryland

Mary Ellen Avery, M.D., Sc.D.(Hon.) Thomas Morgan Rotch Professor of Pediatrics, Harvard Medical School, Boston, Massachusetts

Hans Bachofen, M.D. Professor, Department of Medicine, Inselspital, University of Bern, Bern, Switzerland

Joseph J. Batenburg, Ph.D. Laboratory of Veterinary Biochemistry, Utrecht University, Utrecht, The Netherlands

Richard D. Bland, M.D. Fields Professor of Pediatrics, University of Utah Health Sciences Center, Salt Lake City, Utah

Johannes C. Böck, M.D. Anesthesiology Clinic, Universitätsklinikum Rudolf Virchow, Berlin, Germany

Pinar Boncuk-Dayanikli, M.D. Department of Pediatrics, University of California, San Francisco, San Francisco, California

Kristina Bry, M.D., Ph.D. Associate Professor of Pediatrics, University of California, Irvine School of Medicine, Irvine, California

David P. Carlton, M.D. Assistant Professor of Pediatrics, University of Utah Health Sciences Center, Salt Lake City, Utah

Shoichi Chida, M.D. Associate Professor of Pediatrics, Iwate Medical University, Morioka, Iwate, Japan

John A. Clements, M.D. Julius H. Comroe Professor of Pulmonary Biology, Cardiovascular Research Institute, University of California, San Francisco, San Francisco, California

Ronald I. Clyman, M.D. Professor of Pediatrics, Cardiovascular Research Institute, University of California, San Francisco, San Francisco, California

Jacqueline J. Coalson, Ph.D. Professor of Pathology, University of Texas Health Science Center at San Antonio, San Antonio, Texas

Robert B. Cotton, M.D. Professor of Pediatrics, Vanderbilt University Medical Center, Nashville, Tennessee

Robert A. deLemos, M.D. Hastings Professor of Pediatrics, Department of Pediatrics/Newborn Medicine, LAC+USC Medical Center, Women's and Children's Hospital, Los Angeles, California

Anthony David Edwards, M.A., M.B.B.S., F.R.C.P. Professor of Neonatal Medicine, Department of Pediatrics and Neonatal Medicine, Royal Postgraduate Medical School, Hammersmith Hospital, London, England

David K. Edwards III, M.D. Professor, Departments of Radiology and Pediatrics, University of California, San Diego, San Diego, California

Joanna Floros, Ph.D. Professor, Department of Cellular and Molecular Physiology, The Pennsylvania State University College of Medicine, Hershey, Pennsylvania

Jon Goerke, M.D. Professor, Department of Physiology, Cardiovascular Research Institute, University of California, San Francisco, San Francisco, California

Andreas Günther, M.D. Department of Internal Medicine, Justus-Liebig University, Giessen, Germany

Henry L. Halliday, M.D., F.R.C.P., F.R.C.P.E. Honorary Professor, Department of Child Health, The Queen's University of Belfast, and Consultant Neonatologist, Neonatal Intensive Care Unit, Royal Maternity Hospital, Belfast, Northern Ireland

Mikko Hallman, M.D., Ph.D. Professor, Department of Pediatrics, University of California, Irvine School of Medicine, Irvine, California

Alan H. Jobe, M.D., Ph.D. Professor of Pediatrics, Harbor–UCLA Medical Center, University of California, Los Angeles, School of Medicine, Los Angeles, California

Björn Jonson, M.D., Ph.D., F.C.C.P. Professor, Department of Clinical Physiology, University of Lund, Lund, Sweden

Anne M. Karinch, Ph.D. Assistant Professor, Department of Cellular and Molecular Physiology, The Pennsylvania State University College of Medicine, Hershey, Pennsylvania

Burkhard Lachmann, M.D. Professor, Department of Anesthesiology, Erasmus University, Rotterdam, The Netherlands

Robert J. Mason, M.D. Cetalie and Marcel Weiss Chair and Professor of Medicine, National Jewish Center for Immunology and Respiratory Medicine and the University of Colorado School of Medicine, Denver, Colorado

Francis X. McCormack, M.D. Assistant Professor of Medicine, Division of Pulmonary/Critical Care Medicine, Department of Internal Medicine, University of Cincinnati, Cincinnati, Ohio

David C. McCormick, M.D. Department of Pediatrics, Royal Women's Hospital, Brisbane, Australia

T. Allen Merritt, M.D. Professor of Pediatrics and Chief, Division of Neonatology, University of California, Davis, Medical Center, Sacramento, California

William H. Northway, Jr., M.D. Professor of Radiology and Pediatrics, Department of Radiology, Stanford University School of Medicine, Stanford, and Lucile Packard Children's Hospital, Palo Alto, California

Torsten Olsson, Ph.D. Professor of Medical Electronics, Department of Applied Electronics, Chalmers University of Technology, Gothenburg, Sweden

Sylvia Pietschmann, Ph.D. Department of Anesthesiology, Universitätsklinikum Rudolf Virchow, Berlin, Germany

Ulrich Pison, M.D. Department of Anesthesiology, Universitätsklinikum Rudolf Virchow, Berlin, Germany

Rangasamy Ramanathan, M.D. Assistant Professor of Pediatrics, Department of Pediatrics/Division of Neonatology, LAC+USC Medical Center, Women's and Children's Hospital, Los Angeles, California

E. Osmund R. Reynolds, M.D. Professor, Department of Pediatrics, University College, London Medical School, London, England

Bengt Robertson, M.D. Director, Division of Experimental Perinatal Pathology, Department of Woman and Child Health, Karolinska Institute, Stockholm, Sweden

Ola Didrik Saugstad, M.D., Ph.D. Professor/Director, Department of Pediatric Research, The National Hospital, University of Oslo, Oslo, Norway

Samuel Schürch, Ph.D. Professor of Medical Physiology, Department of Medical Physiology, Health Sciences Centre, The University of Calgary, Calgary, Alberta, Canada

Werner Seeger, M.D. Professor, Department of Internal Medicine, Justus-Liebig University, Giessen, Germany

Steven R. Seidner, M.D. Assistant Professor of Pediatrics, University of Texas Health Science Center at San Antonio, San Antonio, Texas

Jack Sills, M.D. Associate Clinical Professor of Pediatrics, University of California, Irvine School of Medicine, Irvine, California

Klaus Slama, M.D. Anesthesiology Clinic, Universitätsklinikum Rudolf Virchow, Berlin, Germany

Roger F. Soll, M.D. Associate Professor, Department of Pediatrics, University of Vermont College of Medicine, Burlington, Vermont

Christian P. Speer, M.D. Professor of Pediatrics, Department of Neonatology, University Children's Hospital, Tübingen, Germany

Nils W. Svenningsen, M.D., Ph.D. Professor of Pediatrics and Neonatal Medicine, Neonatal Intensive Care Unit, Department of Pediatrics, University Hospital, and Lund University, Lund, Sweden

H. William Taeusch, M.D. Professor of Pediatrics, Department of Pediatrics, University of California, San Francisco, and San Francisco General Hospital, San Francisco, California

Terry Turner, R.N., P.N.P. University of California, Davis, Medical Center, Sacramento, California

Lambert M. G. van Golde, Ph.D. Professor of Biochemistry, Division of Biochemistry, Department of Veterinary Basic Sciences, Utrecht University, Utrecht, The Netherlands

J. Freek van Iwaarden, Ph.D. Utrecht University, Utrecht, and Department of Cell Biology and Immunology, Vrije Universiteit, Amsterdam, The Netherlands

Yvonne Vaucher, M.D., M.P.H. Department of Pediatrics, University of California, San Diego, San Diego, California

Siegfried Veit, M.D. Anesthesiology Clinic, Universitätsklinikum Rudolf Virchow, Berlin, Germany

Frans J. Walther, M.D., Ph.D. Professor of Pediatrics, Department of Pediatrics, Charles R. Drew University and University of California, Los Angeles, Los Angeles, California

Timothy E. Weaver, Ph.D. Associate Professor of Pediatrics, Division of Pulmonary Biology, Children's Hospital Medical Center, Cincinnati, Ohio

Jeffrey A. Whitsett, M.D. Director of Pulmonary Biology, Department of Pediatrics, Children's Hospital Medical Center, Cincinnati, Ohio

Mary Jesse Wilson, M.D., M.P.H. California Children's Services, and Medical Consultant, Department of Health Services, Sacramento, California

Per Wollmer, M.D. Professor, Department of Clinical Physiology, University of Lund, Lund, Sweden

CONTENTS

Part II: PATHOLOGY AND CLINICAL DIAGNOSIS OF SURFACTANT DYSFUNCTION

SURFACTANT THERAPY FOR LUNG DISEASE

Part One

BASIC PHYSIOLOGICAL AND BIOCHEMICAL ASPECTS OF SURFACTANT FUNCTION

1

Biophysical Aspects in the Design of a Therapeutic Surfactant

SAMUEL SCHÜRCH
The University of Calgary
Calgary, Alberta, Canada

HANS BACHOFEN
University of Bern
Bern, Switzerland

I. Introduction

A thorough understanding of the mechanical effects of surfactant in the lung has been hindered by several problems: the behavior of surfactant films in vitro, e.g., in the Langmuir-Wilhelmy balance or in the pulsating bubble surfactometer, is different from that of the alveolar lining layer (1). Although minimum surface tensions below 5 mN/m in the Langmuir-Wilhelmy balance or below 1 mN/m in the pulsating bubble surfactometer can be obtained at a relatively high speed of film compression, these low surface tensions have much less stability (surface tension versus time at minimum tension) than the alveolar film. The alveolar film itself has a far greater stability, as calculated from pressure-volume studies on lungs of intact animals or on excised lungs (2,3). These results are in line with the surface tension stability data obtained by direct measurement of alveolar surface tension by the microdroplet spreading technique (4–6).

An examination of the results on surfactant activity obtained with various methods demonstrates clearly that the criteria for "good" surface activity depend on the instrument employed and for a particular instrument on the way a certain test is performed. Although the therapeutic efficacy of a particular surfactant preparation has to be tested in animal models of surfactant deficiency (7; see also Chapter 12), in vitro studies provide valuable guidelines for choosing or preparing a physiologically active surfactant. A standardized approach with a particular instrument may give results with regard to surface activity that correlate well with physiological parameters measured in animals even if the approach does not mimic the situation in the lung.

Unfortunately, the standardization of a particular approach to measure surface activity for a given instrument is quite difficult. This can be demonstrated for the Wilhelmy-Langmuir balance and the pulsating bubble surfactometer, which are the two most popular methods at present. Goerke and Gonzales (8) carefully primed the Teflon walls and barrier of their balance with long-chain saturated phophatidylcholine and a solution of lanthanum chloride to reduce film leakage. In addition, continuous Teflon ribbons standing on edge were used in the 1960s by Clements in rectangular troughs (9) and with rhombic frames (10).

In our experience, even these ribbon balances do not contain films from natural surfactant or lipid extract surfactant unless they are primed by overcompressing (collapsing) several films of disaturated phosphatidylcholine prior to the experiments. Thus, minimum surface tension and film stability (surface tension versus time at minimum tension) depend on the careful preparation of the surface balance as films that produce low and stable minimum surface tensions in a leak proof system show instability in a leaky balance.

Similarly, special precautions have to be taken when the pulsating bubble surfactometer is used. Putz and coworkers (11) recently improved the performance of the pulsating bubble surfactometer by keeping the capillary of the sample chamber dry. They demonstrated by video observations that this modified instrument performs better than the unmodified version, because keeping the capillary dry prevents surface films from occupying part of the capillary surface during cycling.

It appears that the film area changes, especially in the unmodified pulsating bubble surfactometer, during pulsations are not well defined, which may lead to erroneous interpretations of the results obtained with this instrument. For example, some surfactant films have to be pulsated in the pulsating bubble surfactometer for 10–20 times at 20 cycles/min in order to obtain near zero surface tensions (e.g., see ref. 12), whereas the same surfactant films produce near zero surface tensions on a first quasi-static or dynamic compression in the captive bubble surfactometer (13). The necessity for prolonged pulsations to achieve near zero tension in the pulsating bubble surfactometer for certain films compared with those that only need a few pulsations to obtain low minimum surface tensions is usually interpreted as the necessity to produce refinement of the dipalmitoyl phosphatidylcholine (DPPC) in the former films, whereas the latter films show already a behavior close to that of DPPC. Since the amount of film area compression might be uncertain, especially in the unmodified pulsating bubble surfactometer, the notion of film refinement or squeeze-out or film purification has to be carefully scrutinized.

By comparing the results obtained in the pulsating bubble surfactometer with those in the captive bubble surfactometer, Putz et al. (11) concluded that the captive bubble surfactometer should be used where accurate film area compressions are required to explain the mechanisms that govern surfactant surface activity, near zero surface tension, film stability, film compressibility, and hysteresis.

In this chapter, we will review recent results with regard to physical or surface chemical aspects of some surfactants used for replacement therapy in cases of surfactant deficiency. Particular attention will be given to film formation by adsorption, to film compressibility, and to the effect of overcompressing films at near zero minimum surface tensions. Based on these in vitro observations, we will make suggestions for choosing a particular mode of ventilation for optimal surface activity of a particular surfactant to be used for replacement therapy. In addition, the question of the amount of surfactant associated with the interfacial film, monolayer or multilayer, and its implications for surface activity will be addressed by electron microscopic analysis and investigations in the captive bubble surfactometer.

II. Characteristics of Surfactant Deduced from Studies on Lungs

A. Adsorption

An effective surfactant adsorbs rapidly, within a few seconds to around 25 mN/m, the plateau or equilibrium surface tension (1). Rapid adsorption toward equilibrium means that adsorption will keep the surface tension in the lung near the equilibrium value during inspiration to total lung capacity (TLC). This will keep the surface component of lung recoil pressure as low as possible, which helps to minimize the work of breathing (11). Goerke (14) pointed out that the capacity for surfactant to adsorb rapidly is indirectly observed on ventilated patients in the operating room, where the anesthesiologist sometimes is forced to ventilate a patient at low tidal volumes for prolonged periods. This mode of ventilation is often accompanied by an increase in inflation pressure that is likely due to microcollapse related to film overcompression and loss of surface activity. In this situation, a single breath to TLC restores normal inflation pressure by allowing new surfactant to adsorb within seconds to the depleted film. The restored film is then compressed again to a low tension as the original low pressure at functional residual capacity (FRC) is approached during deflation. In a closely related situation in ventilated dogs, Mead and Collier (2) restored volume at FRC and compliance by a single breath to TLC. The prerequisite of fast adsorption into the air-liquid interface for an effective surfactant is further supported by a recent animal experiments reported by Ogawa et al. (15) indicating that lung surfactants showing faster adsorption rates in vitro produce lower mean airway pressures and larger lung compliancies.

B. Surface Tension, Stability, Hysteresis, and Lung Microstructure

Measurements of surface tension has been made by two methods: (1) by placing microdroplets of a variety of test fluids onto alveolar surfaces (4–6) and (2) by washing procedures involving pressure-volume studies after filling the lungs or covering the alveoli with test liquid films (16–18). The microdroplet method showed that surface tension varied with lung volume.

For excised lungs held at 37°C and deflated to FRC, the minimum surface tension is below 1 mN/m at FRC. Remarkably, this minimum surface tension can be obtained under quasi-static conditions; that is, a minimum compression rate is not required to achieve near zero tension. In addition, this low surface tension is extremely stable (6), similar to values inferred from pressure-volume curves on air-filled lungs where the surface tension rose only 1–2 mN/m during 20 min at FRC (3). The maximum quasi-static surface tension during a pressure-volume loop between FRC and TLC is approximately 30 mN/m (5, 19).

The direct measurements of alveolar surface tension agree well with results obtained by the model of Wilson and Bachofen (20), which is based on an energy analysis of well-defined structure-function relations of isolated, air-filled, and perfused lungs. These studies have been possible because of the excellent preservation for microscopy of the lung microstructure by the perfusion fixation technique in combination with morphometric analysis perfected by Weibel and his associates during the past 20 years.

The combination of morphometric analysis with determination of alveolar surface tension has allowed Bachofen and his coworkers (19) not only to determine the surface tension at FRC (minimum) and TLC (maximum) but also at intermediate lung volumes on the deflation as well as on the inflation limb of the pressure-volume curve. For lungs inflated from zero pressure, the surface tensions on the deflation limb were considerably lower than on the inflation limb: at FRC about 1 mN/m on deflation, whereas on inflation the tension was approximately 6 mN/m. The corresponding alveolar surface areas were 63 and 47%, respectively, of the area at TLC. These values demonstrate that at low volumes, at the surface tension of 6 mN/m, the alveolar surface area is approximately 16% smaller than at the surface tension of 1 mN/m, suggesting that surfactants having minimum surface tensions of 5 or 6 mN/m on deflation will not sufficiently stabilize alveolar surface area. This may have important implications for the quality control for a surfactant to be used for replacement therapy. Only if the minimum surface tension at low volumes can reach a value near zero will there be the optimal alveolar area available for the gas exchange. The correlation studies between lung microstructure and alveolar surface tension further demonstrated that the area compression is about 30% from TLC to FRC, corresponding to surface tensions of about 30 and 1 mN/m, respectively (19). In addition, the studies performed an excised rabbit lungs demonstrated that pressure-volume and surface tension–area hysteresis is substantial only in excised lungs inflated from volumes lower than FRC or from about zero transpulmonary pressure. In healthy, normally breathing lungs, the pressure-volume hysteresis is relatively small (16). This corresponds to the very small hysteresis if the lining film is reexpanded from FRC (19). Thus, a good-quality surfactant investigated in vitro after a few cycles that feature compressions only to minimum surface tension, that is, without overcompression and collapse, should not show appreciable hysteresis during quasi-static or dynamic cycling (21,22).

III. Perfluorocarbon Fluid on Alveolar Surfaces

Bachofen and his coworkers (23) recently conducted a series of experiments with fluorocarbon and hexadecane to study the influence of altered surface tension on alveolar micromechanics. Experiments are in progress in many laboratories to apply fluorocarbon fluids in the clinic for the treatment of the respiratory distress syndrome (24,25). These substances offer the advantage of high oxygen and carbon dioxide solubility and a surface tension reducing effect in case of severe surfactant deficiency or dysfunction. The studies appear to be quite promising, although alterations of lung mechanics in fluorocarbon-filled or fluorocarbon-treated lungs have been well documented (26, 27). Further, fluorocarbons are under consideration as constituent parts in artificial surfactants. Since there is a subtle interplay between microstructure and surface forces at the alveolar level (20), any alteration of surface physics will result in a complex change of the structure-function relationship.

Fig. 1 shows the alveolar morphology of rabbit lungs filled with hexadecane (A) and perfluorocarbon FC77 (B). The lungs were fixed at the same volume: 40% TLC on the deflation limb of the pressure-volume curve. Hexadecane-filled lungs are barely distinguishable from saline-filled lungs. This is not surprising, since the measured plateau interfacial tension between the surfactant solution (1 mg/ml of bovine lipid extract surfactant, bLES, Biochemicals Inc., London, Ontario, Canada) and hexadecane is 0.6 mN/m at 37°C. On the other hand, we concluded that the interfacial tension between FC77 and the alveolar lining layer is about 15 mN/m. This follows from in vitro measurements of surfactant-FC77 interfacial tensions at changing surface areas of the captive bubble. The alveolar

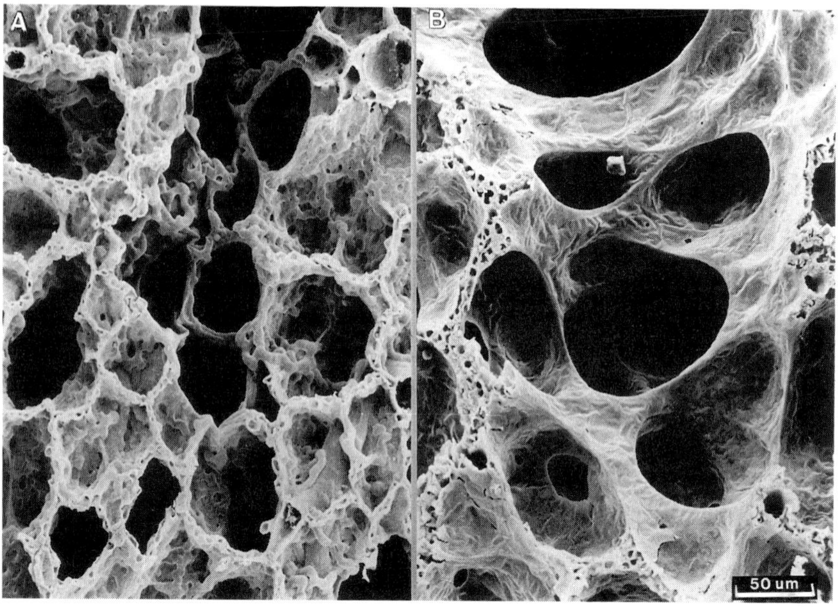

Figure 1 Alveolar morphology of rabbit lungs filled with hexadecane (A) and fluorocarbon FC77 (B). The lungs were fixed by vascular perfusion at 40% total lung capacity on deflation. The hexadecane filled lungs were barely distinguishable from saline filled lungs: The alveolar surfaces are highly corrugated by bulging capillaries. Fluorocarbon filled lungs show relatively wide airspaces with smooth surfaces. The hexadecane-surfactant interfacial tension was 0.6 mN/m, in contrast, the FC77-surfactant interfacial tension was above 10 mN/m. (For discussion, see text.)

surface area for the fluorocarbon-filled lungs was about 1.2 m^2, whereas the surface area of the hexadecane-filled lungs was about 2.7 m^2, or more than twice the area of the FC77-filled lungs.

Hexadecane has a fluid-vapor surface tension of about 26 mN/m at 37°C, whereas that of FC77 is 15 mN/m. For additional results and a discussion of the fluorocarbon- or FC77-rinsed lungs, we refer to the article by Bachofen et al. (23). In conclusion, the effect of foreign fluids introduced into the lung cannot be predicted from their surface tension.

IV. In Vitro Models: The Captive Bubble Surfactometer

As pointed out in the introduction, recent advances in assessing surface properties of pulmonary surfactant films using a leak proof captive bubble system have facilitated the collection of more reliable data describing surface tension–area relations than by using more conventional methods.

In this section, we briefly describe the apparatus depicted in Fig. 2 and surface activity tests frequently performed with the captive bubble system.

The captive bubble method is an in vitro technique developed for the determination of the surface tension, area, and volume of a bubble with a surfactant film at the air-water interface of the bubble. Bubble size and thus the surface tension of any insoluble film at the bubble surface is altered by changing the pressure within the closed chamber. Surfactant films may be formed by using a spreading agent or by adsorption from a surfactant suspension. The design and construction of the apparatus are described at length by Schürch et al. (21). The instrument consists of a sample chamber constructed from cylindrical glass tubing with an inner diameter of either 0.5 or 1.0 cm. A metal piston with a tight O-ring seal is fitted into the glass tubing. The ceiling of the chamber consists of a slightly concave surface of a 1% agarose gel cylinder attached to the metal piston generating a completely hydrophilic surface for contact with the bubble. Under this condition, the bubble surface phase is continuous, there is no tube to interrupt the surface film and adhesion to any kind of support, e.g., hydrophobic plastic is avoided, thus removing the possibility of film leakage. The temperature of the chamber is regulated and maintained at 37°C. The sample chamber, either 0.15 or 1.0 ml volume, is filled with the suspension to be investigated, and a bubble of 1–3 mm (small chamber) or 3–6 mm (large chamber) in diameter is rapidly introduced. The chamber content is stirred with a small magnetic bar. The air bubble within the chamber is compressed by moving the glass chamber upward toward the stationary piston. To expand the bubble, the chamber is moved downward. The chamber is mounted onto the movable stage of a microscopic stand. The microscope focusing knob serves to control the movement.

A second version of the captive bubble system has been described recently by Putz et al. (29). With this instrument, the captive bubble is pressure driven from an exterior pressure reservoir rather than by a piston. Both versions have been further developed for convenience and reliability (11,22,30) and produce equivalent results.

The bubble is recorded continuously throughout the experiment on a video recorder. Video images are printed by a video copier or single frames are stored on a computer's hard disk and loaded into an image processing and analysis program (30). The bubble surface tension is calculated using the method of Malcolm and Elliott (31). With this method, the surface tension can be derived from the maximum height and diameter of the bubble, having a 180-degree contact angle; i.e., the bubble is totally surrounded by aqueous media and does no adhere to the agarose ceiling. Bubble height and diameter can be obtained to any degree of precision depending on the mea-

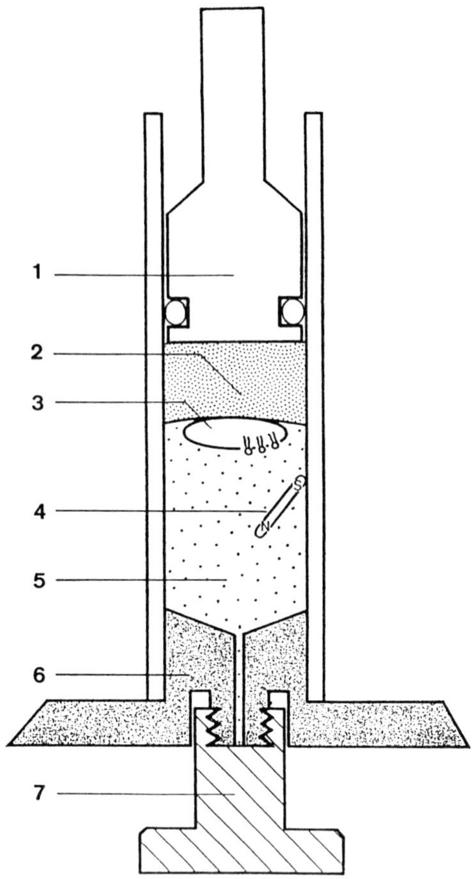

Figure 2 Captive bubble chamber. 1, piston; 2, 1% agarose gel; 3, air bubble with surfactant film; 4, magnetic stir bar; 5, surfactant suspension in sample chamber; 6, chamber base; 7, chamber filling port plug. The chamber is mounted onto a moveable stage of a microscope stand. The microscope focusing knob serves to control the movement.

suring procedure employed. Bubble areas and volumes are calculated by an original algorithm relating bubble height and diameter to areas of revolution (30).

A. Adsorption Measurements

A 20-G needle (flat tip) is introduced through the bottom inlet of the chamber, the needle tip is moved up to within 1 cm of the agarose ceiling, and the needle is held in this position by friction. Stirring is started at this point and continued during the adsorption period. A bubble of 3–7 mm in diameter, depending on the chamber size, is then formed by turning the focusing knob of the microscope stand rapidly by about 60–90 degrees. The transition time for the bubble formation from the first appearance of air at the needle tip to the resting position of the agarose ceiling is about 0.15 sec, which is measured by counting single frames on the TV monitor. After this interval, the bubble shape is Laplacian (time zero for adsorption). The bubble is then continuously recorded during the adsorption period and the following manipulations for quasi-static or dynamic cycling (22).

B. Quasi-static Isotherms

After adsorption to approximately 25 mN/m, the bottom inlet of the bubble chamber is sealed, and the film is compressed stepwise; waiting at each step until the bubble shape no longer changes noticeably within 20–30 sec (this corresponds to a change in surface tension of less than 0.5 mN/m in that period. Approximately 10 steps are taken for each compression and expansion part of the cycle. Film collapse at minimum surface tension is avoided as the bubble area is expanded just after reaching minimum surface tension (22).

The term *Quasi-static* is used here in accordance with physiological manipulations employed for pressure-volume relations for excised lungs. Quasi-static cycling involves a series of small discrete alterations in bubble area where the surface film is allowed to partially "relax" during the compression-expansion process. These processes are not quasi-static processes as defined in thermodynamics where a quasi-static process is an idealized concept that is defined as a succession of equilibrium states (32).

C. Dynamic Hysteresis Loops

The bubble area may be compressed and expanded periodically at cycling speeds up to 100 cycles/min. Film area compressions can be performed with only minimum collapse at near zero minimum tension or with differing amounts of film collapse, creating various amounts of surface tension-area hysteresis (see below). Minimum surface tension is attained when the bubble apex ceases to move upward on further bubble compression.

D. Subphase Depletion and the Surface-Associated Reservoir

The aqueous subphase in the bubble chamber is depleted of surfactant after adsorption to approximately 25 mN/m onto a small bubble. To deplete the surfactant in the aqueous subphase, the aqueous medium is replaced several times with a pure salt solution. A 16-G stainless steel needle, with its tip down, is mounted onto the chamber inlet. As much as possible of the liquid chamber content is removed by moving the chamber upward relative to the piston by turning the focusing knob at the stand. A pure salt solution without any surfactant is then drawn into the chamber by reversing the relative motion between chamber and piston. This washing procedure is repeated at least six times until the subphase consists only of the salt solution and no surfactant. The absence of surfactant in the salt solution is tested in independent measurements by forming an air bubble and by measuring its surface tension. The subphase is taken as "surfactant free" if the bubble surface tension at 37°C is greater than 68 mN/m, which is very close to the surface tension of water, approximately 70 mN/m at 37°C. During the washing procedure, the bubble stays intact and its surface tension remains at the plateau value, which was obtained previously by adsorption.

After sealing off the bottom inlet of the chamber, the bubble is expanded and compressed repeatedly. While the bubble surface area is increased during bubble expansion, the surface tension stays at approximately 25 mN/m indicating surfactant adsorption from a "surface associated reservoir," since all of the surfactant material in the bulk phase had previously been depleted. The expansion process is continued until the surface tension starts to increase to values substantially above 25 mN/m, indicating that most of the surfactant from the reservoir associated with the interface had moved into the surface active film. Fig. 3 illustrates the results obtained from an experiment described above. The surfactant was bLES, and the suspension contained 1 mg/ml of phospholipid in 0.9% NaCl and 1.5 mM $CaCl_2$ at pH 5.5. The filled symbols represent the compression part of a cycle, and the open symbols represent the expansion part. The film area change for the first compression after adsorption to about 23 mN/m was approximately 15%, corresponding to a film compressibility at 15 mN/m of about 0.007 $(mN/m)^{-1}$, close to that for a DPPC film, which is 0.005 $(mN/m)^{-1}$. The low compressibility and low film area change suggest a film already highly enriched in DPPC before the first compression. This is similar to the observations on fresh Curosurf films (see below). The relatively flat part (open circles) represents adsorption from film material that stayed associated with the bubble surface during subphase depletion. We have chosen the term *surface-associated reservoir* to indicate that there is more material at or in the air-liquid interface than just a monolayer. By compressing the film a second time (filled triangles) and then a third time (filled squares), it is possible to determine the amount of film material in the surface-associated reservoir in terms of densely packed "monolayers" of near zero surface tension. The film area at minimum tension on the last compression before the surface tension begins to increase substantially above 25 mN/m is about 1.1 cm^2, or 3.4 times the area at the first minimum (0.3 cm^2). It appears that there is at least an amount of film material for two more monolayers associated with the first film just after adsorption (filled circles). Thus, this first film may not be a monolayer.

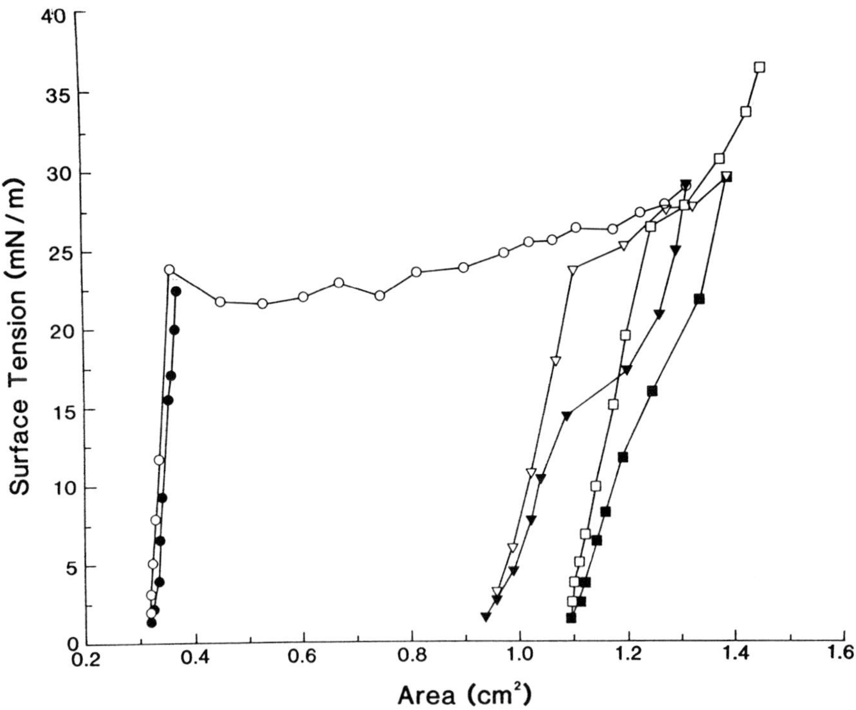

Figure 3 Surface tension–area isotherms of a bovine lipid extract surfactant (bLES) film performed with a captive bubble in 0.9% NaCl, 1.5 mM $CaCl_2$. The surfactant in the subphase was depleted after adsorption to equilibrium, before the first quasi-static compression (filled circles). Note the small film area change required to produced near zero minimum surface tension, indicating a film highly enriched in DPPC. The open circles represent bubble area expansion. The surface tension stays around 25 mN/m because of adsorption from material associated with the interface ("surface-associated reservoir"). Filled triangles, second compression at larger bubble area. Note: Increased film compressibility on second compression because of material other than DPPC moved into surface active film from the reservoir. Filled squares, third compression. Note: Film compressibility appears to decrease on compression after exhaustion of the surface-associated reservoir. (For a discussion, see text.)

E. Electron Microscopy: Film Morphology

The question is whether there is morphological evidence for a surface-associated reservoir at the alveolar liquid-air interface. Since the pioneering work of Weibel and his associates (33–35) numerous studies have been published which have demonstrated an extracellular lining layer covering the alveolar surface. However, the morphological examinations revealed a considerable polymorphism of this layer, and in transmission electron micrographs the postulated continuity of the lining layer could never be proven. In fact, there is evidence that pure monolayers of saturated phospholipids cannot be fixed by the usual fixation techniques, including osmium tetroxide (36). Recent experiments (37,38) have been more successful in preserving and demonstrating the lining layer. By high-pressure perfusion of excised rabbit lungs with 6% albumin solution, alveolar edema was introduced such that the surface film was lifted off the epithelial lining layer. High-power magnification of the film revealed a rather polymorphous structure. At some sites, the lining layer covering the increased volume of the hypophase appears to be an amorphous material, and at other sites, triple layers or even multilayers can be recognized (Figs. 4A–C). In agreement with the in vitro bubble experiments, these observations suggest that there is an excess of surfactant material also at the alveolar surface, and that the well-accepted monolayer theory might not reflect reality.

V. Surfactant Investigated with the Captive Bubble Surfactometer

A. Lipid Extract Surfactants

We have extensively studied the surface chemical properties of bLES and Curosurf (Chiesi Pharmaceutici, Parma, Italy). Briefly, bLES is obtained by organic extraction of bovine lung lavage material. Neutral lipids are removed by acetone solubilization. The material is dried under N_2, made up in chloroform/methanol 9:1, and stored at –20°C. This preparation contains all of the phospholipids of natural surfactant and the two small hydrophobic surfactant-associated proteins, SP-B and SP-C; however, it has been stripped of the hydrophilic surfactant associated protein SP-A. The phospholipid composition [(mean $\pm$ SE, n $=$ 3), phosphatidylcholine (PC), 79.2 $\pm$ 0.65%; phosphatidylglycerol (PG), 14.4 $\pm$ 0.51%; phosphatidylethanolamine, 3.0 $\pm$ 0.18%; sphingomyelin, 2.0 $\pm$ 0.35%; lysophosphatidylcholine, 0.20 $\pm$ 0.03%; lyso-bis-phosphatidic acid, trace] is similar to that previously published (39). The low molecular weight hydrophobic proteins account for ~1% (wt/wt) of bLES when assayed by the procedure of Lowry et al. (40) and are present in an SP-B to SP-C ratio of ~1:3 based on dansylation analysis (41). Before use, the surfactant is dried and suspended in saline solution that contains either 0.9% NaCl or 0.9% NaCl + 1.5 mM $CaCl_2$.

Curosurf is isolated from minced pig lungs by a sequence of steps, including washing, centrifugation, chloroform-methanol extraction, and liquid-gel chromatography (42). The isolated polar lipid fraction is dissolved in chloroform and sterilized by means of a high-pressure filter system (first filter 0.45 μm, second

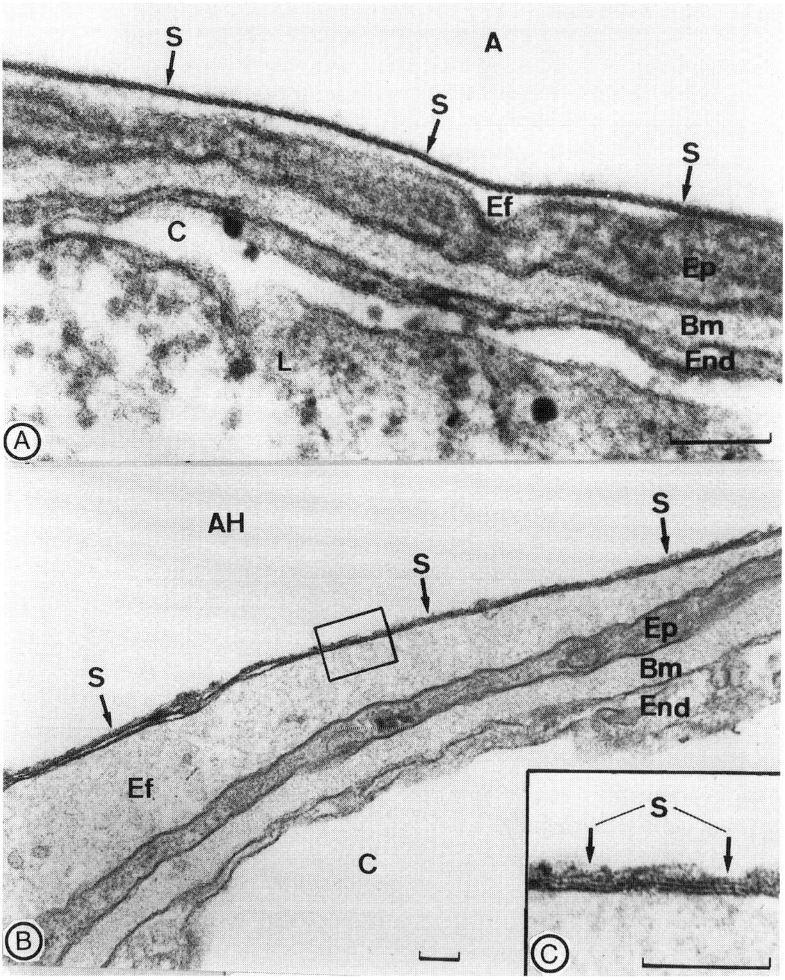

Figure 4 Multilayers of surfactant film (S). (A) Rabbit lung, fixed by vascular perfusion, with discrete alveolar edema (high pressure pulmonary edema) to demonstrate the continuous surface film on the thin part of the blood-gas barrier. Note that the film is thicker than the cell membranes which consist of phospholipid bilayers. (B) Rabbit lung filled with hexadecane to better preserve the surfactant film (fixation by vascular perfusion), and with slight alveolar edema to lift the surfactant film off the epithelial cell layer. (C) inset of B: Higher magnification of the surfactant film, which consists of three layers at least. (A, alveolus filled with air; AH, alveolus filled with hexadecane; Ef, edema fluid; Ep, epithelial cell layer; Bm, fused basement membrane; End, endothelial cell layer; C, capillary lumen; L, leukocyte in capillary; S, surfactant film. Scale markers: 1 μm.)

filter 0.20 μm), and subsequent steps, including evaporation of the solvent and suspension of the surfactant in normal saline by gentle sonication (50 W, 40 kHz) at a phospholipid concentration of 80 mg/ml, are performed under sterile conditions with autoclaved glassware (43). No antioxidant is added. The final product contains about 99% polar lipids (30–35% DPPC) and 1% hydrophobic proteins, the surfactant-associated proteins B and C (SP-B and SP-C in an approximate molar ratio of 1:2). The surfactant-associated hydrophilic protein SP-A is absent. Curosurf was supplied as a suspension in unbuffered normal saline (pH 5–6) with a phospholipid concentration of 80 mg/ml, as verified by phosphorus determination according to Bartlett (44). Ninety percent of the particles in the suspension had a diameter ≤5 μm, 95% ≤10 μm. Both surfactant preparations, bLES and Curosurf were stored at –20°C until use. After opening a vial to remove the amount of surfactant needed for a series of experiments during a period of approximately 4 hr, the vial was immediately capped and stored at 2–3°C. For the experiments phospholipid concentrations in the samples were adjusted to 50 μg/ml, 400 μg/ml, 1 mg/ml, 2 mg/ml, and 3 mg/ml by adding 0.9% NaCl or 0.9% NaCl + 1.5 mM $CaCl_2$. Lipid concentrations above 3 mg/ml could not be studied in the present version of the captive bubble surfactometer, as discerning the edges of the bubbles above that concentration was too difficult because these suspensions are too murky. One independent experiment was performed by using one chamber filling of surfactant at a particular concentration. The measured pH was 5.5.

After an extensive study on Curosurf or bLES stored for several days at 2–3°C after opening a particular vial, we concluded that the surfactant from an opened vial should be used as quickly as possible during a maximum period of 2 days. Experiments on surfactant from a particular vial after 5 days or more of repeated opening and closing for removal of material and storage 2–3°C showed decreased adsorption rates even at concentrations above 1 mg/ml. Typically, the time to reach a plateau value of 23–25 mN/m for 1 mg/ml was 10 sec compared with 2 sec or less for fresh material. In addition, quasi-static compressions demonstrated substantially increased film compressibility, especially for the first and second quasi-static compression. To maintain the best possible in vitro surface activity, including fast adsorption, low compressibility and near zero, stable minimum surface tensions, we have adopted the following procedure: The surfactant in a particular vial is divided immediately after opening the vial into convenient aliquots to be used within 1 day. Typically, one aliquot consists of 1 ml surfactant at 10 mg/ml. These aliquots are filled into small vials and capped under N_2 and stored at –20°C until use.

B. Synthetic Surfactants

The following synthetic surfactants were studied with the captive bubble surfactometer in our laboratory: (1) the most widely used synthetic surfactant,

Exosurf (Burroughs Wellcome, Research Triangle Park, NC), which consists of DPPC, hexadecanol, and tyloxapol, mixed in weight proportions 13.5:1.5:1, and (2) a mixture of DPPC and egg PG (molar ratio 7:3). A similar mixture was developed by Morley et al. [45] and is marketed under the name ALEC (artificial lung expanding compound) by Brittannia Pharmaceuticals, Surrey, U.K.

VI. Adsorption and Film Area Compression to Minimum Surface Tension

Adsorption in a continuously stirred surfactant suspension in the captive bubble surfactometer is measured at maximum bubble size at 37°C. For the lipid extract surfactants, Curosurf or bLES, the plateau or equilibrium surface tension is between 23 and 25 mN/m regardless of the concentration used. The rate of adsorption is strongly dependent on the concentration of the lipid in the bulk suspension. Fig. 5 shows the time course of adsorption for bLES at differing concentrations. Samples at and above 800 μg/ml of phospholipid require less than 5 sec to reach a plateau surface tension of approximately 25 mN/m. At low concentrations, Curosurf appears to adsorb faster than bLES, as Curosurf at 50 μg/ml reached the plateau value of about 25 mN/m in 5 min, whereas bLES at

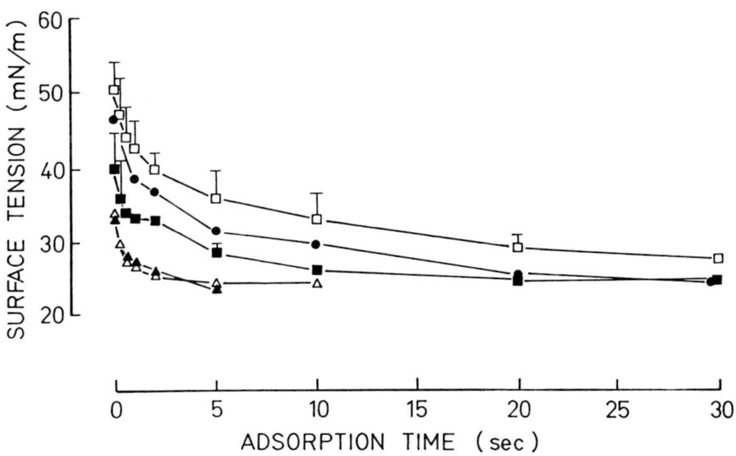

Figure 5 Time courses for adsorption of bovine lipid extract surfactant (bLES) at different concentrations. Samples are suspended in 0.9% NaCl, 1.5 mM $CaCl_2$. Surface tension (mN/m) is plotted versus adsorption time (sec) for bLES 100 (□), 200 (●), 400 (■), 800 (△), and 1,000 (▲) μg/ml. Values are means ± SEM, n = 4. (From ref. 13; used with permission.)

the same low concentration required more than 30 min to reach equilibrium. However, at and above 1 mg/ml of phospholipids, the time courses for adsorption for the two surfactants are similar; both preparations reach the equilibrium surface tension of about 25 mN/m in less than 5 sec, and at and above 2 mg/ml the adsorption time decreases to approximately 1 sec regardless whether or not calcium is added.

Recent work on Curosurf adsorption (22) and studies performed on bLES for the present work demonstrate that fresh lipid extract surfactant, that is, surfactant from a vial opened and used the same day, has the capacity to adsorb by a cooperative movement of large collective units of molecules into interface during adsorption. The phenomenon of adsorption by the transport of lipid aggregates has been discussed previously; e.g., Goerke and Clements (1), Keough and coworkers (46), and again by Keough (47). In contrast to the clicks that characterize a sudden increase in surface tension accompanied by a decrease in surface area (48), the sudden adsorption jumps caused by the movement of lipid aggregates into the interface have been called adsorption clicks (22). These adsorption clicks characterize a stepwise decrease in surface tension which can easily be seen with the captive bubble technique by observing a sudden decrease in the height of the captive bubble. For example, for a bubble of a diameter of about 0.8 cm at a surface tension of 35 mN/m, a large adsorption click of 10 mN/m causes the real bubble apex to move upward by about 0.75 mm. This movement can be observed on the TV monitor magnified by a factor 20; that is, a movement of the bubble apex by approximately 1.5 cm. We found that the frequency and magnitude of these adsorption clicks did not depend on whether or not calcium was added to the surfactant suspensions. Thus, this phenomenon does not depend on the surface-associated protein SP-A, since lipid extract surfactants contain SP-B and SP-C but not SP-A. Further, these adsorption clicks cannot be related to tubular myelin, since these structures contain SP-A. Films at and above 1 mg/ml, which are formed by rapid, gradual adsorption within a few seconds to equilibrium, do not produce squeeze-out or purification plateaus on quasi-static or dynamic compression to near zero minimum surface tension. Curosurf frequently adsorbed by large adsorption clicks to the equilibrium tension between 23 and 25 mN/m in less than 1 sec even at low lipid concentrations of 50 or 200 μg/ml. For bLES, adsorption was generally more gradual and concentrations of approximately 1 mg/ml were needed to obtain the equilibrium tension within 5 sec. Minimum surface tension of about 1 mN/m were obtained on a film area compression of approximately 20% for the first cycle after adsorption and 16% or less for subsequent cycles (Fig. 6) for which the compressibility at 15 mN/m was 0.008 $(mN/m)^{-1}$. This is close to the value for DPPC, 0.005 $(mN/m)^{-1}$, calculated from previous data (48). The low compressibility almost identical to that of a pure DPPC film suggests that the film is already highly enriched in DPPC at the end of film formation by adsorption (22).

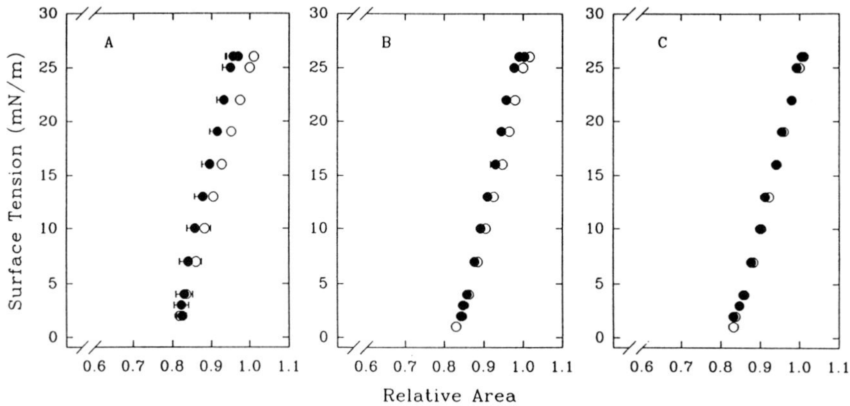

Figure 6 Quasi-static isotherms of porcine lipid extract surfactant (Curosurf). Surface tension (mN/m) is plotted versus relative area for Curosurf at 1 mg/ml. *Open symbols*, measurements made during compression; *filled symbols*, measurements made during expansion. Samples were suspended in 0.9% NaCl. Values are means ± SEM, n = 5. A: first cycle; B: second cycle; C: fourth cycle. Calculated compressibilities at $\gamma = 15$ mN/m are A: 0.008 ± 0.005 $(mN/m)^{-1}$, and B, C: 0.007 ± 0.005 $(mN/m)^{-1}$. (From ref. 22; used with permission.)

We estimated the number of surfactant molecules that enter the interface in collective units to produce moderate (1–5 mN/m) to large (~10 mN/m) sudden decreases in the bubble surface tension. The calculations are based on the assumption that the molecules are DPPC, using the isotherms for DPPC at 37°C (48). This assumption is reasonable, in the view of the low compressibility determined for the first cycles in Fig. 6 (C_{15} = 0.008 ± 0.002 $[mN/m]^{-1}$, mean ± SEM, n = 4). For large adsorption clicks (10 mN/m at 35 mN/m), the estimated number of DPPC molecules entering the interface as an aggregate is 10^{14}. An aggregate of 10^{14} molecules corresponds to approximately 120 ng of phospholipid or a particle with a diameter of about 3 μm. Assuming the content of hydrophobic proteins in Curosurf is 1% (by weight), the aggregate would contain 10^{11} protein molecules with 2:1 molar proportion between SP-C and monomeric SP-B (49). The structure of these rapidly absorbing large molecular aggregates is unknown, but recent ultrastructural studies of reconstituted preparations indicate that mixtures of surfactant lipids (DPPC and phosphatidylglycerol) generate both membraneous layers and discoid particles in the presence of SP-B and SP-C (50).

In contrast to the lipid extract surfactants, adsorption for the synthetic surfactants was much slower, Exosurf of 1 mg/ml reached approximately 38 mN/m, and the mixture DPPC/egg PG reached about 35 mN/m at 37°C in 5-min adsorption time.

Exosurf films required 80% compression (quasi-static) to achieve a minimum surface tension below 1 mN/m. If the cycling rate was increased (e.g., to 15 cycles/min), always avoiding collapse at minimum surface tension, the area compression required to reach near zero tension was about 60%. At 50 cycles/min, minimum surface tension was achieved after 40% compression (Fig. 7). For Exosurf, increasing the cycling rate resulted in a film enriched in DPPC. At lower rates of cycling, a squeeze-out or purification plateau is evident. It appears that at lower rates of cycling, tyloxapol or hexadecanol must be squeezed out before minimum surface tension can be obtained. For fast cycling (>50 cpm) with continuous total film area compressions of 80%, area compressions to 1 mN/m were also close to 80%. Thus, the mode of cycling is important to optimize Exosurf surface activity.

After adsorption to approximately 25 mN/m within 5 min, films from DPPC/egg PG at 1 mg/ml, pH 6.5, had to be compressed by about 40% for the first quasi-static cycle to reach a minimum tension of 1 mN/m. With repeated,

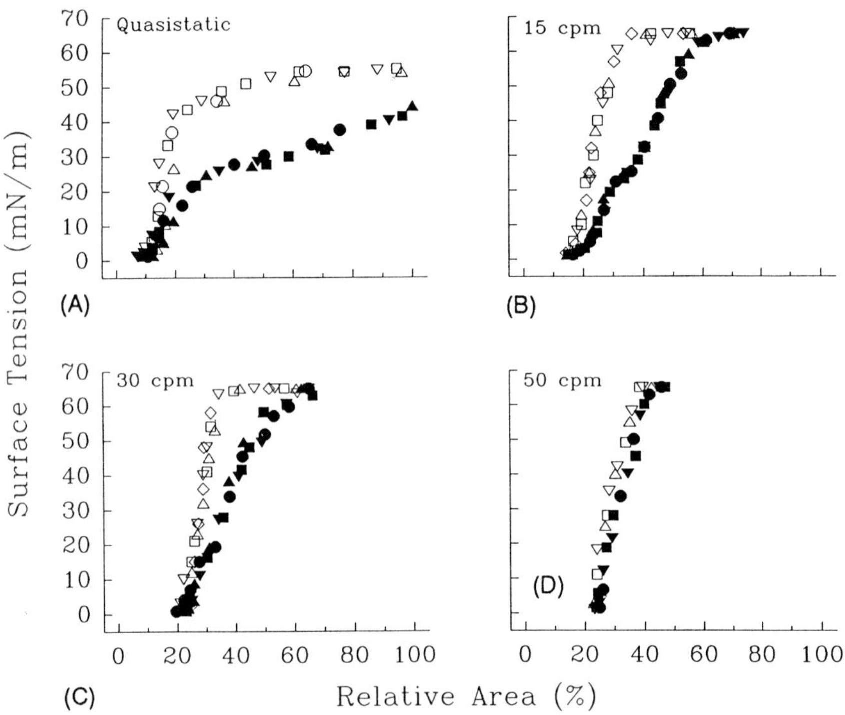

Figure 7 Effect of cycling speed on film area compressions of Exosurf needed to achieve near zero minimum surface tensions. A: Quasi-static conditions, B–D: dynamic cycling at 15, 30, and 50 cycles per min (cpm), respectively. *Filled symbols*, film compressions, *open symbols*, film expansions. (Adapted from ref. 53; used with permission.)

quasi-static cycling, the film area compression required to obtain near zero minimum tension tended to decrease. At the fourth cycle, only about 25% compression was needed. With dynamic cycling (20–30 cpm), initially with a total film area compression of about 50% to obtain near zero surface tension, the surface activity deteriorated; that is, maximum surface tension after 20 dynamic cycles was close to 70 mN/m. For these curves, the area compressions required to reach near zero tension was about 80% compared with only about 25% area compression if collapse at near zero minimum surface tension was avoided. Again, this demonstrates that the mode of cycling is important.

VII. Dynamic Cycles: Influence of Film Collapse

A. Hysteresis Loops

Fig. 8 shows average curves of four consecutive dynamic cycles centering on the 20th cycle: Fig. 8A, for a total film area compression of approximately 80% and Fig. 8B, for a total film area compression of approximately 50%. For these experiments Curosurf was used, the concentration of lipid extract surfactant was 1 mg/ml in 1.5 mM $CaCl_2$ and 0.9% NaCl. When the surfactant film is cycled with 80% total area compression, a plateau at about 20 mN/m is observed (Fig.

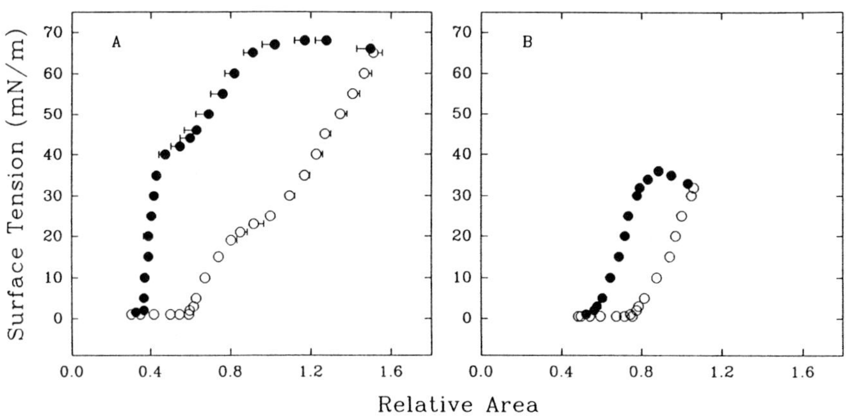

Figure 8 Dynamic (20–30 cycles/min) surface tension versus area relations of porcine lipid extract surfactant (Curosurf). Surface tension (mN/m) is plotted versus relative area for Curosurf at 1 mg/ml. *Open symbols*, measurements during compression; *filled symbols*, measurements made during expansion. Samples were suspended in 0.9% NaCl, 1.5 mM $CaCl_2$. Values are means ± SEM, n = 4. Plots are summaries of four consecutive dynamic cycles, centering on the 20th cycle. (A) Total film area compression 80%; area compression from γ = 25 mN/m to <1 mN/m, 40%. (B) Total film area compression 50%; area compression from γ = 25 mN/m to <1 mN/m, 28%. (From ref. 22; used with permission.)

8A). The compressibility at 15 mN/m was 0.045 $(mN/m)^{-1}$, which is about 10 times the value observed for pure DPPC. The compression part of the loop demonstrates that the film had to be compressed by 60% to reach the minimum surface tension below 1 mN/m. After the end of the collapse plateau at minimum tension, there was a small delay in the rise of surface tension upon expansion of the film (22). For large film area compressions, in the presence of calcium, a shoulder above 40 mN/m is observed (Fig. 8A).

For a total area compression of only 50% in Fig. 8B, the loops have a very different shape. Only 30% film area compression was required to produce a minimum surface tension below 1 mN/m. Similar to Fig. 8A, there was a delay in the rise of surface tension at the beginning of film area expansion. This delay in the rise of surface tension was not observed for quasi-static cycling (see Fig. 6). There was no shoulder at about 40 mN/m and the maximum surface tension was only 35 mN/m as opposed to about 68 mN/m for Fig. 8A. The compressibilities for the curves (Fig. 8B) at 15 mN/m were 0.011 $(mN/m)^{-1}$ or only 25% of the value in Fig. 8A.

In the following series of experiments, the possible consequences of film collapse were studied for surfactant at 1 mg/ml without added calcium. The films were dynamically cycled at 20–30 cpm for 50 consecutive cycles and the total area compression was always 80%. The first cycle, starting after adsorption to 25 mN/m, is shown in Fig. 9A, the second cycle is plotted in Fig. 9B, and the 20th cycle in Fig. 9C. After adsorption, the film had to be compressed by only 20% to reach a minimum tension below 1 mN/m (Fig. 9A). The second hysteresis loop (Fig. 9B) demonstrates a distinct plateau just below 25 mN/m. It appears that this plateau is related to film collapse at minimum surface tension (collapse plateau) as shown in Fig. 9A. The film area compression in Fig. 9B required to reach a minimum surface tension below 1 mN/m was close to 60%. With increasing numbers of consecutive cycles, the film area compression required to reach minimum tension was increased, and after 10–15 cycles, collapse plateaus at minimum tension were no longer observed and the shape of the curves was identical to that for cycle 20 (Fig. 9C). The area changes required to reach tensions below 1 mN/m were close to 80%, the total film area compression provided in the experiment. There was no noticeable change in shape during continuous cycling from cycle 20 to cycle 50. Minimum surface tension below 1 mN/m was still observed. However, as pointed out above, the film area compressions required were approximately 80%, identical to the total film area compression. The maximum surface tensions tended to approach 70 mN/m as the cycling number increased. In addition, there was no shoulder above 35 mN/m for these cycles.

Increasing the concentration can improve the surface activity of dynamically cycled films, but even at 3 mg/ml without added calcium, the performance is not as good as that of the films with calcium at 1 mg/ml (22).

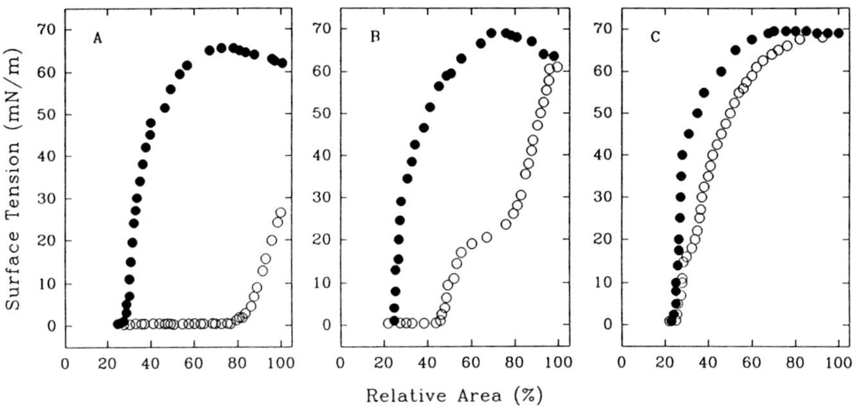

Figure 9 Dynamic (20–30 cycles/min) surface tension versus area relations of porcine lipid extract surfactant (Curosurf). Surface tension (mN/m) is plotted versus relative area for Curosurf at 1 mg/ml suspended in 0.9% NaCl. *Open symbols*, measurements made during compression, *filled symbols*, measurements made during expansion. Curves are typical examples from a series of consecutive dynamic cycles. (A) First dynamic cycle after adsorption to 24–25 mN/m. Note: relatively large collapse plateau at minimum tension, total area compression is 80%. (B) Second dynamic cycle. Note: Apparent squeeze-out plateau at 20 mN/m as a consequence of film collapse in A. (C) 20th dynamic cycle. Note: Collapse plateau at minimum tension has disappeared. Film area compression required to obtain minimum surface tension 80%, equal to total film area compression. (From ref. 22; used with permission.)

B. Adsorption After Film Collapse

In order to clarify the role of calcium in the surface activity of dynamically cycled films with collapse plateaus at surface tensions near 1 mN/m, adsorption was examined after the completion of different numbers of hysteresis loops. The chamber contents were continuously stirred during cycling and adsorption. The total film area compression was 80%, and cycling was stopped at maximum film area to measure adsorption versus time. The phospholipid concentration was 1 mg/ml.

Fig. 10 demonstrates adsorption after the completion of 1, 20, and 50 cycles. Compared with the initial adsorption where the time to reach the equilibrium value of 23–25 mN/m was 2–3 sec, a considerable delay in the adsorption rate was observed. Fig. 10 shows that increasing adsorption times were required with increasing numbers of consecutive hysteresis loops. After 1 loop it took about 50 sec to reach 25 mN/m, and after 50 loops it took 100 sec to reach 25 mN/m. Fig. 11 demonstrates that the addition of calcium accelerated adsorption after dynamic hysteresis loops with collapse plateaus. After 1 cycle, the adsorption time to 25 mN/m was 20 sec, and after 20–50 cycles it took 40–50 sec to reach 25 mN/m, or approximately half the time required compared with the samples without added calcium.

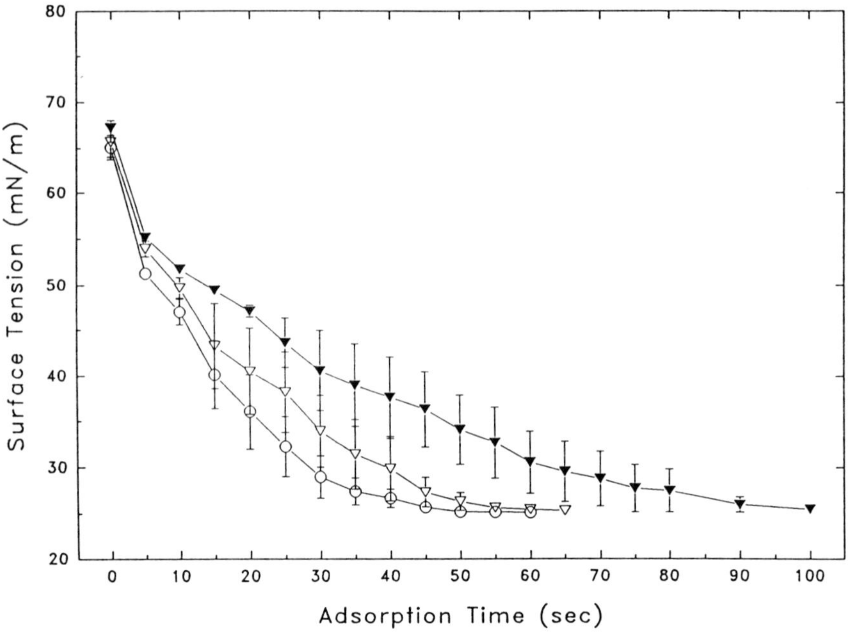

Figure 10 Time course for adsorption of porcine lipid extract surfactant (Curosurf) (1 mg/ml) without calcium added at maximum bubble area after differing numbers of consecutive dynamic cycles (20–30 cycles/min) with total film area compression of 80% which included collapse at minimum tension. Samples were suspended in 0.9% NaCl. Values are means ± SEM, n = 4. *Open circles*: Adsorption after one completed cycle with collapse at minimum tension. *Open triangles*: Adsorption after 20 completed cycles with collapse at minimum tension. *Filled triangles*: Adsorption after 50 completed cycles with collapse at minimum tension. (From ref. 22; used with permission.)

VIII. What Can We Learn from the In Vitro Studies?

A. Lipid Extract Surfactants

Under ideal conditions, that is, if inhibitory substances are absent, fresh lipid extract surfactants (bLES or Curosurf) have the capacity to form a film highly enriched in DPPC by selective adsorption from a well-stirred suspension. Therefore, the combination of surfactant lipids with SP-B and SP-C for a phospholipid concentration at and above 1 mg/ml appears to promote selective adsorption such that the resulting film behaves as a film highly enriched in DPPC. Further purification by selective squeeze-out does not appear necessary for such films. In a previous paper (13), based on experiments with low lipid concentrations, it was suggested that SP-A may promote selective adsorption. The conclusions from that report and others was that SP-A has an essential function

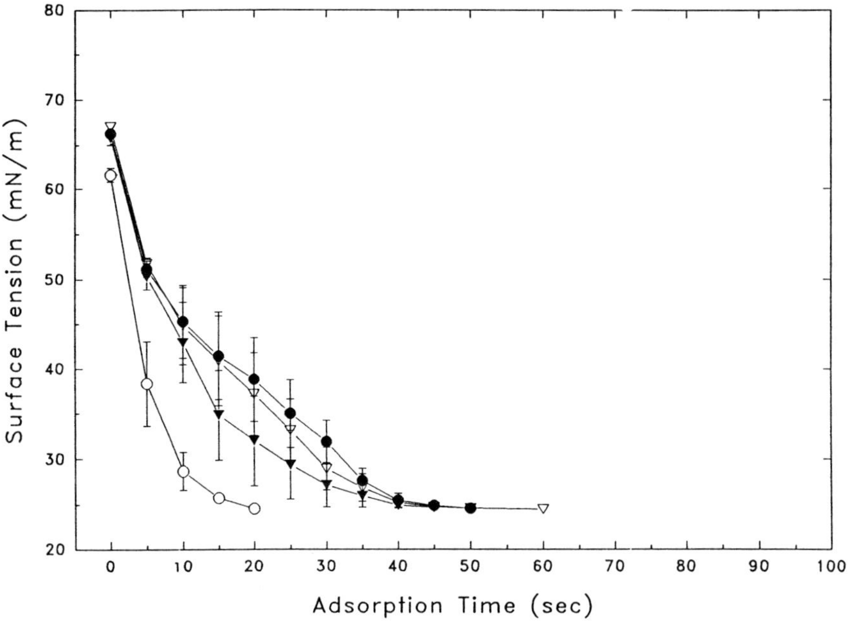

Figure 11 Time course for adsorption of porcine lipid extract surfactant (Curosurf) (1 mg/ml) with calcium added at maximum bubble area after differing numbers of consecutive dynamic cycles (20–30 cycles/min) with total film area compressions of 80% which included collapse at minimum tension. Samples were suspended in 0.9% NaCl, 1.5 mM $CaCl_2$. Values are means ± lSEM, n = 4. *Open circles*: Adsorption after one completed cycle with collapse at minimum tension. *Filled circles*: Adsorption after 50 completed cycles with collapse at minimum tension. *Open triangles*: Adsorption after 20 completed cycles with collapse at minimum tension. *Filled triangles*: Adsorption after 5 completed cycles with collapse at minimum tension. Note: Faster adsorption times in presence of added calcium. (From ref. 22; used with permission.)

when the surface activity of surfactant is limited owing to a variety of causes. It appears that the lack of SP-A in lipid extract surfactants can partially be compensated for by increasing their phospholipid concentration to at least 1 mg/ml (22). Fresh Curosurf and to a lesser extent bLES frequently adsorb into the air-water interface in quantities of up to 10^{14} phospholipid and 10^{11} protein molecules. These adsorption clicks are observed regardless of the bulk phospholipid concentration, even at 50 μg/ml, provided the subphase is well stirred. The film area compressions needed after adsorption to 23–25 mN/m are only 20% or less.

Stable minimum surface tensions below 1 mN/m can easily be obtained in the captive bubble surfactometer for Curosurf even at 50 μg/ml of phospholipids.

For bLES, the minimum concentrations required are generally about 200 μg/ml. This may be related to less frequent adsorption clicks observed during bLES adsorption.

If films are compressed in quasi-static or dynamic fashion beyond the point of collapse at minimum surface tension, a collapse phase consisting of a bilayer or multilayers of unknown structure are formed and remain associated with the monolayer unless the film area compression is reduced. Reducing the film area compression promotes the recovery of the collapse phase into the surface active phase. This recovery is greatly enhanced by calcium.

Repeated cycling with the formation of a collapse phase has a profound influence on the film surface activity. (1) An apparent squeeze-out plateau is formed at about 20 mN/m. The film compressibility is substantially increased; that is, the film area compressions needed to achieve near zero surface tensions is much greater than in the absence of a collapse phase. (2) Adsorption which may include adsorption from the bulk suspension and/or from the collapse phase is much slower after expansion of overcompressed films, but adsorption is considerably faster in the presence of added calcium. This is in line with the observation of Possmayer et al. (51), who found faster rates of adsorption in the presence of added calcium using the pulsating bubble technique. Adsorption was measured under dynamic 50% compression of film area; that is, adsorption was likely measured in the presence of a collapse phase due to overcompression. In addition, Kobayashi et al. (52) recently found that near zero surface tensions in the pulsating bubble surfactometer were not possible unless the concentration was at least 3 mg/ml, whereas in our study, even concentrations below 1 mg/ml produced minimum tensions less than 1 mN/m. Again, this discrepancy can likely be explained by the presence of a collapse phase increasing the film compressibility.

B. Synthetic Surfactants

Adsorption of Exosurf or phospholipid mixtures of DPPC and egg PG in molar ratio 7:3, pH 6.5 (DPPC/egg PG) is much slower than that of the lipid extract surfactants, even at concentrations above 2 mg/ml of phospholipid. After 5 min adsorption time, the plateau surface tensions of 38 and 35 mN/m, respectively, also indicate that much less lipid has been transported to the air-liquid interface than for the lipid extract surfactants where the plateau or equilibrium tensions were 23–25 mN/m within a few seconds.

The high plateau tensions for synthetic films means that these films have to be compressed more than lipid extract films to reach the closely packed state at near zero minimum tension. Under quasi-static conditions, Exosurf films have to be compressed by about 80% and the DPPC/egg PG films by 45% to obtain near zero minimum tensions. There is no evidence for selective adsorption into these films. However, their surface activity can be greatly improved by squeeze-out or surface sorting on compression.

On consecutive quasi-static or dynamic cycling, and by avoiding over-compression at near zero minimum tension, the compressibility of the DPPC/PG films decreases. This is reflected in a decreasing film area compression needed (~25% after four cycles) to achieve stable near zero minimum surface tension. Although the cycling rate for DPPC/PG films do not appear to be important for surface activity, this is quite different for Exosurf. The film area compression required to achieve near zero surface tensions decreases dramatically from 80% (quasi-static) to approximately 40% at 50–60 cycles/min.

The lipid extract surfactants can tolerate slight overcompression on repeated cycling; however, the synthetic surfactants will lose their surface activity within a few cycles if overcompressed at near zero minimum tension. It appears that the collapse material in the absence of surface-associated proteins will remain excluded from the surface active film. For example, films from the DPPC/PG mixture with initial film area compressions of 50% demonstrated maximum surface tensions near 70 mN/m and required film area compressions near 80% to achieve near zero surface tensions after 20 cycles at 20–30 cycles/min.

IX. What Can We Learn from the Structure-Function Studies?

From the correlation studies of lung microstructure and surface tension measurements, we know that an alveolar air-liquid surface tension of 6 mN/m at 40% TLC stabilizes a considerably lower alveolar surface area than a minimum surface tension of 1 mN/m (see Section II.B).

A good surfactant in vitro should produce a minimum surface tension of less than 5 mN/m on the first compression after adsorption (11). In view of the structure-function studies, a minimum surface tension of 5 mN/m is probably too high, and thus lower values, about 1 mN/m, should be achieved within very few cycles. In addition, the film area compression needed to achieve near zero tension should not substantially exceed 30% (19,22).

The lipid extract surfactants investigated in this chapter fulfill these requirements easily under quasi-static or dynamic conditions. The two synthetic surfactants approach these requirements closely if the mode of cycling (speed, area compression) is chosen such that surface activity is optimized. If foreign fluids are considered to be introduced into lungs to improve gas exchange, their performance should be scrutinized by structure-function studies, since their interfacial properties cannot be predicted from their surface tension properties.

A. The Surfactant Film: Monolayer or Multilayer?

Recent experiments on excised rabbit lungs, fixed by vascular perfusion, suggest a variable and rather complex structure of the alveolar air-liquid film. Invariably, the osmiophilic film appears to be wider than a monolayer, and at many sites a triple layer or even a multilayer can be recognized.

These findings appear to correlate well with in vitro findings in the captive bubble from experiments conducted for the present study. It is interesting to note that lipid extract surfactant, having SP-B and SP-C but not SP-A, has the capacity to transport more material than what is needed for one monolayer to the bubble interface. At present, we do not know whether this additional material (the surface-associated reservoir) at the interface is in the form of well-organized multilayers or in a more amorphous state. We can speculate that the relatively large amount of film material at the very interface in situ might be important in modulating the harmful effect of inhibitory agents.

X. Summary

A. General Guidelines

For all of the surfactants tested, film collapse at near zero minimum surface tension should be avoided, because of the creation of a collapse phase that will increase film compressibility and decrease adsorption during cycling.

The in vitro surface activity of a particular surfactant can be optimized by choosing a "customized" approach to testing surface activity; e.g., fast dynamic cycling for Exosurf or adding calcium to lipid extract surfactant suspensions.

Concentration requirements may have to be established from in vitro studies on surfactant inhibition and from model experiments on animals, since in the captive bubble surfactometer concentrations at and above 1 mg/ml of phospholipid give equivalent results, provided the surfactant is fresh and there are no inhibitors in the suspensions studied.

B. Lipid Extract Surfactants

Good surfactants have the capacity to form a film already enriched in DPPC on adsorption. Less than 20% film area compression upon the first quasi-static or dynamic cycle after adsorption to equilibrium produces near zero surface tension. There is no evidence of a distinguished squeeze-out plateau in the surface tension-area relations.

C. Synthetic Surfactants

In contrast to the lipid extract surfactants, the two surfactants investigated demonstrate substantial squeeze-out and purification toward a purer DPPC film on repeated cycling.

D. Implications for Choosing a Particular Mode of Ventilation

Suggestions for choosing a particular mode of ventilation may be considered from the in vitro tests. For all of the surfactants studied, avoiding film overcompression at minimum surface tension is important. Thus, the application of positive end-expiratory pressure might be beneficial from the point of view of maintaining optimal surface activity. By increasing the lung's resting volume, the formation of a collapse phase might be reduced. This appears particularly important for surfactants that show poor respreading after film collapse.

Acknowledgments

This work was supported by the Medical Research Council of Canada, grant MT6435, the Alberta Heritage Foundation for Medical Research, and the Swiss National Foundation for Scientific Research. The excellent technical assistance by Stanley Cheng, Karl Babl, Ursula Gyger, Barbara Krieger, and Dr. Michael Schoel are acknowledged. We also thank Dr. Jon Goerke and Dr. Fred Possmayer for helpful suggestions.

References

1. Goerke J, Clements JA. Alevolar surface tension and lung surfactant. In: Handbook of Physiology. The Respiratory System. Mechanics of Breathing. Bethesda: Am Physiol Soc, 1986, Sect. 3, Vol. III, Part 1: 247–261.
2. Mead J, Collier C. Relation of volume history of lungs to respiratory mechanics in anesthetized dogs. J Appl Physiol 1959; 14:669–678.
3. Horie T, Hildebrandt J. Dynamic compliance, limit cycles, and static equilibria of excised cat lung. J Appl Physiol 1971; 31:423–430.
4. Schürch S, Goerke J, Clements JA. Direct determination of surface tension in the lung. Proc Natl Acad Sci USA 1976; 73:4698–4702.
5. Schürch S, Goerke J, Clements JA. Direct determination of volume- and time-dependence of alveolar surface tension in excised lungs. Proc Natl Acad Sci USA 1978; 75:3417–3421.
6. Schürch S. Surface tension at low lung volumes: Dependence on time and alveolar size. Respir Physiol 1982; 48:339–355.
7. Fujiwara T, Robertson B. Pharmacology of exogenous surfactant. In: Robertson B, Van Golde LMG, Batenburg JJ. eds. Pulmonary Surfactant: From Molecular Biology to Clinical Practice. Amsterdam: Elsevier, 1992:561–592.
8. Goerke J, Gonzales J. Temperature dependence of dipalmitoyl phosphatidylcholine monolayer stability. J Appl Physiol 1971; 51:1108–1114.
9. Clements JA. Sixth Bowditch lecture: Surface phenomena in relation to pulmonary function. Physiologist 1962; 5:11–28.
10. Schoedel W, Slama H, Hansen E. Zeitabhängiges Verhalten von Filmen von

oberflächenaktivem Material aus Lungenalveolen, Pfluegers Arch 1971; 322:336–346.
11. Putz G, Goerke J, Taeusch HW, Clements JA. Comparison of captive- and pulsating-bubble surfactometers using lung surfactant. J Appl Physiol 1994; 76:1425–1431.
12. Yu S-H, Possmayer F. Adsorption, compression and stability of surface films from natural, lipid extract and reconstituted pulmonary surfactants. Biochim Biophys Acta 1993; 1167:264–271.
13. Schürch S, Possmayer F, Cheng S, Cockshutt AM. Pulmonary SP-A enhances adsorption and appears to induce surface sorting of lipid extract surfactant. Am J Physiol 1992; 263:L210–L218.
14. Goerke J. Surfactant and lung mechanics. In: Robertson B, Van Golde LMG, Batenburg JJ, eds. Pulmonary Surfactant: From Molecular Biology to Clinical Practice. Amsterdam: Elsevier, 1992:165–192.
15. Ogawa A, Brown CL, Schlueter MA, Benson BJ, Clements JA, Hawgood S. Lung function, surfactant apoprotein content and level of PEEP in prematurely delivered rabbits. J Appl Physiol 1994; 77:1840–1849.
16. Bachofen H, Hildebrandt J, Bachofen M. Pressure-volume curves of air- and liquid-filled excised lungs—surface tension in situ. J Appl Physiol 1970: 29:422–431.
17. Stamenovic D, Smith JC. Surface forces in lungs. II. Microstructural mechanics and lung stability. J Appl Physiol 1986; 60:1351–1357.
18. Ganesan S, Lai-Fook SJ, Schürch S. Alveolar liquid pressure in nonedematous and kerosene-washed rabbit lungs by micropuncture. Respir Physiol 1989; 78:281–296.
19. Bachofen H, Schürch S, Urbinelli M, Weibel ER. Relations among alveolar surface tension, surface area, volume and recoil pressure. J Appl Physiol 1987; 62:1878–1887.
20. Wilson TA, Bachofen H. A model for mechanical structure of the alveolar duct. J Appl Physiol 1982; 52:1064–1070.
21. Schürch S, Bachofen H, Goerke J, Green F. Surface properties of rat pulmonary surfactant studied with the captive bubble method: Adsorption, hysteresis, stability. Biochim Biophys Acta 1992; 1103:127–136.
22. Schürch S, Schürch D, Curstedt T, Robertson B. Surface activity of lipid extract surfactant in relation to film area compression and collapse. J Appl Physiol 1994; 77:974–986.
23. Bachofen H, Schürch S, Possmayer F. Disturbance of alveolar lining layer: Effects on alveolar microstructure. J Appl Physiol 1994; 76:1983–1992.
24. Curtis SE, Fuhrmann BP, Howland DF. Airway and alveolar pressures during perfluorocarbon breathing in infant lambs. J Appl Physiol 1990; 68:2322–2328.
25. Fuhrmann BP, Paczan PR, De Francisis M. Perfluorocarbon-associated gas exchange. Crit Care Med 1991; 19:712–718.
26. Kylstra JA, Schoenfisch WH. Alveolar surface tension in fluorocarbon-filled lungs. J Appl Physiol 1972; 33:32–35.
27. Lowe CA, Shaffer TH. Pulmonary vascular resistance in the fluorocarbon-rinsed lungs. J Appl Physiol 1986; 60:154–159.
28. Oldmixon EH, Suzuki S, Butler JP, Hoppin Jr FG. Perfusion dehydration fixes elastin and preserves lung airspace dimensions. J Appl Physiol 1985; 58:105–113.

29. Putz G, Goerke J, Schürch S, Clements JA. Evaluation of a pressure-driven captive bubble surfactometer. J Appl Physiol 1994; 76:1417–1424.
30. Schoel WM, Schürch S, Goerke J. The captive bubble method for the evaluation of pulmonary surfactant: Surface tension, area and volume calculations. Biochim Biophys Acta 1994; 1200:286–290.
31. Malcolm JD, Elliott CD. Interfacial tension from height and diameter of a single profile drop or captive bubble. Can J Chem Eng 1980; 58:151–153.
32. Callen HB. Thermodynamics. New York: John Wiley, 1960:1–376.
33. Weibel ER, Gil J. Electron microscopic demonstration of an extracellular lining layer of alveoli. Respir Physiol 1968; 4:42–57.
34. Gil J, Weibel ER. Improvements in demonstration of lining layer of lung alveoli by electron microscopy. Respir Physiol 1969/70; 8:13–36.
35. Untersee P, Gil J, Weibel ER. Visualization of extracellular lining layer of lung alveoli by freeze etching. Respir Physiol 1971; 13:171–185.
36. Chapman D, Fluck DJ. Physical studies of phospholipids. III. Electron microscope studies of some pure fully saturated 2,3-diacyl-DL-phosphatidyl-ethanolamines and phosphatidylcholines. J Cell Biol 1966; 30:1–11.
37. Bachofen H, Schürch S, Michel RP, Weibel ER. Experimental hydrostatic pulmonary edema in rabbit lungs. Morphology. Am Rev Respir Dis 1993; 147:989–996.
38. Bachofen H, Schürch S, Weibel ER. Experimental hydrostatic pulmonary in rabbit lungs. Barrier lesions. Am Rev Respir Dis 1993; 147:997–1004.
39. Yu S-H, Harding PGR, Smith N, Possmayer F. Bovine pulmonary surfactant: Chemical composition and physical properties. Lipids 1983; 18:522–529.
40. Lowry OH, Rosebrough NJ, Farr AL, Randall RJ. Protein measurement with Folin phenol reagent. J Chem Eng 1951; 193:265–275.
41. Yu S-H, Possmayer F. Comparative studies on the biophysical activities the low-molecular-weight hydrophobic proteins purified from bovine pulmonary surfactant. Biochim Biophys Acta 1988; 961:337–350.
42. Robertson B, Curstedt T, Johansson J, et al. Structural and functional characterization of porcine surfactant isolated by liquid-gel chromatography. Progr Respir Res 1990; 25:237–246.
43. Collaborative European Multicenter Study Group. Surfactant replacement therapy for severe respiratory distress syndrome: An international randomized clinical trial. Pediatrics 1988; 82:683–691.
44. Bartlett GR. Phosphorus assay in column chromatography. J Biol Chem 1959; 234:466–468.
45. Morley CJ, Greenough A, Miller NG, et al. Randomized trial of artificial surfactant (ALEC) given at birth to babies from 23 to 34 weeks gestation. Early Hum Dev 1988; 17:41–54.
46. Keough KMW, Farrell E, Cox M, et al. Physical, chemical and physiological characteristics of isolates of pulmonary surfactant from adult rabbits. Can J Physiol Pharmacol 1985; 63:1043–1051.
47. Keough KMW. Physical chemistry of pulmonary surfactant in the terminal air spaces. In: Robertson B, Van Golde LMG, Batenburg JJ, eds. Pulmonary Surfactant: From Molecular Biology to Clinical Practice. Amsterdam: Elsevier, 1992:109–164.

48. Schürch S, Bachofen H, Goerke J, Possmayer F. A captive bubble method reproduces the in situ behavior of lung surfactant monolayers. J Appl Physiol 1992; 67:2389–2396.
49. Curstedt T, Johansson J, Robertson B, et al. Structure and function of hydrophobic surfactant-associated proteins. In: Bevilacqua G, Parmigiani S, Robertson B, eds. Surfactant in Clinical Practice. Chur: Harwood, 1993:55–60.
50. Williams MC, Hawgood S, Hamilton RL. Changes in lipid structure produced by surfactant proteins SP-A, SP-B, and SP-C. Am J Respir Cell Mol Biol 1991; 5:41–50.
51. Possmayer F, Yu S-H, Weber JM, Harding PGR. Pulmonary surfactant. Can J Biochem Cell Biol 1984; 62:1121–1133.
52. Kobayashi T, Robertson B. Surface adsorption of pulmonary surfactant in relation to bulk-phase concentration and presence of $CaCl_2$. Respiration 1983; 44:63–70.
53. Schürch FS. Surface tension properties of surfactant. In: Long WA, Tilson HH, eds. Proceedings of the Exosurf Neonatal Treatment IND Investigator's Meeting, Nov 13–14, 1991. Longhorn, PA: Adis International, 1991:95–102.

2

Surfactant and Lung Fluid Balance

DAVID P. CARLTON and RICHARD D. BLAND
University of Utah Health Sciences Center
Salt Lake City, Utah

I. Introduction

Two pioneers in the study of surfactant, Pattle (1) and Clements (2), called attention to the theoretical importance of alveolar surface tension in the development of pulmonary edema and suggested a possible benefit of surface-active material in preventing liquid from shifting out of the lung circulation into the terminal air spaces. The discovery that surfactant deficiency was responsible for the respiratory distress syndrome following premature birth and the recognition that pulmonary edema was a consistent feature of this disease provided sufficient rationale to pursue the relationship between surfactant function and edema formation (3–5).

The purpose of this chapter is to review experimental evidence regarding the relationship between pulmonary surfactant and edema formation in the lung. Such evidence derives from studies in vivo and in vitro in lungs from a variety of animal species. This presentation will emphasize recent work that we have done to examine postnatal changes in lung fluid dynamics associated with premature birth and surfactant deficiency, with and without surfactant replacement therapy at birth.

II. Fluid Balance in the Lung

A number of factors determine fluid balance in the lung. Transmural hydrostatic and protein osmotic pressures, vascular surface area, and vascular barrier permeability regulate the magnitude of fluid flux into the lung interstitium (6). An increase in the difference between the microvascular and perimicrovascular hydrostatic pressures or a decrease in the difference between microvascular and perimicrovascular protein osmotic pressures will enhance leakage of fluid from the pulmonary microcirculation. Likewise, an increase in microvascular surface area or an increase in lung microvascular permeability will promote fluid flux into the lung. Several of these factors contribute to the effect of surfactant on lung fluid balance.

III. Effect of Surface Tension on Fluid Filtration Forces

Surface-active material in the distal air spaces acts to lower surface tension at the air-liquid interface (7). Studies in which changes in pulmonary vascular perfusion were measured in response to alterations in surface tension provided the initial evidence that changes at the air-liquid interface might affect transvascular fluid filtration. Lloyd and Wright (8) studied pulmonary vascular perfusion under conditions in which surface tension forces in the lung were eliminated by filling the alveoli with liquid. They found that vascular perfusion was enhanced when surface tension forces were high. Bruderman et al. (9) and Pain and West (10) performed experiments in excised lungs in which they studied vascular perfusion during inflation and deflation, which are conditions that are associated with different alveolar surface tensions. They found that pulmonary vascular perfusion was increased under conditions in which surface tension was elevated. These experiments established a role for the air-liquid interface in regulating pulmonary vascular resistance, and they suggested that an increase in surface tension might increase transmural hydrostatic force, perhaps by decreasing perimicrovascular pressure. Hida and Hildebrandt (11) used a wick technique to measure directly the perimicrovascular pressure in isolated lungs at varied surface tension. These studies confirmed that as surface tension increases, perimicrovascular pressure falls.

IV. Surfactant Deficiency and Lung Fluid Balance

The link between surfactant deficiency and lung edema derives from histological observations of lungs from premature infants and animals (5,12). Premature infants and animals that have respiratory distress following premature birth show pathological features of excess lung water. Terminal respiratory units typically are filled with protein-containing fluid, and lymphatic vessels are distended with liquid. The respiratory distress that often occurs after premature birth is a direct result of incomplete development of the pulmonary surfactant system.

In addition to the histological evidence of pulmonary edema, physiological studies show excess lung water in infants and animals with respiratory distress after premature birth (4,13–15). Troug et al. (13) found that lung water was increased in primates with respiratory distress after premature birth compared with more mature primates without respiratory distress. Using an indicator dilution method, Sundell et al. (14) found similar results in premature lambs: Extravascular lung water was significantly greater in preterm lambs with respiratory distress compared with more mature lambs without respiratory distress.

Bland et al. (15) studied two groups of chronically catheterized preterm lambs (131 ± 1 day gestation) for 8 hr after birth and found that postmortem extravascular lung water was greater in preterm lambs with respiratory distress than it was in preterm lambs without respiratory distress. Postnatally, lymph flow increased more than twofold, and lymph protein clearance increased more than threefold in lambs with respiratory distress. There were no changes in lymph flow or protein clearance in lambs without respiratory distress. Pulmonary arterial and left atrial pressures were similar between the two groups of lambs; plasma protein concentrations were less in lambs that had respiratory distress compared with lambs without lung disease.

As in respiratory failure after premature birth, pulmonary edema and plasma proteins within the air spaces typically accompany abnormalities of surfactant function in adult respiratory distress syndromes (ARDS) (16–19). The specific contribution of surfactant dysfunction to excess lung water in ARDS is unclear, as conditions that trigger respiratory failure may cause pulmonary edema without necessarily affecting surfactant function. The apparent benefit of surfactant replacement in patients with ARDS supports the notion that impaired surfactant function may contribute to the pathophysiology of adult respiratory failure (20,21).

To simulate the defective surfactant activity in ARDS, several investigators have studied lung fluid balance after instillation of detergent into the lungs of adult animals. This procedure impairs normal surfactant activity and yields stiff lungs with abnormal surface tension (22–24). These studies have shown that detergent-mediated loss of surfactant activity increases lung water content. Bredenberg et al. (22) found that bronchoalveolar lavage with detergent increased extravascular lung water on average by nearly 35% in lungs from adult dogs. Lung water content was even greater in dogs that received detergent by aerosol inhalation (24). Others have shown that detergent-induced surfactant dysfunction increases lung lymph flow (23,25). Surfactant inactivation from intrapulmonary detergent had no significant effect on lung vascular pressures, cardiac output, or protein osmotic pressure in plasma (22,24). Thus, studies with both preterm animals and mature animals with surfactant deficiency have demonstrated an increase in fluid movement from the pulmonary circulation into the interstitium, with resultant pulmonary edema.

The physiological mechanisms responsible for enhanced fluid filtration and excess lung water in the absence of surfactant remain unclear. Surfactant deficiency has a variable effect on pulmonary vascular pressures. Pulmonary arterial pressure remains elevated after birth in preterm lambs with respiratory distress, whereas lung vascular pressure tends to fall in lambs without respiratory distress (15). Left atrial pressure is similar regardless of respiratory status after birth. Whether the relative elevation in pulmonary arterial pressure in those lambs with respiratory failure is a direct result of the absence of surfactant, or simply related to the accompanying hypoxemia, is unclear. Whereas, in vivo studies of surfactant deficiency from lung lavage with detergent have demonstrated no effect on either pulmonary arterial or left atrial pressure, other studies of in situ adult lungs have shown that pulmonary arterial pressure increases as surfactant is washed out with detergent (22,24,26).

Surfactant deficiency also might influence lung water balance by affecting the protein osmotic pressure in plasma. Plasma protein concentration is lower in preterm lambs with respiratory failure than it is in lambs without disease (15), and respiratory distress in human infants is often associated with hypoproteinemia (27). In studies of surfactant washout in adult lungs, however, plasma protein concentration did not change (22, 24).

Changes in vascular surface area could contribute to excess fluid filtration and lung edema in the absence of surfactant. When surfactant function is disturbed by intrapulmonary instillation of detergent, the number of perfused alveolar capillaries more than doubles (26). This vascular recruitment may be a result of the lower perimicrovascular pressure following detergent treatment, an interpretation supported by studies in excised lungs in which perimicrovascular pressure is lower in the absence of adequate surfactant function. Albert et al. (28) studied excised dog lungs and showed that isogravimetric pressure relative to alveolar pressure fell when surfactant was inactivated by overventilation with cold gas. Isogravimetric pressure is the intravascular pressure at which the lung neither gains nor loses weight, and it is considered to be equivalent to perimicrovascular pressure in isolated lungs. Beck and Lai-Fook (29) measured alveolar liquid pressure, which approximates perimicrovascular pressure (30), following surfactant inactivation by detergent lavage or by overventilation with cold gas. They showed that surfactant dysfunction was associated with a decrease in alveolar liquid pressure. Raj (31) measured alveolar liquid pressure in isolated lungs of premature fetal rabbits with surfactant deficiency, and she found a direct relationship between endogenous alveolar phospholipid content and alveolar liquid pressure: Lungs that had little or no alveolar phospholipid had a low alveolar liquid pressure.

An additional consequence of surfactant deficiency is a decrease in the barrier function of the respiratory epithelium. Jobe et al. (32) found that protein yield from lung lavage was increased in preterm lambs that were mechanically ventilated for 3 hr after birth compared with mature newborn lambs that were managed in a similar fashion. Jefferies et al. (33) aerosolized small solutes into the lungs of premature infants and found that particles disappeared faster from the lungs of premature infants with hyaline membrane disease compared with infants without lung disease. Studies with adult dogs that were rendered surfactant deficient by detergent washout also showed more rapid clearance of small solutes across the lung epithelium (34).

Our studies of preterm lambs demonstrated abnormal postnatal lung vascular protein permeability in the absence of surfactant (15). Protein clearance was nearly fourfold greater in preterm lambs with respiratory failure than it was in preterm lambs without lung disease. Whether lung vascular permeability increases in adult animals with surfactant dysfunction is uncertain. Some investigators have found that detergent-induced surfactant dysfunction has no effect on vascular permeability; others have reported that vascular permeability is increased (23,25).

V. Surfactant Replacement and Lung Fluid Balance

If surfactant deficiency leads to lung edema, does surfactant replacement prevent edema formation? Early studies of surfactant replacement in premature animals failed to show an effect on lung water content, but these studies were of brief duration and may not have allowed sufficient time for postnatal drainage of fetal lung liquid (35–37). In more recent studies, we extended the period of observation to 8 hr after birth and found that surfactant replacement inhibited lung vascular injury and edema (38).

In these studies, we surgically prepared fetal lambs at 121–125 days gestation (term 147 days) for subsequent measurement of systemic and pulmonary vascular pressures, lung lymph flow, and pleural liquid drainage (the sum of which reflects net fluid movement from the pulmonary circulation into the lung). Three to 7 days after surgery, we studied the lambs for 2–4 hr before and 8 hr after delivery by cesarean section. At the time of study, the lambs averaged 127–128 days gestation. Four lambs received calf-lung surfactant at the time of birth and eight received saline placebo. After birth the lambs were mechanically ventilated with oxygen for 8 hr at a rate of 30 breaths per minute and end-expiratory pressure at 4–6 cmH_2O. We adjusted the peak inflation pressure to maintain $Paco_2$ between 35 and 45 mmHg. At the end of these studies, we removed the lungs for subsequent microscopy and measurement of extravascular lung water.

After birth systemic and pulmonary vascular pressures were similar in both groups of lambs (Table 1). By 6–8 hr after birth, seven of the eight control lambs, but none of the surfactant-treated lambs, had hypoxemia ($Pa_{O_2} < 50$ mmHg). Peak inflation pressure at 0–2 hr and 6–8 hr after birth was greater in control lambs. By 6–8 hr after birth, total lung liquid drainage (the sum of lymph and pleural liquid flows) was threefold greater than prenatal values in control lambs, but it did not change significantly after birth in surfactant-treated lambs (Fig. 1). Total protein drainage during the 6–8 hr after birth more than doubled in control lambs, but it tended to fall or remain constant in surfactant-treated lambs. Extravascular lung water was significantly less in lambs treated with surfactant. Edema, hyaline membranes, and abundant neutrophils were typically present in the air spaces of control lambs (Fig. 2).

Surfactant replacement also influences lung water content in animal models of lung injury that are associated with surfactant inactivation. Matalon et al. (39) studied the effect of surfactant replacement on lung water content of adult rabbits that had abnormal surfactant function from prolonged oxygen breathing. After development of hyperoxic lung injury, the rabbits received either intrapulmonary surfactant or saline; 24 hr later, lung water was less in rabbits that received surfactant compared with saline-treated controls. In a subsequent study of similar design, Loewen et al. (40) treated adult rabbits with surfactant before the start of oxygen breathing, and then they repeated surfactant treatment daily during oxygen exposure. Surfactant treatment did not reduce lung water to normal

Table 1 Physiological Variables Before and After Birth in 12 Preterm Lambs (127–128 Days Gestation) Treated at the Time of Operative Delivery with Either Placebo (Control, n = 8) or Surfactant (Surfactant Treated, n = 4)

	Control		Surfactant treated	
Time period	before birth[a]	after birth[a]	before birth	after birth
Vascular pressures (mmHg)				
Aorta	44 ± 1	56 ± 3[b]	42 ± 2	54 ± 3[b]
Pulmonary artery	45 ± 1	54 ± 4	45 ± 2	42 ± 3
Left atrium	2 ± 1	3 ± 1[b]	1 ± 1	4 ± 1
Blood values				
pH	7.38 ± 0.01	7.25 ± 0.05[b]	7.34 ± 0.03	7.38 ± 0.03
Pa_{O_2}, mmHg	20 ± 1	36 ± 10	21 ± 1	279 ± 50[b]
Pa_{CO_2}, mmHg	46 ± 1	49 ± 4	44 ± 2	40 ± 2
Hematocrit (%)	35 ± 1	39 ± 2[b]	34 ± 1	37 ± 2

[a]Before birth and after birth refer to 2–4 hr before and 6–8 hr after birth, respectively.
[b]Significantly different from before birth, $p < 0.05$.
Source: From ref. 38; used with permission.

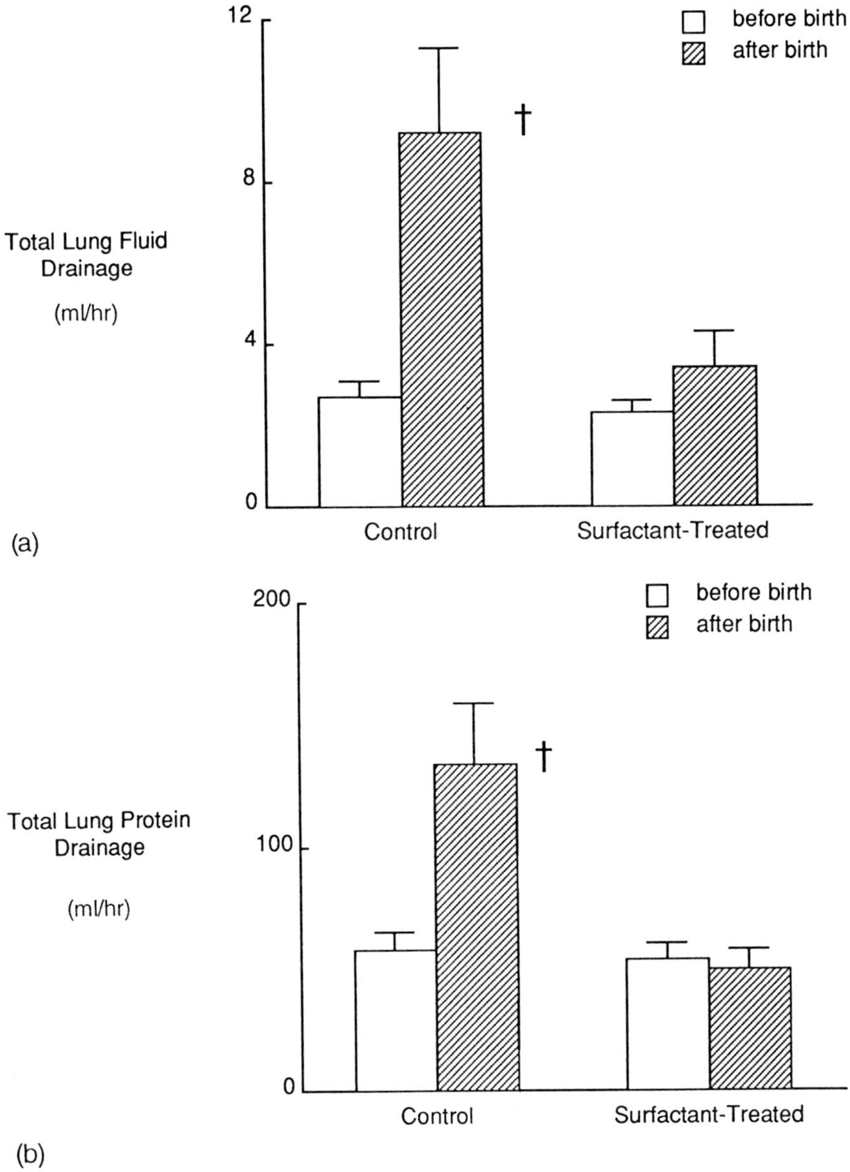

Figure 1 Total lung fluid drainage (a), total lung protein drainage (b), and extravascular lung water (c) measured 8 hr after birth in 12 preterm lambs that were treated at delivery with either intrapulmonary saline (n = 8, control) or surfactant (n = 4). Mean ± SE. † Significantly different from before birth, $p < 0.05$. * Significantly different from control, $p < 0.05$. (From ref. 38; used with permission.)

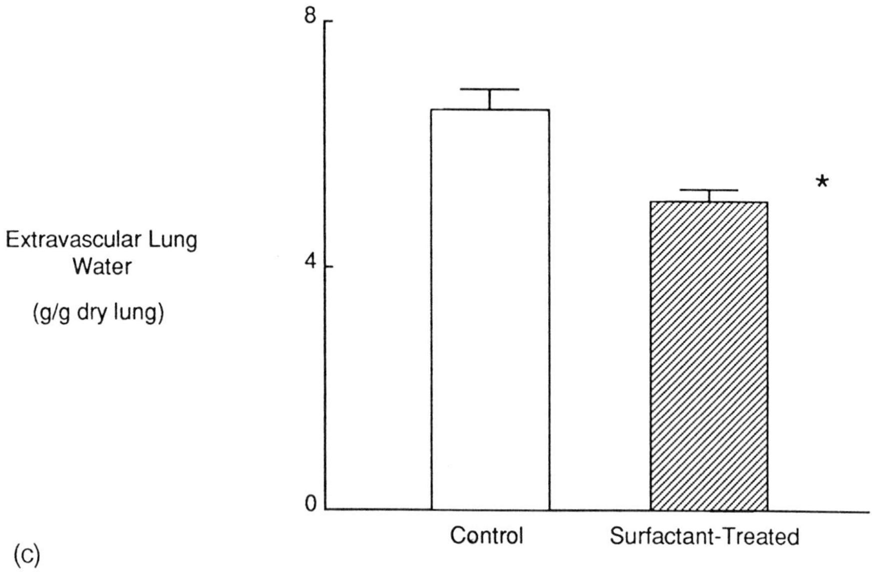

Figure 1 *(Continued)*

(compared with controls that breathed room air), but lung edema was less than it was in saline-treated controls.

Surfactant replacement probably reduces transvascular fluid movement and lung edema by influencing transmural filtration forces and barrier permeability. Our studies with premature lambs showed that fluid filtration decreases after surfactant replacement, but this effect was not a result of changes in pulmonary vascular pressures (38). Pulmonary arterial and left atrial pressures were unaffected by surfactant administration, a result that is consistent with earlier studies of surfactant administration after premature birth (41,42). It is possible, however, that surfactant replacement may alter pulmonary vascular pressures under different experimental conditions. In studies of adult sheep with lung injury induced by bronchoalveolar lavage with saline, surfactant administration reduced pulmonary arterial pressure without affecting pulmonary arterial wedge pressure (43). Likewise, surfactant treatment reduces pulmonary arterial pressure in premature human infants with respiratory distress (44). In our studies of preterm lambs, surfactant administration probably decreased lung edema, at least in part, by altering perimicrovascular pressure. Raj (31) measured alveolar liquid pressure by micropuncture in lungs from premature rabbits following surfactant administration and found that surfactant increased alveolar liquid pressure.

Surfactant replacement after premature birth also inhibits lung edema by preventing a postnatal increase in lung vascular protein permeability (38). In

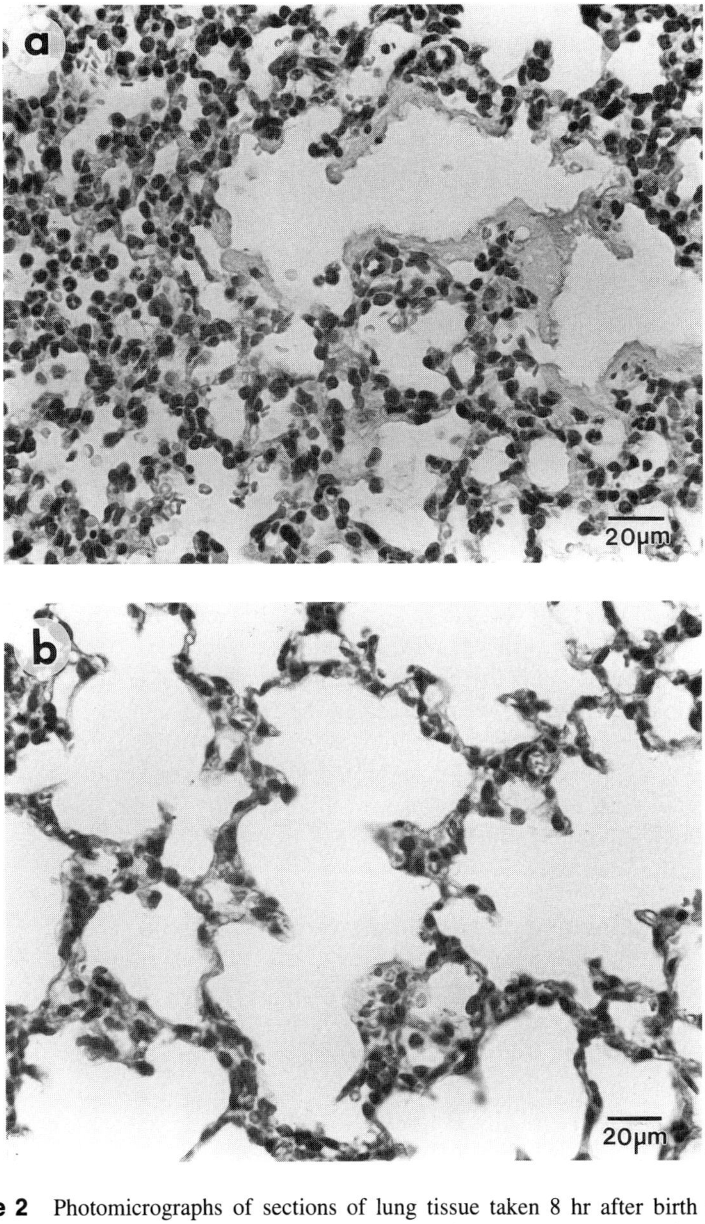

Figure 2 Photomicrographs of sections of lung tissue taken 8 hr after birth from a preterm lamb that received either intrapulmonary saline (a, control) or surfactant (b, treated) at the time of delivery. Tissue sections are stained with hematoxylin and eosin. (From ref. 38; used with permission.)

lambs that did not receive surfactant at delivery, lung protein drainage increased significantly, whereas lung protein drainage did not change after birth in lambs that received surfactant. This result resembles the postnatal course of lung protein drainage that occurs in healthy term lambs (45).

Jobe et al. (46) and Robertson et al. (47) demonstrated a similar beneficial effect of surfactant on the integrity of the lung epithelial barrier. When they administered surfactant to premature lambs or rabbits at the time of delivery, protein recovery in alveolar lavage decreased. Surfactant administration also preserves the barrier function of the respiratory epithelium when normal surfactant is inactivated. Following sustained hyperoxia, adult rabbits become surfactant dificient and show evidence of increased lung epithelial permeability; surfactant replacement in this model of lung injury reduced protein recovery in alveolar lavage (48).

Maintenance of epithelial and endothelial protein permeability following surfactant administration may be a consequence of reduced ventilator support. Jobe et al. (46) showed that recovery of protein in lung lavage of newborn sheep was directly related to inflation pressure: Preterm lambs that were treated with surfactant at birth required less inflation pressure and had less epithelial protein leak when compared with lambs that did not receive surfactant. Carlton et al. (49) showed that lung vascular injury occurred in lambs that were mechanically ventilated with large tidal volumes. Recently, the same investigators (38) found that lung water and lung protein drainage measured 8 hr after birth were directly related to peak inflation pressure during the first 2 hr after delivery (Fig. 3). Surfactant administration consistently lowered peak inflation pressure, extravascular lung water, and lung vascular protein leak. These observations underscore the notion that therapeutic measures adopted early in the course of acute respiratory failure might induce lung injury many hours later.

VI. Conclusions and Unanswered Questions

In the four decades since Pattle (1) and Clements (2) postulated that surfactant may regulate lung fluid balance, a variety of experiments have provided evidence for such an effect. We now know that surfactant deficiency increases fluid filtration from the pulmonary circulation into the lung interstitium (15), an observation that is usually attributed to reduced hydrostatic pressure around microvessels within the lung tissue (28,29,31). We also know that surfactant deficiency impairs respiratory gas exchange and thereby may increase hydrostatic pressure in the pulmonary circulation (15). It is, therefore, not surprising that lung water content is greater than normal in both human infants (4) and preterm animals with respiratory distress from surfactant deficiency (13–15).

What happens to fluid balance in surfactant-deficient lungs when surfactant

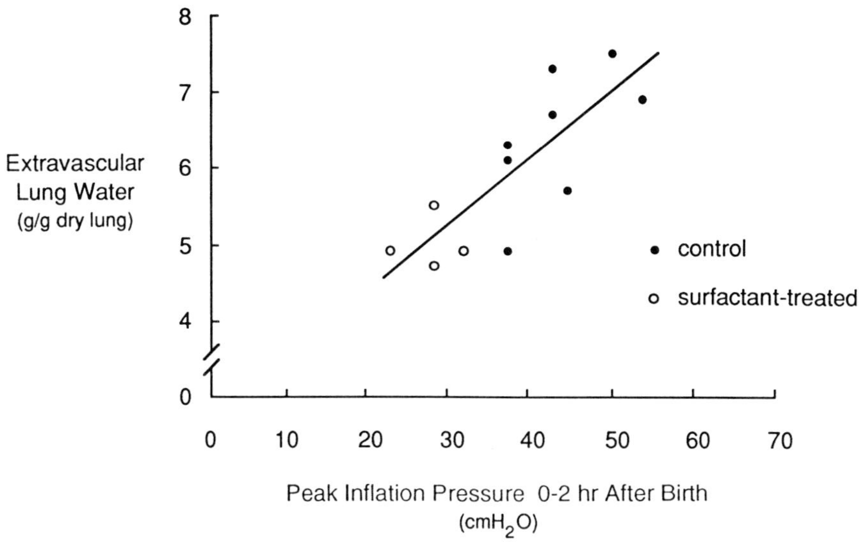

Figure 3 Relationship between extravascular lung water measured 8 hr after delivery and peak inflation pressure 0–2 hr after delivery in 12 preterm lambs treated with saline (control, n = 8) or surfactant (n = 4). (From ref. 38; used with permission.)

is replenished? We know that surfactant replacement improves respiratory gas exchange, which tends to reduce pulmonary vascular filtration pressure (38). We know that surfactant replacement increases alveolar liquid pressure (31), which approximates the hydrostatic pressure within the lung interstitium (30). This reduction in net filtration pressure decreases the flow of fluid from the pulmonary circulation into the lungs. Other studies have shown that surfactant therapy reduces pulmonary epithelial protein leak and lung vascular fluid and protein leak, perhaps as a result of lower inflation pressures (38,46,47,50). The net outcome of surfactant therapy in surfactant-deficient lungs is to lessen fluid and protein entry into the lungs. The mechanisms that are responsible for these effects remain obscure and merit further inquiry. Regardless of mechanisms, however, the bottom line is that surfactant inhibits edema formation in the immature lung and in the mature lung with abnormal surfactant function.

It is unclear if surfactant treatment improves lung fluid balance directly or indirectly. Gas exchange and lung compliance improve following surfactant treatment, each of which may affect lung fluid balance by influencing vascular surface area and hydrostatic pressure within and immediately surrounding the microcirculation. The role of surfactant replacement in reducing lung inflamma- tion is unexplored, particularly as it relates to the development of lung vascular injury in the presence of high inflation pressure. This last possibility is most intriguing, especially in light of evidence that inflammatory cells may play a role in the lung vascular injury that follows premature birth (51,52).

Acknowledgments

This work was supported in part by National Heart, Lung, and Blood Institute Grants HL-25816 and HL/HD-40802. We thank P. Davis for her technical assistance and S. Marron for preparing the manuscript.

References

1. Pattle RE. Properties, function and origin of the alveolar lining layer. Proc R Soc Lond Ser B 1958; 148:217–240.
2. Clements JA. Pulmonary edema and permeability of alveolar membranes. Arch Environ Health 1961; 2:280–283.
3. Avery ME, Mead J. Surface properties in relation to atelectasis and hyaline membrane disease. Am J Dis Child 1959; 97:517–523.
4. DeSa DJ. Pulmonary fluid content in infants with respiratory distress. J Pathol 1969; 97:469–479.
5. Lauweryns JM. Hyaline membrane disease: A pathological study of 55 infants. Arch Dis Child 1965; 40:618–625.
6. Staub NC. Pulmonary edema. Physiol Rev 1974; 54:678–811.
7. Pattle RE. Properties, function and origin of the alveolar lining layer. Nature 1955; 175:1125–1126.
8. Lloyd TC Jr., Wright GW. Pulmonary vascular resistance and vascular transmural gradient. J Appl Physiol 1960; 15:241–245.
9. Bruderman I, Somers K, Hamilton WK, et al. Effect of surface tension on circulation the excised lungs of dogs. J Appl Physiol 1964; 19:707–712.
10. Pain MCF, West JB. Effect of the volume history of the isolated lung on distribution of blood flow. J Appl Physiol 1966; 21:1545–1550.
11. Hida W, Hildebrandt J. Alveolar surface tension, lung inflation, and hydration affect interstitial pressure [Px(f)]. J Appl Physiol 1984; 57:262–270.
12. Stahlman M, LeQuire VS, Young WC, et al. Pathophysiology of respiratory distress in newborn lambs. Am J Dis Child 1964; 108:375–393.
13. Truog WE, Standaert TA, Murphy JH, et al. Effects of prolonged high-frequency oscillatory ventilation in premature primates with experimental hyaline membrane disease. Am Rev Respir Dis 1984; 130:76–80.
14. Sundell HW, Harris TR, Cannon JR, et al. Lung water and vascular permeability-surface area in premature newborn lambs with hyaline membrane disease. Circ Res 1987; 60:923–932.
15. Bland RD, Carlton DP, Scheerer RG, et al. Lung fluid balance in lambs before and after premature birth. J Clin Invest 1989; 84:568–576.
16. Ashbaugh DG, Bigelow DB, Petty TL, Levine BE. Acute respiratory distress in adults. Lancet 1967; 2:319–323.

17. Petty TL, Reiss OK, Paul GW, et al. Characteristics of pulmonary surfactant in adult respiratory distress syndrome associated with trauma and shock. Am Rev Respir Dis 1977; 115:531–536.
18. Petty TL, Silvers GW, Paul GW, Stanford RE. Abnormalities in lung elastic properties and surfactant function in adult respiratory distress syndrome. Chest 1979; 75:571–574.
19. Hallman M, Spragg R, Harrell JH, et al. Evidence of lung surfactant abnormality in respiratory failure. J Clin Invest 1982; 70:673–683.
20. Heikinheimo M, Hynynen M, Rautiainen P, et al. Successful treatment of ARDS with two doses of synthetic surfactant. Chest 1994; 105:1263–1264.
21. Spragg RG, Gilliard N, Richman P, et al. Acute effects of a single dose of porcine surfactant on patients with the adult respiratory distress syndrome. Chest 1994; 105:195–202.
22. Brendenberg C, Paskanik A, Nieman G. High surface tension pulmonary edema. J Surg Res 1983; 34:515–523.
23. Bredenberg CE, Nieman GF, Paskanik AM, Hart AKE. Microvascular membrane permeability in high surface tension pulmonary edema. J Appl Physiol 1986; 60:253–259.
24. Nieman GF, Bredenberg CE. High surface tension pulmonary edema induced by detergent aerosol. J Appl Physiol 1985; 58:129–136.
25. Wang CZ, Barrow RE, Cox CS, et al. Influence of detergent aerosol on lung microvascular permeability. J Appl Physiol 1993; 74:1016–1023.
26. Nieman G, Hakim T, Bredenberg C. Effect of increased alveolar surface tension on segmental pulmonary vascular resistance. J Appl Physiol 1988; 64:154–161.
27. Bland RD. Cord-blood total protein level as a screening aid for the idiopathic respiratory distress syndrome. N Engl J Med 1972; 287:9–13.
28. Albert RK, Lakshminarayan S, Hildebrandt J, Kirk W. Increased surface tension favors pulmonary edema formation in anesthetized dogs' lungs. J Clin Invest 1979; 63:1015–1018.
29. Beck KC, Lai-Fook SJ. Alveolar liquid pressure in excised edematous dog lung with increased static recoil. J Appl Physiol 1983; 55:1277–1283.
30. Fike CD, Lai-Fook SJ, Bland RD. Alveolar liquid pressures in newborn and adult rabbit lungs. J Appl Physiol 1988; 64:1629–1635.
31. Raj JU. Alveolar liquid pressure measured by micropuncture in isolated lungs of mature and immature fetal rabbits. J Clin Invest 1987; 79:1579–1588.
32. Jobe A, Jacobs H, Ikegami M, Berry D. Lung protein leaks in ventilated lambs: Effect of gestational age. J Appl Physiol 1985; 58:1246–1251.
33. Jefferies AL, Coates G, O'Brodovich H. Pulmonary epithelial permeability in hyaline-membrane disease. N Engl J Med 1984; 311:1075–80.
34. Nieman G, Ritter-Hrncirik C, Grossman Z, et al. High alveolar surface tension increases clearance of technetium 99m diethylenetriamine-pentaacetic acid. J Thorac Cardiovasc Surg 1990; 100:129–133.
35. Adams FH, Towers B, Osher AB, et al. Effects of tracheal instillation of natural surfactant in premature lambs. I. Clinical autopsy findings. Pediatr Res 1978; 12:84–848.

36. Derechin NM, Schlueter MA, Brown CL, et al. Controlled trial of a protein-free synthetic surfactant in preterm rabbits. Pediatr Res 1984; 18:387A.
37. Notter RH, Egan EA, Kwong MS, et al. Lung surfactant replacement in premature lambs with extracted lipids from bovine lung lavage: effects of dose, dispersion technique, and gestational age. Pediatr Res 1985; 19:569–577.
38. Carlton DP, Cho SC, Davis P, et al. Surfactant treatment at birth reduces lung vascular injury and edema in preterm lambs. Pediatr Res 1995; 37:1–6.
39. Matalon S, Holm B, Notter R. Mitigation of pulmonary hyperoxic injury by administration of exogenous surfactant. J Appl Physiol 1987; 62:756–761.
40. Loewen G, Holm B, Milanowski L, et al. Alveolar hyperoxic injury in rabbits receiving exogenous surfactant. J Appl Physiol 1989; 66:1087–1092.
41. Clyman RI, Jobe A, Heymann M, et al. Increased shunt through the patent ductus arteriosus after surfactant replacement therapy. J Pediatr 1982; 100:101–107.
42. Durand DJ, Clyman RI, Heymann MA, et al. Effects of a protein-free, synthetic surfactant on survival and pulmonary function in preterm lambs. J Pediatr 1985; 107:775–780.
43. Lewis JF, Tabor B, Ikegami M, et al. Lung function and surfactant distribution in saline-lavaged sheep given instilled vs. nebulized surfactant. J Appl Physiol 1993; 74:1256–1264.
44. Kaapa P, Kero P, Saraste M. Synthetic surfactant replacement therapy decreases estimated pulmonary artery pressure in respiratory distress syndrome. Am J Dis Child 1992; 146:961–964.
45. Bland RD, Hansen TN, Haberkern CM, et al. Lung fluid balance in lambs before and after birth. J Appl Physiol 1982; 53:992–1004.
46. Jobe A, Ikegami M, Jackobs H, et al. Permeability of premature lamb lungs to protein and the effect of surfactant on that permeability. J Appl Physiol 1983; 55:169–176.
47. Robertson B, Berry D, Curstedt T, et al. Leakage of protein in the immature rabbit lung; effect of surfactant replacement. Respir Physiol 1985; 61:265–276.
48. Engstrom PC, Holm BA, Matalon S. Surfactant replacement attenuates the increase in alveolar permeability in hyperoxia. J Appl Physiol 1989; 67:688–693.
49. Carlton DP, Cummings JJ, Scheerer RG, et al. Lung overexpansion increases pulmonary microvascular protein permeability in young lambs. J Appl Physiol 1990; 69:577–583.
50. Carlton DP, Cho S-C, Davis P, Bland RD. Inflation pressure and lung vascular injury in preterm lambs. Chest 1994; 105:115S–116S.
51. Albertine K, Carlton D, Lont M, et al. Pulmonary sequestration of neutrophils in preterm lambs with lung vascular injury. Pediatr Res 1994; 35:389A.
52. Carlton DP, Cho SC, Albertine KH, et al. Neutrophil depletion inhibits lung vascular injury and edema in preterm lambs. Pediatr Res 1994; 35:327A.

3

Biosynthesis, Secretion, and Recycling of Surfactant Components

JOSEPH J. BATENBURG
Utrecht University
Utrecht, The Netherlands

I. Introduction

Pulmonary surfactant is a lipid-protein mixture that coats the inside of the lungs. The presence of the lipids as a monolayer at the air-liquid interface in the alveoli reduces the surface tension. Thereby it diminishes the tendency of alveoli to collapse during expiration (1,2) and perhaps also the transudation of fluid into the air space (3,4).

Lipids constitute the major part (~90%) of pulmonary surfactant (5,6). Analyses of the lipid composition of surfactant for a large number of animal species (6–8) have shown that of the lipids in surface-active material 80–90% are phospholipids, whereas cholesterol comprises the largest amount of neutral lipid. Phosphatidylcholine (PC) constitutes the major part (70–80%) of the phospholipids in surfactant. Generally around 60% of the PC molecules contain two saturated fatty-acyl moieties. This disaturated PC (DSPC) is largely dipalmitoyl PC (DPPC). In many species, including humans and the rat and rabbit, the second major phospholipid in adult surfactant is phosphatidylglycerol (PG), which constitutes up to 10% of the surfactant phospholipids. This is an unusually high percentage. In most tissues, PG serves primarily as precursor for cardiolipin and occurs only in very small quantities. The remainder of the surfactant phospholipids includes among others phosphatidylinositol (PI). Immature mammalian surfactants contain a high percentage of PI instead of PG (9–13). In humans and the rat, a low PG/PI ratio in surfactant is a sign of immaturity (9,11–13). However, this appears not to be true for all mammals (for review, see refs. 12 and 13).

In addition to the lipids, the surfactant contains several specific proteins, nowadays termed surfactant protein (SP)-A, SP-B, SP-C, and SP-D (14–16).

The surfactant lipids are produced by the alveolar type II epithelial cells (4,12,17). The proteins are also synthesized in these cells, but with the exception of SP-C, they are also formed in bronchiolar epithelial cells (see later section). In the type II cells, the surfactant is stored as closely packed bilayers in storage organelles, the lamellar bodies. The contents of these lamellar bodies can be secreted into the aqueous lining layer of the alveolar air space, upon which the bilayers are transformed into a lattice-like structure known as tubular myelin (Fig. 1). This tubular myelin probably serves as the precursor of the phospholipid monolayer at the air-water interface (for review, see refs. 4 and 17). The monolayer becomes enriched in DPPC, probably by a process of squeeze-out of non-DPPC components during the contraction and expansion due to the breathing movements of the lung. Worn-out surfactant and material not included in or squeezed out of the monolayer can eventually be taken back into the type II cell (4,18).

II. The Role of the Various Surfactant Components

A. Lipids

It is generally agreed that DPPC, the most abundant lipid in pulmonary surfactant, is also its major surface-active component. The physiological function of this compound is thought to be the provision of alveolar stability by lowering of the surface tension at the alveolar surface to values less than 10 mN/m at end expiration (1,2) (see also Chapter 1). The role of the other surfactant lipids is less certain. They may aid in rapid adsorption and spreading of surfactant at the air-liquid interface (5,18). If acidic phospholipids are necessary for normal surfactant function, then PI may substitute for PG. This follows from experiments in which adult rabbits were fed myo-inositol. The surface properties of the surfactant were unchanged despite the fact that the inositol administration resulted in an increased proportion of PI and a decreased proportion of PG in the surfactant (19,20). The observation that in surfactant of newborn rabbits PG starts to appear in the first few hours after birth with a concomitant decline in the percentage of PI (10), whereas despite the extremely low proportion of PG at birth, the neonatal rabbits do not exhibit respiratory distress, also suggests that PG is not essential to the surface activity of surfactant. In addition, a very low percentage of PG is found in the surfactant of the adults of some species (12,13).

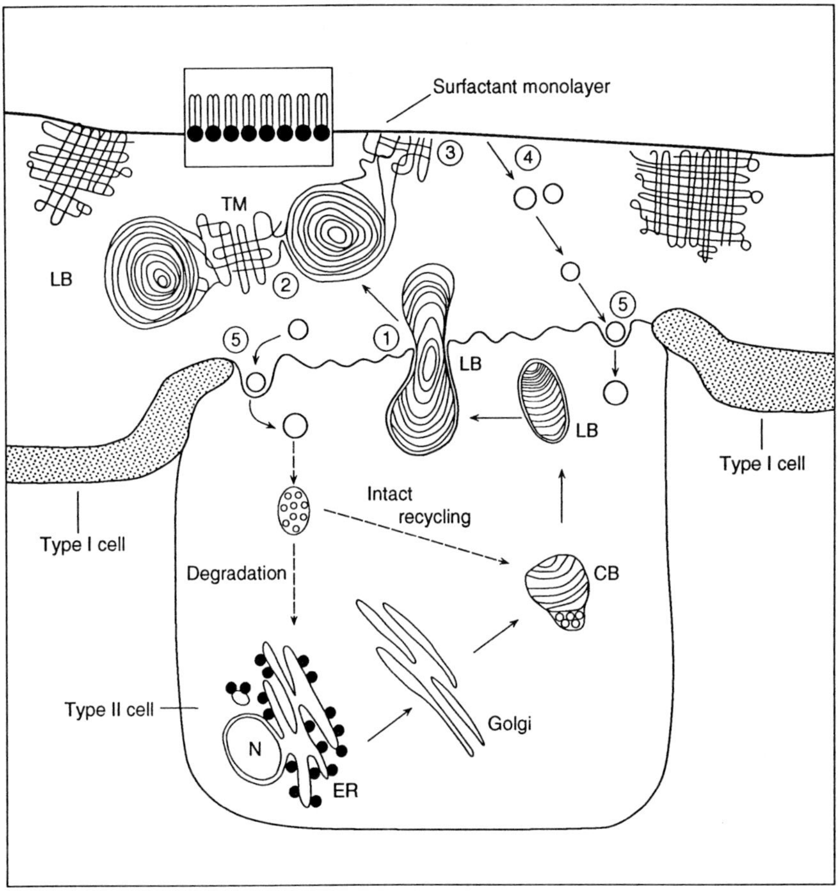

Figure 1 Schematic diagram of surfactant metabolism. Generally accepted pathways are indicated by solid arrows. Less well-substantiated pathways are indicated by broken arrows. N, nucleus; ER, endoplasmic reticulum; CB, composite body; LB, lamellar body; TM, tubular myelin; 1, secretion of LB; 2, conversion of LB into TM; 3, generation of monolayer from TM material; 4, formation of small aggregate material from monolayer; 5, reuptake of surfactant material.

B. Proteins

A great number of physiological roles have been proposed for the surfactant proteins, but at present there is very little support from studies with intact animals for any of these functions.

SP-A is known to bind lipids (14,21), particularly DPPC (22), and to cause aggregation of phospholipid vesicles in the presence of Ca^{2+} (14,21).

These properties may be required for one of its proposed functions: to play a role in the formation of tubular myelin from secreted lamellar body material. Reconstitution experiments in vitro showed that the formation of tubular myelin depended on the presence of surfactant lipids (DPPC and PG), SP-A, SP-B, and Ca^{2+} (23). The preferential localization of SP-A in the corners of the tubular myelin lattice (24) suggests that it provides the framework for this structure.

Another physiological role of SP-A may be the regulation of surfactant homeostasis. Based on experiments in vitro it was reported that SP-A decreases the secretion of lamellar bodies from type II cells (25,26) and increases the uptake of DPPC into these cells (27,28). However, the reported enhancement by SP-A of DPPC endocytosis by type II cells was recently challenged (29).

The third function of SP-A, suggested by its being a C-type lectin and by experiments in vitro, is a role in pulmonary defense mechanisms. As described in Chapter 4, there is evidence that SP-A stimulates phagocytosis of bacteria and viruses as well as oxygen radical production by alveolar macrophages, enhances the chemotaxis of these cells, and scavenges lipopolysaccharide (endotoxin) from gram-negative bacteria.

SP-D, like SP-A a C-type lectin, is also thought to be involved in defense mechanisms. It activates alveolar macrophages and binds to lipopolysaccharide (for further details, see Chapter 4).

The importance of SP-B in surfactant function is indicated by the observation that in neonatal rabbits intratracheal instillation of antibodies to SP-B led to decreased lung compliance and respiratory failure (30). The reconstitution experiments of Suzuki et al. (23), referred to above, indicated that, besides SP-A, SP-B is required for the formation of tubular myelin from secreted lamellar body material. In addition to that role, SP-B is probably involved in the formation of the surfactant monolayer. This is indicated by the observations (31–35) that SP-B promotes the adsorption of phospholipid molecules from suspended membranes to an air-liquid interface. The involvement of SP-B in transformation of lamellar bodies into tubular myelin and in the subsequent formation of the phospholipid monolayer may be related to the induction of lipid mixing by SP-B (36). The absorption of phospholipids to an air-liquid interface is also promoted by SP-C, but less actively than by SP-B (31,33–35). SP-A alone has little effect on the phospholipid adsorption, but accelerates the adsorption promoted by SP-B even further (32,35). SP-B may exhibit a specific interaction with the acidic phospholipid PG (35,37). It has been proposed that SP-B not only enhances phospholipid adsorption, but also promotes the removal of PG and other non-DPPC molecules from the monolayer during repeated expansion and compression (as during breathing), thereby enriching the film in DPPC (35,38). Also this effect may be enhanced by SP-A (38).

III. Biosynthesis of Surfactant Lipids

A. Substrates

Glucose from the circulation is the major source of glycerol backbone for surfactant lipid synthesis in adult type II cells, whereas glycerol plays only a minor role (39). However, glycerol may be an important substrate for PC synthesis in the early neonatal period (40). In the late fetal period glycogen, which has previously been accumulated in type II cells, may be an important source of carbon atoms for pulmonary phospholipid synthesis (12,13,41).

The fatty acids required for surfactant lipid synthesis may be obtained from the circulation as free fatty acids or in the form of triacylglycerols in lipoproteins. Fatty acid uptake from the blood into the type II cells is probably mediated by a membrane fatty acid–binding protein (42). Fatty acids are also formed in type II cells by hydrolysis of phospholipids when these are taken up from the alveoli (43). In addition, type II cells can synthesize fatty acids de novo at a high rate (44,45). They prefer lactate over glucose as substrate for this process (45). In the late fetal period, glycogen may be an important fatty acid precursor (12,41), whereas acetoacetate may constitute an important precursor of the fatty acids for surfactant lipid synthesis in neonates (46). The relative contribution of the various sources of fatty acids is incompletely known and probably varies with development and nutritional status. However, a number of observations point to the importance of fatty acid synthesis de novo for surfactant phospholipid formation in the perinatal period: (1) in fetal rat lung, the rate of fatty acid synthesis and the specific activities of fatty acid synthase and acetyl-CoA carboxylase, which together convert acetyl-CoA via malonyl-CoA to fatty acid, show a developmental increase in the period when surfactant production is accelerated (12,13,47); (2) inhibitors of fatty acid biosynthesis decrease the rate of DSPC synthesis in explants of fetal rat lung even when palmitate is added (48); and (3) compared with exogenous palmitate, fatty acid synthesized from acetate is preferentially incorporated into surfactant PC and DSPC in lungs of newborn rabbits (49). In rat and mouse lung, the activities of acetyl-CoA carboxylase and fatty acid synthase are depressed on fasting and increased on refeeding, similar to what occurs in liver under the same conditions. However, Batenburg and Whitsett (50) recently showed that on fasting and subsequent refeeding with a carbohydrate-rich fat-free diet, the mRNAs encoding acetyl-CoA carboxylase and fatty acid synthase in adult rat lungs changed to a lesser extent than those in the livers of the same rats. The same observation was made for ATP-citrate lyase and malic enzyme, two cytosolic enzymes involved in the transport of acetyl-CoA formed in the mitochondrial matrix to the cytosol where it is converted to fatty acid (50).

Choline required for PC synthesis in the type II cells is probably derived mainly from the diet (51). Type II cells can accumulate choline against a concentration gradient by an energy-dependent saturable transport process (52).

The myo-inositol necessary for the formation of surfactant PI, but also of PI involved in signal transduction, can be synthesized by various body tissues, but additional supplementation of inositol by the diet is sometimes required (53). The administration of inositol to premature infants with respiratory distress syndrome who are receiving parenteral nutrition leads to increased survival without bronchopulmonary dysplasia (53). Rabbit lung tissue can produce inositol from glucose (54). Type II cells can take up inositol by a saturable sodium- and energy-dependent (54,55) and by a nonsaturable sodium- and energy-independent (55) mechanism. This indicates that these cells obtain the inositol needed for PI formation at least partly from outside, either from other pulmonary cells or from the blood.

B. Pathways for Phosphatidylcholine Synthesis

The synthesis de novo of surfactant phospholipids begins with the formation of phosphatidic acid (PA) by acylation of glycerol-3-phosphate. The fatty acids needed for the acylation steps are converted to acyl-CoAs by acyl-CoA synthetase. The first step in PA synthesis is the formation of 1-acylglycerol-3-phosphate by glycerol-3-phosphate acyltransferase (Fig. 2, reaction 1). In adult type II cells, this enzyme is located predominantly in the endoplasmic reticulum (12). Its activity in type II cell microsomes is considerably higher than in microsomes from whole lung (12). The second acylation step is catalyzed by 1-acylglycerol-3-phosphate acyltransferase (Fig. 2 reaction 2).

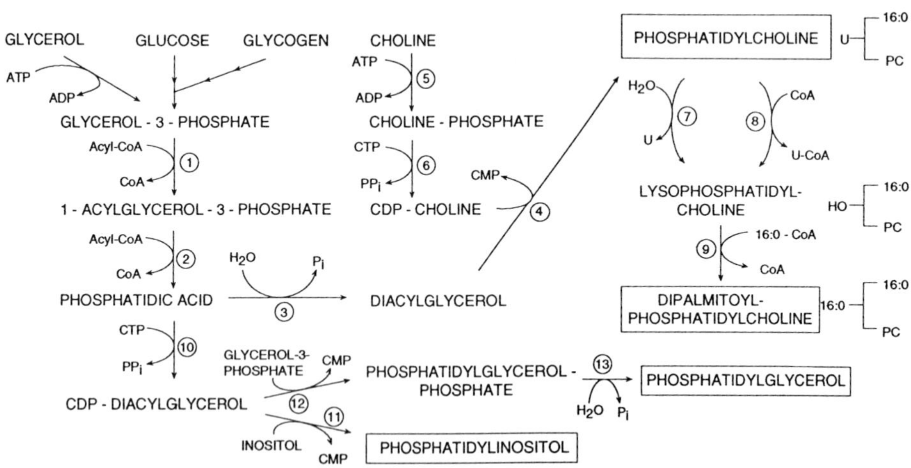

Figure 2 Pathways involved in the synthesis of phosphatidylcholine, phosphatidylglycerol and phosphatidylinositol. The names of the enzymes indicated by numbers are given in the text. U, unsaturated fatty acid.

The routes for the biosynthesis of PC on the one hand and of PG and PI on the other hand diverge after the formation of PA. On the way to PC, the PA is hydrolyzed to diacylglycerol by the action of phosphatidate phosphatase (Fig. 2, reaction 3). In lung tissue, several different forms of this enzyme have been identified, which differ in their subcellular localization (cytosolic or membrane-associated) and required physical form of the substrate (membrane-bound or aqueously dispersed PA) (56).

In the lung, PC is synthesized from diacylglycerol and CDPcholine by the enzyme cholinephosphotransferase (reaction 4). The CDPcholine is formed from choline by the sequential action of choline kinase (reaction 5) and choline-phosphate cytidylyltransferase (reaction 6). Choline kinase is a cytosolic enzyme. In the cytosol of type II cells, its specific activity was found to be fivefold that in cytosol from whole lung (57), which may enable type II cells to take up choline very efficiently. Choline-phosphate cytidylyltransferase shows a bimodal subcellular distribution: It is found both in the soluble fraction and membrane bound (8,58,59). The soluble fraction prepared from lung and from alveolar type II cells contains two forms of the enzyme. The L-form, a dimer of the M_r 45,000 catalytic subunit, is inactive when assayed in the absence of lipids. The H-form, the predominant soluble form in whole lung and type II cells, which appears to be a high molecular weight lipoprotein consisting of L-form apoprotein complexed with lipids, may be the physiologically active soluble form of the enzyme (60). The membrane-bound form of choline-phosphate cytidylyltransferase is similar, if not identical, to the soluble H-form (58). Although it is generally thought that the soluble enzyme forms are cytosolic and the membrane-bound form is located at the endoplasmic reticulum, it was recently reported that in Chinese hamster ovary cells the membrane-bound form is associated with the nuclear envelope (61), whereas in various nonpulmonary cell types the soluble form is located within the nucleus (62). These unexpected results require further investigation. The interaction of the cytidylyltransferase with membranes may be mediated by the hydrophobic side of a 58-residue amphipathic helix (63). Conversion of one form of the enzyme into another may have significance with respect to the regulation of PC formation (see Section V.B).

The last step of PC synthesis, catalyzed by cholinephosphotransferase, takes place at the endoplasmic reticulum (8,12).

Direct synthesis de novo from dipalmitoyl PA accounts for only 25–45% of total DPPC formation (64,65). The remodeling mechanism, which accounts for the formation of 55–75% of DPPC, involves removal of the unsaturated fatty acid from the 2-position of initially synthesized PC having a palmitoyl group at the 1-position and an unsaturated fatty acyl group at the 2-position (reaction 7 or 8 in Fig. 2), followed by reacylation of the resultant 1-palmitoyl-lysophosphatidylcholine with palmitoyl CoA by the microsomal enzyme lysophosphatidylcholine acyltransferase (reaction 9). The latter enzyme is highly enriched in type II cells and has a preference for palmitoyl CoA (12,66). Formation of DPPC by transacylation between two molecules of 1-palmitoyl-lysophosphatidylcholine is quantitatively unimportant (for review, see ref. 12). Classically, the deacylation of PC in the remodeling process is thought to occur through the action of phospholipase A_2 (reaction 7) (4,12). This enzyme, of which Ca^{2+}-dependent and Ca^{2+}-independent forms are known, was found in many subcellular fractions (for review, see ref. 12). Support for the involvement of phospholipase A_2 in the remodeling process came from observations that in type II cells phospholipase A_2 inhibitors decreased the degree of saturation of PC synthesized form various radioactive precursors (67), whereas activation of the enzyme led to an increase (68). However, there are indications that the deacylation can also be brought about by lysophosphatidylcholine acyltransferase acting in retrograde direction (reaction 8) (4,12).

C. Synthesis of Other Surfactant Lipids

The acidic lipids PG and PI are synthesized from CDPdiacylglycerol, which in turn is produced from PA by phosphatidate cytidylyltransferase (Fig. 2, reaction 10). It is probably the microsomal and not the mitochondrial activity of this enzyme that is involved in surfactant PG and PI biosynthesis (10).

PI can be made from CDPdiacylglycerol by a reaction with myo-inositol. CDPdiacylglycerol-inositol phosphatidyltransferase, the enzyme catalyzing this reaction (reaction 11), is located in the endoplasmic reticulum of type II cells (69,70).

Alternatively, CDPdiacylglycerol can be converted by glycerolphosphate phosphatidyltransferase (reaction 12) into phosphatidylglycerolphosphate, which is subsequently dephosphorylated to PG by phosphatidylglycerophosphatase (reaction 13). Glycerolphosphate phosphatidyltransferase is associated primarily with the mitochondria in both adult (70) and fetal (69) type II cells. However, there are strong indications that it is the microsomal glycerolphosphate phosphatidyltransferase activity which is involved in surfactant PG formation (10,69).

Studies with isolated perfused rat lungs indicated that endogenous synthesis in the lung accounts for less than 1% of cholesterol present in surfactant and that most of the cholesterol is taken up from low-density lipoproteins or high-density lipoproteins (71). The levels of these lipoproteins in the circulation probably regulate the endogenous synthesis of cholesterol in type II cells (71).

IV. Structure and Biosynthesis of Surfactant Proteins

SP-A, the most abundant hydrophilic surfactant protein, has a monomeric molecular mass of 28–36 kDa, depending on the degree of glycosylation (14,16). Analyses of the primary structure of SP-A for a number of species have shown that this protein is highly conserved (14,16). A 7–10 amino acid long N-terminal region contains a cysteine that is probably important for interchain disulfide bridge formation on oligomerization (72). Next to the N-terminal region comes a collagen-like domain consisting of 23–24 Gly-X-Y repeats, where Y is frequently hydroxyproline (14,16,72). Based on similarity to the collagen family of proteins, it is thought that this part of the SP-A molecule is folded into a triple helix (73,74). A kink in the triple helix is probably caused by the insertion of the sequence Pro-Cys-Pro-Pro after the 13th Gly-X-Y repeat in each polypeptide chain (73). A stretch of approximately 30–40 amino acids links the collagen-like domain to the C-terminal region. This linking region may constitute or contribute to the lipid-binding domain of SP-A (75). The globular carboxyterminus of SP-A is a carbohydrate recognition domain of approximately 130 amino acids, which has structural and functional similarities to other C-type lectins, such as C1q, mannose-binding protein, conglutinin, and SP-D (14,16,21,76). A complex, sialated high-mannose oligosaccharide is attached to asparagine 187 in this carbohydrate-recognition domain (14,21). The functional form of SP-A is probably an oligomeric complex of 18 monomers (6 trimers), held together by interchain disulfide bridges and noncovalent interactions of the collagenous domains, similar to the structure reported earlier for C1q (73,74).

The aminoterminal end of the primary translation product of SP-A consists of a 17–20 (depending on the species) amino acid signal peptide (72,77,78), which probably directs SP-A cotranslationally into the secretory pathway of the cell and is cleaved off during or after translocation of the SP-A into the lumen of the endoplasmic reticulum. Glycosylation at asparagine 187 with a high-mannose oligosaccharide in the endoplasmic reticulum probably occurs cotranslationally (16,21,79). After trimming of the oligosaccharide, it is sialated in the Golgi complex (80).

Although in experimental animals no evidence has been obtained for the presence of more than one SP-A gene (16,21), the human genome contains at least two distinct functional SP-A genes (81,82) and an SP-A pseudogene (83), all localized together in a cluster on chromosome 10q (14,16,21,84). The physiological significance of the existence of distinct SP-A genes in humans is not clear.

SP-A is synthesized in type II alveolar epithelial cells (14,16,21), in nonciliated bronchiolar epithelial cells (14,16,21), and in a few bronchial epithelial cells (85). The bronchiolar epithelial cells expressing SP-A are often assumed to be Clara cells, although this has recently been questioned (86). The relative contribution of the type II cells and the bronchiolar epithelial cells to the pool of SP-A in the alveolar space is unknown.

Mature SP-B (monomeric molecular mass 8 kDa) is a hydrophobic basic peptide that consists of 79 amino acids, of which 7 are cysteines (16,87,88). Six of these cysteins are involved in the formation of intrachain disulfide bridges

(88). That these are important for the structure of the active peptide is indicated by the observation that in all species investigated so far the positions of the cysteines are conserved (89). Under nonreducing conditions, SP-B occurs usually as a dimer but sometimes as an oligomer (16,87).

In humans, the SP-B gene is located on chromosome 2 (90,91). SP-B is expressed in alveolar type II cells and in bronchiolar epithelial cells (16,92). Its primary translation product has a molecular mass of 40 kDa (93). From this preproSP-B a signal sequence of 20–23 amino acid residues is cleaved off to yield proSP-B. This is glycosylated at an asparagine residue in a region flanking the C-terminal end of the mature form of SP-B, bringing the molecular mass to 42 kDa (79). Subsequent removal from the proSP-B of approximately 176 amino acids at the N-terminal end and 102–107 amino acids (depending on the species) at the C-terminal end yields mature SP-B (79). From immunoelectron microscopy studies, it was concluded that in type II cells precursor SP-B is proteolytically processed in an endosomal/lysosomal compartment, most probably in multivesicular bodies, while moving from the Golgi complex to the lamellar bodies (94). The enzyme responsible for the N-terminal processing is cathepsin-D or a similar protease (95).

SP-C, an extremely hydrophobic protein with a molecular mass of 4 kDa, contains a continuous, 23 amino acid long, hydrophobic domain, rich in valine residues (16,87,96). Mature SP-C from species containing two cysteines near the N-terminus contains two palmitoyl groups attached to these amino acids (97), whereas one palmitoyl group is attached to the only cysteine in canine SP-C (98). Palmitoylation of the SP-C increases the hydrophobicity of the molecule even further. In humans, the SP-C gene is located on chromosome 8p (99). SP-C is synthesized by alveolar type II cells but not by bronchiolar epithelial cells (100–102). Like SP-B, SP-C is processed from a much larger precursor protein. This proSP-C has a molecular mass of 21 kDa (16,79,96). The aminoterminal flanking region of SP-C, unlike that of SP-A and SP-B, does not contain a classic signal sequence to direct its insertion into the endoplasmic reticulum and there are no sites for asparagine-linked glycosylation (16,79,96). The region of the proSP-C that constitutes the future mature SP-C may act as signal sequence and membrane-anchoring domain (103). Processing of proSP-C to mature SP-C involves palmitoylation of proSP-C, conversion to higher molecular mass proSP-C by an unidentified modification and cleavage of amino- and carboxylterminal peptides (79,96,104).

SP-D is, like SP-A, a hydrophilic collagenous glycoprotein (105). The human SP-D gene is located close to the SP-A gene cluster on chromosome 10q (84,106). SP-D is synthesized by alveolar type II cells (107,108) and by Clara cells (107). Its primary translation product (39 kDa) undergoes posttranslational N-linked glycosylation, as well as hydroxylation and glycosylation of lysine residues within the collagenous domain (108), resulting in a 43-kDa monomer.

The monomers form disulfide-bonded trimers that are associated via their N-termini to form a multimer containing 12 identical 43-kDa polypeptides (109). SP-D is also similar to SP-A in that it is a Ca^{2+}-dependent carbohydrate-binding protein that is structurally and functionally related to other C-type mammalian lectins (110). The majority of SP-D is not associated with the surfactant pellet but is recovered from the supernatant fraction of bronchoalveolar lavage (111). SP-D, unlike SP-A, could not be detected in lamellar bodies (107).

V. Developmental Regulation of Surfactant Synthesis

A. Hormonal Regulation

Experiments with several animal species have shown that the production of surfactant phospholipids (8,9,13) and proteins (9,13,16,112,113) in the fetal lung increases toward the end of gestation. In this period, the activity of various enzymes involved in pulmonary lipid synthesis shows a rise (for review, see refs. 9 and 13). Ample evidence indicates that endogenous glucocorticoids and thyroid hormones are involved in the regulation of this phenomenon (9,114–116). Estrogens also stimulate pulmonary PC synthesis, but their physiological role in the regulation of surfactant formation is in doubt (9,114–116). Androgens produced in the male fetal testis probably slow down the onset of surfactant phospholipid formation (9,115,116). The delay in surfactant PC and PG synthesis in infants of diabetic mothers may be due to fetal hyperinsulinemia (9,114–117). Studies in vivo and in vitro indicated that the glucocorticoid-induced increase in fetal lung DSPC is potentiated by excess inositol (118). This may be due to an increased amount of inositol-containing compounds important in signal transduction.

The effects of the hormones on surfactant lipid synthesis in the type II cells involve epithelial-mesenchymal interactions. Glucocorticoids stimulate fetal lung fibroblasts to produce a polypeptide called fibroblast pneumonocyte factor (FPF). This FPF in turn stimulates the synthesis of PC, DSPC, and PG but not that of other phospholipids in the fetal type II cells (12,115,116,119). Thyroid hormones were suggested to increase fetal type II cell responsiveness to FPF, insulin inhibits the formation of FPF in the lung fibroblasts, while androgens inhibit the cortisol-induced formation of FPF by fetal lung fibroblasts and block the response of fetal type II cells to FPF (12,115,116,119). Sofar FPF has not been isolated and sequenced. It was recently reported (120) that at the end of gestation the production of FPF by rat lung fibroblasts increases, whereas at the same time the fibroblasts diminish the production of a transforming growth factor β (TGF-β) homologue that blocks the action of FPF. TGF-β inhibits the synthesis of DSPC in fetal type II cells (121). It appears, therefore, that a developmental increase in the FPF/TGF-β homologue ratio is involved in the developmental increase of DSPC synthesis in fetal type II cells.

Other hormones, in addition to the ones already mentioned, that have been reported to increase surfactant lipid synthesis include prolactin and epidermal growth factor (EGF), whereas müllerian-inhibiting substance was found to reduce fetal pulmonary DSPC synthesis (116). (For a complete compilation of all effects of various hormones on pulmonary phospholipids and lipid synthesizing enzymes observed in vivo and in vitro and for a more extensive discussion of interactions between hormones, see refs. 9 and 114–117).

Hormones also influence the perinatal expression of surfactant proteins. In most cases, a change in the amount of a surfactant protein is accompanied by a parallel change in the amount of its mRNA. Glucocorticoids increase or decrease the production of SP-A in the lung depending on the dose, the developmental age, and the animal species (16,21,112,122,123). The expression of SP-B and SP-C is increased by glucocorticoids and cAMP (16,87,112,122). Glucocorticoids also stimulate the production of SP-D (124). SP-A synthesis is increased by cAMP, EGF, and interferon-γ, and is decreased by TGF-β and insulin (16,21,122). Androgens and estrogens were found to have no influence on the expression of SP-A, SP-B, and SP-C (16). Thyroid hormone decreases SP-A and SP-B mRNA content in rat lung but may increase SP-A and its mRNA in human lung (122).

B. Regulation of Phosphatidylcholine Synthesis

Pulse-label and pulse-chase experiments with labeled choline (125,126), measurements of pool sizes of choline and its metabolites (126,127), and studies with isolated type II cells showing that increased rates of PC synthesis are correlated with enhanced activities of choline-phosphate cytidylyltransferase (for review, see refs. 12 and 115) indicated that the cytidylyltransferase catalyzes the rate-limiting step in the flux of choline into PC in type II cells. Hormonal and developmental studies on whole lung tissue pointed in the same direction (8,9,13).

On the basis of experiments with various cell types, Vance and Pelech (128) proposed that the activity of the cytidylyltransferase is modulated by translocation of the enzyme from the cytosol, where it is inactive, to the endoplasmic reticulum, where it is active. This translocation was suggested to be controlled by reversible phosphorylation of the cytidylyltransferase and by fatty acids (128). Although the concept of regulation of the cytidylyltransferase via a translocation mechanism is supported by whole lung studies (59), no such support has sofar been obtained in studies with isolated type II cells. In type II cells exposed to fatty acid (129), in type II cells developing in vivo (130), and in type II cells from fetuses of dexamethasone-treated rats (131) enhanced PC synthesis was accompanied by increased activity of microsomal cytidylyltransferase, but there was no concomitant decrease in cytosolic activity. The results of these studies indicate that the rate of PC synthesis is controlled by the activity of microsomal cytidylyltransferase. However, there are also many indications that the cytosolic form of the enzyme regulates pulmonary PC metabolism (for review, see ref. 8). Interconversion of the cytosolic H- and L-forms (60) may be involved in this regulation.

Although choline-phosphate cytidylyltransferase has received most attention among the enzymes involved in PC synthesis, it is probably not the only regulatory enzyme. Under specific conditions glycerol-3-phosphate acyltransferase (57) and choline kinase (127) may become rate-limiting. Moreover, phosphatidate phosphatase may also be involved in regulation of pulmonary PC formation (8,9,13). In addition, regulation of enzymes involved in substrate supply for pulmonary phospholipid synthesis may also contribute to the late-fetal acceleration of surfactant synthesis (for review, see refs. 9 and 13). In rat lung late-prenatal increases in activity, brought about via pretranslational regulation (50), have been found for the lipogenic enzymes fatty acid synthase, acetyl-CoA carboxylase, and ATP-citrate lyase.

Glucocorticoids enhance the activity of fatty acid synthase in fetal rat lung in vivo (47) and of both fatty acid synthase and fatty acid synthesis in explant cultures of fetal lung (47,132). In rat lung explants, the synthesis of fatty acid synthase is increased by glucocorticoid at a pretranslational level (133,134). In fetal type II cells, the rate of fatty acid synthesis is increased by exposure to fibroblast-conditioned cortisol-containing medium (135). This involves a rise in the mRNAs of fatty acid synthase, acetyl-CoA carboxylase, and ATP-citrate lyase, which requires both the glucocorticoid and the fibroblast conditioning (136). The FPF that stimulates DSPC formation and choline-phosphate cytidylyltransferase activity in fetal type II cells may therefore also be involved in the stimulation of fatty acid synthesis in these cells (Fig. 3). Although glucocorticoids increase the activity of the cytidylyltransferase in fetal rat lung explants, the amount of enzyme was found to be unchanged (137). Based (1) on this observation, (2) on the observation that glucocorticoids enhance fatty acid synthesis in lung explants and type II cells, (3) on the knowledge that the activity of the cytidylyltransferase can be increased by fatty acids and by some phospholipids (for review, see refs 12 and 137), and (4) on the observation that inhibition of fatty acid synthesis abolishes the stimulatory effect of glucocorticoids on the cytidylyltransferase in fetal lung (138), it has been suggested that the stimulatory effect of glucocorticoids on the cytidylyltransferase activity in fetal lung is secondary to the increased synthesis of fatty acids which, either as free fatty acids or after incorporation into phospholipids, activate the cytidylyltransferase (137,138). It is, therefore, very well possible that the stimulation of the cytidylyltransferase in fetal type II cells by FPF results, at least partly, from increased fatty acid synthesis brought about by this factor (Fig. 3). However, pretranslational regulation of the cytidylyltransferase itself (Fig. 3) may also be involved (136).

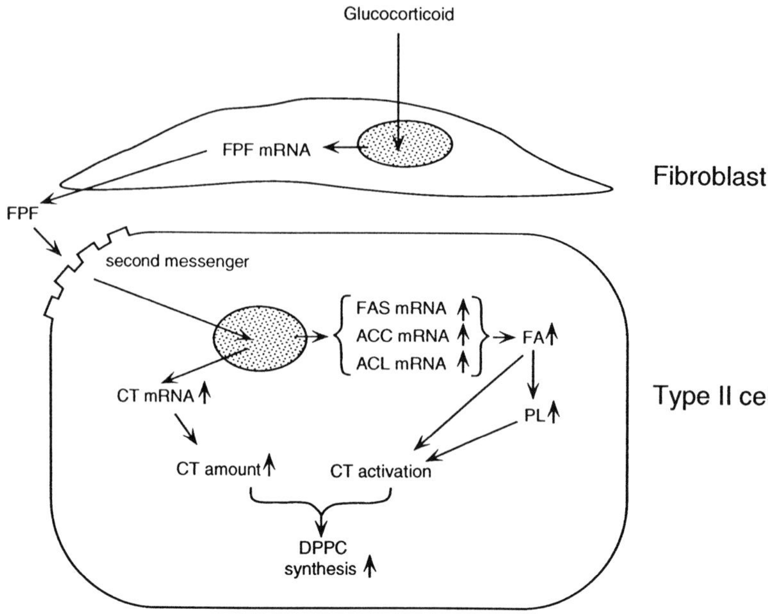

Figure 3 The mechanisms via which glucocorticoids stimulate DPPC synthesis in fetal type II cells. FPF, fibroblast-pneumonocyte factor; CT, choline-phosphate cytidylyltransferase; FAS, fatty acid synthase; ACC, acetyl-CoA carboxylase; ACL, ATP-citrate lyase; FA, fatty acids; PL, phospholipids.

C. Regulation of Phosphatidylglycerol and Phosphatidylinositol Synthesis

The percentage of PI among phospholipids in human amniotic fluid starts to rise after 28 weeks gestation. After 35 weeks, this percentage diminishes again, whereas at the same time the percentage PG rises (11). This pattern reflects changes in the phospholipid pattern of surfactant secreted by the fetal lung. A similar pattern is observed in lamellar bodies isolated from human amniotic fluid (139). A rise in the percentage of PI in the prenatal period, followed by a decrease around birth which was accompanied by a rise in the percentage PG, was also found in the surfactant of various experimental animals (9,13). The switchover from PI to PG synthesis is probably at least partly caused by a decrease in serum inositol at the end of gestation (140) and a developmental decrease in the permeability of type II cells to inositol (55), together with the fact that the availability of inositol plays an important role in the partitioning of CDPdiacylglycerol between PG and PI synthesis (55,141,142). A rise in intracellular cytidine-monophosphate resulting from enhanced PC synthesis (143) and increased activity of microsomal glycerophosphate phosphatidyltransferase around term (10) may also be involved in the stimulation of PG synthesis.

VI. Intracellular Transport and Storage of Surfactant

Prior to its secretion from type II cells, pulmonary surfactant is stored in the lamellar bodies (17,144). These organelles lack a number of enzymes needed for the synthesis de novo of PC and PG and for the remodeling of PC to DPPC (4,12), which makes it unlikely that they contribute significantly to the synthesis of surfactant lipids. Therefore, lipids must somehow be transported to the nascent lamellar bodies (Fig. 1). The details of this process are poorly understood. It may involve vesicular transport or transport by phospholipid-transfer proteins (12,145,146) and/or fusion of small vesicles to lamellar bodies by phospholipid-binding proteins (147). In type II cells, several phospholipid-transfer proteins have been described and there is circumstantial evidence that they play a role in intracellular surfactant transport (for review, see refs. 12, 145, and 146). Evidence for vesicular transport was first obtained from the classic autoradiographic experiments by Chevalier and Collet (144). These studies, involving [^{3}H]-choline injection into mice, indicated that the bulk of surfactant PC synthesized in the endoplasmic reticulum of the type II pneumocytes is transferred from the Golgi system to the lamellar bodies by so-called small lamellar bodies. The suggestion that the small lamellar bodies are intermediates between the Golgi system and the mature lamellar bodies in the transport of surfactant lipids is supported by studies in which labeling in vivo was followed by cell fractionation (148,149). These studies indicated that dense particles with a low phospholipid/protein ratio developed into mature lamellar bodies. Immunoelectron microscopy studies suggest that in type II cells SP-B, SP-C, and that portion of SP-A which is secreted with the lamellar bodies (see Section VII) are transported to the lamellar bodies together through the same biosynthetic pathway via multivesicular bodies (150). The multivesicular bodies that are involved in the transport of surfactant proteins from the Golgi system to the lamellar bodies probably have no role in phospholipid transport (144).

VII. Surfactant Secretion

The surfactant lipids are secreted together from the type II cells by exocytosis of lamellar bodies (Fig. 1). In this secretion process, microtubules and microfilaments appear to be involved (4,17,151). The secretion of surfactant lipids is stimulated by hyperventilation (17,151,152). Type II cell distortion or altered intracellular pH may be involved in this stimulation (17,151). In addition, surfactant phospholipid secretion is stimulated by agonists for β-adrenergic, purinergic, and vasopressin receptors (4,151,152). This stimulation is accompanied by increases in the intracellular cAMP level and the cytosolic Ca^{2+} concentration and involves activation of cAMP-dependent protein kinase and of protein kinase C (4,17,151,152). Also inhibitory mechanisms may be involved in the regulation of surfactant secretion (4,151,152). A recent publication (153) showed that PC secretion from isolated type II cells is inhibited by saturated PCs below their transition temperature (e.g., DPPC at 37°C). Therefore, when vesicles of nearly pure DPPC are formed in vivo, they might act as inhibitory regulators of surfactant. Moreover, as mentioned before, PC release from isolated type II cells is inhibited by SP-A (25,26).

It is not clear whether SP-A is secreted via the lamellar bodies together with the surfactant lipids. Although a number of studies indicate that this is the case (17,151), there are also observations (151,154,155) suggesting that SP-A is secreted by a pathway independent of lamellar bodies. The apparent absence of SP-D from lamellar bodies (107) indicates that this protein is secreted independently from DPPC secretion. The observation that SP-B and SP-C are highly enriched in lamellar bodies (156) suggests that these hydrophobic proteins are secreted together with the surfactant lipids.

VIII. Intra-alveolar Metabolism of Surfactant

After their secretion into the alveolus, the lamellar bodies expand and form the lattice-like structure called tubular myelin (17,157) (Fig. 1). As mentioned before, SP-A, SP-B, and Ca^{2+} are probably involved in this rearrangement of the phospholipids (23). Tubular myelin is probably the precursor of the surfactant monolayer at the air-liquid interface (4,17). As mentioned earlier, SP-B, SP-C, and SP-A may be involved in the introduction of phospholipids from tubular myelin into the monolayer. This surface film is enriched in DPPC, probably due to repeated expansion and compression resulting in the removal of non-DPPC molecules. SP-B (35,38) and perhaps also SP-A (38) may be involved in this enrichment (see also Chapter 1).

Surfactant obtained by lung lavage can be separated by centrifugation into different subfractions (17,157). The heavy large-aggregate forms that contain tubular myelin are precursors to the lighter small-aggregate forms that are predominantly vesicular (17,157). The light forms contain less surfactant proteins, are adsorbed less easily to an air-liquid interface than the heavier forms (17,157), and may represent waste surfactant (Fig. 1). The heavy form can also be converted to the light form in vitro. This conversion requires repeated expansion and contraction of the surface area of the surfactant suspension and the action of a serine protease that is closely associated with surfactant phospholipid and that may be a product of alveolar type II cells (158). Recent evidence (159) indicates that SP-B is degraded during this process. It was hypothesized that in large aggregates the SP-B was inaccessible to the serine protease, but during the increase in surface area, when surfactant absorbes to the air-liquid interface, the SP-B could be degraded by the protease. During the subsequent decrease in surface area, the SP-B–depleted surfactant would form small aggregates (159).

IX. Recycling of Surfactant

Surfactant lipids are removed from the alveoli with a turnover time of 5–10 hr (4,157). This may result from degradation by alveolar macrophages, ciliary transport up the airways, or movement through epithelium and endothelium into blood or lymph. However, it is now clear that a large part of the phospholipids is taken up again and reutilized by the type II cells (4,157,160) (Fig. 1). The efficiency of this reutilization, which may vary with age, may be up to 85% (4,157). A part of the internalized phospholipids is degraded, possibly in lysosomes, after which the degradation products are used for phospholipid formation at the endoplasmic reticulum (4,152,157). However, another part is recycled intact into the lamellar bodies (4,152,157).

SP-A is taken up by the type II cells, probably via receptor-mediated endocytosis (152,161,162), and deposited in lamellar bodies without being degraded (163). SP-B is likewise internalized by type II cells, recycled without degradation into lamellar bodies, and secreted again with the contents of these organelles (164). Part of the SP-B is degraded inside the type II cells, however (165). Although binding and uptake of phospholipid-poor SP-B by type II cells is probably not receptor mediated (164,166), there are indications that in the presence of phospholipids SP-B can bind to specific sites on the type II cell membrane (166). Label from radioactive SP-C was recently also found to appear rapidly in lamellar bodies after intratracheal instillation of the protein into rat lungs (167).

For a steady state, the secretion of surfactant into the alveoli and its removal have to be in balance. A regulatory link between these processes may be provided by β-adrenergic agonists. These do not only stimulate surfactant secretion (see above), but also reuptake (4,152,157). It has been suggested that another such link is provided by SP-A, which reportedly inhibits secretion (see above) and has been proposed to be a recognition signal for uptake of alveolar phospholipids by type II cells (27,28,152,157). However, as mentioned before, the latter role is in doubt (29). At present, it is unknown how the regulation of the synthesis of new surfactant material is coupled with the control of secretion and clearance. In alveolar proteinosis, excess surfactant material is present in the alveolar air spaces. Whether this is caused by excessive production, defective intra-alveolar metabolism, or a defect in reuptake remains to be determined.

Acknowledgments

The author's research is supported in part by the Netherlands Foundation for Chemical Research (SON) with financial aid from the Netherlands Organization of Scientific Research (NWO) and by the Dutch Asthma Foundation (Nederlands Astma Fonds).

References

1. Clements JA. Function of the alveolar lining. Am Rev Respir Dis 1977; 115(Suppl): 67–71.
2. Goerke J, Clements JA. Alveolar surface tension and lung surfactant. In: Handbook of Physiology. The Respiratory System. Mechanics of Breathing. Bethesda: Am Physiol Soc, 1986, Sect. 3, Vol. III, Part 1:247–261.
3. Pattle RE. Surface lining of lung alveoli. Physiol Rev 1965; 45:48–79.
4. Van Golde LMG., Batenburg JJ, Robertson B. The pulmonary surfactant system: Biochemical aspects and functional significance. Physiol Rev 1988; 68:374–455.
5. King RJ, Clements JA. Surface active materials from dog lung II. Composition and physiological correlations. Am J Physiol 1972; 223:715–726.
6. Sanders RL. The composition of pulmonary surfactant. In: Farrell PM, ed. Lung Development: Biological and Clinical Perspectives, Vol. 1 New York: Academic Press, 1982:193–210.
7. King RJ. Pulmonary surfactant. J Appl Physiol 1982; 53:1–8.
8. Rooney SA. The surfactant system and lung phospholipid biochemistry. Am Rev Respir Dis 1985; 131:439–460.
9. Batenburg JJ, Hallman M. Developmental biochemistry of alveoli. In: Scarpelli EM, ed. Pulmonary Physiology: Fetus, Newborn, Child and Adolescent. Philadelphia: Lea & Febiger, 1990:106–139.
10. Hallman M, Gluck L. Formation of acidic phospholipids in rabbit lung during perinatal development. Pediatr Res 1980; 14:1250–1259.
11. Hallman M, Kulovich M, Kirkpatrick E, et al. Phosphatidylinositol and phosphatidylglycerol in amniotic fluid: indices of lung maturity. Am J Obstet Gynecol 1976; 125:613–617.
12. Batenburg JJ. Surfactant phospholipids: Synthesis and storage. Am J Physiol 1992; 262:L367–L385.
13. Cockshutt AM, Possmayer F. Metabolism of surfactant lipids and proteins in the developing lung. In: Robertson B, Van Golde LMG, Batenburg JJ, eds. Pulmonary Surfactant: From Molecular Biology to Clinical Practice. Amsterdam: Elsevier, 1992:339–377.
14. Hawgood S. Pulmonary surfactant apoproteins: a review of protein and genomic structure. Am J Physiol 1989; 257:L13–L22.
15. Possmayer F. The role of surfactant-associated proteins. Am Rev. Respir Dis 1990; 142:749–752.
16. Weaver TA, Whitsett JA. Function and regulation of expression of pulmonary surfactant-associated proteins. Biochem J 1991; 273:249–264.

17. Wright JR, Clements JA. Metabolism and turnover of lung surfactant. Am Rev Respir Dis 1987; 135:426–444.
18. Keough KMW. Physical chemistry of pulmonary surfactant in the terminal air spaces. In: Robertson B, Van Golde LMG, Batenburg JJ, eds. Pulmonary Surfactant: From Molecular Biology to Clinical Practice. Amsterdam: Elsevier, 1992:109–164.
19. Beppu OS, Clements JA, Goerke J. Phosphatidylglycerol-deficient lung surfactant has normal properties. J Appl Physiol 1983; 55:496–502.
20. Hallman M, Enhorning G, Possmayer F. Composition and surface activity of normal and phosphatidylglycerol-deficient lung surfactant. Pediatr Res 1985; 19:286–292.
21. Hawgood S. The hydrophilic surfactant protein SP-A: Molecular biology, structure and function. In: Robertson B, Van Golde LMG, Batenburg JJ, eds. Pulmonary Surfactant: From Molecular Biology to Clinical Practice. Amsterdam: Elsevier, 1992:33–54.
22. Kuroki Y, Akino T. Pulmonary surfactant protein A (SP-A) specifically binds dipalmitoylphosphatidylcholine. J Biol Chem 1991; 266:3068–3073.
23. Suzuki Y, Fujita Y, Kogishi K. Reconstitution of tubular myelin from synthetic lipids and proteins associated with pig pulmonary surfactant. Am Rev Respir Dis 1989; 140:75–81.
24. Voorhout WF, Veenendaal T, Haagsman HP, et al. Surfactant protein A is localized at the corners of the pulmonary tubular myelin lattice. J Histochem Cytochem 1991; 39:1331–1336.
25. Dobbs LG, Wright JR, Hawgood S, et al. Pulmonary surfactant and its components inhibit secretion of phosphatidylcholine from cultured rat alveolar type II cells. Proc Natl Acad Sci USA 1987; 84:1010–1014.
26. Rice WR, Ross GF, Singleton FM, et al. Surfactant-associated protein inhibits phospholipid secretion from type II cells. J Appl Physiol 1987; 63:692–698.
27. Wright JR, Wager RE, Hawgood S, et al. Surfactant apoprotein Mr = 26,000–36,000 enhances uptake of liposomes by type II cells. J Biol Chem 1987; 262:2888–2894.
28. Tsuzuki A, Kuroki Y, Akino T. Pulmonary surfactant protein A-mediated uptake of phosphatidylcholine by alveolar type-II Cells. Am J Physiol 1993; 265:L193–L199.
29. Haagsman HP, Casals C, De Haas CGM, et al. Endocytosis of surfactant protein A (SP-A) and lipids by type II cells studied by laser flow cytometry. Am Rev Respir Dis 1993; 147:A145.
30. Robertson B, Kobayashi T, Ganzuka M, et al. Experimental neonatal respiratory failure induced by a monoclonal antibody to the hydrophobic surfactant-associated protein SP-B. Pediatr Res 1991; 30:239–243.
31. Curstedt T, Jörnvall H, Robertson B, et al. Two hydrophobic low-molecular-mass protein fractions of pulmonary surfactant—Characterization and biophysical activity. Eur J Biochem 1987; 168:255–262.
32. Hawgood S, Benson BJ, Schilling J, et al. Nucleotide and amino acid sequences of pulmonary surfactant protein SP18 and evidence for cooperation between SP18 and SP28-36 in surfactant lipid adsorption. Proc Natl Acad Sci USA 1987; 84:66–70.

33. Oosterlaken-Dijksterhuis MA, Haagsman HP, Van Golde LMG, Demel RA. Interaction of lipid vesicles with monomolecular layers containing lung surfactant proteins SP-B or SP-C. Biochemistry 1991; 30:8276–8281.
34. Revak SD, Merritt TA, Degryse E, et al. Use of human low molecular weight apoprotein in the reconstitution of surfactant biologic activity. J Clin Invest 1988; 81:826–833.
35. Yu SH, Possmayer F. Role of bovine pulmonary surfactant-associated proteins in the surface-active property of phospholipid mixtures. Biochim Biophys Acta 1990; 1046:233–241.
36. Oosterlaken-Dijksterhuis MA, Van Eijk M, Van Golde LMG, Haagsman HP. Lipid mixing is mediated by the hydrophobic surfactant protein SP-B but not by SP-C. Biochim Biophys Acta 1992; 1110:45–50.
37. Baatz JE, Elledge B, Whitsett JA. Surfactant protein SP-B induces ordering at the surface of model membrane bilayers. Biochemistry 1990; 29:6714–6720.
38. Schürch S, Possmayer F, Cheng S, Cockshutt AM. Pulmonary SP-A enhances adsorption and appears to induce surface sorting of lipid extract surfactant. Am J Physiol 1992; 263:L210–L218.
39. Batenburg JJ, Longmore WJ, Van Golde LMG. The synthesis of phosphatidylcholine by adult rat lung alveolar type II epithelial cells in primary culture. Biochim Biophys Acta 1978; 529:160–170.
40. Mims LC, Zee P. Utilization of glycerol by the newborn mammalian lung. Biol. Neonate 1971; 18:356–362.
41. Farrell PM, Bourbon JR. Fetal lung surfactant lipid synthesis from glycogen during organ culture. Biochim Biophys Acta 1986; 878:159–167.
42. Maniscalco WM, Stremmel W, Heeney-Campbell M. Uptake of palmitic acid by rabbit alveolar type II cells. Am J Physiol 1990; 259:L206–L212.
43. Chander A, Reicherter J, Fisher AB. Degradation of dipalmitoyl phosphatidylcholine by isolated rat granular pneumocytes and reutilization for surfactant synthesis. J Clin Invest 1987; 79:1133–1138.
44. Geppert EF, Elstein KH. Short-term regulation of fatty acid synthesis in isolated alveolar type II cells from adult rat lung: effects of free fatty acids and hormones. Exp Lung Res 1983; 4:281–291.
45. Maniscalco WM, Finkelstein JN, Parkhurst AB. De novo fatty acid synthesis by freshly isolated alveolar type II epithelial cells. Biochim Biophys Acta 1983; 751:462–469.
46. Yeh YY. Substrate utilization for phosphatidylcholine synthesis by type II pneumocytes of neonatal rats. Pediatr Res 1991; 30:55–61.
47. Rooney SA. Fatty acid biosynthesis in developing fetal lung. Am J Physiol 1989; 257:L195–L201.
48. Patterson CE, Davis KS, Rhoades RA. Regulation of fetal lung disaturated phosphatidylcholine synthesis by de novo palmitate supply. Biochim Biophys Acta 1988; 958:60–69.
49. Jobe A, Ikegami M, Sarton-Miller I. The in vivo labeling with acetate and palmitate of lung phospholipids from developing and adult rabbits. Biochim Biophys Acta 1980; 617:65–75.
50. Batenburg JJ, Whitsett JA. Levels of mRNAs coding for lipogenic enzymes in rat

lung upon fasting and refeeding and during perinatal development. Biochim Biophys Acta 1989; 1006:329–334.
51. Zeisel SH. Dietary choline: biochemistry, physiology, and pharmacology. Ann Rev Nutr 1981; 1:95–121.
52. Fisher AB, Chander A, Dodia C, et al. Choline transport by lung epithelium. Am J Respir Cell Mol Biol 1989; 1:455–462.
53. Hallman M, Bry K, Hoppu K, et al. Inositol supplementation in premature infants with respiratory distress syndrome. N Engl J Med 1992; 326:1233–1239.
54. Bleasdale JE, Maberry MC., Quirk JG. Myo-inositol homeostasis in foetal rabbit lung. Biochem J 1982; 206:43–52.
55. Hallman M, Slivka S, Wozniak P, Sills J. Perinatal development of myoinositol uptake into lung cells: Surfactant phosphatidylglycerol and phosphatidylinositol synthesis in the rabbit. Pediatr Res 1986; 20:179–185.
56. Walton PA, Possmayer F. The role of Mg^{2+}-dependent phosphatidate phosphohydrolase in pulmonary glycerolipid biosynthesis. Biochim Biophys Acta 1984; 796:364–372.
57. Haagsman HP, Schuurmans EAJM, Batenburg JJ, Van Golde LMG. Synthesis of phosphatidylcholine in ozone-exposed alveolar type II cells isolated from adult rat lung. Is glycerolphosphate acyltransferase a rate-limiting enzyme? Exp Lung Res 1988; 14:1–17.
58. Feldman DA, Rounsifer ME, Charles L, Weinhold PA. CTP: Phosphocholine cytidylyltransferase in rat lung: Relationship between cytosolic and membrane forms. Biochim Biophys Acta 1990; 1045:49–57.
59. Weinhold PA, Rounsifer ME, Williams SE, et al. CTP:phosphorylcholine cytidylyltransferase in rat lung. The effect of free fatty acids on the translocation of activity between microsomes and cytosol. J Biol Chem 1984; 259:10315–10321.
60. Weinhold PA, Rounsifer ME, Charles L, Feldman DA. Characterization of cytosolic forms of CTP:choline-phosphate cytidylyltransferase in lung, isolated alveolar type II cells, A549 cell and Hep G2 cells. Biochim Biophys Acta 1989; 1006:299–310.
61. Watkins JD, Kent C. Immunolocalization of membrane-associated CTP-Phosphocholine cytidylyltransferase in phosphatidylcholine-deficient Chinese hamster ovary cells. J Biol Chem 1992; 267:5686–5692.
62. Wang YL, Sweitzer TD, Weinhold PA, Kent C. Nuclear localization of soluble CTP:phosphocholine cytidylyltransferase. J Biol Chem 1993; 268:5899–5904.
63. Kalmar GB, Kay RJ, Lachance A, et al. Cloning and expression of rat liver CTP:phosphocholine cytidylyltransferase: An amphipathic protein that controls phosphatidylcholine synthesis. Proc Natl Acad Sci USA 1990; 87:6029–6033.
64. Mason RJ, Nellenbogen J. Synthesis of saturated phosphatidylcholine and phosphatidylglycerol by freshly isolated rat alveolar type II cells. Biochim Biophys Acta 1984; 794:392–402.
65. Den Breejen JN, Batenburg JJ, Van Golde LMG. The species of acyl-CoA in subcellular fractions of type II cells isolated from adult rat lung and their incorporation into phosphatidic acid. Biochim Biophys Acta 1989; 1002:277–282.
66. Batenburg JJ, Longmore WJ, Klazinga W, Van Golde LMG. Lysolecithin acyltransferase and lysolecithin: lysolecithin acyltransferase in adult rat lung alveolar type II epithelial cells. Biochim Biophys Acta 1979; 573:136–144.

67. Post M, Schuurmans EAJM, Batenburg JJ, Van Golde LMG. Mechanisms involved in the synthesis of disaturated phosphatidylcholine by alveolar type II cells isolated from adult rat lung. Biochim Biophys Acta 1983; 750:68–77.
68. Chander A, Fisher AB, Strauss JF. Role of an acidic compartment in synthesis of disaturated phosphatidylcholine by rat granular pneumocytes. Biochem J 1982; 208:651–658.
69. Batenburg JJ, Klazinga W, Van Golde LMG. Regulation and location of phosphatidylglycerol and phosphatidylinositol synthesis in type II cells isolated from fetal rat lung. Biochim Biophys Acta 1985; 833:17–24.
70. Bleasdale JE, Tyler NE, Snyder JM. Subcellular sites of synthesis of phosphatidylglycerol and phosphatidylinositol in type II pneumonocytes. Lung 1985; 163:345–359.
71. Hass MA, Longmore WJ. Regulation of lung surfactant cholesterol metabolism by serum lipoproteins. Lipids 1980; 15:401–406.
72. Benson B, Hawgood S, Schilling J, et al. Structure of canine pulmonary surfactant apoprotein: cDNA and complete amino acid sequence. Proc Natl Acad Sci USA 1985; 82:6379–6383.
73. Voss T, Eistetter H, Schäfer K, Engel J. Macromolecular organization of natural and recombinant lung surfactant protein SP 28-36: Structural homology with the complement factor C1q. J Mol Biol 1988; 201:219–227.
74. Haagsman HP, White RT, Schilling J, et al. Studies of the structure of lung surfactant protein SP-A. Am J Physiol 1989; 257:L421–L429.
75. Ross GF, Notter RH, Meuth J, Whitsett JA. Phospholipid binding and biophysical activity of pulmonary surfactant- associated protein (SAP)-35 and its non-collagenous COOH- terminal domains. J Biol Chem 1986; 261:14283–14291.
76. Haagsman HP, Hawgood S, Sargeant T, et al. The major lung surfactant protein, SP 28-36, is a calcium-dependent carbohydrate-binding protein. J Biol Chem 1987; 262:13877–13880.
77. White RT, Damm D, Miller J, et al. Isolation and characterization of the human pulmonary surfactant apoprotein gene. Nature 1985; 317:361–363.
78. Sano K, Fisher J, Mason RJ, et al. Isolation and sequence of a cDNA clone for the rat pulmonary surfactant-associated protein (PSP-A). Biochem Biophys Res Commun 1987; 144:367–374.
79. Weaver TE. Biosynthesis and intracellular processing of surfactant proteins. In: Robertson B, van Golde LMG, Batenburg JJ, eds. Pulmonary Surfactant: From Molecular Biology to Clinical Practice. Amsterdam: Elsevier, 1992:283–293.
80. Whitsett JA, Ross G, Weaver T, et al. Glycosylation and secretion of surfactant-associated glycoprotein A. J Biol Chem 1985; 260:15273–15279.
81. Floros J, Steinbrink R, Jacobs K, et al. Isolation and characterization of cDNA clones for the 35-kDa pulmonary surfactant-associated protein. J Biol Chem 1986; 261:9029–9033.
82. Katyal SL, Singh G, Locker J. Characterization of a second human pulmonary surfactant-associated protein SP-A gene. Am J Respir Cell Mol Biol 1992; 6:446–452.
83. Korfhagen TR, Glasser SW, Bruno MD, et al. A portion of the surfactant protein A (SP-A) gene locus consists of a pseudogene. Am J Respir Cell Mol Biol 1991; 4:463–469.

84. Kölble K, Lu JH, Mole SE, et al. Assignment of the human pulmonary surfactant protein-D gene (SFTP4) to 10q22-q23 close to the surfactant protein-A gene cluster. Genomics 1993; 17:294–298.
85. Broers JLV, Jensen SM, Travis WD, et al. Expression of surfactant associated protein-A and Clara cell 10 kilodalton mRNA in neoplastic and non-neoplastic human lung tissue as detected by in situ hybridization. Lab Invest 1992; 337:337–346.
86. Ten Have-Opbroek AAW, De Vries ECP. Clara cell differentiation in the mouse: Ultrastructural morphology and cytochemistry of surfactant protein A and Clara cell 10 kD protein. Microsc Res Techn 1993; 26:400–411.
87. Whitsett JA, Baatz JE. Hydrophobic surfactant proteins SP-B and SP-C: Molecular biology, structure and function. In: Robertson B, Van Golde LMG, Batenburg JJ, eds. Pulmonary Surfactant: From Molecular Biology to Clinical Practice. Amsterdam: Elsevier, 1992:55–75.
88. Johansson J, Curstedt T, Jörnvall H. Surfactant protein-B–disulfide bridges, structural properties, and kringle similarities. Biochemistry 1991; 30:6917–6921.
89. D'Amore-Bruno MA, Wikenheiser KA, Carter JE, et al. Sequence, ontogeny, and cellular localization of murine surfactant protein-B messenger RNA. Am J Physiol 1992; 262:L40–L47.
90. Emrie PA, Jones C, Hofmann T, Fisher JH. The coding sequence for the human 18,000-Dalton hydrophobic pulmonary surfactant protein is located on chromosome 2 and identifies a restriction fragment length polymorphism. Somatic Cell Mol Genet 1988; 14:105–110.
91. Pilot-Matias TJ, Kister SE, Fox JL, et al. Structure and organization of the gene encoding human pulmonary surfactant proteolipid SP-B. DNA 1989; 8:75–86.
92. Phelps DS, Floros J. Localization of surfactant protein synthesis in human lung by in situ hybridization. Am Rev Respir Dis 1988; 137:939–942.
93. Glasser SW, Korfhagen TR, Weaver T, et al. cDNA and deduced amino acid sequence of human pulmonary surfactant-associated proteolipid SPL(Phe). Proc Natl Acad Sci USA 1987; 84:4007–4011.
94. Voorhout WF, Veenendaal T, Haagsman HP, et al. Intracellular processing of pulmonary surfactant protein-B in an endosomal/lysosomal compartment. Am J Physiol 1992; 263:L479–L486.
95. Weaver TE, Lin S, Bogucki B, Dey C. Processing of surfactant protein-B proprotein by a cathepsin-D–like protease. Am J Physiol 1992; 263:L95–L103.
96. Beers MF, Fisher AB. Surfactant protein-C—A review of its unique properties and metabolism. Am J Physiol 1992; 263:L151–L160.
97. Curstedt T, Johansson J, Persson P, et al. Hydrophobic surfactant-associated polypeptides—SP-C is a lipopeptide with 2 palmitoylated cysteine residues, whereas SP-B lacks covalently linked fatty acyl groups. Proc Natl Acad Sci USA 1990; 87:2985–2989.
98. Johansson J, Persson P, Löwenadler B, et al. Canine hydrophobic surfactant polypeptide SP-C—A lipopeptide with one thioester-linked palmitoyl group. FEBS Lett 1991; 281:119–122.
99. Fischer JH, Emrie PA, Drabkin HA, et al. The gene encoding the hydrophobic surfactant protein SP-C is located on 8p and identifies an EcoRI RFLP. Am J Hum Genet 1988; 43:436–441.

100. Glasser SW, Korfhagen TR, Wert SE, et al. Genetic element from human surfactant protein SP-C gene confers bronchiolar-alveolar cell specificity in transgenic mice. Am J Physiol 1991; 261:L349–L356.
101. Wohlford-Lenane CL, Durham PL, Snyder JM. Localization of surfactant-associated protein C (SP-C) mRNA in fetal rabbit lung tissue by in situ hybridization. Am J Respir Cell Mol Biol 1992; 6:225–234.
102. Kalina M, Mason RJ, Shannon JM. Surfactant protein-C is expressed in alveolar type-II cells but not in Clara cells of rat lung. Am J Respir Cell Mol Biol 1992; 6:594–600.
103. Keller A, Eistetter HR, Voss T, Schäfer KP. The pulmonary surfactant protein-C (SP-C) precursor is a type II transmembrane protein. Biochem J 1991; 277:493–499.
104. Vorbroker DK, Dey C, Weaver TE, Whitsett JA. Surfactant protein-C precursor is palmitoylated and associates with subcellular membranes. Biochim Biophys Acta 1992; 1105:161–169.
105. Persson A, Rust K, Chang D, et al. CP4: A pneumocyte-derived collagenous surfactant-associated protein. Evidence for heterogeneity of collagenous surfactant proteins. Biochemistry 1988; 27:8576–8584.
106. Crouch E, Rust K, Veile R, et al. Genomic organization of human surfactant protein-D (SP-D)—SP-D is encoded on chromosome 10q22.2-23.1. J Biol Chem 1993; 268:2976–2983.
107. Voorhout WF, Veenendaal T, Kuroki Y, et al. Immunocytochemical localization of surfactant protein-D (SP-D) in type-II cells, Clara cells, and alveolar macrophages of rat lung. J Histochem Cytochem 1992; 40:1589–1597.
108. Crouch E, Rust K, Persson A, et al. Primary translation products of pulmonary surfactant protein-D. Am J Physiol 1991; 260:L247–L253.
109. Lu JH, Wiedemann H, Holmskov U, et al. Structural similarity between lung surfactant protein-D and conglutinin—2 distinct, C-type lectins containing collagen-like sequences. Eur J Biochem 1993; 215:793–799.
110. Persson A, Chang D, Crouch E. Surfactant protein-D is a divalent cation-dependent carbohydrate-binding protein. J Biol Chem 1990; 265:5755–5760.
111. Persson A, Chang D, Rust K, et al. Purification and biochemical characterization of CP4 (SP-D), a collagenous surfactant-associated protein. Biochemistry 1989; 28:6361–6367.
112. Mendelson CR, Boggaram V. Hormonal control of the surfactant system in fetal lung. Annu Rev Physiol 1991; 53:415–440.
113. Ogasawara Y, Kuroki Y, Shiratori M, et al. Ontogeny of surfactant apoprotein-D, SP-D, in the rat lung. Biochim Biophys Acta 1991; 1083:252–256.
114. Ballard PL. Hormones and Lung Maturation. Berlin: Springer, 1986.
115. Post M, Van Golde LMG. Metabolic and developmental aspects of the pulmonary surfactant system. Biochim Biophys Acta 1988; 947:249–286.
116. Post M, Smith BT. Hormonal control of surfactant metabolism. In: Robertson B, Van Golde LMG, Batenburg JJ, eds. Pulmonary Surfactant: From Molecular Biology to Clinical Practice. Amsterdam: Elsevier, 1992:397–424.
117. Bourbon JR, Farrell PM. Fetal lung development in the diabetic pregnancy. Pediatr Res 1985; 19:253–267.

118. Hallman M. Effect of extracellular myo-inositol on surfactant phospholipid synthesis in the fetal rabbit lung. Biochim Biophys Acta 1984; 795:67–78.
119. Smith BT, Post M. Fibroblast-pneumonocyte factor. Am J Physiol 1989; 257:L174–L178.
120. Torday JS, Kourembanas S. Fetal rat lung fibroblasts produce a TGFβ homolog that blocks alveolar type-II cell maturation. Dev Biol 1990; 139:35–41.
121. Caniggia I, Tseu I, Han RNN, et al. Spatial and temporal differences in fibroblast behavior in fetal rat lung. Am J Physiol 1991; 261:L424–L433.
122. Gross I. Regulation of fetal lung maturation. Am J Physiol 1990; 259:L337–L344.
123. Liley HG, White RT, Benson BJ, Ballard PL. Glucocorticoids both stimulate and inhibit production of pulmonary surfactant protein A in fetal human lung. Proc Natl Acad Sci USA 1988; 85:9096–9100.
124. Ogasawara Y, Kuroki Y, Tsuzuki A, et al. Pre- and postnatal stimulation of pulmonary surfactant protein D by in vivo dexamethasone treatment of rats. Life Sci 1992; 50:1761–1767.
125. Post M, Batenburg JJ, Schuurmans EAJM, Van Golde LMG. The rate-limiting step in the biosynthesis of phosphatidylcholine by alveolar type II cells from adult rat lung. Biochim Biophys Acta 1982; 712:390–394.
126. Post M, Batenburg JJ, Van Golde LMG, Smith BT. The rate-limiting reaction in phosphatidylcholine synthesis by alveolar type II cells isolated from fetal lung. Biochim Biophys Acta 1984; 795:558–563.
127. Post M, Batenburg JJ, Smith BT, Van Golde LMG. Pool sizes of precursors for phosphatidylcholine formation in adult rat lung type II cells. Biochim Biophys Acta 1984; 795:552–557.
128. Vance DE, Pelech SL. Enzyme translocation in the regulation of phosphatidylcholine biosynthesis. Trends Biochem Sci 1984; 9:17–20.
129. Burkhardt R, Von Wichert P, Batenburg JJ, Van Golde LMG. Fatty acids stimulate phosphatidylcholine synthesis and CTP:choline-phosphate cytidylyltransferase in type II pneumocytes isolated from adult rat lung. Biochem J 1988; 254:495–500.
130. Zimmermann LJ, Hogan M, Carlson KS, et al. Regulation of phosphatidylcholine synthesis in fetal type II cells by CTP:phosphocholine cytidylyltransferase. Am J Physiol 1993; 264:L575–L580.
131. Post M. Maternal administration of dexamethasone stimulates choline-phosphate cytidylyltransferase in fetal type II cells. Biochem J 1987; 241:291–296.
132. Gonzales R, Ertsey R, Ballard PL, et al. Glucocorticoid stimulation of fatty acid synthesis in explants of human fetal lung. Biochim Biophys Acta 1990; 1042:1–12.
133. Xu Z-X, Stenzel W, Sasic SM, et al. Glucocorticoid regulation of fatty acid synthase gene expression in fetal rat lung. Am J Physiol 1993; 265:L140–L147.
134. Fraslon C, Batenburg JJ. Pre-translational regulation of lipid synthesizing enzymes and surfactant proteins in fetal rat lung in explant culture. FEBS Lett 1993; 325:285–290.
135. Batenburg JJ, Den Breejen JN, Geelen, MJH, et al. Phosphatidylcholine synthesis in type II cells and regulation of the fatty acid supply. Prog Respir Res 1990; 25:96–103.
136. Batenburg JJ, Elfring RH. Pre-translational regulation by glucocorticoid of fatty

acid and phosphatidylcholine synthesis in type-II cells from fetal rat lung. FEBS Lett 1992; 307:164–168.
137. Rooney SA, Smart DA, Weinhold PA, Feldman DA. Dexamethasone increases the activity but not the amount of choline-phosphate cytidylyltransferase in fetal rat lung. Biochim Biophys Acta 1990; 1044:385–389.
138. Xu Z-X, Smart DA, Rooney SA. Glucocorticoid induction of fatty-acid synthase mediates the stimulatory effect of the hormone on choline-phosphate cytidylyltransferase activity in fetal rat lung. Biochim Biophys Acta 1990; 1044:70–76.
139. Oulton M, Martin TR, Faulkner GT, et al. Developmental study of a lamellar body fraction isolated from human amniotic fluid. Pediatr Res 1980; 14:722–728.
140. Burton LE, Wells WW. Studies on the developmental pattern of the enzymes converting glucose 6-phosphate to myo-inositol in the rat. Dev Biol 1974; 37:35–42.
141. Batenburg JJ, Klazinga W, Van Golde LMG. Regulation of phosphatidylglycerol and phosphatidylinositol synthesis in alveolar type II cells isolated from adult rat lung. FEBS Lett 1982; 147:171–174.
142. Bleasdale JE, Tyler NE, Busch FN, Quirk JG. The influence of myo-inositol on phosphatidylglycerol synthesis by rat type II pneumonocytes. Biochem J 1983; 212:811–818.
143. Bleasdale JE, Thakur NR, Rader GR, Tesan M. Cytidine monophosphate-dependent synthesis of phosphatidylglycerol in permeabilized type II pneumonocytes. Biochem J 1985; 232:539–545.
144. Chevalier G, Collet AJ. In vivo incorporation of choline-^{3}H, leucine-^{3}H and galactose-^{3}H in alveolar type II pneumocytes in relation to surfactant synthesis. A quantitative radioautographic study in mouse by electron microscopy. Anat Rec 1972; 174:289–310.
145. Funkhouser JD, Read RJ. Phospholipid transfer proteins from lung, properties and possible physiological functions. Chem Phys Lipids 1985; 38:17–27.
146. Lumb RH. Phospholipid transfer proteins in mammalian lung. Am J Physiol 1989; 257:L190–L194.
147. Tsao FHC. Purification and characterization of two rabbit lung Ca^{2+}-dependent phospholipid-binding proteins. Biochim Biophys Acta 1990; 1045:29–39.
148. Jobe A, Ikegami M, Sarton-Miller I, et al. Characterization of phospholipids and localization of some phospholipid synthetic and subcellular marker enzymes in subcellular fractions from rabbit lung. Biochim Biophys Acta 1981; 666:47–57.
149. Magoon MW, Wright JR, Baritussio A, et al. Subfractionation of lung surfactant—Implications for metabolism and surface activity. Biochim Biophys Acta 1983; 750:18–31.
150. Voorhout TE, Weaver TE, Haagsman P, et al. Biosynthetic routing of pulmonary surfactant proteins in alveolar type II cells. Microsc Res Techn 1993; 26:366–373.
151. Chander A, Fisher AB, Regulation of lung surfactant secretion. Am J Physiol 1990; 258:L241–L253.
152. Wright JR, Dobbs LG. Regulation of pulmonary surfactant secretion and clearance. Annu Rev Physiol 1991; 53:395–414.
153. Suwabe A, Mason RJ, Smith D, et al. Pulmonary surfactant secretion is regulated by the physical state of extracellular phosphatidylcholine. J Biol Chem 1992; 267:19884–19890.

154. Rooney SA, Gobran LI, Umstead TM, Phelps DS. Secretion of surfactant protein A from rat type II pneumocytes. Am J Physiol 1993; 265:L586–L590.
155. Ikegami M, Lewis JF, Tabor B, et al. Surfactant protein-A metabolism in preterm ventilated lambs. Am J Physiol 1992; 262:L765–L772.
156. Oosterlaken-Dijksterhuis MA, Van Eijk M, Van Buel BLM, et al. Surfactant protein composition of lamellar bodies isolated from rat lung. Biochem J 1991; 274:115–119.
157. Wright JR. Clearance and recycling of pulmonary surfactant. Am J Physiol 1990; 259:L1–L12.
158. Gross NJ, Schultz RM. Requirements for extracellular metabolism of pulmonary surfactant—Tentative identification of serine protease. Am J Physiol 1992; 262: L446–L453.
159. Veldhuizen RAW, Inchley K, Hearn SA, et al. Degradation of surfactant-associated protein-B (SP-B) during in vitro conversion of large to small surfactant aggregates. Biochem J 1993; 295:141–147.
160. Rider ED, Ikegami M, Jobe AH. Localization of alveolar surfactant clearance in rabbit lung cells. Am J Physiol 1992; 263:L201–L209.
161. Ryan RM, Morris RE, Rice W, et al. Binding and uptake of pulmonary surfactant protein (SP-A) by pulmonary type II epithelial cells. J Histochem Cytochem 1989; 37:429–440.
162. Kuroki Y, Mason RJ, Voelker DR. Alveolar type II cells express a high-affinity receptor for pulmonary surfactant protein. Proc Natl Acad Sci USA 1988; 85:5566–5570.
163. Young SL, Wright JR, Clements JA. Cellular uptake and processing of surfactant lipids and apoprotein SP-A by rat lung. J Appl Physiol 1989; 66:1336–1342.
164. Breslin JS, Weaver TE. Binding, uptake, and localization of surfactant protein-B in isolated rat alveolar type II cells. Am J Physiol 1992; 262:L699–L707.
165. Bates SR, Fisher AB. Degradation of surfactant protein-B by alveolar type II cells. Am J Physiol 1993; 265:L448–L455.
166. Bates SR, Beers MF, Fisher AB. Binding and uptake of surfactant protein-B by alveolar type II cells. Am J Physiol 1992; 263:L333–L341.
167. Pinto RA, Wright JR, Lesikar D, et al. Uptake of pulmonary surfactant protein-C into adult rat lung lamellar bodies. J Appl Physiol 1993; 74:1005–1011.

4

Pulmonary Surfactant and Lung Defense

Interactions of Surfactant Proteins with Phagocytic Cells and Pathogens

J. FREEK VAN IWAARDEN
Utrecht University
Utrecht
and Vrije Universiteit
Amsterdam, The Netherlands

LAMBERT M. G. VAN GOLDE
Utrecht University
Utrecht, The Netherlands

I. Introduction

Pulmonary surfactant is a complex material that confers mechanical stability to the alveoli. It consists of approximately 90% of lipids and 5–10% of proteins. The surfactant lipids and proteins are synthesized by the type II pneumocytes and secreted by these cells into the fluid layer that lines the alveolar epithelium (see Chapter 3). The surfactant lipids can subsequently spread as a monolayer at the air-liquid interface and, by lowering surface tension, prevent alveolar collapse at low lung volumes (1,2). In addition to lipids, pulmonary surfactant contains two hydrophilic proteins, SP-A and SP-D, and two extremely hydrophobic proteins, SP-B and SP-C (3). Three of these proteins (SP-A, SP-B, and SP-C) play key roles in the dynamics and intra-alveolar metabolism of the surfactant system (for review, see refs. 3–7). So far, there is no evidence supporting a role for SP-D in the adsorption of surfactant lipids to the air-liquid interfaces of the lungs. In that respect, it is even questionable whether SP-D should be designated as a true surfactant protein.

Although stabilizing the lungs is undoubtedly the major physiological function of pulmonary surfactant, there is accruing evidence that components of the surfactant system may interact with inhaled microorganisms and with phagocytic cells, and thus contribute to the lung defense system. In the upper and central airways, infiltrated pathogens are largely removed by sneezing, coughing, and mucociliary clearance. In the alveolar region, which is not equipped with such mechanisms, phagocytic cells are responsible for the inactivation and elimination of inhaled pathogens. Alveolar macrophages, which, for example, rapidly clear inhaled bacteria (8,9), play a central role in the alveolar defense system. In addition, monocytes and polymorphonuclear leukocytes originating from the bloodstream participate in the inactivation of pathogens during pulmonary inflammation (10).

The first indications for a role of surfactant in the host-defense system were obtained by La Force and colleagues (11), who reported enhanced killing of *Staphylococcus aureus* by alveolar macrophages in the presence of surfactant. Since then, several investigators found stimulating effects of either whole surfactant or surfactant lipids on the phagocytosis and killing of bacteria by alveolar macrophages (12,13) and on the activation of these cells (14). However, other investigators found no (15) or even an inhibitory effect (16) on the phagocytosis of bacteria by alveolar macrophages. Interpretation of these older studies (for review, see ref. 17) is complicated by the fact that they were carried out with either whole surfactant or the lipid fraction of surfactant. As will be discussed in this chapter, more recent studies have provided evidence for a potentially important role of the surfactant proteins SP-A and SP-D in the interactions of pulmonary surfactant with phagocytic cells and pathogens. In the following section, we will first briefly describe the structure of these two hydrophilic surfactant proteins, with some emphasis on their structural resemblance to defense proteins in the circulation.

II. The Hydrophilic Surfactant Proteins SP-A and SP-D

A. SP-A

SP-A is the most abundant hydrophilic surfactant protein. In its monomeric form, it has a molecular mass of 28–36 kDa, depending on the degree of glycosylation. The primary structure of SP-A has been established for a variety of species, including the human protein (5,6,18), and it appears to be highly conserved. The monomeric SP-A has several distinct structural domains (Fig. 1). A short NH_2-terminal region of 7–10 amino acids contains a cysteine that forms an interchain disulfide bond, which is important in aligning the SP-A monomers for oligomerization. The aminoterminal part is flanked by a collagen-like domain containing 24 Gly-X-Y repeats, where X is any amino acid and Y is hydroxyproline in 13 of the 24 triplets. This structural motif suggests that this region of the molecule is folded into a triple helix. The sequence of repeating triplets is interrupted between the 13th and 14th repeat by the sequence pro-cys-pro-pro.

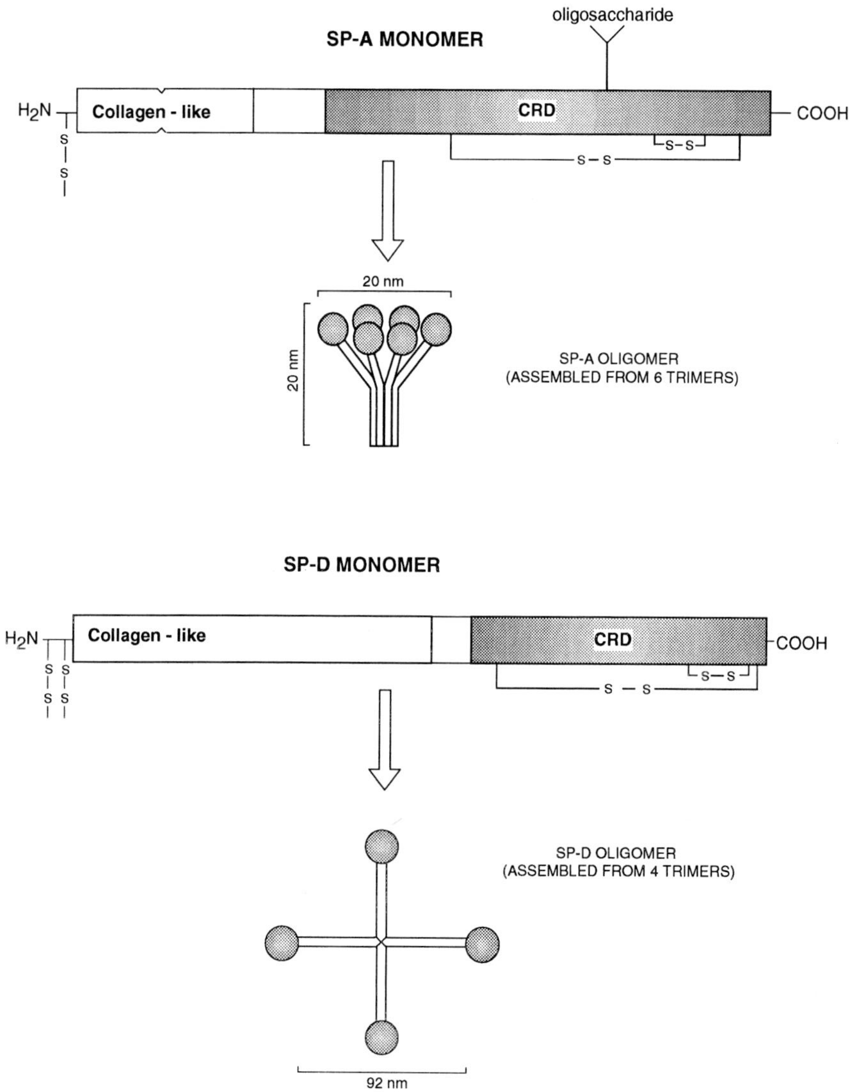

Figure 1 Structures of the hydrophilic surfactant proteins SP-A and SP-D.

The carboxyterminal carbohydrate recognition domain (CRD), which is encoded by a single exon (18), has sequence similarity with a number of Ca^{2+}-dependent or C-type lectins, such as the plasma proteins mannose-binding protein and conglutinin (19–21). A complex sialated oligosaccharide is attached to SP-A at asparagine-187 (5).

Rotary shadowing electron microscopy (22) suggested that in its functional form SP-A consists of 18 monomeric subunits (6 trimers) that are assembled through interchain disulfide bridges and noncovalent interactions via the collagenous domain to the characteristic funnel-shaped structure reported earlier for C1q (23). The break in the collagen-like sequence introduces a flexible kink in the collagen rods allowing the six individual triple helices to fan out radially from the tightly associated stem (Fig. 1). Its lectin property of binding to mannose residues (24) and its structural similarities with important plasma defense molecules such as C1q, conglutinin, and mannose-binding proteins were indeed important indications that SP-A may have a similar function in the alveoli.

B. SP-D

The second hydrophilic surfactant protein is SP-D. Like SP-A, it is a collagenous glycoprotein (25,26) that is synthesized by type II cells and Clara cells (27,28). Its primary translation product in the rat and human is a 39-kDa protein that undergoes posttranslational N-linked glycosylation as well as hydroxylation and glycosylation of lysine residues within the collagenous domain (29). The primary structure of SP-D has been established for several species, including the human protein (29–33). The protein comprises a short aminoterminal region, a collagen-like domain of 59 Gly-X-Y repeats, a short linking domain, and the carboxyterminal carbohydrate recognition domain (CRD) (Fig. 1). The collagen-like domain of SP-D is much longer than that of SP-A, and its 59 Gly-X-Y repeats are not interrupted. The carbohydrate recognition domain has sequence similarity with the corresponding domain in other members of the C-type lectins. In its functional form the protein is probably assembled as multimers of disulfide-bonded trimers comprised of 12 apparently identical 43-kDa proteins. Rotary shadowing electron microscopy showed that SP-D has a similar cruciform structure as conglutinin, although the majority of the preparation consisted of single stalks with globular heads (34). The shape of SP-D seems ideal for agglutination reactions. The molecule spans a distance of 92 nm and consists of four globular carbohydrate-binding heads each connected to 46-nm long rods that are associated via the free end.

In the following sections, we will subsequently discuss the influence of the hydrophilic surfactant proteins on pathogens and on the interactions of these proteins with alveolar macrophages.

III. Influence of SP-A and SP-D on Pathogens

A. Interactions of SP-A and SP-D with Gram-Negative Bacteria and Lipopolysaccharides

Lipopolysaccharide (LPS), or endotoxin, is a component of the outer membrane of gram-negative bacteria and consists of lipid A (the biologically active constituent of endotoxin), a relatively conserved core region, and a terminal polysaccharide of variable length and composition that comprises the O-specific antigen domain (35). LPS causes a wide variety of toxic and immunomodulatory effects in the body (for review, see refs. 36 and 37). Recently, evidence was provided that both SP-A and SP-D associate with gram-negative bacteria and with LPS.

Kuan et al (38) reported time and concentration dependent binding of ^{125}I-labeled SP-D to *Escherichia coli*, as well as aggregation of these bacteria in the presence of calcium and SP-D. No binding or aggregation of the bacteria was observed when maltose was present, indicating that association of SP-D with *E. coli* is mediated via the carbohydrate-binding domain of SP-D. The part of the LPS molecule that is involved in the interaction with SP-D is probably the carbohydrate-rich core region. This was strongly suggested by the observation that labeled SP-D bound only to LPS derived from bacteria that contained lipid A and part of the core region (rough LPS), whereas it did not associate with purified lipid A. Interestingly, SP-D did not aggregate *E. coli* containing LPS with a complete core region and O-antigen domain (smooth LPS). To explain the observation that SP-D associated with bacteria with rough LPS but not with those containing smooth LPS, the authors suggested that the SP-D–binding core region of smooth LPS is shielded from interaction with SP-D by the oligosaccharide-rich O-antigen domain (38).

Binding studies performed with fluorescein isothiocyanate (FITC)–labeled SP-A and LPS of various chain lengths coupled to beads indicated that SP-A also binds to LPS (39). In analogy with SP-D, SP-A bound only to rough LPS and not to smooth LPS. However, in contrast to SP-D, SP-A associated with the lipid A moiety of LPS and not with the core region. Binding of SP-A to lipid A required the presence of both calcium and sodium cations and could not be inhibited by carbohydrates, such as mannose oligomers. In addition, deglycosylation of SP-A by enzymatic digestion did not affect the binding of SP-A to LPS. These results suggest that neither the carbohydrate-binding region nor the carbohydrate moieties of SP-A are involved in the binding of SP-A to LPS. The nature of the domain of SP-A that is responsible for the interaction with LPS is not known at present, but the lipid-binding region of SP-A (5) may be an attractive candidate (39).

Association of LPS with phagocytes such as polymorphonuclear leukocytes (PMNs), monocytes, and macrophages leads to stimulation of these cells to produce, for instance, oxygen radicals and cytokines such as tumor necrosis factor (TNF). The effect of complex formation of rough LPS with SP-A could affect these LPS-mediated processes. Binding studies performed with alveolar macrophages and PMNs with FITC-labeled LPS complexed to SP-A indicated that the complex formation with SP-A altered the interaction of LPS with these phagocytes (40). Binding of LPS to the alveolar macrophages was enhanced, whereas the binding of LPS to PMNs was inhibited when LPS was complexed to SP-A. Since SP-A alone can bind to alveolar macrophages but not to PMNs (40), these observations may be explained by the following hypothesis: LPS-SP-A complexes may bind to alveolar macrophages either via the LPS receptor or the SP-A receptor, whereas the binding of LPS to its receptor on PMNs is blocked by the presence of SP-A in the complex. This hypothesis is supported by the observations that the LPS-mediated production of oxygen radicals by PMNs was inhibited by SP-A, whereas the LPS-mediated TNF production by alveolar macrophages was not influenced by SP-A, SP-A alone had no effect on these processes.

Whether binding of either SP-A and/or SP-D to LPS plays a role in the pathogenesis of gram-negative pneumonia is not known. However, it is of interest to note that the SP-A levels in patients with gram-negative pneumonia were lower than in healthy volunteers (41), which may suggest a connection between SP-A and gram-negative pneumonia.

B. Influence of SP-A on Viruses

Van Iwaarden et al. (42) demonstrated enhanced binding of FITC-labeled SP-A to herpes simplex virus type 1–infected cells over noninfected cells. These observations suggested interaction of SP-A with the viral proteins. In the presence of calcium ions, SP-A also induced aggregation of the virus, which was recorded spectrophotometrically as an increase in turbidity (17). After removal of the carbohydrate moiety of SP-A by enzymatic digestion, no more binding of SP-A to the herpes simplex virus was observed, whereas other properties of SP-A such as the binding to lipids (43) or the stimulation of alveolar macrophages (42) were not affected. These findings indicated that the association of SP-A to herpes virus is mediated via the carbohydrate moiety of SP-A. It is not known whether binding of SP-A to the membrane-associated proteins of herpes simplex virus or the SP-A–mediated aggregation of the virions influences the infection of cells by this virus.

Influenza viruses are important agents of seasonally occurring epidemics of respiratory disease (44). We were able to demonstrate interaction of SP-A with influenza A viruses (45). Binding studies with FITC-SP-A and influenza A–infected cells indicated concentration and time-dependent binding of SP-A to the influenza A proteins. Enzymatic digestion of SP-A with neuraminidase abolished the interaction of SP-A with the virus, whereas blocking of the carbohydrate-binding domain of SP-A with mannose-oligosaccharides did not prevent this interaction. This strongly suggests that SP-A binds via sialic acid residues of its carbohydrate moiety to influenza A virus. Association of SP-A with influenza A also affected the infectivity of the virus (45). Preincubation of influenza A with SP-A markedly reduced the amount of viral proteins on the outer membrane of cells when the cells were incubated with this mixture, as was determined by monoclonal antibodies directed against one of the viral proteins. Not only the amount of virus proteins associated with the host cells was diminished in the presence of SP-A, but also the number of cells infected by the virus, as was shown using an immunoplaque assay specific for influenza A virus. The infection of cells by other viruses such as influenza B and mumps, which are known to interact with sialated glycoproteins (46,47), was not influenced by SP-A. The sialic acid residues of SP-A probably have the specific conformation required for the inhibition of the infection of cells by influenza A viruses but not for inhibiting the infection by the other viruses that were tested. Interestingly, though SP-A could not prevent infection of cells by influenza B virus (Fig. 2),

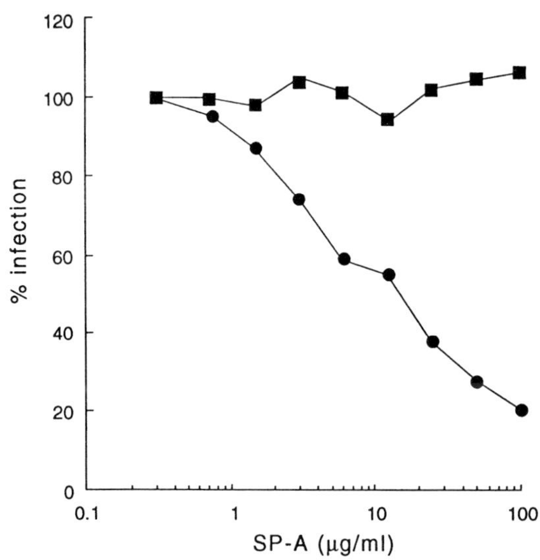

Figure 2 Influence of SP-A on the infection of cells by influenza A and B viruses. Influenza A (H3N2) virus (circles) or influenza B virus (squares) were preincubated with the indicated concentrations of human SP-A. Subsequently, the virus SP-A mixtures were added to LLC-monkey kidney (MK2D) cells (LLC cells) and incubated for 22 hr at 37°C (45). The cell-associated viral proteins, a measure for the infection of cells, were visualized with monoclonal antibodies directed against either influenza A or influenza B. The infection of cells was expressed as percentage of cells infected with virus in the absence of SP-A. Data from four representative experiments are shown.

it did bind with high affinity and in a concentration-dependent manner to cells infected by this virus (Fig. 3). In this way, SP-A may assist in the clearance of the virus from the lungs by, for instance, opsonization of the virus for phagocytosis by alveolar macrophages.

C. Influence of SP-A on Pneumocystis Carinii

Pneumocystis carinii is a major cause of pneumonia in immunocompromised hosts, particularly those with the acquired immunodeficiency syndrome (AIDS) (48). Severe *P. carinii* pneumonia is often associated with respiratory distress characterized by poor oxygenation and pulmonary compliance (49). Hence, a connection between *P. carinii* pneumonia and the pulmonary surfactant system seemed likely. Indeed, a marked decreased was observed in the concentrations of the surfactant lipids in a rat model for *P. carinii* pneumonia (50), as well as in the bronchoalveolar lavages of patients with human immunodeficiency virus (HIV) infection and *P. carinii* pneumonia (51) compared with controls. Not only the surfactant lipids may be involved in the pathogenesis of the disease, but also SP-A. Phelps et al. (52) detected elevated levels of SP-A in the bronchoalveolar lavages of HIV-infected patients with *P. carinii* pneumonia and non–*P. carinii*

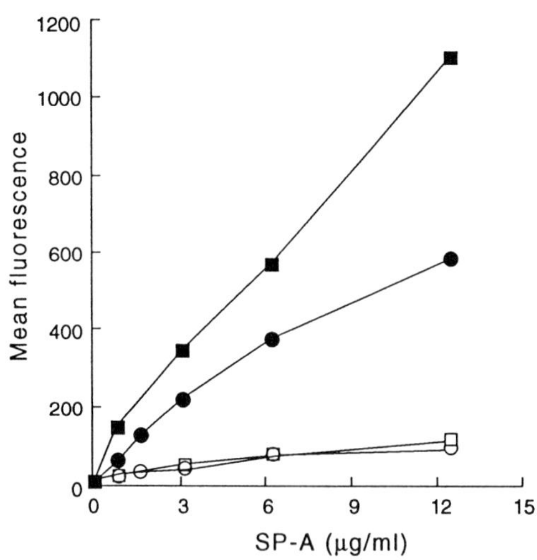

Figure 3 Binding of FITC-labeled SP-A to cells infected with influenza A or influenza B virus. LLC cells, infected with influenza A virus (closed circles), influenza B virus (closed squares) or incubated with buffer (open symbols), were exposed to the indicated concentrations of FITC-SP-A for 1 hr at 37°C (45). The cell-associated fluorescence, a measure for the amount of SP-A bound to the cells, was determined by flow-cytometry. Data from three representative experiments are shown.

pneumonia. In addition, Zimmerman et al. (53) demonstrated specific, time- and concentration-dependent binding of ^{125}I-SP-A to *P. carinii* in the presence of calcium ions. The binding of SP-A to *P. carinii* could be inhibited by mannose coupled to albumin, indicating involvement of the carbohydrate-binding domain of SP-A in the interaction with *P. carinii*. Blotting of the membrane proteins of *P. carinii* showed binding of SP-A to a mannose-rich membrane-associated glycoprotein of 120 kDa (GP-120). GP-120 may be involved in the attachment of the organism to the alveolar epithelium. The authors suggested that SP-A may enhance adherence of *P. carinii* to alveolar epithelium, thereby facilitating infection (53). However, an interesting alternative could be that coating of *P. carinii* with SP-A may lead to opsonization for phagocytosis by alveolar macrophages and perhaps prevent infection.

IV. Interaction of SP-A and SP-D with Alveolar Macrophages

Alveolar macrophages originate from the bone marrow. The progenitor cells are the blood monocytes, although there are indications that local replication of alveolar macrophages may also occur in the lung (10). A wide variety of defense mechanisms is available to the alveolar macrophages. These include phagocytosis, intracellular and extracellular killing of microorganisms, recruitment of polymorphonuclear granulocytes and other phagocytic cells by the production and secretion of chemotactic substances, and the production and secretion of cytokines. The effects of SP-A and SP-D on these processes will be briefly discussed below.

A. Influence of SP-A on Migration of Alveolar Macrophages

Wright et al. (54) reported concentration-dependent stimulation of chemotaxis of rat alveolar macrophages by SP-A reaching a maximum at approximately 100 μg/ml. The SP-A–mediated chemotaxis was partially inhibited when SP-A was subjected to heat treatment and completely abolished after enzymatic digestion with collagenase. These results suggest that the collagen-like domain of SP-A is involved in the stimulation of migration by alveolar macrophages. Interestingly, SP-A also stimulated the migration of peritoneal macrophages.

B. Influence of SP-A and SP-D on the Production of Toxic Oxygen Metabolites by Alveolar Macrophages

The killing of microorganisms by phagocytes can be initiated by various reaction mechanisms such as, for instance, the secretion of proteolytic enzymes and the production of toxic oxygen metabolites. So far there is only information about the effects of SP-A and SP-D on the production of oxygen metabolites by phagocytes but not on the other processes involved in the killing of bacteria.

The initial step in the generation of oxygen metabolites is reduction of oxygen by NADPH-oxidase complex leading to superoxide (O_2^-). Following superoxide formation, other oxygen metabolites may then appear including H_2O_2, $^{\cdot}OH$, $^1O_2$, and HOCl, with the latter being formed by myeloperoxidase from H_2O_2 and Cl^- (55). During the formation of superoxide and HOCl by the phagocytes, light is generated, which is the so-called chemiluminescence (for review see, ref. 56). Chemiluminescent probes such as luminol and lucigenin can enhance the weak natural chemiluminescence. The chemiluminescence enhanced by luminol or lucigenin can be measured and used as an indication for the production of oxygen metabolites by phagocytes. The specificities for oxygen metabolites of lucigenin and luminol differ. Luminol has been shown to be highly sensitive to HOCl, whereas lucigenin is specific for superoxide (57–59). Since alveolar macrophages contain little or no myeloperoxidase (60,61), determination of oxygen radical production by alveolar macrophages should be performed using lucigenin-dependent chemiluminescence.

We were able to show that rat surfactant enhances the lucigenin-dependent chemiluminescence response by rat alveolar macrophages (62). The component in surfactant responsible for this effect appeared to be SP-A, as antibodies directed against this particular surfactant protein could abolish the surfactant-induced chemiluminescence. Furthermore, purified human SP-A isolated from alveolar proteinosis patients could also elicit a lucigenin-dependent chemiluminescence response. These results indicate that SP-A stimulates the production of superoxide by alveolar macrophages. Interestingly, peritoneal macrophages, monocytes, and polymorphonuclear leukocytes were not stimulated by SP-A to produce oxygen radicals, indicating that the SP-A–mediated production of oxygen radicals is restricted to alveolar macrophages only. However, no stimulation of the lucigenin-dependent chemiluminescence response was found by Weber et al. (63) when canine bronchoalveolar phagocytes were incubated with canine SP-A. In addition, Katsura et al. (64) also did not detect an enhancement of the oxygen radical production of rat alveolar macrophages by rat SP-A using a ferricytochrome *c* reduction assay. One possible explanation for the discrepancy between their and our results may be the fact that different procedures were used for the isolation of SP-A. We recently obtained evidence (J.F. van Iwaarden, unpublished observations) that butanol extraction of canine and rat surfactant, the method used by Weber et al. (63) and Katsura et al. (64) to separate SP-A from the lipid fraction, destroys the alveolar macrophage-stimulating properties of SP-A.

Also, rat SP-D can elicit a lucigenin-dependent chemiluminescence response by rat alveolar macrophages (65). In analogy with SP-A, no chemiluminescence response could be evoked in peritoneal macrophages. However, the concentrations of SP-A and SP-D needed for a maximal response differed. Approximately 10 times less SP-D (0.1 μg/ml) was needed. Furthermore, the SP-A–mediated response was inhibited by surfactant lipids, whereas the SP-D–mediated oxygen radical production by alveolar macrophages was not. These results may suggest that the SP-A– and SP-D–induced stimulation of oxygen metabolites production by alveolar macrophages is mediated by different mechanisms.

C. Influence of SP-A on Complement- and Immunoglobulin-Mediated Phagocytosis by Alveolar Macrophages

Phagocytosis of microorganisms and particles by alveolar macrophages occurs after interaction(s) with receptors present on the macrophage (for review, see ref. 66). The presence of surface receptors for the Fc part of several immunoglobulins (Igs) and for the complement fragment C3b on the alveolar macrophage is probably essential for the phagocytosis of bacteria and particles coated (opsonized) with immunoglobulins and/or complement. After interaction with receptors on the macrophage, the receptor-particle (or microorganism) complex is internalized and directed to the lysosome where it is subjected to the action of lysosomal enzymes.

We were able to demonstrate that SP-A enhanced the phagocytosis of *S. aureus* by rat alveolar macrophages (62). However, SP-A only showed this effect when the bacteria had been opsonized with serum. SP-A alone had no effect on the phagocytosis of *S. aureus* by the macrophages, suggesting that SP-A may stimulate complement and/or immunoglobulin mediated phagocytosis. This suggestion is in agreement with observations by Tenner et al. (67), who reported enhanced phagocytosis of sheep erythrocytes coated with IgG or IgM and complement by macrophages. In contrast to these findings, McNeely et al. (68) reported that the phagocytosis of serum-opsonized heat-killed *S. aureus* by rabbit alveolar macrophages was not stimulated by SP-A. This discrepancy could be due to species differences or to variations in the preparation of bacteria. Manz-Keinke et al. (69) demonstrated that the ability of SP-A to opsonize *S. aureus* depended on the growth phase of the bacteria. SP-A stimulated phagocytosis of serum-opsonized *S. aureus* by rat alveolar macrophages when the bacteria were in their stationary growth phase, whereas SP-A acted as an opsonin for the phagocytosis of these bacteria only when they were in their logarithmical growth phase.

D. Opsonic Activities of SP-A and SP-D

SP-A enhanced the phagocytosis of FITC-labeled herpes simplex virus type 1 by rat alveolar macrophages as was demonstrated using flow cytometry (70). The enhancement of the phagocytosis was time and concentration dependent, and it did not require opsonization of the virus by, for instance, rat serum, indicating that

SP-A alone mediated herpes phagocytosis. Preincubation of the alveolar macrophages with SP-A and subsequent addition of $F(ab')_2$ fragments of a polyclonal antiserum specific for SP-A abolished the SP-A–mediated phagocytosis of this virus. Furthermore, deglycosylation of SP-A, which inhibited the binding of SP-A to the virus but not the binding of SP-A to alveolar macrophages and the stimulation of these cells (42), prevented SP-A–mediated phagocytosis of the virus. Hence, phagocytosis of herpes simplex virus requires binding of SP-A to the alveolar macrophages followed by binding of virus to the attached SP-A. These observations strongly suggest that SP-A acts as an opsonin in the phagocytosis of herpes simplex virus by alveolar macrophages. Whether SP-A can act as an opsonin for phagocytosis of other viruses by alveolar macrophages such as, for instance, influenza A or influenza B viruses, is not known at present, but seems likely, since both viruses associate with SP-A (Fig. 3).

In a preceding section, we mentioned that both SP-A and SP-D bind and aggregate gram-negative bacteria with rough LPS (38,39). Fluorescence-binding studies performed with the J5 mutant of *Escherichia coli*, a bacterium which contains rough LPS, and O111 *E. coli*, which contains smooth LPS, showed that SP-A mediated the attachment of J5 but not that of O111 to rat alveolar macrophages (71). Using immunoelectron microscopy, we were able to demonstrate that SP-A increased phagocytosis of J5 by alveolar macrophages approximately six times over the control incubations.

Manz-Keinke et al. (69) reported enhanced SP-A–mediated phagocytosis of *E. coli* in the logarithmic growth phase but not when the bacteria were in their stationary growth phase. This could be explained by the fact that the synthesis and assembly of LPS are dependent on the growth phase of the bacteria and that the LPS formed in this phase is predominantly of the rough type (72,73), which would facilitate interaction with SP-A.

Although SP-D bound and aggregated J5 bacteria and stimulated alveolar macrophages, SP-D did not increase the attachment of these bacteria to alveolar macrophages or their phagocytosis even at SP-D concentrations of 5 μg/ml, which are far above the concentrations needed for either stimulation of alveolar macrophages (0.1 μg/ml (65)) or aggregation of J5 (0.5 μg/ml (71)). In addition, SP-D did not influence the SP-A–mediated phagocytosis of J5 by alveolar macrophages. These observations suggest that the interactions of SP-D with J5 and with alveolar macrophages may take place via other mechanisms than the SP-A interactions with J5 and alveolar macrophages.

E. Receptors for SP-A and SP-D on Alveolar Macrophages

The nature of the SP-A receptor on alveolar macrophages is controversial. Wintergerst et al. (74) reported that mannose bound to albumin inhibited the uptake of SP-A coupled to gold particles by alveolar macrophages, suggesting that SP-A associates via its carbohydrate binding domain to alveolar macrophages. However, only partial inhibition of the uptake of SP-A was observed when the macrophages were preincubated with a mannose oligosaccharide (75). On the other hand, Malhotra et al. (76) reported binding of SP-A to U937 cells, which express the C1q receptor. The binding of SP-A to these cells was inhibited in the presence of C1q. In addition, these investigators demonstrated that SP-A inhibited the binding of an isolated and purified C1q receptor to immobilized C1q (77). Although the latter results favour binding of SP-A to the C1q receptor, and therefore indicate that the SP-A receptor on alveolar macrophages could be the C1q receptor, binding studies with SP-A should be interpreted with great care. Oosting et al. (78) reported that the binding of alveolar macrophages to SP-A coupled to magnetic beads was inhibited in the presence of either SP-A, SP-D, or C1q. However, after preincubation of the alveolar macrophages with either SP-A, SP-D, C1q, or mannose oligosaccharides, only the alveolar macrophages preincubated with SP-A did not bind to SP-A-coated beads. Binding studies performed with ^{125}I–SP-A showed that SP-D, C1q, and mannose oligosaccharides all bound to SP-A. The authors suggested that the inhibition of binding of SP-A to alveolar macrophages in the presence of either SP-D, C1q, or mannose oligosaccharides is caused by binding of these compounds to SP-A, thereby preventing binding of SP-A to its receptor on the alveolar macrophages. In conclusion, more studies will be needed to determine exactly the nature of the SP-A and SP-D receptors on alveolar macrophages.

V. Conclusions

The research on possible roles of the hydrophilic surfactant proteins in the pulmonary defense system is a relatively new field. The work that has been done so far indicates that the surfactant proteins may be active in the defense system at least at two levels: (1) interaction of the proteins with pathogens leading to aggregation of the pathogens and, in the case of influenza A virus, neutralization; and (2) stimulation of alveolar macrophages leading to serum-mediated or SP-A–mediated (and perhaps SP-D–mediated) phagocytosis. Although it is obvious that much research remains to be done before a complete picture will be obtained on the putative role of these proteins in defense against pulmonary infections, the results so far do justify the conclusion that the role of pulmonary surfactant is probably not limited to conferring mechanical stability to the lungs. (The interaction between bacteria and different exogenous surfactants is further discussed in Chapter 12.)

Acknowledgments

The work carried out in L. M. G. van Golde's laboratory was supported by the Dutch Asthma Foundation (Nederlands Astma Fonds), by the Dutch Praeventiefonds, and by the Netherlands Foundation for Chemical Research (SON).

References

1. Clements JA. Function of the alveolar lining. Am Rev Respir Dis 1977; 115:67–71.
2. Van Golde LMG, Batenburg JJ, Robertson B. The pulmonary surfactant system: Biochemical aspects and functional significance. Physiol Rev 1988; 68:374–455.
3. Possmayer F. The role of surfactant-associated proteins. Am Rev Respir Dis 1990; 142:749–752.
4. Haagsman HP, van Golde LMG. Synthesis and assembly of lung surfactant. Annu Rev Physiol 1991; 53:441–464.
5. Weaver TA, Whitsett JA. Function and regulation of expression of pulmonary surfactant-associated proteins. Biochem J 1991; 273:249–264.
6. Hawgood S. Pulmonary surfactant apoproteins: A review of protein and genomic structure. Am J Physiol 1989; 257:L13–L22.
7. Wright JR, Clements JA. Metabolism and turnover of lung surfactant. Am Rev Respir Dis 1987; 135:426–444.
8. Green GM, Kass EH. The role of the alveolar macrophage in the clearance of bacteria from the lung. J Exp Med 1964; 119:167–175.
9. Hocking WG, Golde DW. The pulmonary alveolar macrophage. N Engl J Med 1979; 301:580–587.
10. Sibille Y, Reynolds HY. Macrophages and polymorphonuclear neutrophils in lung defense and injury. Am Rev Respir Dis 1990; 141:471–501.
11. LaForce FM, Kelley WJ, Huber GL. Inactivation of staphylococci by alveolar macrophages with preliminary observations on the importance of alveolar lining material. Am Rev Respir Dis 1973; 108:783–790.
12. Juers JA, Rogers RM, McCurdy JB, Cook WW. Enhancement of bactericidal capacity of alveolar macrophages by human alveolar lining material. J Clin Invest 1976; 58:271–275.
13. O'Neill S, Lesperance E, Klass DJ. Rat lung lavage surfactant enhances bacterial phagocytosis and intracellular killing by alveolar macrophages. Am Rev Respir Dis 1984; 130:225–230.
14. Webb DSA, Jeska EL. Enhanced luminol-dependent chemiluminescence of stimulated rat alveolar macrophages by pretreatment with alveolar lining material. J Leukocyte Biol 1986; 40:55–64.
15. Jonsson S, Musher DM, Goree A, Lawrence EC. Human alveolar lining material and antibacterial defenses. Am Rev Respir Dis 1986; 133:136–140.
16. Coonrod DJ, Jarrells MC, Yoneda K. Effect of rat surfactant lipids on complement and Fc receptors of macrophages. Infect Immun 1986; 54:371–378.
17. Van Iwaarden JF. Surfactant and the pulmonary defense system. In: Robertson B, van Golde LMG, Batenburg JJ, eds. Pulmonary Surfactant. From Molecular Biology to Clinical Practice. Amsterdam: Elsevier, 1992:215–227.
18. White RT, Damm D, Miller J, et al. Isolation and characterization of the human pulmonary surfactant apoprotein gene. Nature 1985; 317:361–363.
19. Drickamer K, Dordal MS, Reynolds L. Mannose-binding proteins isolated from rat liver contain carbohydrate-recognition domains linked to collagenous tails. Complete primary structures and homology with pulmonary surfactant apoprotein. J Biol Chem 1986; 261:6878–6887.

20. Drickamer K. Two distinct classes of carbohydrate-recognition domains in animal lectins. J Biol Chem 1988; 263:9557–9560.
21. Thiel S, Reid KBM. Structures and functions associated with the group of mammalian lectins containing collagen-like sequences. FEBS Lett 1989; 250:78–84.
22. Voss T, Eistetter H, Schäfer K, Engel J. Macromolecular organization of natural and recombinant lung surfactant protein SP 28-36: Structural homology with the complement factor C1q. J Mol Biol 1988; 201:219–227.
23. Brodsky-Doyle BKR, Leonard KR, Reid KBM. Circular-dichroism and electron microscopy study of human subcomponent Ciq before and after limited proteolysis by pepsin. Biochem J 1976; 159:279–286.
24. Haagsman HP, Hawgood S, Sargeant T, et al. The major lung surfactant protein, SP 28-36, is a calcium-dependent, carbohydrate-binding protein. J Biol Chem 1987; 262:13877–13880.
25. Persson A, Rust K, Chang D, et al. CP4: A pneumocyte-derived collagenous surfactant-associated protein. Evidence for heterogeneity of collagenous surfactant proteins. Biochemistry 1988; 27:8576–8584.
26. Persson A, Chang D, Rust K, et al. Purification and biochemical characterization of CP4 (SP-D): A collagenous surfactant-associated protein. Biochemistry 1989; 28:6361–6367.
27. Voorhout WF, Veenendaal T, Kuroki Y, et al. Immunocytochemical localization of surfactant protein-D (SP-D) in type-II cells, Clara cells, and alveolar macrophages of rat lung. J Histochem Cytochem 1992; 40:1589–1597.
28. Crough E, Parghi D, Kuan S-F, Persson A. Surfactant protein D: Subcellular localization in nonciliated bronchiolar epithelial cells. Am J Physiol 1992; 263:L60–L66.
29. Rust K, Grosso L, Zhang V, et al. Human surfactant protein D: SP-D contains a C-type lectin carbohydrate recognition domain. Arch Biochem Biophys 1993; 290:116–126.
30. Lu J, Willis AC, Reid KBM. Purification, characterization and cDNA cloning of human lung surfactant protein D. Biochem J 1992; 284:795–802.
31. Crouch E, Rust K, Veile R, et al. Genomic organization of human surfactant protein D (SP-D). SP-D is encoded on chromosome 10q22.2-23.1 J Biol Chem 1993; 268:2976–2983.
32. Shimizu H, Fisher JH, Papat P, et al. Primary structure of rat pulmonary surfactant protein D. cDNA and deduced amino acid sequence. J Biol Chem 1992; 267:1853–1857.
33. Lim BL, Lu J, Reid KBM. Structural similarity between bovine conglutinin and bovine lung surfactant protein D and demonstration of liver as a site of synthesis of conglutinin. Immunology 1993; 78:159–165.
34. Lu J, Wiedemann H, Holmskov U, et al. Structural similarity between lung surfactant protein D (SP-D) and conglutinin: Two distinct, C-type lectins containing collagen-like sequences. Eur J Biochem 1993; 215:793–799.
35. Raetz CRH, Ulevitch RJ, Wright SD, et al. Gram-negative endotoxin: An extraordinary lipid with profound effects on eukaryotic signal transduction FASEB J 1991; 5:2652–2660.
36. Brigham KL, Meyrick B. Endotoxin and lung injury. Am Rev Respir Dis 1986; 133:913–927.

37. Burrell, R. Immunomodulation by bacterial endotoxin. Crit Rev Microbiol 1990; 17:189–208.
38. Kuan S-F, Rust K, Crouch E. Interactions of surfactant protein D with bacterial lipopolysaccharides. Surfactant protein D is an Escherichia coli–binding protein in bronchoalveolar lavage. J Clin Invest 1992; 90:97–106.
39. Van Iwaarden JF, Pikaar JC, Storm J, et al. Binding of surfactant protein A to the lipid A moiety of bacterial lipopolysaccharides. Biochem J 1994; 303:407–411.
40. Corrales I, van Iwaarden JF, van Golde LMG, et al. Complex formation of surfactant protein A with bacterial lipopolysaccharides alters the interactions of lipolysaccharides with phagocytes. Submitted for publication.
41. Baughman RP, Sternberg RI, Hull W, et al. Decreased surfactant protein-A in patients with bacterial pneumonia. Am Rev Respir Dis 1993; 147:653–657.
42. Van Iwaarden JF, van Strijp JAG, Visser H, et al. Binding of surfactant protein A (SP-A) to Herpes simplex virus type 1–infected cells is mediated by the carbohydrate moiety of SP-A. J Biol Chem 1992; 267:25039–25043.
43. Haagsman HP, Elfering RH, van Buel BLM, Voorhout WF. The lung lectin surfactant protein A aggregates phospholipid vesicles via a novel mechanism. Biochem J 1991; 275:273–276.
44. McIntosh K, Hallonen P, Ruuskanen O. Report of a workshop on respiratory viral infections: Epidemiology, diagnosis, treatment and prevention. Clin Infect Dis 1993; 16:151–164.
45. Benne CA, Kraaijeveld CA, van Strijp JAG, et al. Interactions of surfactant protein A with influenza A viruses: Binding and neutralization. J Infect Dis. In press.
46. Wiley DC, Skehel JJ. The structure and function of the haemagglutinin membrane glycoprotein of influenza virus. Ann Rev Biochem 1987; 56:365–394.
47. Markwell M, Portner A, Schwarz E. An alternative route of infection for viruses: Entry by means of an asialoglycoprotein receptor for a Sendai virus mutant lacking its attachment protein. Proc. Natl Acad Sci USA 1985; 85:978–982.
48. Masur H, Lane HC, Kovacs JA, et al. Pneumocystis pneumonia: From bench to clinic. Ann Intern Med 1989; 111:813–826.
49. Maxfield RA, Sorkin IB, Fazzini EP, et al. Respiratory failure in patients with acquired immunodeficiency syndrome and Pneumocystis carinii pneumonia. Crit Care Med 1986; 14:443–449.
50. Sheenan PM, Stokes DC, Yeh YY, Hughes WT. Surfactant phospholipids and lavage phospolipase A_2 in experimental Pneumocystis carinii pneumonia. Am Rev Respir Dis 1986; 134:526–531.
51. Hoffman AGD, Lawrence MG, Ognibene FP, et al. Reduction of pulmonary surfactant in patients with human immunodeficiency virus infection and Pneumocystis carinii pneumonia. Chest 1992; 102:1730–1736.
52. Phelps DS, Rose RM. Increased recovery of surfactant protein A in AIDS-related pneumonia. Am Rev Respir Dis 1991; 143:1072–1075.
53. Zimmerman PE, Voelker DR, McCormack FX, et al. 120-kD surface glycoprotein of Pneumocystis carinii is a ligand for surfactant protein A. J Clin Invest 1992; 89:143–149.

54. Wright JR, Youmans DC. Pulmonary surfactant protein A stimulates chemotaxis of alveolar macrophage. Am J Physiol 1993; 264:L338–L344.
55. Fantone JC, Ward PA. Role of oxygen-derived free radicals and metabolites in leukocyte-dependent inflammatory reactions. Am J Pathol 1982; 107:397–418.
56. Schadelin J, Schadelin R, Mandell GL. Chemiluminescence of phagocytic cells. Crit Rev Clin Lab Sci 1981; 13:1–19.
57. Aniansson H, Stendahl O, Dahlgren C. Comparison between luminol- and lucigenin-dependent chemiluminescence of polymorphonuclear leukocytes. Acta Pathol Microbiol Immunol Scand [C] 1984; 92:357–361.
58. Edwards, SW. Luminol- and lucigenin-dependent chemiluminescence of neutrophils: Role of degranulation. J Clin Lab Immunol 1987; 22:35–39.
59. Gyllenhammar, H. Lucigenin chemiluminescence in the assessment of neutrophil superoxide production. J Immunol Meth 1987; 97:209–213.
60. Biggar WD, Sturgess JM. Peroxidase activity of alveolar macrophages. Lab Invest 1976; 34:31–34.
61. Devalon ML, Elliott GR, Regelmann WE. Oxidative response of human neutrophils, monocytes and alveolar macrophages induced by an opsonized surface-adherent Staphylococcus aureus. Infect Immun 1987; 55:2398–2403.
62. Van Iwaarden F, Welmers B, Verhoef J, et al. Pulmonary surfactant protein A enhances the host-defense mechanism of rat alveolar macrophages. Am J Respir Cell Mol Biol 1990; 2:91–98.
63. Weber H, Heilmann P, Meyer B, Maier KL. Effect of canine surfactant protein (SP-A) on the respiratory burst of phagocytic cells. FEBS Lett 1990; 270:90–94.
64. Katsura H, Kawada H, Konno K. Rat surfactant apoprotein A (SP-A) exhibits antioxidant effects on alveolar macrophages. Am J Respir Cell Mol Biol 1993; 9:520–525.
65. Van Iwaarden JF, Shimizu H, van Golde PHM, et al. Rat surfactant protein D enhances the production of oxygen radicals by rat alveolar macrophages. Biochem J 1992; 286:5–8.
66. Kaplan J, McVey Ward D. Movement of receptors and ligands through the endocytic apparatus in alveolar macrophages. Am J Physiol 1990; 258:L263–L270.
67. Tenner AJ, Robinson SL, Borchelt J, Wright JR. Human pulmonary surfactant protein (SP-A), a protein structurally homologous to C1q, can enhance FcR- and CR1-mediated phagocytosis. J Biol Chem 1989; 264:13923–13928.
68. McNeely TB, Coonrod JD. Comparison of the opsonic activity of human surfactant protein A for Staphylococcus aureus and Streptococcus pneumoniae with rabbit and human macrophages. J Infect Dis 1993; 167:91–97.
69. Manz-Keinke H, Plattner H, Schlepper-Schäfer J. Lung surfactant protein A (SP-A) enhances serum-independent phagocytosis of bacteria by alveolar macrophages. Eur J Cell Biol 1992; 57:95–100.
70. Van Iwaarden JF, van Strijp JAG, Ebskamp MJM, et al. Surfactant protein A is an opsonin in the phagocytosis of herpes simples virus type 1 by rat alveolar macrophages. Am J Physiol 1991; 61:L204–L209.
71. Pikaar JC, van Strijp JAG, Voorhout WF, et al. Comparison of the opsonic activities of surfactant protein A and surfactant protein D for Escherichia coli phagocytosis by alveolar macrophages. Submitted for publication. J Infect Dis 1995. In press.
72. Hancock REW, Mutharia LM, Chan L, et al. Pseudomonas aeuginosa isolates from

patients with cystic fibrosis: a class of serum sensitive, non-typable strains deficient in lipopolysaccharide O side chain. Infect Immun 1983; 42:170–177.

73. McCallus DE, Norcross NL. Antibody specific for Escherichia coli cross-reacts to various degrees with an Escherichia coli clinical isolate grown for different lengths of time. Infect Immun 1987; 55:1042–1046.
74. Wintergerst E, Manz-Keinke H, Plattner H, Schlepper-Schäfer J. The interaction of a lung surfactant protein (SP-A) with macrophages is mannose dependent. Eur J Cell Biol 1989; 50, 291–298.
75. Manz-Keinke H, Egenhofer C, Plattner H, Schlepper-Schäfer J. Specific interaction of lung surfactant protein A (SP-A) with rat alveolar macrophages. Exp Cell Res 1991; 192:597–603.
76. Malhotra R, Haurum J, Thiel S, Simm RB. Interaction of C1q receptor with lung surfactant protein A. Eur J Immunol 1992; 22:1437–1445.
77. Malhotra R, Thiel S, Reed KBM, Sim RB. Human leukocyte C1q receptor binds other soluble proteins with collagen domains. J Exp Med 1990; 172:955–959.
78. Oosting RS, Wright JR. Characterization of the surfactant protein A receptor: Cell- and ligand-specificity. Am J Physiol. In press.

Part Two

PATHOLOGY AND CLINICAL DIAGNOSIS OF SURFACTANT DYSFUNCTION

5

Genetics of Neonatal Lung Disease in Relation to the Surfactant Protein Genes

JOANNA FLOROS and ANNE M. KARINCH
The Pennsylvania State University College of Medicine
Hershey, Pennsylvania

I. Genetic Evidence for Respiratory Distress Syndrome

Respiratory distress syndrome (RDS) primarily affects prematurely born babies. It is a respiratory disease of the neonatal period that results in considerable mortality and morbidity among newborns (1). Several factors appear to contribute to the development of RDS (2). In addition to factors such as premature birth, which clearly are of importance, a variety of epidemiological studies have strongly hinted at a genetic component in the development of the disease, and thus the etiology of RDS is considered multifactorial and/or multigenic. In 1965, Graven and Mesenheimer (3) reported that mothers who delivered low birth weight (LBW) babies could be divided into two groups; one group whose LBW babies rarely develop RDS and one group whose LBW infants have a very high incidence of RDS. Since the groups did not differ in the progress of the pregnancy, labor, or delivery, the authors suggested that an unknown genetic factor is involved in the development of the disease. A study by Lankenau (4) also provided evidence for a genetic component of RDS. Nagourney and colleagues (5) found that singleton preterm babies born to women who had previously delivered a premature baby with RDS had a significantly increased chance of developing RDS compared with those who did not have a previously affected sibling. Studies of twins (6,7) show a higher incidence of RDS among monozygotic (MZ) twins than among dizygotic (DZ) twins. However, in one study (7), the authors attributed the higher incidence of RDS among MZ twins to the greater degree of immaturity of MZ compared with DZ twins.

A different type of evidence for a genetic component of RDS comes from a study that found linkage between incidence of RDS and two HLA antigens, HLA-A3 and HLA-B14 (8). There is no linkage disequilibrium between HLA-A3 and HLA-B14 antigens among the general population in the study group. The authors suggested that a "susceptibility gene" that is linked to HLA-A3 and HLA-B14 plays a role in development of RDS. The well-documented effect of race (prematurely born black infants are less likely to develop RDS than their weight-matched white counterparts) (9,10) may also reflect the impact of genotype on susceptibility to the condition.

In all the studies cited above, epidemiological analysis suggests the involvement of genetic elements in the development of RDS, but the affected genes are unknown. The involvement of "genetic factors" in the development of, or predisposition to, a disease implies the presence of susceptibility genes or of defective genes. Since the ultimate product of a gene is a specific protein, genetic factors must be proteins that in some way predispose an individual to develop a particular disease or, alternatively, be a defective version of a protein that is essential for the synthesis, structure, or function of some necessary cellular product. Proteins in the former category may be difficult to identify, but identification of the latter class of proteins can be more readily approached.

In 1959, Avery and Mead (11) suggested that RDS in newborn infants was caused by lack of surfactant in their lungs and 2 years later surfactant was described by a number of investigators as a lipoprotein complex (12,13). Defective surfactant activity leading to RDS could result from a decrease in the level of surfactant or from functionally impaired surfactant. Since surfactant is a complex mixture of lipid and protein, a defect of either its lipid or protein component has the potential to compromise its surface tension–lowering properties. Defects in enzymes essential for lipid metabolism could affect the lipid component of surfactant. To date, no such defects have been linked to RDS. This observation is not surprising, since the enzymes of lipid metabolism are present throughout the body. Defects in the pathways of lipid metabolism would most probably be pleiotropic, leading to multiple metabolic and physiological complications or be lethal very early in development and therefore rarely be seen in neonates. However, the major surfactant-associated proteins (SP-A, SP-B, and SP-C) are known to play important roles in the structure, function, and metabolism of surfactant. These proteins are lung specific, and there is evidence that variation in the level of their expression (14–17) or genetic variation in their genes is associated with RDS (18) and congenital pulmonary alveolar proteinosis (19).

II. Molecular Characterization of the Surfactant Protein Genes

The focus in this section is on the genomic characteristics of the major human surfactant protein genes (SP-A, SP-B, SP-C) for two reasons. The products of these genes play important roles in many aspects of surfactant and alteration in the expression of some of them has been associated with respiratory diseases in neonates. For information on the structural characteristics of the surfactant proteins, their function, and regulation, the reader may consult a recent review by Floros and Phelps (20).

A. SP-A

The human SP-A locus has been mapped on chromosome 10 (21,22) and consists of a pseudogene sequence (23) and of two classes of functional genes, represented by the published genomic SP-A gene I (24) and SP-A gene II (25) sequences. Each functional SP-A gene encodes a precursor (26) that undergoes a number of posttranslational modifications (20) to give rise to a sialoglycoprotein. The product of each functional SP-A gene appears to be required for stable mature SP-A (27). Corresponding cDNA sequences for gene I and gene II have been published and have been denoted 6A and 1A, respectively (26). An allelic variant sequence for SP-A 6A (or gene I), termed $6A^1$, has also been identified (28).

The genomic structural organization of both SP-A functional genes is depicted in Fig. 1. It consists of four exons containing in their entirety or in part, coding sequences. The last coding exon contains a long 3′-untranslated region (3′-UT). Among humans, the sequence of the 3′-UT exhibits genetic variation (28,29) that appears to be meiotically stable over a three-generation family (30). In addition, the SP-A gene contains a number of untranslated exons at the 5′ end. Three of the untranslated exons have been reported previously (24,25), but recently additional 5′-untranslated exons have been identified for both functional SP-A genes (31,32).

Within coding sequences the major differences between the functional SP-A genes appear to be amino acid substitutions that alter the position of the hydroxyproline residues (leucine to proline) and formation of disulfide bonds (cysteine to arginine) (25). The main difference between the SP-A gene I allelic variants, 6A and $6A^1$, is a change from leucine to valine in exon 1 and an insertion/deletion in the 3′ UT (28). Evolutionarily the SP-A genomic sequences appear to have arisen from a single primordial primate sequence that duplicated, giving rise to SP-A gene I (6A) and an ancestral sequence. The latter sequence underwent a further duplication event to give rise to SP-A gene II (1A) and the pseudogene sequence (29).

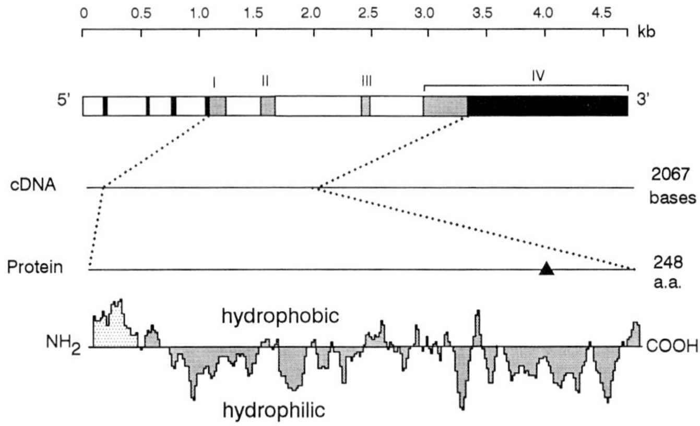

Figure 1 Genomic organization of SP-A. A schematic representation of the SP-A gene is shown along with a size scale. Regions with black fill are untranslated portions of the gene and those with dark stipple encode portions of the mature protein. The dotted lines delineate the relative positions of the translated portion of the cDNA. The lengths of the cDNA and protein are given. The triangle represents a potential N-linked glycosylation site in the protein. The bottom tracing shows a hydropathicity plot of the protein based on the amino acid sequence (50). Within the hydropathicity plot, dark stipple represents the mature protein and light stipple indicates portions of the precursor that are cleaved during processing.

B. SP-B

Both genomic and cDNA SP-B sequence have been published (33,34). The SP-B locus is located on chromosome 2 (35) on the proximal short arm (2p12-p11.2) (36). Its genomic structural organization, depicted in Fig. 2, consists of 11 exons, 10 of which contain coding sequences, whereas the eleventh exon encodes a 3′-UT region. A small 5′-UT region has also been identified as part of the first coding exon. This gene includes a number of distinct structural features, such as Alu sequences and $(CA)_n$ repeats (33). The SP-B large precursor protein undergoes amino- and carboxyterminal cleavages to give rise to mature SP-B, which is the form found in bronchoalveolar lavage material. Mature SP-B, as shown in Fig. 2, is encoded by exons 6 and 7 and is very hydrophobic.

C. SP-C

The SP-C gene is located on chromosome 8p (37) and consists of six exons (Fig. 3). A portion of exon 1 contains a small 5′-UT region. Part of exon 5 and the entire exon 6 contain the 3′-UT region (38). Alternative splicing results in several classes of mRNAs in human (38,39). Unlike the highly variable SP-A, SP-C is

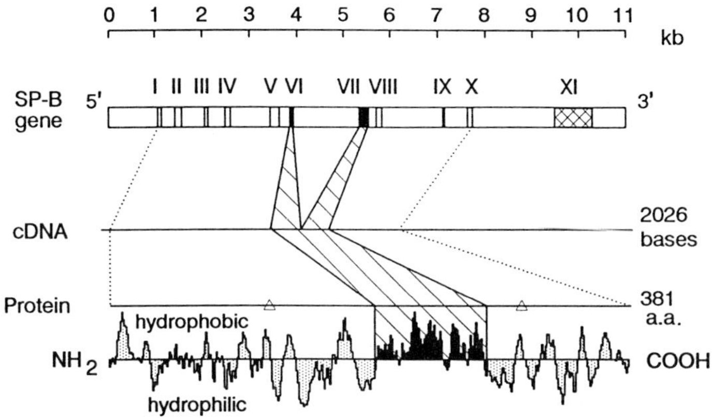

Figure 2 Genomic organization of SP-B. Details of this figure are identical to those described for Fig. 1 and light stippled exons encode portions of the precursor protein that are cleaved during processing. The hatched areas trace the portions of the cDNA and protein that are included in the mature protein. (From ref. 20; used with permission.)

quite conserved among humans (40). Like SP-B, the SP-C precursor protein undergoes posttranslational amino- and carboxyterminal cleavages to form mature SP-C, encoded by exon 2. The hydropathicity plot (Fig. 3) shows that the mature SP-C is very hydrophobic. Unlike both SP-A and SP-B, the aminoterminus of the mature SP-C protein varies (41).

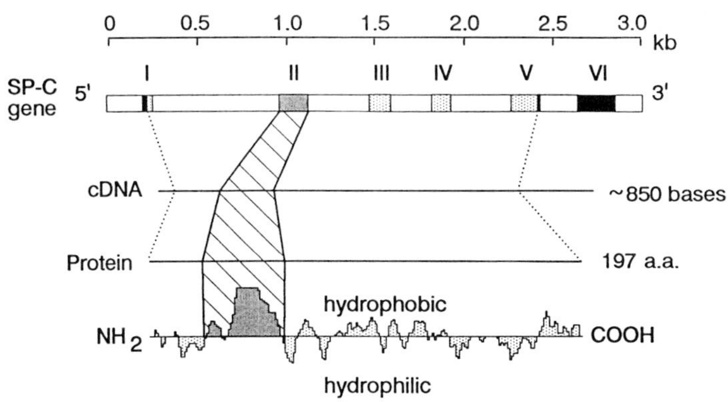

Figure 3 Genomic organization of SP-C. Details are as described in the legends of Figs. 1 and 2. (From ref. 20; used with permission.)

D. SP-D

SP-D is designated as a surfactant-associated protein and its gene is located on chromosome 10q (42), like that of SP-A (21,22). To date, it has not been shown to contribute to the surface tension–lowering properties of surfactant in the lung. Moreover, its role during neonatal disease, if any, is currently unknown and therefore it will not be discussed any further in this chapter.

III. Genetic Variation in the Surfactant Protein Genes and Potential Contribution to Neonatal Disease

A. SP-A

Immunological postmortem examination of lung tissue from babies who died from RDS showed that the levels of SP-A and SP-B/SP-C proteins were all reduced compared with their levels in lung tissue of babies who died from other causes (15–17). SP-A was particularly affected, being absent from some specimens. As noted in the previous section, considerable genetic heterogeneity has been observed in SP-A (28,29,31,32). Based on insight gained from other systems, it seems possible that some of the heterogeneity has the potential for altering the level of expression of SP-A. Splicing variability in the 5′-UT region (31,32) is found in both functional SP-A genes. It is not currently known whether the splicing variants differ in their efficiency of translation in vivo or in their regulation during development and/or in response to various agents or disease states.

A nucleotide base change (C to G) in coding exon 1 of the SP-A I (6A) gene changes the encoded amino acid from leucine to valine and represents the allelic variant, $6A^1$ (28). The frequency of the 6A genotypes in three different populations was determined and showed that the frequency of some SP-A genotypes was higher in Nigerians (28,30). The significantly higher incidence of the 6A/6A genotype among the black Nigerian population, compared with whites, is of particular interest because RDS is almost unknown in Nigeria (43). This observation is consistent with findings from epidemiological studies where the incidence of RDS was shown to be lower in prematurely born black babies than among their white counterparts. However, the distribution of 6A genotypes does not differ among American blacks or whites (30), suggesting that other or additional factors contribute to the lower incidence of RDS in blacks.

Regulation of gene expression can also be accomplished by alteration in mRNA stability, most frequently achieved through elements found in the 3′-UT region of the gene. SP-A expression has been shown to be regulated, at least in part, by changes in message stability (44,45), although the responsible elements have yet to be identified. The high degree of heterogeneity in the 3′-UT region of SP-A (Fig. 4) could result in individuals having SP-A mRNAs of varying stability. Another prominent variation in the 3′-UT region that may affect mRNA

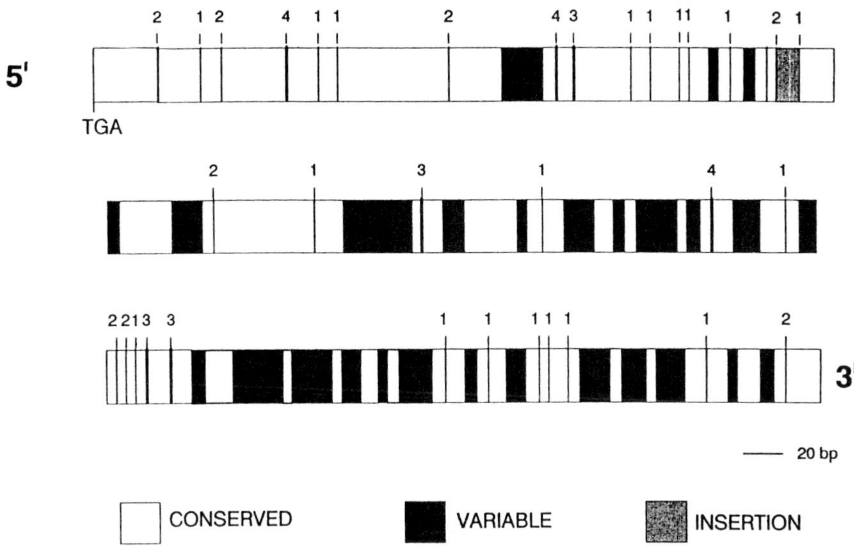

Figure 4 Conserved and variable regions of the (3′UT) of the human SP-A locus. The diagram represents an overview of the analysis of 3′UT sequences from 16 clones derived from eight genomic specimens (two clones/genomic specimen). Regions containing 5 or more base changes are shown in solid bars and conserved regions in open bars. The numbers indicate the size of the smaller regions (less than five bases) that contain changes. Numbers 1 and 2 indicate the presence of one and two base changes, respectively. Numbers 3 and 4 indicate that in a region of three or four bases one can observe two to three and two to four base changes, respectively. Occasional changes found only in one of the 16 clones are omitted from this analysis. The 11-base insertion present in the $6A^1$ allele is shown in stippled bar.

stability is the presence or absence of an 11-base segment at about 407 bases past the translation termination codon (28,29). The 3′-UT heterogeneity appears to have arisen in part as a result of gene conversion-like events during evolution of the human SP-A genes (29).

In summary, considerable heterogeneity has been identified at the SP-A locus. Fig. 5 illustrates the locations within the SP-A gene where genetic diversity has been described. Whether this heterogeneity correlates with or contributes to the pathogenesis of neonatal disease remains to be determined. It is possible, however, that the variability observed in the SP-A mRNA level among humans (46) reflects the genetic variability seen in the SP-A locus (28,29). On the other hand, the SP-C mRNA level does not vary significantly among humans (46), and a recent study (40) showed that there is very little variation in the SP-C locus. Taken together, these findings suggest that variability in the expression of the surfactant proteins reflects the degree of genetic variation of the respective genes.

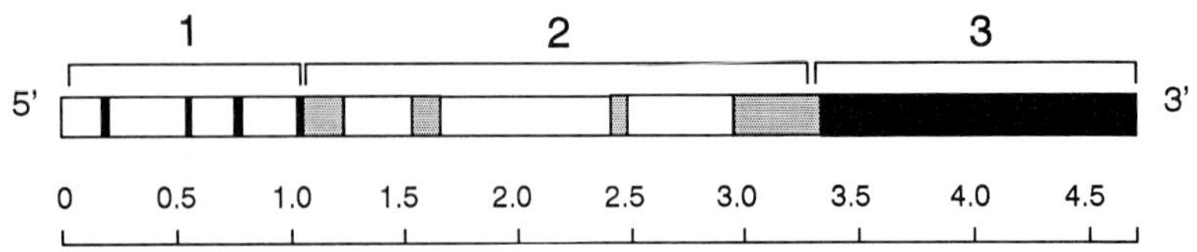

Figure 5 Genetic heterogeneity of SP-A locus. This figure illustrates the location of the genetic variability that occurs in human SP-A. Exons with black fill are untranslated portions of the gene and those with light stipple encode portions of the mature protein. The scale is in kilobases. Location 1 designates the 5′UT which undergoes alternative splicing; location 2 designates coding regions where genotypic differences occur among SP-A alleles; location 3 is the 3′UT which contains extensive sequence heterogeneity.

B. SP-B

Defective expression of the SP-B gene has been clearly implicated in congenital pulmonary alveolar proteinosis (19). Lung tissue of three siblings who died of the disease lacked both SP-B protein and mRNA. The defect is a frameshift mutation in exon 4 that is predicted to cause premature termination of translation, resulting in lack of SP-B protein. The affected siblings were homozygous for the defect and their parents and two unaffected siblings were all heterozygous. Two unrelated infants with SP-B deficiency and alveolar proteinosis were homozygous for the same defect, whereas a third was heterozygous for this and another uncharacterized mutation on the other allele (47). Another variation in the SP-B gene that involves insertion or deletion of motifs containing $(CA)_n$ repeats in intron 4 appears to be correlated with RDS (18,48).

C. SP-C

The SP-C gene appears to be conserved and to date there are no identifiable mutations that correlate with any neonatal disease. The conservation of this locus (40) and the early appearance of SP-C during lung development (49) suggest an important function of this gene product in addition to its involvement in surfactant action. If this is so, most, if not all, mutations in SP-C are lethal and therefore not detectable. Posttranslational heterogeneity at the aminoterminus of the mature SP-C protein has been identified and the relative abundance of the various SP-C forms varies in fetal and adult lung (41). However, the significance of this observation in normal and disease states is not known.

IV. Future Directions

It is clear from the discussion in the preceding sections of this chapter that genetic heterogeneity occurs in the surfactant protein genes. The significance of most of this heterogeneity has yet to be determined. In the future, a thorough understanding of the genetic variation may be gained through extensive haplotype analysis. The frequency of various haplotypes within and between different groups can then be determined and links between markers and disease states forged. Since the etiology of RDS and of other neonatal diseases is likely most often to be multifactorial and/or multigenic, a systematic search for additional disease-contributing factors may be carried out.

Acknowledgments

This work is supported by National Institutes of Health grants HL34788 and HL49823. The authors would also like to thank Beth Tyrpin for typing the manuscript for this chapter.

References

1. Perelman RH, Farrell PM. Analysis of causes of neonatal death in the United States with specific emphasis on fatal hyaline membrane disease. Pediatrics 1982; 70:570–575.
2. Farrell PM, Avery ME. Hyaline membrane disease. Am Rev Respir Dis 1975; 111:657–688.
3. Graven SN, Mesenheimer HR. Respiratory distress syndrome and the high risk mother. Am J Dis Child 1965; 109:489–494.
4. Lankenau HM. A genetic and statistical study of the respiratory distress syndrome. Eur J Pediatr 1976; 123:167–177.
5. Nagourney BA, Usher RH, Kramer MS. Is there a familial tendency in the etiology of respiratory distress syndrome (abstr). Pediatr Res 1990; 27:1288.
6. Myrianthopoulos NC, Churchill JA, Baszynski AJ. Respiratory distress syndrome in twins. Acta Genet Med Gemellol 1971; 20:199–204.
7. de la Verduczo R, Rosario R, Rigatto H. Hyaline membrane disease in twins. Am J Obstet Gynecol 1976; 125:668–671.
8. Hafez M, El-Sallab SH, Khashaba M, et al. Evidence of HLA-linked susceptibility gene(s) in respiratory distress syndrome. Dis Markers 1989; 7:201–208.
9. Fujikawa T, Froehlich LA. The influence of race and other factors on pulmonary hyaline membranes. Am J Obstet Gynecol 1966; 95:572–578.
10. Farrell PM, Wood RE. Epidemiology of hyaline membrane disease in the United States: Analysis of national mortality statistics. Pediatrics 1976; 58:167–176.
11. Avery ME, Mead J. Surface properties in relation to atelectasis and hyaline membrane disease. Am J Dis Child 1959; 97:517–523.
12. Buckingham S. Studies on the identification of an antiatelectasis factor in normal sheep lung. Am J Dis Child 1961; 102:521–522.
13. Pattle RE, Thomas LC. Lipoprotein composition of the film lining the lung. Nature 1961; 189:844.

14. deMello DE, Chi EY, Doo E. Lagunoff D. Absense of tubular myelin in lungs of infants dying with hyaline membrane disease. Am J Pathol 1987; 127:131–139.
15. deMello DE, Phelps DS, Patel G, et al. Expression of the 35kDa and low molecular weight surfactant-association proteins in the lungs of infants dying with respiratory distress syndrome. Am J Pathol 1989; 134:1285–1293.
16. Floros J, Phelps DS, deMello DE, et al. Surfactant proteins and respiratory distress syndrome. In: von Wichert P, Müller B, eds. Basic Research on Lung Surfactant. Progress in Respiration Research. Vol. 25. Basel: Karger, 1990:231–236.
17. deMello DE, Heyman S, Phelps DS, Floros J. Immunogold localization of SP-A in lungs of infants dying from respiratory distress syndrome. Am J Pathol 1993; 142:1631–1640.
18. Floros J, Veletza V, Kotikalapudi P, Krizkova L, Karinch AN, Friedman C, Buchter S, Marks K. Dinucleotide repeats in the human surfactant protein B gene and respiratory distress syndrome. Biochem J 1995; 305:583–590.
19. Nogee LM, deMello DE, Dehner LP, Colten HR. Deficiency of pulmonary surfactant protein B in congenital alveolar proteinosis. N Engl J Med 1993; 328:406–410.
20. Floros J, Phelps DS. Pulmonary Surfactant. In: Biebuyck JF, Lynch III C, Maze M, et al., eds. Anesthesia: Biologic Foundations. New York: Raven Press.
21. Bruns G, Stroh H, Velman GM, et al. The 35kd pulmonary surfactant-associated protein is encoded on chromosome 10. Hum Genet 1987; 76:58–62.
22. Fisher JH, Kao FT, Jones C, et al. The coding sequence for the 32,000-dalton pulmonary surfactant-associated protein A is located on chromosome 10 and identifies two separate restriction-fragment-length polymorphisms. Am J Hum Genet 1987; 40:503–511.
23. Korfhagen TR, Glasser SW, Bruno MD, et al. A portion of the human surfactant protein A (SP-A) gene locus consists of a pseudogene. Am J Respir Cell Mol Biol 1991; 4:463–469.
24. White RT, Damm D, Miller J, et al. Isolation and characterization of the human pulmonary surfactant apoprotein gene. Nature 1985; 317:361–363.
25. Katyal SL, Singh G, Locker J. Characterization of a second human pulmonary surfactant-associated protein SP-A gene. Am J Respir Cell Mol Biol 1992; 6:446–452.
26. Floros J, Steinbrink R, Jacobs K, et al. Isolation and characterization of cDNA clones for the 35kDa pulmonary surfactant associated protein (PSP-A). J Biol Chem 1986; 261:9029–9033.
27. Voss T, Melchers K, Scheirle G, Schäfer KP. Structural comparison of recombinant pulmonary surfactant protein SP-A derived from two human coding sequences: Implications for the chain composition of natural human SP-A. Am J Respir Cell Mol Biol 1991; 4:88–94.
28. Rishi A, Hatzis D, McAlmon K, Floros J. An allelic variant of the 6A gene for human surfactant protein A. Am J Physiol 1992; 262 (Lung Cell Mol Physiol 6):L566–573.
29. Floros J, Rishi A, Veletza SV, Rogan PK. Concerted and independent genetic events in the 3′untranslated region of the human surfactant protein A genes. Am J Hum Genet 1993; 53:A683.

30. Krizkova K, Sakthivel R, Olowe SA, et al. Human SP-A: Genotype and single strand conformation polymorphism analysis. Am J Physiol 266 (Lung Cell Mol Physiol 10), 1994; L519–L527.
31. McCormick SM, Mendelson CR. The human surfactant (SP)-A1 and SP-A2 genes are differentially regulated during development and by cyclic AMP and glucocorticoids (abstr). Am J Respir Dis 1993; 147:249.
32. Karinch AM, Floros J. 5′ splicing and allelic variants of the human pulmonary surfactant protein A genes. Am J Respir Cell Mol Biol 1995; 12:77–78.
33. Pilot-Matias TJ, Kister SE, Fox JL, et al. Structure and organization of the gene encoding human pulmonary surfactant proteolipid SP-B. DNA 1989; 8:75–86.
34. Jacobs KA, Phelps DS, Steinbrink R, et al. Isolation of a cDNA clone encoding a high molecular weight precursor to a 6kDa pulmonary surfactant-associated protein. J Biol Chem 1987; 262:9808–9811.
35. Emrie PA, Jones C, Hofman T, Fisher JH. The coding sequence for the human 18,000-dalton hydrophobic pulmonary surfactant protein is located on chromosome 2 and identifies a restriction fragment length polymorphism. Somat Cell Mol Genet 1988; 14:105–110.
36. Vamvakopoulos NC, Modi WS, Floros J. Mapping the human pulmonary surfactant-associated protein B (SFTP3) gene on the proximal short arm of chromosome 2 (2p12-p11.2). Cytogen Cell Genet 1995; 58:8–10.
37. Fisher JH, Emrie PA, Drabkin HA, et al. The gene encoding the hydrophobic surfactant protein SP-C is located on 8p and identifies an EcoRI RFLP. Am J Hum Genet 1988; 43:436–441.
38. Glasser SW, Korfhagen TR, Perme CM, et al. Two SP-C genes encoding human pulmonary surfactant proteolipid. J Biol Chem 1988; 263:10326–10331.
39. Warr RG, Hawgood S, Buckley DI, et al. Low molecular weight human pulmonary surfactant protein (SP-5): Isolation, characterization, and cDNA and amino acid sequences. Proc Natl Acad Sci USA 1987; 84:7915–791.
40. Hatzis D, Dieter G, deMello D, Floros J. Human surfactant protein-C: Genetic homogeneity and expression in RDS; comparison with other species. Exp Lung Res 1994; 20:57–72.
41. Johansson J, Jörnvall H, Eklund A, et al. Hydrophobic 3.7 kDa surfactant polypeptide: Structural characterization of the human and bovine forms. FEBS Lett 1988; 232:61–64.
42. Crouch E, Rust K, Veile R, et al. Genomic organization of human surfactant protein-D (SP-D)—SP-D is encoded on chromosome 10q22.2-23.1. J Biol Chem 1993; 268:2976–2983.
43. Olowe SA, Akinkugbe A. Amniotic fluid lecithin/sphingomyelin ratio: Comparison between an African and a North American community. Pediatrics 1978; 62:38–41.
44. Boggaram V, Smith ME, Mendelson CR. Regulation of expression of the gene encoding the major surfactant protein (SP-A) in human fetal lung *in vitro*. J Biol Chem 1989; 264:11421–11427.
45. Iannuzzi DM, Ertsey R, Ballard PL. Biphasic glucocorticoid regulation of pulmonary SP-A: Characterization of inhibitory process. Am J Physiol 1993; 264:L236–L244.
46. Floros J, Phelps DS, deMello DE, et al. The utility of post-mortem lung for RNA

studies: Variability and correlation of the expression of surfactant proteins in human lung. Exp Lung Res 1991; 17:91–104.
47. Nogee LM, Murphy AM, Dietz HC. Identification of a common mutant allele in the pulmonary surfactant protein B (SP-B) gene in patients with neonatal alveolar proteinosis (abstr). Am J Hum Genet 1993; 53:93.
48. Veletza SV, Floros J. Genetic variation in $(CA)_n$ repeats in the human surfactant protein B (abstr). Am J Respir Crit Care Med 1994; 149:500.
49. Liley HG, White RT, Warr RG, et al. Regulation of mRNAs for the hydrophobic surfactant proteins in human lung. J Clin Invest 1989; 83:1191–1197.
50. Kyte J, Doolittle RF. A simple method for displaying the hydropathic character of a protein. J Mol Biol 1982; 157:105–132.

6

A Stable Microbubble Test for Antenatal and Early Neonatal Diagnosis of Surfactant Deficiency

SHOICHI CHIDA
Iwate Medical University
Morioka, Iwate, Japan

I. Introduction

Since the introduction of the amniotic fluid lecithin/sphingomyelin (L/S) ratio test by Gluck and associates in 1971 (1), the prenatal assessment of fetal lung maturity has gained wide acceptance, and a number of additional tests have been proposed. Although these tests offer advantages in predicting the development of respiratory distress syndrome (RDS), the methodologies required make the urgent performance of the tests inconvenient in some institutions.

With the recent advent of surfactant replacement therapy, there is an increasing need for a rapid and reliable test to predict RDS immediately before or at birth. The stable microbubble (SM) test developed by Pattle et al. (2) is a rapid and simple test that is performed on amniotic fluid and reflects the adequacy of pulmonary surfactant. Although the SM test is based on the finding of foam in acute lung edema (3), which resulted in the discovery of surfactant, this test has received little attention.

The purpose of this chapter is to describe the SM test as it is currently performed to identify a population that is surfactant deficient immediately before or at birth. (For review of other predictors of fetal lung maturity, see refs. 4 and 5.)

II. Methodology of the SM Test

The SM test is based on the biophysical capacity of pulmonary surfactant to generate SMs that are less than 15 μm in diameter [2]. The stability of bubbles <15 μm in diameter depends on the "surpellic" property of the surfactant; namely, its capacity to reduce the net surface tension to a small fraction of its equilibrium value. The SM test is performed according to the method described by Pattle et al. (2).

To generate bubbles, the uncentrifuged test sample is swirled to resuspend the sediment. An aliquot (around 40 μl) is aspirated up to 5 cm of the stem of a Pasteur pipette (lumen diameter 1.0 mm; stem length 11.5 cm) with a 2-ml rubber cap, and placed on a 50-mm × 35-mm microscope slide. For investigational purposes, a 40-μl aliquot is placed on a slide with an Eppendorf (Hamburg, Germany) pipette. The drop is then sucked into and expelled from the pipette in quick succession, 20 times in 6 sec, with the pipette tip touching the slide vertically in the drop. This process has to be performed as strongly as is possible without splashing the aliquot all over the slide. If correctly done, a characteristic sound is made, as when squirting a small amount of fluid in and out quickly between the front teeth. If done incorrectly, very few bubbles will be formed. The slide is then immediately inverted over a hollow slide, so that a hanging drop is formed. After 4 min, the slide is examined under a microscope at a magnification of 10 × 10, using a 1-mm^2 field and a 15-μm scale (Tokyo Tanabe, Tokyo, Japan). Counts are made in five regions, in the four quadrants of and at the center of the bubble field. All SMs <15 μm in diameter are counted. The mean count of SM/mm^2 of the five regions is calculated (Figs. 1 and 2).

Pattle et al. [2] originally proposed the following SM rating according to the number of SMs formed using amniotic fluid: strong, >20 SM/mm^2; medium, 10–20 SM/mm^2; weak, 2–10 SM/mm^2; very weak, <2 SM/mm^2; zero, no SM. A strong rating indicates that RDS will not occur, whereas a weak or lower rating suggests a high risk of RDS.

III. Characteristics of the SM Test

A. Bubble Size and Distribution

The distribution of different bubble sizes in a representative sample of mature amniotic fluid was examined on photographs taken in the five regions after 4 min of bubble generation. The diameter of each bubble and the number of bubbles per surface unit of each photograph were computed, using National Institutes of Health (NIH) image software (NIFTY-serve, Tokyo, Japan) (Fig. 3). The bubbles ranged in diameter from <3 to 250 μm. The distribution of microbubbles <15 μm and of relatively large bubbles of ≥15 μm was uneven for each field on

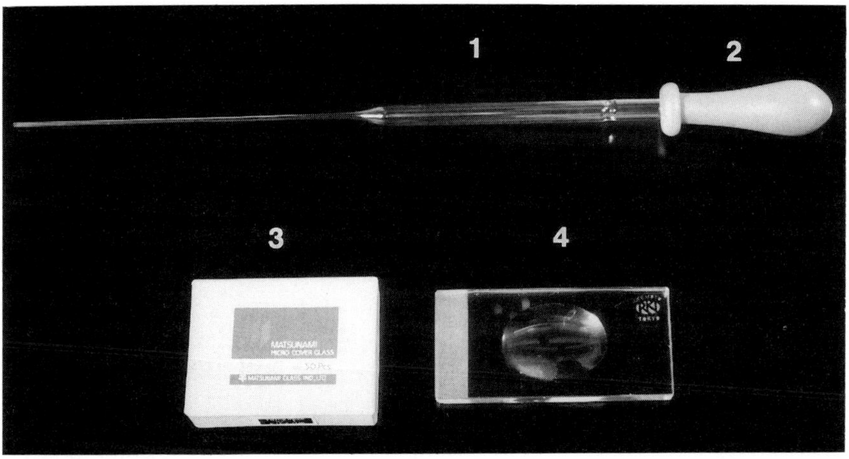

Figure 1 Equipment used to generate bubbles: 1, Pasteur pipette; 2, 2-ml rubber cap; 3, microscope slide contained in a box; 4, hollow slide.

the same slide. Therefore, counts were made in five regions and the mean count was calculated for the SM test.

B. Stability of Bubbles

The behavior of individual bubbles from amniotic fluid and gastric aspirate was observed using a computer-aided image analyzer (IBAS-2000, Zeiss, Ober-Kochen, Germany) (Fig. 4) (6). The number and size of microbubbles $<15\ \mu m$ in diameter in samples of both amniotic fluid and gastric aspirate remained unchanged from 2 to 30 min after the production of the bubbles (it took at least 2 min to set up and start the image analyzer). In contrast, bubbles $\geq 15\ \mu m$ in diameter were unstable; a significant number of the bubbles disappeared after 8–12 min, and the remainder contracted significantly during the observation period. These findings confirmed those in the original report by Pattle et al. (2), in showing that microbubbles $<15\ \mu m$ in diameter are stable, and further indicated that the time between bubble generation and counting could be shortened to 2 min.

The question may be raised regarding the substances that determine the bubble size in the SM test. According to Freer et al. (7), the capacity of a given substance to form a stable foam is largely related to its own surface tension characteristics. If the surface tension of a bubble formed from protein shaken in water is lower than that of the existing air-liquid interface, then the bubble structure may remain stable for a long period. Conversely, if the surface tension of the bubble is higher, the bubble tends to collapse. Therefore, it seems that

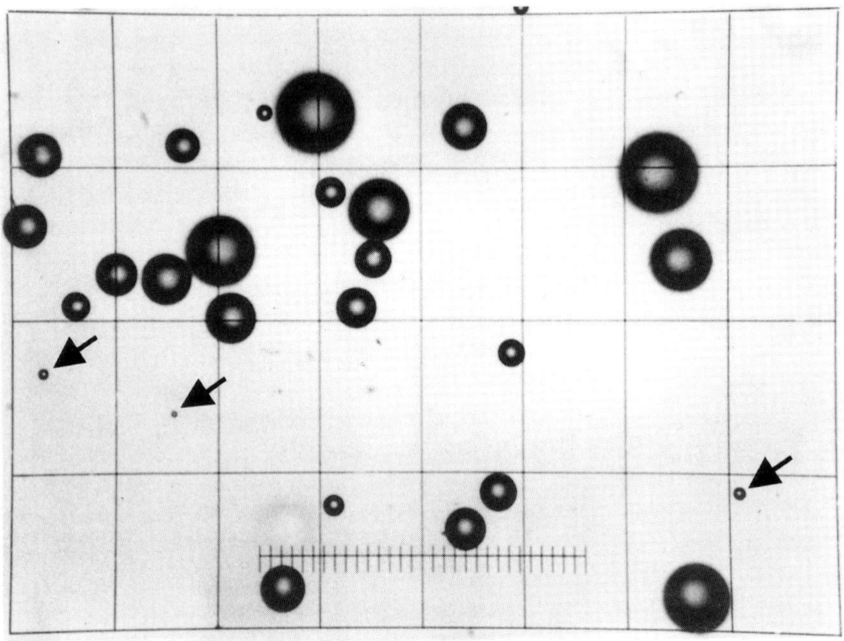

Figure 2 Microscopic view of bubble crop in amniotic fluid with 3 SM/mm^2 (arrows). The large rectangular field indicates 1 mm^2 and the scale is 15 μm wide. The 1-mm^2 field is subdivided into 4 × 8 fields.

the larger unstable bubbles described above could be formed by inadequate amounts of surfactant, by surfactant with abnormal function, by other substances present in the biological fluid, or by a combination of these factors.

C. Dose-Response Relationship

The dose-response relationship between the concentration of surfactant phospholipid and the number of SMs was examined with different surfactant preparations (8). The surfactants studied were Surfactant-TA, crude natural surfactant lipid of porcine lung lavage, purified natural surfactant of porcine lung lavage, phospholipid fraction of minced porcine lung, and a mixture of dipalmitoylphosphatidylcholine and phosphatidylglycerol (7:3).

All surfactant preparations showed linear regression relationships (Fig. 5). However, the concentrations of phospholipid needed to produce SMs and the slopes of the regression line differed among the surfactants. Surfactant-TA produced many SMs at the lowest concentration of phospholipid. This finding was consistent with its in vitro surface properties (8). The results of this study

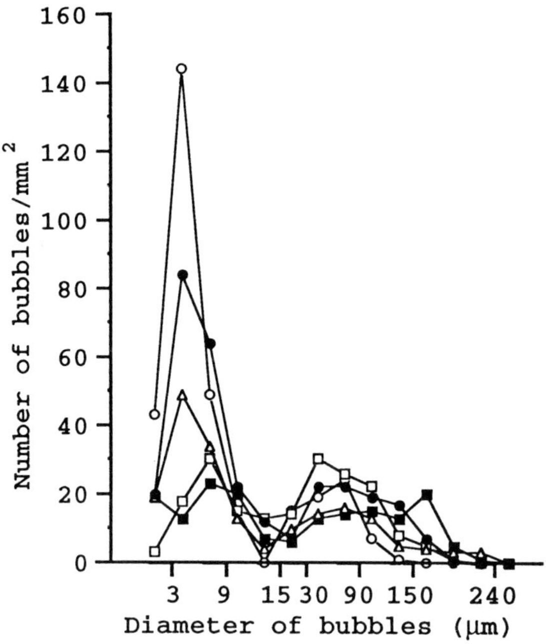

Figure 3 Number of bubbles counted according to bubble diameter in five regions indicated by different symbols. (Courtesy Dr. K. Cho, Morioka, Japan.)

lead us to speculate that the relationship between the dose (phospholipid) and response (SM) might reflect the quality of surfactant activity.

To assess surfactant inhibition, Berggren et al. (9) measured bubble diameters in a suspension of modified porcine surfactant (Curosurf) and in a mixture of this suspension with albumin or fibrinogen, using a computer-aided image analyzer. Since the diameter of bubbles generated in the presence of albumin or fibrinogen was four to five times larger than that of bubbles in the original suspension alone, they concluded that the evaluation of bubble size provided an objective and rapid assessment of surfactant inhibition. This measurement could be used to evaluate the quality of surfactant. However, the samples were vortexed to generate bubbles, producing rather few microbubbles in a 5 mg/ml suspension of Curosurf. The original method (2) to generate bubbles appears to be much more sensitive, since a similar number of microbubbles was formed at surfactant concentrations of only 10–50 μg/ml (Fig. 5).

D. Effect of Contaminants

Blood or meconium in amniotic fluid interferes with the biochemical measurement of surfactant. The effect of blood on the biophysical SM test was reported

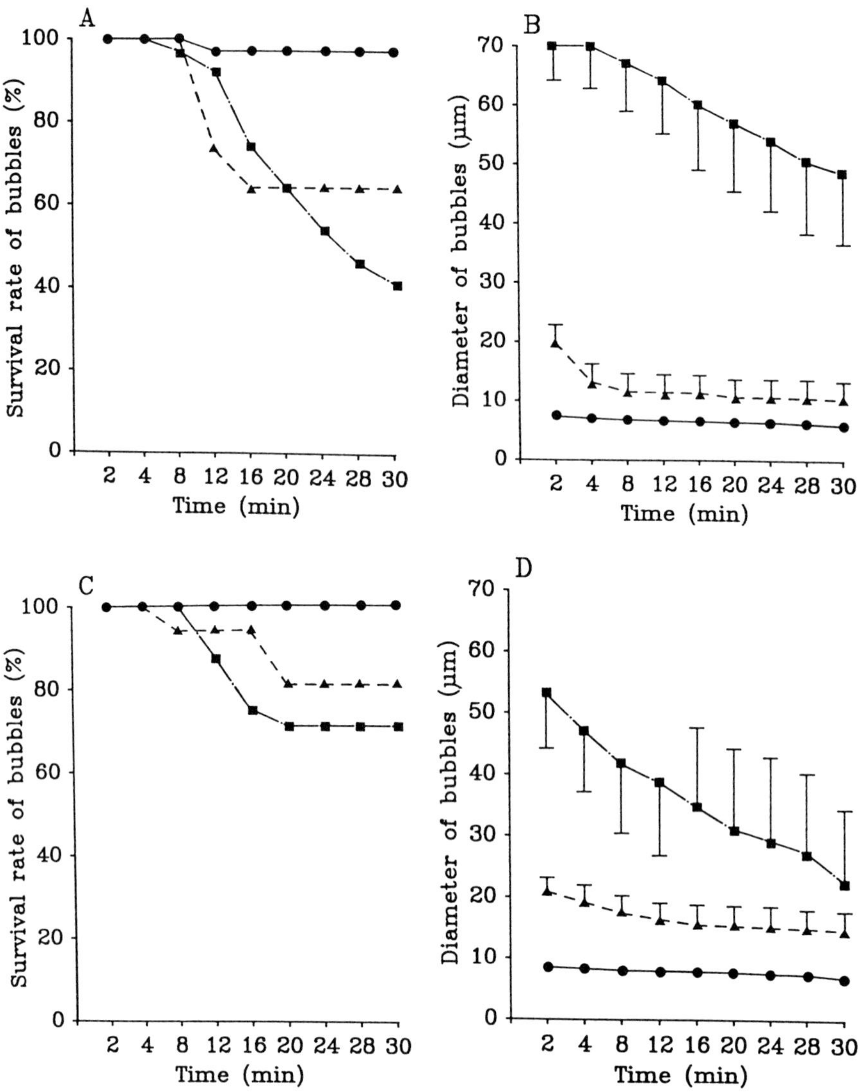

Figure 4 Time-course of number and size of bubbles in amniotic fluid (A, B) and gastric aspirate (C, D). The initial number of bubbles (A and C), and the number of stable bubbles (B, D), given in parenthesis according to bubble diameter as indicated by different symbols were: ● bubbles <15 μm (A, n = 76; B, n = 74; C, n = 62; D, n = 62); ▲ bubbles 15–30 μm (A, n = 22; B, n = 14; C, n = 16; D, n = 13); ■ bubbles 31–100 μm (A, n = 39; B, n = 16; C, n = 24; D, n = 17). Bars indicate 95% confidence intervals. The 95% confidence intervals of bubbles <15 μm in diameter are smaller than the symbol and therefore not shown. (From ref. 6; used with permission)

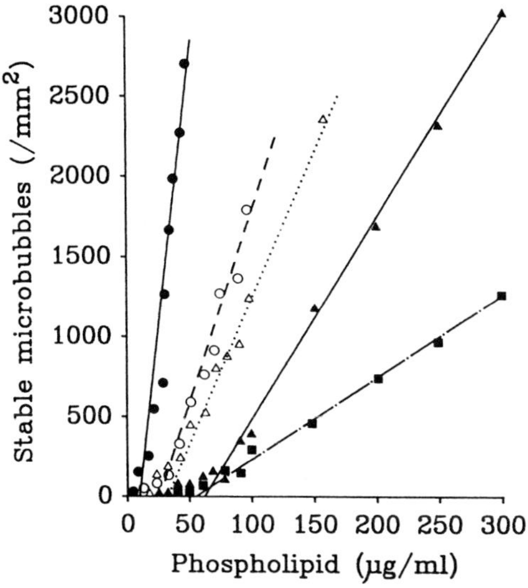

Figure 5 Relationship between the concentration of surfactant phospholipid and the number of SM in different surfactant preparations. ● Surfactant-TA; ○ purified natural surfactant of porcine lung lavage; ▲ crude natural surfactant lipid of porcine lung lavage; ■ phospholipid fraction of minced porcine lung; △ mixture of dipalmitoylphosphatidylcholine and phosphatidylglycerol (7:3) (From ref. 8; used with permission.)

by Pattle et al. (2), who found that 10% citrated blood produced no significant reduction in bubble count. The effect of meconium on SM count has not been evaluated systematically. Pattle et al. (2) examined four samples of meconium that were all rated "strong" (>20 SM/mm^2). Since no consistent results were obtained after some dilution, they concluded that samples stained with meconium were suspect. Although meconium-stained amniotic fluid or gastric aspirate is rare in the preterm delivery of very low birth weight infants, this aspect needs to be further elucidated.

Other possible contaminants have been examined to determine whether they formed SMs. Urine and saliva from neonates and povidone-iodine solution and chlorhexidine gluconate, which are used as antiseptics for pregnant women, produced no SMs (10).

E. Effects of Storage

Thus far, we have performed the SM test immediately after obtaining the samples for clinical evaluation. We have therefore not determined the storage conditions that might affect the test results. Whether frozen samples give the same results as unfrozen ones has not been evaluated. In the original study, Pattle et al. (2)

did not use samples that had been stored frozen for more than 3 months, stored for more than 2 weeks in liquid form at 3°C, or kept for more than 12 hr at room temperature.

F. Precision and Reliability

The results of the SM test may be influenced by other variables entering the methodology. In addition to interanalyst variation, sampling per se might influence the test results, since the pulmonary surfactant present in amniotic fluid, unlike other biochemical constituents in biological fluids, is heterogeneous with respect to density and surface activity (11).

To assess the precision and reliability of the measurement methodology of the SM test, we had three analysts with little experience perform the test. This was done in blind experiments in quadruplicate on nine different amniotic fluid samples (12). On completion of each analysis by the first analyst, the bubbles on the same slide were counted by two observers. One of the observers in turn became the analyst and the remaining two became the observers. Three-way analysis of variance revealed that there were significant differential effects of the analyst, observer, and sampling on the SM values, and also that there were statistically significant interactions between the analyst and observer, as well as between the analyst and sampling. However, the magnitude of these effects was not large enough to modify the interpretation of the test results.

IV. Other Factors Affecting the Test Results

To evaluate the value of the SM test for identifying neonates with surfactant deficiency, we must discuss some other factors that affect the test results.

A. Surfactant Deficiency and RDS

The laboratory diagnosis of surfactant deficiency, or RDS, is usually made by measuring surfactant components in amniotic fluid or in other biological sources. These measurements are greatly affected by many confounding variables, including the methodology of the test, its diagnostic accuracy, the definition of RDS, time of sampling, and quality of perinatal care. In addition, the pathophysiology of RDS is complex, depending on factors other than surfactant deficiency alone. Functional surfactant deficiency might form part of the spectrum of RDS. It could be caused by lower amounts of surfactant, an inactivation of surfactant, or suboptimal function of surfactant (5).

It is therefore not surprising that surfactant deficiency indicated by laboratory tests may not necessarily signify the development of RDS. Nor does surfactant deficiency predict problems related to structural lung immaturity.

B. Diagnosis of RDS

The diagnostic accuracy of the test result depends on the definition of the disease. The clinical features of RDS have changed greatly, particularly in very low birth weight infants, who often require intubation and subsequent mechanical ventilation, and who are treated with exogenous surfactant. The severity of RDS is also modified by the intubation itself, by the mode of ventilation (slow or rapid rate or high-frequency oscillation), and by the type of ventilator. Thus, different management protocols influence the criteria used for the diagnosis of RDS at each institution. Our criteria for the diagnosis of RDS are listed in Table 1. It is possible that a few neonates with very mild RDS might not meet our criteria, since early intubation and respiratory support, even with lower pressure, might modify the severity of RDS and the chest radiographic appearance. However, these neonates would be managed without surfactant treatment, and they could be diagnosed retrospectively from their clinical course.

C. Predictive Value of the Tests

The positive predictive value is defined as the proportion of patients reported positive who have the disease, whereas the negative predictive value is the proportion of patients reported negative who do not have the disease. Formulae are available to calculate the positive and negative predictive values in populations with different prevalences of the disease (13).

In a clinical trial of prophylactic surfactant treatment, we consider that the use of a test with high positive (immature) predictive value is extremely important. Such a test will prevent neonates without RDS from being eligible for the trial.

V. Comparison Between SM Test and Other Predictors of Lung Maturity

We evaluated the clinical value of the SM test in the prediction of RDS by comparisons with other tests on amniotic fluid obtained within 12 hr before

Table 1 Criteria for Diagnosis of RDS

Positive x-ray findings (reticulogranular pattern with air bronchogram)
Ventilatory requirements at 3–6 hr of age after initial stabilization[a]:
1. Oxygen ≥40% and/or
2. Mean airway pressure ≥7 cmH_2O

[a]Our initial settings with pressure preset ventilators for noncompliant lung disease were: rate 30–60 breaths/min, inspiration time 0.5–1.0 sec, pressure 20–30/4 cmH_2O. These settings are based on maintaining Pa_{O_2} between 60 and 80 mmHg and Pa_{CO_2} <50 mmHg.

delivery from 40 pregnancies of 23–35 weeks' gestation (14). These tests included determinations of the L/S ratio, the disaturated phosphatidylcholine/sphingomyelin (DSPC/S) ratio, and levels of lecithin, DSPC, and surfactant-associated proteins A, B and C (SP-A, SP-B, SP-C). Amniotic fluid samples were obtained by anterior amniotomy (n = 9), cesarean section (n = 5), and vaginal collection after rupture of membranes (n = 26). None of the samples were heavily contaminated with blood or meconium. Samples from patients with diabetes or with polyhydramnios or oligohydramnios were excluded. The diagnosis of RDS was made according to the criteria presented in Table 1 and the clinician was unaware of the test results. The cut-off value of each test for predicting RDS was determined at a point of maximum diagnostic accuracy. Fourteen of 40 neonates (35%) were diagnosed as having RDS. The overall diagnostic accuracy of the SM test, defined as percentage of correct results, was similar to that of the other tests (Table 2). However, both the SM test and the SP-B, SP-C concentration showed positive predictive values of 100%. This study showed that the SM test was as reliable as the immunological measurement of SP-B, SP-C in identifying a population of infants that developed RDS if they were born within 12 hr after the amniotic fluid was sampled.

We did not compare the SM test with the other rapid biophysical test, the foam stability test described by Clements et al. (15). The SM test is quite distinct from the foam stability test, where the observed bubbles were reported to be 50–500 μm in diameter (2). Although the foam stability test has proven extremely

Table 2 Comparison of Amniotic Fluid Tests for Predicting RDS

Test	Cut-off value	Sensitivity (%)	Specificity (%)	Positive predictive value (%)	Negative predictive value (%)	Overall accuracy (%)
Lecithin	<2.0 mg/dl	64	85	69	81	78
	<3.0 mg/dl	79	77	65	87	78
DSPC	<0.5 mg/dl	64	96	90	83	85
L/S ratio	<2.0	86	88	80	92	88
DSPC/S ratio	<0.7	71	92	83	86	85
SP-A	<0.35 μg/ml	64	88	75	82	80
	<0.60 μg/ml	79	81	69	88	80
SP-B, SP-C	<0.02 μg/ml	79	100	100	90	93
SM	0/mm^2	50	100	100	79	83
	<5/mm^2	57	96	89	81	83

Source: From ref. 14; used with permission.

valuable for reliably identifying infants with mature lungs (no RDS), it produces a high incidence of false-positive results (i.e., the prediction of RDS in an infant who remains healthy) (16). The high negative (mature) predictive value of the foam stability test suggests that this can be used in combination with the SM test to confirm lung maturity.

VI. Prospective Evaluation of the SM Test

Since amniocentesis is not performed in many neonates, alternative biological fluids, such as oropharyngeal aspirates and gastric aspirates obtained at birth have been used for evaluation of pulmonary surfactant.

We determined, prospectively, if the SM test on gastric aspirate obtained at birth was as useful as that on amniotic fluid in predicting RDS. We studied 105 paired samples of amniotic fluid, obtained at delivery from 105 consecutive women with a gestation of 35 weeks or less, and gastric aspirates from their neonates obtained within 30 min of birth (17). No samples were heavily contaminated with blood or meconium. Amniotic fluid samples were obtained within 24 hr before delivery (median 0 hr, range 0–24 hr) by anterior amniotomy (n = 48), cesarean section (n = 21), amniocentesis (n = 1), and vaginal collection (n = 35). Five neonates were not included for the following reasons; diabetes (n = 1), multiple pregnancies (n = 2), and polyhydramnios (n = 1) and oligohydramnios (n = 1). The diagnosis of RDS was made in accordance with the criteria shown in Table 1. The total of 105 neonates was divided into three groups: RDS (n = 35), other respiratory difficulties (n = 23), and normal (n = 47). Other respiratory difficulties included apnea (n = 6), transient tachypnea (n = 5), asphyxia (n = 6), and pneumonia (n = 6).

Fig. 6 shows scatter diagrams of the SM counts of amniotic fluid and gastric aspirate in relation to the clinical outcome. Table 3 shows the test results for a range of possible cut-off values. An SM test with the predefined cut-off value of less than 5 SM/mm^2 for amniotic fluid and less than 10 SM/mm^2 for gastric aspirate signified a risk of RDS with a positive predictive value of 100 and 96%, respectively, and a negative predictive value of 91 and 84%, respectively. These values indicated that this was an excellent test for identifying neonates with surfactant deficiency immediately before or at birth. This study confirmed the value of the amniotic fluid SM test originally described by Pattle et al. (2) in predicting the development of RDS, and it further showed that gastric aspirate obtained at birth could be used as an alternative biological fluid for this test.

This test has the disadvantage of missing some neonates who develop RDS. The sensitivity of this test in predicting RDS was 80% for amniotic fluid and 63% for gastric aspirate. When both samples were taken into consideration, the sensitivity increased to 89%. Therefore, if the clinician wishes to detect as many neonates as possible at risk of developing RDS in a clinical trial of surfactant

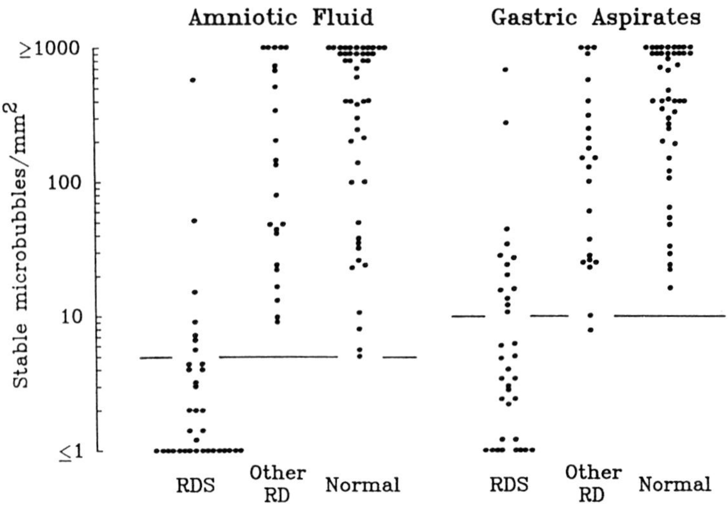

Figure 6 SM counts in amniotic fluid and gastric aspirate in relation to the clinical outcome classified into three groups. Values were plotted on a semilogarithmic scale. The horizontal lines indicate the predefined cut-off values for each source of samples. Other RD, other respiratory difficulties (From ref. 17; used with permission.)

therapy, it is advisable to perform an SM test on both amniotic fluid and gastric aspirate obtained at birth (Table 3).

The SM test on gastric aspirates was used in two controlled trials of rescue surfactant therapy (18,19) and in a controlled trial of prophylactic surfactant therapy (20) in Japan to define a population of neonates with surfactant deficiency. Only neonates whose SM value was $<10/mm^2$ in gastric aspirates obtained at birth were included in these trials. All of the neonates included in rescue trials and all those in the rescue arm of the prophylactic trial developed moderate to severe RDS.

VII. Conclusions

The overall diagnostic accuracy of the SM test on amniotic fluid compares favorably with that of other biochemical or immunological tests; however, the advantage is that this test can supply results within 10 min. In a prospective study, this test was found to be a reliable procedure when performed on either amniotic fluid or gastric aspirate, identifying a group of neonates who will develop RDS. This test can be used by the attending physician in a bedside setting to define a population of neonates with surfactant deficiency in clinical trials of prophylactic surfactant replacement therapy.

Table 3 Test Results in Relation to Sample Source and Different Cut-off Values

Sample source and cut-off value (SM/mm^2)	Sensitivity (%)	Specificity (%)	Positive predictive value (%)	Negative predictive value (%)	Overall accuracy (%)
Amniotic fluid					
0	31	100	100	74	77
2	54	100	100	81	85
4	69	100	100	86	90
5	80	100	100	91	93
6	83	97	94	92	92
8	89	97	94	94	94
10	91	93	86	96	90
20	94	89	80	97	90
50	94	70	61	96	78
Gastric aspirate					
0	9	100	100	69	70
2	29	100	100	74	76
4	49	100	100	80	83
7	63	100	100	84	88
10	63	99	96	84	87
15	71	97	93	87	89
20	77	96	90	89	90
40	91	81	71	95	85
50	94	80	70	97	85
Both samples					
5 or 10	89	99	97	95	95

Acknowledgment

The author wishes to thank Dr. Tetsuro Fujiwara for his valuable suggestions.

References

1. Gluck L, Kulovich MV, Borer RC, et al. Diagnosis of the respiratory distress syndrome by amniocentesis. Am J Obstet Gynecol 1971; 109:440–445.
2. Pattle RE, Kratzing CC, Parkinson CE, et al. Maturity of fetal lungs tested by production of stable microbubbles in amniotic fluid. Br J Obstet Gynaecol 1979; 86:615–622.
3. Pattle RE. Properties, function and origin of the alveolar lining layer. Nature 1955; 175:1125–1126.
4. Hallman M. Antenatal diagnosis of lung maturity. In: Robertson B, van Golde LMG, Batenburg JJ, eds. Pulmonary Surfactant: From Molecular Biology to Clinical Practice. Amsterdam, Elsevier Science, 1992:423–458.

5. Jobe A. Surfactant and the developing lung. In: Thibeault DW, Gregory GA, eds. Neonatal Pulmonary Care. 2nd ed. Norwalk, CT, Appleton-Century-Crofts, 1986: 75–99.
6. Kaneko J, Maeta H. Evaluation of microbubble stability in amniotic fluid and gastric aspirate with computer-aided image analysis. J Iwate Med Assoc 1993; 45:407–414 [in Japanese].
7. Freer DE, Statland BE, Sher G. Rational basis for foam-stability assays of amniotic surfactant. Clin Chem 1978; 24:1980–1984.
8. Sasaki M. Comparison of five pulmonary surfactants: in vitro surface properties and ultrastructures. J Iwate Med Assoc 1990; 42:883–896 [in Japanese].
9. Berggren P, Eklind J, Linderholm B, Robertson B. Bubbles and computer-aided image analysis for evaluation of surfactant inhibition. Biol Neonate 1992; 61(suppl 1):15–20.
10. Takahashi H. Stable microbubble rating in amniotic fluid and gastric aspirate in predicting respiratory distress syndrome. J Iwate Med Assoc 1990; 42:219–225 [in Japanese].
11. Fujiwara T, Higuchi M. Isolation, purification, and quantitation of a surface-active material from human amniotic fluid: Correlation with gestational age and the surfactant titer. Proc Jpn Soc Biol Interface 1973; 4:200–207 [in Japanese].
12. Chida S, Fujiwara T, Takahashi A, Kanehama S, Kaneko J. Precision and reliability of stable microbubble test as a predictor of respiratory distress syndrome. Acta Paediatr Jpn 1991; 33:15–19.
13. Freedman LS. Evaluating and comparing imaging techniques: A review and classification of study designs. Br J Radiol 1987; 60:1071–1081.
14. Chida S, Fujiwara T. Stable microbubble test for predicting the risk of respiratory distress syndrome: I. Comparisons with other predictors of fetal lung maturity in amniotic fluid. Eur J Pediatr 1993; 152:148–151.
15. Clements JA, Platzker ACG, Tierney DE, et al. Assessment of the risk of the respiratory-distress syndrome by a rapid test for surfactant in amniotic fluid. N Engl J Med 1972; 286:1077–1081.
16. Farrell PM, Avery ME. Hyaline membrane disease. Am Rev Respir Dis 1975; 111:657–688.
17. Chida S, Fujiwara T, Konishi M, Takahashi H, Sasaki M. Stable microbubble test for predicting the risk of respiratory distress syndrome: II. Prospective evaluation of the test on amniotic fluid and gastric aspirate. Eur J Pediatr 1993; 152: 152–156.
18. Konishi M, Fujiwara T, Naito T, et al. Surfactant replacement therapy in neonatal respiratory distress syndrome. A multi-center, randomized clinical trial: comparison of high- versus low-dose of Surfactant-TA. Eur J Pediatr 1988; 147:20–25.
19. Fujiwara T, Konishi M, Chida S, et al. Surfactant replacement therapy with a single postventilatory dose of a reconstituted bovine surfactant in preterm neonates with respiratory distress syndrome: Final analysis of a multicenter, double-blind, randomized trial and comparison with similar trials. Pediatrics 1990; 86:753–764.
20. Konishi M, Fujiwara T, Chida S, et al. A prospective, randomized trial of early versus late administration of a single dose of Surfactant-TA. Early Hum Dev 1992; 29:275–282.

7

Lung Mechanics in Respiratory Distress Syndrome

ROBERT B. COTTON
Vanderbilt University Medical Center
Nashville, Tennessee

TORSTEN OLSSON
Chalmers University of Technology
Gothenburg, Sweden

I. Introduction

The term *lung mechanics* refers to the analysis of the mechanical response by the lung to a force which is usually applied as a pressure gradient between the airway opening and pleural surface. When a pressure differential is applied between the airway opening and pleural surface, part of the pressure is used to overcome elastic recoil in order to increase lung volume and part is dissipated in the process of overcoming resistance offered by the lung to the movement of air. When lung mechanics are analyzed, the elastic recoil of the lung is quantitatively expressed as lung compliance (C_L) and the resistance to flow ($\dot{V}$) is quantitatively expressed as lung resistance (R_L). In order to understand the implications of a given measurement of C_L or R_L reported for a premature infant with respiratory distress syndrome (RDS), it is important to know the physiological and physical basis of these properties and how they are affected by the conditions under which they are measured.

The mechanical properties of the respiratory system in premature infants with RDS are highly abnormal. In addition to the direct biophysical consequences of surfactant deficiency, major disturbances in the mechanical behavior of the respiratory system also occur as a result of factors such as the injury to the lung accompanying surfactant deficiency and pulmonary edema due to left-to-right shunting through a patent ductus arteriosus. In this chapter, we will consider (1) the physiological basis of the mechanical indices compliance and resistance, (2) how these indices are assessed and why the results may be affected by the measurement method, (3) the results of these measurements in RDS, and (4) the pathophysiological basis for the disturbances observed in the mechanical properties of the respiratory system in RDS.

II. Physiological Background

A. Elastic Recoil

General Considerations

The elastic recoil of the lung over its entire range of volume is described by a plot of volume (V) as a function of pressure (P) measured under static conditions at various points during inflation and deflation (Fig. 1). When normalized for

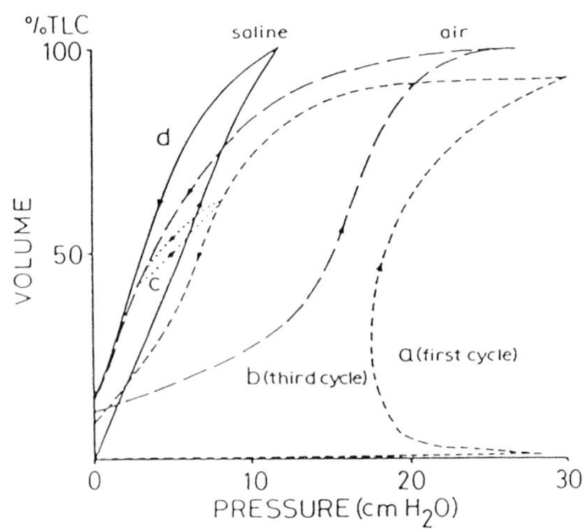

Figure 1 Four inflation-deflation maneuvers in excised rabbit lung generating characteristic volume-pressure loops. a, Inflation from degassed state shows transpulmonary pressures in excess of 20 cmH_2O required before there is substantial opening. On deflation to 0 cmH_2O, emptying is incomplete, with substantial air trapped in lung. b, Repeated cycles between 0 and 30 cmH_2O show stable loops. Lung is now much more easily opened than in a, but still becomes relatively stiff near 30 cmH_2O. c, Small volume cycles (such as in tidal breaths in vivo) run between ~3 and 8 cmH_2O. d, With air removed and saline introduced, lung shows much less recoil over same volume range. (From Ref. 1; used with permission.)

total lung capacity (TLC), composition of the filling medium, prior volume history, and temperature, the PV relationships of the normal lung are almost precisely reproducible (1). Compliance is an index of the elastic recoil of the lung which in the static case is expressed as the tangent slope, $\Delta V/\Delta P$, at one point on the complete PV curve (which is not a straight line), or as the chord slope from a given point on the PV curve to the origin at $P = 0$ and $V = 0$. By either calculation, C_L is a limited index of the elastic recoil of the lung which characterizes only one point or interval on a curve which itself is influenced by numerous factors.

Since C_L describes the elastic recoil over only a limited segment of the entire PV curve, the location of this segment relative to the entire PV curve must be specified or controlled. A change in measured C_L can appear to occur when the overall lung PV characteristics are unchanged if C_L is not measured over the same volume interval. In the normal lung, C_L can be standardized for TLC by expressing it as specific compliance ($sC_L = C_L/FRC$ or C_L/TLC). When FRC or TLC is unknown, or in abnormal lungs such as in RDS, it may be more appropriate to normalize C_L to body weight when one is comparing elastic recoil across patients with different body sizes. Because of the major effect of volume history on elastic recoil illustrated in Fig. 1, this factor also must be standardized in order to compare C_L from measurement to measurement.

Elastic recoil pressure can be regarded as the sum of the forces which occur at the interface between alveolar gas and alveolar lining liquid and the forces resulting from lung tissue elastic properties. The recoil pressure due to tissue elastic properties can be demonstrated by a PV curve obtained from a lung which is saline filled, and therefore has no gas-liquid interfaces (Fig. 1). The degree to which the PV curve of a gas-filled lung is shifted and tilted to the right compared with the saline-filled lung indicates the added elastic recoil pressure attributed to surface forces at gas-liquid interfaces. Note that the gas-liquid interface generates a major part of the overall recoil force.

Surface Elastic Properties

As seen in Fig. 1, there is minimal added elastic recoil in the normal lung due to surface forces at low lung volume, reflecting the effective surface tension lowering property of surfactant as alveolar volume decreases. A greater elastic recoil in the gas-filled lungs compared with the saline-filled lungs in Fig. 1 is observed at high lung volume where surfactant has the least surface tension–lowering effect. In the absence of surfactant, surface tension on the walls of terminal air spaces would be constant and similar in magnitude to the high values seen near TLC. This condition, which might be regarded in some ways as analogous mechanically to RDS, can be produced by replacing surfactant with a surface layer of material which exhibits a constant surface tension. The effect of this manipulation on lung elastic recoil pressure can be seen in Fig. 2, in which gas deflation PV characteristics of lungs previously rinsed with one of two detergents are compared with that of a normal lung and a saline-filled lung. In regard to the limitations described above when compliance measurements are used to assess elastic recoil pressure, note that the increased elastic recoil pressure of the Tween 80 lung would not have been detected by a tangent slope measurement of C_L at mid lung volume. Only below 5 cmH_2O does the increased elastic recoil of the Tween 80 lung appear to be detectable by a tangent slope measurement of C_L.

Tissue Elastic Properties

The airways and vasculature, pleural and interlobular septa, and alveolar septa are the structures which contribute to the tissue elastic recoil of the lung (1). Because the lung parenchyma is so dominated by the network of alveolar septa, it is assumed that fibrous structural elements at the alveolar level are the principal source of tissue elastic recoil in the fully developed lung. Since alveolarization is incomplete in the lung of a premature infant, the principal site of tissue elastic recoil in infants with RDS is assumed to be at the level of the respiratory bronchioles and the alveolar ducts. The structural elements thought to determine tissue elastic properties are elastin and collagen (1). Collagen has great tensile strength but low compliance. In contrast, elastin fibers have lower tensile strength

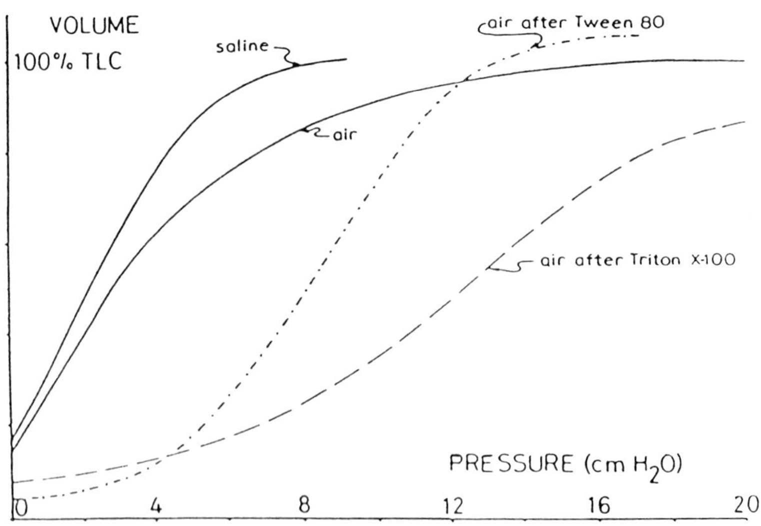

Figure 2 Deflation volume-pressure characteristics of lungs filled with different substances. (From Ref. 1; used with permission.)

but a higher compliance than collagen fibers. It is thought that the elastin network dominates lung tissue elastic recoil at low and middle volume ranges, and that collagen dominates at high lung volume (1).

B. Flow Resistance

Lung airflow resistance, R_L, is the sum of airway resistance, R_{aw}, and lung tissue resistance. R_{aw} is directly proportional to length and inversely proportional to the square of the cross-sectional area of the airways. Like compliance, resistance is also a function of lung volume in normal subjects (2). The reciprocal of R_{aw}, airway conductance (G_{aw}), is directly proportional to lung volume as measured by thoracic gas volume in infants and adults, although the slope of the relationship changes with age (3). Specific airway conductance ($sG_{aw} = G_{aw}/TGV$ or G_{aw}/FRC) decreases with postconceptual age between 30 and 40 weeks, implying that the rate of growth of terminal air spaces is greater than the rate of growth of conducting airways during this period (3).

Airway resistance is measured as the pressure drop between the terminal air spaces and the airway opening divided by flow. At the relatively low flows in peripheral airways, flow is laminar and the pressure drop across the airways is a linear function of flow. In the treachea and glottis where flow is greatest, it may become turbulent, so that greater pressure gradients are required for a given flow than if the flow was laminar. In contrast to adults, a substantial portion of R_{aw} in infants is contributed by the most peripheral airways, which may contribute nearly as much as the larger airways (4). Lung tissue resistance in infants is reported to contribute almost 40% of total R_L, which is considerably greater than the 18% estimated for adults (5,6).

III. Measurement of Compliance and Resistance

A. Quantitative Relationships

During breathing, a quantitative relationship between the applied pressure and the resulting volume and flow can be described by the following equation:

$$P = \left(\frac{1}{C}\right)V + R\dot{V}$$

In this equation, which is a shortened form of the equation of motion, P is the applied pressure, V is volume, $\dot{V}$ is flow, and C and R are the properties compliance and resistance, respectively (2).

When this equation is used to estimate C and R, the anatomical structures included in the analysis are determined by where P is measured. When P is measured between the airway opening and the pleural surface, C and R represent lung compliance (C_L) and lung resistance (R_L), and reflect the respective properties of the lungs. When P is measured at the airway opening during positive-pressure mechanical ventilation, C and R reflect the respective properties of the total respiratory system, and as such are designated C_{rs} and R_{rs}. Chest wall compliance (C_W) is five times greater than C_L in premature infants (7,8). Since $(1/C_{rs}) = (1/C_L) + (1/C_W)$, C_{rs} is almost the same as C_L when $C_W >> C_L$, justifying the use of C_{rs} as a surrogate for C_L in premature infants.

Resistance in the equation includes both resistance to gas flow through airways and resistance offered by tissue movement. In normal lungs, tissue resistance is small compared with airflow resistance, and R_L is reported to be 74% of R_{rs} in infants (9). For these reasons, R_{rs} is regarded as an acceptable estimate of both R_L and of airflow resistance.

B. Effects of Respiratory Muscle Activity on Measurements

The chest wall is both friend and foe of those who want to measure C and R in premature infants. As pointed out above, a highly compliant chest wall makes it possible to use C_{rs} as an estimate of C_L in premature infants, thereby avoiding the need to rely on esophageal pressure changes to reflect pleural pressure changes. On the other hand, a highly compliant chest wall is also susceptible to distortion during spontaneous breathing. With chest wall distortion, regional differences in pleural surface pressure may invalidate the assumption that changes in esophageal pressure, measured either with an esophageal balloon or a liquid-filled catheter, are representative of mean changes in pleural surface pressure (10,11).

Uncertainty about the validity of the esophageal pressure signal during spontaneous breathing is not the only problem faced when attempting to assess the mechanical properties of the lung in the presence of respiratory muscle activity. Chest wall distortion may also lead to an inhomogeneity in peripheral airway resistance, causing an underestimation of C when measured during uninterrupted spontaneous breathing (12). Although the complications caused by chest wall distortion are mostly limited to inspiration, muscle activity present during expiration can cause an overestimation of both C_{rs} and R_{rs}. Postinspiratory activity of the inspiratory muscles can oppose lung recoil, causing C_{rs} to be overestimated. Laryngeal adduction during expiration will increase measured airway resistance (13).

Unless one is specifically studying the mechanical properties of the respiratory system as influenced by muscle activity, it is highly desirable, and in many applications mandatory, to carry out measurements of C and R under passive conditions. Passive conditions can be achieved several ways. Not only can muscle paralysis be used to eliminate activity during mechanical ventilation, but active respiratory efforts can also be suppressed by increasing mechanical ventilation to overcome the ventilatory drive of CO_2 and other stimuli (13).

During either mechanical ventilation or spontaneous breathing, relaxation of the inspiratory muscles can be achieved by activating the Hering-Breuer inflation reflex with an occlusion of the airway during expiration while the volume of the lung is greater than its relaxation volume (14). The relaxation produced by this maneuver during a brief occlusion will persist sufficiently long following release of the occlusion to allow measurement of the expiratory time constant of the respiratory system during passive conditions (see below). Since most interest in assessing lung mechanical properties in the RDS will involve infants who are intubated and receiving mechanical ventilation, it should be possible to achieve passive conditions by one of these tactics.

C. Dynamic Versus Static Conditions

Compliance and resistance may be evaluated in premature infants with RDS under either dynamic or quasi-static conditions. When the evaluation is carried out during uninterrupted breathing, either spontaneous or during mechanical ventilation, the results are qualified as being "dynamic"; e.g., dynamic compliance (Cdyn). Except for special circumstances such as during extracorporeal membrane oxygenation (ECMO), it is not possible to carry out these measurements in newborn infants under truly static conditions. However, static conditions can be approached by occluding the airway briefly so that a pressure plateau is observed at the airway opening while $\dot{V} = 0$. Under such quasi-static conditions, the results are qualified as being "static"; e.g., static compliance of the respiratory system ($C_{rs}st$).

In newborns, Cdyn underestimates Cst, and the ratio of Cdyn/Cst decreases with increasing frequency of ventilation (12,15,16). Two mechanisms are involved in the frequency dependence of Cdyn (12). Owing to lung viscoelasticity, there is a decay in transpulmonary pressure following inflation to a constant volume. Since lung viscoelasticity is greater in newborns than in adults (17,18), this effect will cause a greater underestimation of Cst by Cdyn in newborns than in adults, in whom Cdyn is almost the same as Cst (13). In addition to lung viscoelasticity, lung mechanics are also affected by inhomogeneity of ventilation such that measured Cdyn and R_L both decrease with increasing frequency even though there is no change in the physical properties of the lung (19). Ventilatory inhomogeneity occurs in otherwise normal newborn infants (20) and in premature infants with RDS (21,22).

Measurements During Uninterrupted Breathing

Dynamic compliance and resistance measurements are based on the equation given above. Two methods are commonly used to evaluate the coefficients C and R from P, V, and $\dot{V}$. In the 2-point method, compliance is derived by dividing tidal volume by the difference between P measured at end inspiration when $\dot{V}$

$= 0$ and P measured at end expiration when $\dot{V} = 0$. Resistance is evaluated at 2 time points in the ventilatory cycle when lung volumes are equal, one in inspiration and the other in expiration. By assuming that the elastic recoil at a given volume during inspiration is equal to the elastic recoil at the same volume during expiration, resistance can be determined by dividing the difference in P by the difference in $\dot{V}$ between these 2 points. A second method uses multivariate linear regression analysis to estimate C and R in the equation given above in which P is regarded as a dependent variable and V and $\dot{V}$ are regarded as independent variables (23–25). All data points in a single breath are used for this analysis. This method is often referred to as the least mean squares error method, because the regression process selects the C and R combination which results in the smallest value of the sum of $(Pm - Pp)^2$ evaluated at each point in the breath, where Pm is the measured P and Pp is the P predicted by C and R. Theoretically, these two methods will give similar results. But since all data points during the breath are used by the regression analysis, this method has the advantage of being less sensitive to data noise than the 2-point method (25).

Measurements Based on Flow Interruption

There are two methods based on flow interruption which have been established and validated for use in premature infants with RDS. The multiple occlusion method (15,26,27) involves an occlusion at different volumes during expiration in multiple breaths and provides a measurement of $C_{rs}st$. The other method, the passive expiratory flow-volume technique (14,26,28), involves the occlusion of a single breath at end inspiration and provides measurements of $C_{rs}st$, R_{rs}, and time constant of the respiratory system (τ_{rs}). Although the two methods are similar in that they rely on flow interruption by airway occlusion to provide quasi-static and passive conditions, they are conceptually different.

With the multiple occlusion method, the volume above end-expiratory volume and pressure are measured at each occlusion over as wide a range as possible within tidal volume. Each occlusion must last at least 50 msec to achieve respiratory muscle relaxation from the Hering-Breuer reflex. Static compliance is equal to the slope ($\Delta V/\Delta P$) of the volume versus pressure plot and can be estimated using linear regression analysis. Either $C_{rs}st$ or $C_{L}st$ can be measured depending on whether Pao is measured in reference to ambient or esophageal pressure (13). This method can be applied either during spontaneous breathing without an endotracheal tube or during positive pressure mechanical ventilation with an endotracheal tube in place.

The passive expiratory flow-volume technique is based on estimating the time constant of the respiratory system, τ_{rs}, from the slope of the linear portion of the volume versus flow plot following occlusion of a single breath at end inspiration, during which $\Delta V/\Delta\dot{V} = \tau_{rs} = R \times C$. Compliance is derived as C_{rs}

$= V_E/Pao$, where V_E is the volume intercepted at $\dot{V} = 0$ by extrapolation of the linear portion of the V versus $\dot{V}$ plot, and Pao is the pressure at the airway opening. Resistance is derived as $R_{rs} = \tau_{rs}/C_{rs}$ or as $R_{rs} = Pao/\dot{V}_0$, where $\dot{V}_0$ is the flow intercepted at $V = 0$ by extrapolation of the linear portion of the V versus $\dot{V}$ plot. Both C_L or C_{rs} and R_L or R_{rs} can be measured with this method depending on which pressures are measured (14,28). As with the multiple occlusion method, infants can be assessed with this method during either spontaneous breathing or mechanical ventilation. However, the passive expiratory flow-volume technique is unsatisfactory for unintubated infants in the immediate neonatal period, since these infants may exhibit marked laryngeal braking of expiratory airflow (28).

IV. Results of Compliance and Resistance Measurements in RDS

A. Results in Newborn Infants Without Lung Disease

$C_L$dyn in normal newborn infants and otherwise healthy premature infants during spontaneous breathing is approximately 1 to 2 ml · cmH_2O^{-1} · kg^{-1} (29–32). Specific $C_L$dyn during spontaneous breathing has been reported to be 0.044 ± 0.016 ml/cmH_2O per milliliter FRC in newborn infants without lung disease who weighed between 980 and 3840 g (31), 0.058 ± 0.004 ml/cmH_2O per milliliter FRC following recovery after tachypnea of unknown cause (33), and 0.047 ± 0.013 ml/cmH_2O per milliliter FRC in healthy premature infants up to 30 weeks' postnatal age (15). Passive C_{rs} measured by the multiple occlusion technique has been reported as 1.12 ± 0.30 (34) and 1.00 ± 0.22 ml · cmH_2O^{-1} · kg^{-1} in normal newborn infants, and as 1.11 ± 0.32 ml · cmH_2O^{-1} · kg^{-1} (35) in newborn preterm infants without lung disease who weighed between 1375 and 2980 g at birth. Passive s$C_L$dyn in healthy preterm infants has been reported to be 0.06 ml/cmH_2O per milliliter FRC (15).

R_L measured in spontaneously breathing newborn infants without lung disease has been reported as 29 ± 11 cmH_2O · ml^{-1} · s (29) and as 42 ± 16 cmH_2O · ml^{-1} · s (32).

B. Results in Newborn Infants with RDS

Studies in Era Prior to Routine Use of Mechanical Ventilation

Compared with newborn infants without lung disease, lung compliance is decreased in infants with RDS when measured as $C_L$dyn, C_{rs}dyn or when measured by the multiple occlusion technique or by single breath occlusion as quasi-static passive C_{rs}. Among the earliest quantitative assessments of reduced lung compliance in RDS was the work of Karlberg et al. (36), who observed that spontaneous ventilation in these infants required esophageal pressure changes that were two to five times the pressure changes required by normal infants. Cooke et al. (29) measured $C_L$dyn values of 0.43 and 0.22 ml · cmH_2O^{-1} · kg^{-1} during spontaneous breathing in two infants with RDS. Since then numerous studies of lung compliance in RDS have been conducted in which the average values of $C_L$dyn reported have ranged from 0.35 to 0.54 ml · cmH_2O^{-1} · kg^{-1} (31,32,37–39).

Measurements of lung resistance were made by Hjalmarson (32) in spontaneously breathing premature infants with RDS using a face-out whole body plethysmograph to measure airway flow. Average R_L for 18 infants during RDS was 69 cmH_2O · ml^{-1} · s (range, 27–200). Average R_L for 16 infants after recovery from RDS was 54 cmH_2O · ml^{-1} · s (range, 30–113).

Studies in Infants Receiving Mechanical Ventilation

In the past 10 years, interest in the effect of surfactant treatment on the mechanical properties of the lung and the availability of rapid data acquisition and analysis using computer-based pulmonary function systems have led to many reports of studies of lung compliance in RDS. Even though the patients studied over the past decade have been smaller and more immature than those from the early era, and even though the methods and study conditions are quite different, the results of compliance measurements from the more recent studies have been similar to those obtained in the early era. In these more recent studies, average reported compliance values have ranged from 0.26 to 0.53 ml · cmH_2O^{-1} · kg^{-1}.

Measurements of dynamic compliance made early in the course of RDS prior to surfactant treatment have been reported by Davis et al. (40), Couser et al. (41), Bhat et al. (42), Edberg et al. (43), Goldsmith et al. (44), Bhutani et al. (45), and Cotton et al. (46). The lowest reported compliance, 0.26 ± 0.06 ml · cmH_2O^{-1} · kg^{-1}, was measured in infants who had been paralyzed with pancuronium bromide (46). The unusually low compliance in these infants may have been the result of an exceptionally low FRC, which was documented to have decreased following paralysis (47). None of the other reports of dynamic compliance involved the use of muscle relaxants. The highest value reported, 0.53 ± 0.06 ml · cmH_2O^{-1} · kg^{-1}, was obtained from measurements made during spontaneous breaths (39). $C_L$dyn measured from ventilator breaths in the same patients was significantly lower: 0.38 ± 0.05 ml · cmH_2O^{-1} · kg^{-1}. These investigators suggested that under the conditions of mechanical ventilation, the patients were operating on the "flattened" upper portion of the pressure-volume curve, causing $C_L$dyn measured during mechanical breaths to be lower than when measured during spontaneous breaths.

Measurements of compliance under quasi-static conditions early in the course of RDS prior to surfactant treatment have been reported as 0.53 ml · cmH_2O^{-1} · kg^{-1} using a multiple occlusion technique (48) and as 0.28 to 0.41

$ml \cdot cmH_2O^{-1} \cdot kg^{-1}$ using the single breath occlusion technique (16,49–51). In one study (16), measurements of $C_{rs}dyn$ also were made on the same patients and found to be significantly lower than $C_{rs}st$ (0.29 ± 0.02 versus 0.41 ± 0.02). Part of the difference between $C_{rs}st$ and $C_{rs}dyn$ observed in this study may have been due to the frequency dependence of Cdyn discussed above. In addition, the measurement of $C_{rs}dyn$ was based on a sample of the pressure volume curve that was constrained to the pressure range imposed by the ventilator. The measurement of $C_{rs}st$ by the single breath occlusion technique was based on a sample of the pressure volume curve that was obtained during expiration from peak to ambient pressure. In infants with RDS, passive deflation compliance decreases as airway pressure increases above 6 cmH_2O (52). During mechanical ventilation with positive end-expiratory pressure (PEEP), the measurement of $C_{rs}dyn$ may fail to incorporate the more compliant lower volume region of the PV curve between a typical PEEP of 4–6 cmH_2O and ambient pressure. This zone is included in the measurement of $C_{rs}st$ by the single breath occlusion technique.

Most reports of specific compliance in RDS show that this index is decreased (0.018–0.022 cmH_2O^{-1}) when compared with values of 0.04–0.06 cmH_2O^{-1} obtained from newborn infants without lung disease (32,37,39,43). Except for the study by Edberg et al. (43), these reports were based infants who were studied in the era prior to the routine use of mechanical ventilation. High values for specific compliance, 0.077 ± 0.029 and 0.078 ± 0.045 cmH_2O, were found in two studies (44,46) involving infants receiving mechanical ventilation. A low specific compliance implies an increased elastic recoil per ventilated alveolus, i.e., that there is a decrease in compliance which is not accounted for by a decrease in the number of ventilated alveoli. High values of specific compliance might be measured in RDS if unstable alveoli are being recruited and derecruited with each tidal volume. In this hypothetical case, a compliance measurement would include a larger number of alveoli than would be reflected by the measured FRC.

Serial measurements in RDS show that abnormally low lung compliance increases to near normal values with time (37,38) and a correlation with gas exchange as assessed by the ratio of arterial to alveolar oxygen tension (50). In another longitudinal study of infants with RDS, a doubling of C_Ldyn between 2 and 7 days, and further increases by 14 and 28 days was observed, by which time C_Ldyn for the group had reached a low normal value of 1.03 ± 0.14 $ml \cdot cmH_2O^{-1} \cdot kg^{-1}$ (45).

Resistance in RDS measured during mechanical ventilation is three to six times greater than in normal newborn infants during spontaneous breathing. Average results of R_L measurements range from 90 to 160 $cmH_2O \cdot ml^{-1} \cdot s$ (41,42,44,45,54). Average results of R_{rs} measured during ventilator breaths range from 95 to 182 $cmH_2O \cdot ml^{-1} \cdot s$ (43,46), with the higher values obtained from infants who were paralyzed (46). Resistance has been shown to increase following muscle paralysis (55). Average results of R_{rs} measured by the single breath occlusion technique range from 100 to 180 $cmH_2O \cdot ml^{-1} \cdot s$ (49–51).

C. Effect of Distending Airway Pressure

When distending airway pressure is applied to infants with RDS during expiration, there is a prompt improvement in arterial oxygen tension. In the original study of the beneficial effect of continuous positive airway pressure (CPAP) in RDS (55), no significant change in lung compliance was detected. This observation led the investigators to argue that the improvement in oxygenation with CPAP resulted from the inflation of atelectatic areas, since increased inflation of only the terminal airways that were already being ventilated before CPAP would have caused dynamic compliance to decrease. In subsequent studies, however, dynamic compliance was observed to decrease following the application of distending airway pressure. A decrease in Cdyn was detected when the distending pressure was applied as either continuous positive pressure (57), continuous negative pressure (58), or as positive end-expiratory pressure (59,60). However, a decrease in Cdyn when distending airway pressure is applied in RDS does not necessarily mean that atelectatic areas have not been inflated. Any potential increase in Cdyn due to recruitment of atelectatic areas could be offset by forcing the tidal volume excursions to take place at a higher, less compliant volume on the PV curve. The studies cited above often involved the use of distending airway pressures greater than 6 cmH_2O, a level above which passive deflation compliance decreases as airway pressure increases (52). For example, the study by Phillips et al. (60) demonstrated a progressive decrease in Cdyn as positive end-expiratory pressure was increased from 0 to 10 cmH_2O. It is also possible that a potential increase in Cdyn due to recruitment of atelectatic areas could have been offset by the stabilization of a population of alveoli above their critical closing pressures so that they would not collapse with each expiration (see below).

D. Effect of Pulmonary Edema

The low lung compliance characteristic of RDS may be further influenced by lung water status. Lung compliance is low in association with pulmonary edema (61) and lung water content is increased in RDS (62). Infants with RDS have a spontaneous diuresis near the time in the natural course of the disease when gas exchange rapidly improves and when breathing becomes less labored. The improvement in lung function implied clinically at this time is confirmed by an increase in FRC and $C_L$dyn (63). Early diuretic therapy with furosemide in premature infants with RDS will enhance the spontaneous diuresis, resulting in a further decrease in ventilatory support (64,65). In a study of the effect of furosemide on lung compliance in premature infants 1 week of age recovering from RDS, $C_L$dyn increased 2 hrs after each of four daily doses of furosemide (66). This effect was transient in that $C_L$dyn returned to baseline by 6 hrs following each dose, and no sustained improvement in $C_L$dyn was observed over the study period, although there was a significant improvement in oxygenation when compared with a control group. No diuresis occurred following furosemide, leading the investigators to conclude that the beneficial effect of furosemide on lung compliance and oxygenation resulted from an effect on lymph flow or on pulmonary and systemic vascular capacitance.

Symptomatic patent ductus arteriosus (PDA) is a common complication of recovery from RDS which is characterized clinically by progressive respiratory failure and pulmonary edema in association with left-to-right shunting through the PDA. Following improvement after resolution of the acute phase of RDS, C_{rs}st has been shown to decrease significantly by 40% in association with the appearance of a clinically detectable PDA and increase 66% 24–48 hrs after successful treatment with indomethacin to close the ductus (67). Other studies have also demonstrated an increase in $C_L$dyn in patients with symptomatic PDA following closure of the ductus either by ligation (68) or by indomethacin treatment (69). These clinical findings of decreased lung compliance in association with a PDA could not be reproduced in an experimental model of PDA in premature lambs (70,71). No difference in C_{rs}dyn or FRC was detected over 12 hrs between animals maintained with ductus patency and animals maintained with the ductus closed. Nor were there acute effects of ductus patency on C_{rs}dyn or FRC detected 40 mins after opening or closing the ductus. In these studies, C_{rs}dyn and FRC decreased during ductus patency only when challenged with a rapid saline infusion (50 ml $\cdot$ kg^{-1} over 3 min). Since extravascular lung water or blood volume was not measured in these studies, the results of these experiments could only be interpreted in regard to the functional consequences of ductus patency.

E. Predictive Value of Lung Mechanics of Outcome in RDS

Lung compliance and resistance measured in the first week after birth in infants with RDS have been shown to be predictive of outcome; that is, of both survival and subsequent development of bronchopulmonary dysplasia (BPD). Dynamic compliance has been shown to be predictive of either death (72) or BPD (72,73) as separate outcome variables. Using stepwise logistic regression modeling, C_{rs}dyn, measured on the first day after birth, and either birth weight or gestational age were shown by Freezer and Sly (74) to be significant independent predictors of BPD in patients with RDS, birth weight $\leq$ 1500 g, who could be classified with or without BPD at 28 days' postnatal age. By using logistic discriminant analysis, Bhutani and Abbasi (75) demonstrated that dynamic compliance measured 4–7 days after birth, when included in a statistical model with birth weight and gestational age, was a significant independent predictor of BPD among a group of RDS survivors. However, when C_{rs}st and conductance of the respiratory system (G_{rs}) measured by single breath airway occlusion 6–48 hrs after birth were included in a stepwise linear regression analysis with birth weight and a ventilatory index (product of mean airway pressure and FIO_2), neither C_{rs}st nor G_{rs} was a statistically significant predictor of death or oxygen dependence at 28 days' postnatal age (76). It would appear that the common denominator of risk in all these studies is severity of the initial lung disease. Whether the antecedent of BPD is the initial lung injury, or the secondary lung injury resulting from barotrauma and oxygen toxicity, or both, cannot be determined from these results.

Lung resistance, but not $C_L$dyn, measured by the 2-point method during mechanical ventilation within 7 days after birth has also been shown to be significantly associated with the later development of BPD in infants with severe RDS (54). In addition, R_{rs} has been significantly linked to the magnitude of improvement in oxygenation following treatment of RDS with synthetic surfactant (77). These investigators demonstrated a significant inverse correlation between pretreatment R_{rs} and improvement in the arterial/alveolar oxygen tension ratio at 24 and 48 hr after treatment. Pretreatment C_{rs} was not correlated with improvement in oxygenation following treatment.

V. Pathophysiology of Changes in Lung Mechanics in RDS

In this section, we will attempt to relate the changes in lung compliance and resistance seen in RDS to the pathophysiology of the disorder. First, mechanisms which explain why compliance is reduced in RDS will be discussed.

The decrease in lung compliance in RDS can be considered as the consequence of two factors: (1) a decrease in the number* of ventilated terminal airspaces, i.e., derecruitment; and (2) an increase in the recoil pressure of ventilated terminal air spaces. These two factors are closely interrelated, since the reduced number of ventilated air spaces is at least in part a result of increased recoil pressure. For purposes of discussion, however, it is helpful to consider these factors separately. In addition, dynamic, but not static, compliance is further reduced in RDS owing to viscoelastic properties of lung tissue and the presence of inhomogeneity in ventilation.

---

*There is no direct confirmation that the number of ventilated terminal air spaces is reduced in vivo in RDS. However, this concept, which is inferred from histopathological findings, is useful as a model.

A. Derecruitment

A decrease in number of ventilated alveoli will result in a decrease in compliance, even if the elastic recoil per ventilated alveolus is normal. In this case, specific compliance would be normal. As already mentioned, in RDS we consider the number of terminal air spaces to be reduced (compared with comparable premature infants without RDS) and also the elastic recoil per ventilated terminal air space to be increased. In this section, events leading to the reduction in number of air spaces is discussed. In the next section, factors underlying increased recoil of ventilated air spaces are discussed.

Decreased lung volume is a hallmark of RDS (78–81). Functional residual capacity (FRC) in newborn infants without lung disease is approximately 30 ml/kg. In RDS, reported measurements of FRC have ranged from 4 to 20 ml/kg (43,44,46,82). Since lung compliance is a function of lung volume, decreased compliance in RDS can be explained in part by the loss of FRC which is characteristic of this disorder. Loss of FRC, or derecruitment, can be considered to occur as a result of the collapse of unstable terminal air spaces or as a result of alveolar flooding and tissue injury. How much of the loss of FRC is due to essentially liquid-free collapsed air spaces and how much is due to alveolar flooding by proteinaceous liquid is debated (83).

Collapse Due to Instability

Based on classic theory, surfactant-deficient alveoli will collapse during deflation because of instability (84). However, the lung in premature infants differs considerably from the model on which this theory is based in that the alveoli are far from fully developed, either in structure or in number. In addition, alveolar ducts are not rigid tubes leading to distensible spheres. Furthermore, the classic model does not include the influence of mechanical interdependence between the alveolus and adjacent structures. Questions about the role of alveolar collapse as the predominant cause of reduced lung gas volume in RDS have been raised by a recent morphometric study demonstrating that liquid-filled alveoli and alveolar ducts, rather than collapsed air spaces, are the most predominant histological finding in premature monkeys with surfactant-deficient lungs (83). In any case, whether the reduced lung volume in RDS is due to collapsed terminal air sacs, to liquid-filled terminal air sacs, or to terminal air sacs operating at a reduced volume remains subject to investigation. In the meantime, the concept that reduced lung volume in RDS is in part accounted for by the collapse of unstable terminal airways continues to be consistent with many of the experimental and clinical observations of pulmonary function in this disorder.

The term *alveolar instability* refers to the tendency for an alveolus to switch abruptly between the inflated state and the collapsed state (85). Inflation of an unstable alveolus occurs suddenly when transalveolar pressure exceeds the critical opening pressure. During deflation, an unstable alveolus collapses abruptly when transalveolar pressure falls below the critical closing pressure (which is lower than the opening pressure). If capillary perfusion of unstable alveoli continues while they are collapsed, the resulting venous admixture will contribute to the overall intrapulmonary shunt and arterial hypoxemia. When unstable alveoli have been stabilized by surfactant repletion, they deflate progressively without collapse so that they retain gas volume at end-expiratory pressures below their previous critical closing pressures (84,85). In stabilized alveoli, effective gas exchange should be able to take place during expiration as well as during inspiration.

The stabilizing effect of surfactant treatment on a surfactant deficient alveolus is illustrated by Fig. 3, in which data taken from Clements et al. (84) are plotted to show the pressure-volume (PV) characteristics of a model of an isolated alveolus lined by extract from a premature infant's lung and the PV characteristics of the same model after it has been "treated" with surfactant by mathematically replacing its lining with extract from an adult human lung. During deflation, the surfactant-deficient model has collapsed at approximately 7 cmH_2O, but the surfactant treated model still retains about half of its maximal volume at this pressure. At maximal volume there is only a small difference in the distending pressure between the model lined with extract from a premature infant's lung and the model lined with extract from an adult human lung. This difference corresponds to the relatively small difference in surface tension between lung extract from a premature infant's lung when maximally expanded and lung extract from an adult human lung when maximally expanded. The deflation limb of the PV curve of the surfactant-deficient model is steeper than the deflation limb of the PV curve from the surfactant-treated model, so that compliance calculated over the mid-volume range of the deflation limbs is actually lower in the surfactant-treated model (1.28 $\mu ml/cmH_2O$ versus 2.31 $\mu ml/cmH_2O$).

Given that the dimensions of the terminal air spaces are not uniform throughout the lung, one would not expect all air spaces to behave uniformly in surfactant deficiency. Instead, there would be a range of critical opening and closing pressures, so that at any time under fixed conditions of mechanical ventilation of a patient with RDS, one population or compartment of terminal air spaces might remain collapsed throughout inspiration and expiration, another might be ventilated during inspiration, but collapsed during each expiration, and another might be ventilated and stable to the extent that gas volume were retained at end expiration.

The net effect of changes in the relative size of these three compartments on end-expiratory lung volume, tidal volume, and compliance of total lung is illustrated in Fig. 4 by a model of a hypothetical 12-alveolus lung with surfactant deficiency (86). As illustrated by the model, one effect of surfactant treatment, i.e., alveolar stabilization, leads to a decrease in compliance and an increase in

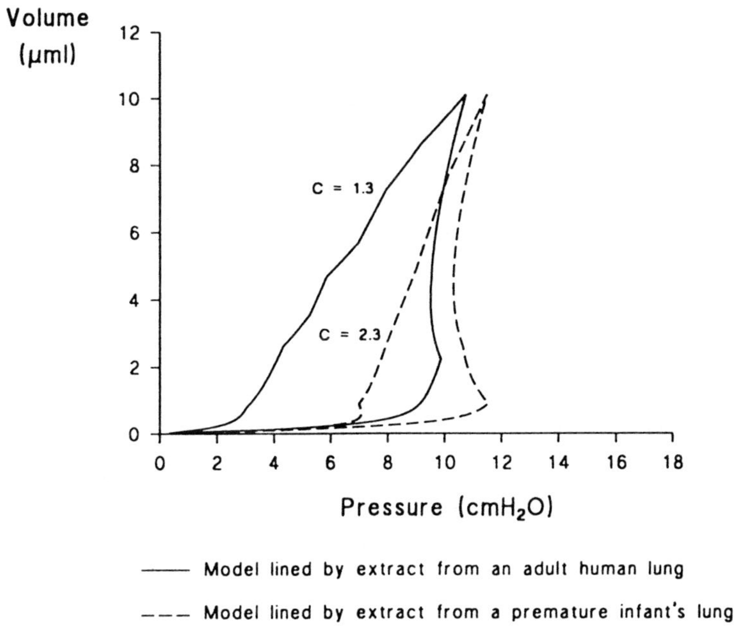

Figure 3 Pressure volume characteristics of a model alveolus when lined by extract from a premature infant's lung (broken line) or when lined by extract from an adult human lung (solid line). The data and model used to construct these PV curves were taken from Clements et al. (82). Pressure is calculated as the sum of Ps and PT. Ps is the pressure required to overcome surface forces (Ps = $2\gamma/R$, where γ = surface tension and R = radius of a spherical alveolar unit). PT is the pressure required to overcome tissue elastic forces (PT = E · (V/Vmax), where E is the coefficient of tissue elasticity, V is the volume of the alveolar unit, and Vmax is the maximal volume of the unit). The alveolar unit is modeled as a bubble on the end of a rigid tube. The radius of the tube is 60 μm and E = 5000 dynes/cm^2. Compliance (C) was estimated using linear regression analysis of the mid-volume range of the deflation limb of each PV loop. (From Ref. 86; used with permission.)

end-expiratory lung volume. Another effect of surfactant treatment, i.e., alveolar recruitment, results in an increase in both compliance and end-expiratory lung volume in this hypothetical 12-alveolus lung ventilated with the same airway pressures from panel to panel.

This model is an oversimplification, since it ignores many additional factors contributing to abnormal lung mechanics in RDS. It does not take into consideration factors such as tissue and surfactant elastance and mechanical interdependence which also act to stabilize terminal air spaces (85). Nevertheless,

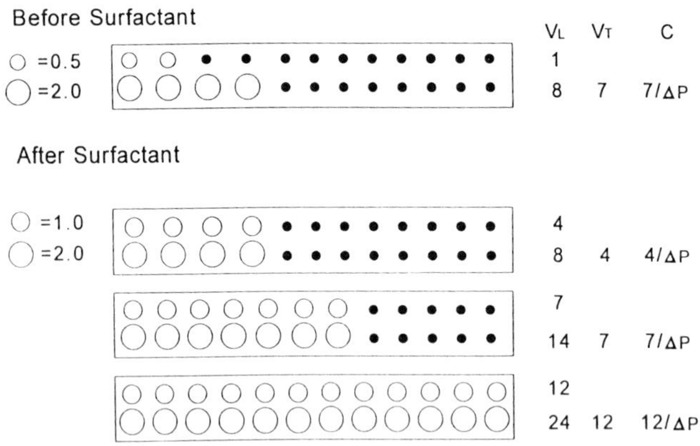

Figure 4 Model of a 12-alveolus lung in which the top row of each panel represents the volume of each alveolus at end expiration and the bottom row represents the volume of each alveolus at end inspiration. The solid circles indicate alveolar collapse. The open circles indicate alveoli which are not collapsed. The end-expiratory volume and end-inspiratory volume of an individual alveolus are shown to the left of panels 1 and 2. Before surfactant treatment, there are 2 ventilated alveoli which are stable, two ventilated alveoli which are unstable, and eight collapsed alveoli which comprise an unventilated compartment. In panel 2, after surfactant, the two ventilated alveoli which were unstable before surfactant have become stabilized. The unventilated compartment of eight collapsed alveoli remains the same as before surfactant. In panel 3, three alveoli from the unventilated compartment have been recruited and stabilized. In panel 4, the unventilated compartment has been fully recruited and all alveoli are ventilated and stable. The stepwise effect of this process of stabilization and recruitment on lung volume (V_L), tidal volume (V_T), and compliance (C) is shown to the right of the panels. (From Ref. 86; used with permission.)

it does serve as an hypothesis to explain some unexpected observations in infants with RDS discussed above such as the effect of distending airway pressure on compliance and the finding of high values for specific compliance in some patients with RDS. This hypothesis is also consistent with the observed effects of surfactant treatment on lung volume and compliance (44,46,53).

Derecruitment Due to Alveolar Flooding and Tissue Injury

Histopathological findings of the lung in experimental RDS and human premature infants dying with RDS provide clear evidence of lost alveolar volume occurring in association with the lung injury of this disorder (87,88). Marked capillary and venous congestion is apparent. Interstitial edema is widespread and dilated lymphatic spaces are frequently seen adjacent to respiratory bronchioles and arterioles. Hyaline membrane formation, which represents a coagulum of sloughed cell debris in a protein matrix, occurs characteristically at the junction of respiratory bronchioles and alveolar ducts. Hyaline membranes are visible evidence that this disease involves the exudation of plasma proteins occurring in association with a destructive injury of the epithelial lining of the terminal conducting airways. In some cases, the respiratory bronchioles and alveolar ducts may be filled with protein-rich edema fluid in association with membrane formation which in some cases totally obstructs the respiratory bronchiole. The histological evidence of edema and vascular congestion is confirmed by direct measurements in premature lambs. When compared with control animals, lambs with RDS have over twice as much extravascular water and 50% more intravascular blood volume (62).

In addition to reducing the number of ventilated terminal air spaces by displacement of gas and obstruction of the terminal conducting airways by a coagulum of hyaline membrane, alveolar flooding and protein leak also interfere with surfactant function (see below).

B. Increased Recoil Pressure of Ventilated Terminal Air Spaces

Elastic recoil pressure in the lung can be regarded as the sum of surface forces at the interface between alveolar gas and alveolar lining liquid and the forces resulting from lung tissue elastic properties. An increase in elastic recoil pressure due to an increase in surface forces is considered to be the keystone of the pathophysiology of RDS. Surface elastic forces are increased in RDS as a result of surfactant deficiency, inhibited surfactant function, or both. Inadequate production and release of surfactant by type II cells is a maturational phenomenon. In some cases, decreased surfactant availability may be further aggravated by ischemic injury to terminal airway epithelium which includes the type II cell.

Inhibition of surfactant function may be caused by protein leaked into airways (89,90). Nearly complete inhibition of a porcine surfactant has been demonstrated both in vitro and in vivo by edema fluid sampled from the airways of hyperoxia-exposed adult rabbits (91). Fibrinogen, a major component of the hyaline membrane, is said to be the plasma protein with the greatest inactivating potency yet described (92). In addition to protein effects, ion effects, lipid effects, and pH effects have also been shown to be involved in mechanisms of surfactant inactivation (92). Synthetic surfactant-associated proteins SP-B and SP-C peptides in surfactant lipids have been shown to permit resistance to inhibition by several plasma constituents that inactivate surfactant (93). Surfactant function in the neonatal period can also be inhibited experimentally by a monoclonal antibody to SP-B (94). In addition, clinically impaired surfactant function occurs in association with congenital SP-B deficiency (95).

Alveolar flooding may increase surface elastic forces. Cook et al. (61) observed a marked decrease in lung compliance during induced pulmonary edema in anesthetized dogs. Their findings suggested that surface phenomena were responsible for the mechanical behavior of edematous lungs rather than vascular congestion, per se, or intrinsic tissue changes. Their conclusion was borne out by experiments in the same study on excised lungs which showed that the elastic properties of edematous lungs were not significantly different from normal lungs when surface forces were minimized. In a study of mature rabbits with lungs containing large amounts of instilled saline, a marked improvement in oxygenation was demonstrated following the administration of exogenous surfactant, a result which was similar to the increase in arterial oxygen tension following surfactant treatment of premature infants with RDS (96). These investigators suggested that the excess liquid would be equivalent to a large hypophase, decreasing the amount of surfactant at the air-liquid interface.

Increased elastic recoil due both to surface forces and to tissue elastic forces will occur in the infant with RDS who is ventilated high on the volume axis of the lung's PV curve either inadvertently or out of necessity. In RDS, there is a large compartment of terminal air spaces which are unventilated or only poorly ventilated (97,98). To achieve acceptable gas exchange, the remaining air spaces must provide more than their normal share of ventilation. The smaller the ventilated compartment, the more distended will its terminal air spaces become at end inspiration for a given tidal volume. At high volume, surface forces are minimally reduced by surfactant (even when present) and tissue elastance increases as the elastin network, which dominates at low and middle volume ranges, gives way to the structural influence of poorly compliant collagen (1).

The extent to which abnormal lung tissue mechanical properties contribute to increased recoil pressure of ventilated terminal air spaces in RDS is not well documented. One might expect interstitial edema to cause increased tissue elastic recoil, but the evidence cited above obtained from acute studies of mongrel dogs did not substantiate this possibility. Whether these findings also apply to ongoing pulmonary edema in a premature infant with incomplete lung development is conjectural. In another study of the interrelations between pulmonary liquid volumes and lung compliance in an isolated perfused and ventilated rabbit lung preparation, the fall in compliance following elevation of left atrial pressure was thought to result from increases in pulmonary blood volume, but not from accumulation of interstitial edema (99). These investigators suggested two possible mechanisms to explain the reduced compliance with increased pulmonary blood volume: (1) that an increased competition for space between blood and gas could lead to a decrease in FRC and reduced caliber of terminal airways, or (2) that an increased rigidity of the lung vasculature caused by elevated transmural pressures could be the source of an increase in tissue elastic recoil. These mechanisms may be involved in the decrease in compliance observed when significant left-to-right ductus shunting occurs in association with RDS. Although Clyman et al. (70) did not observe a significant effect of left-to-right ductus shunting on lung compliance in premature lambs, it is unknown whether pulmonary blood volume was increased when the ductus was open in these studies, since neither this factor nor left atrial pressure was measured.

Another possible source of increased tissue elastic recoil in RDS is the injury to the terminal conducting airways and the ensuing repair process. The formation of hyaline membranes at the junction of respiratory bronchioles and alveolar ducts places these eschar splints at a location which could effectively stiffen terminal airways. Decreased compliance might also be expected from increased tissue recoil when fibrosis occurs following injury in those infants who go on to develop bronchopulmonary dysplasia.

C. Increased Lung Resistance

As noted earlier in this chapter, lung resistance measured in RDS in spontaneously breathing infants prior to the era of routine use of mechanical ventilation was not markedly different from values obtained from newborn infants without lung disease, but more recent measurements made in infants with RDS requiring mechanical ventilation have resulted in values of R_L and R_{rs} which are three to six times greater than in normal newborn infants. Some of the increased R in these infants may have included the resistance of the endotracheal tube. Although it is difficult in practice to determine how much of the increase in R measured during mechanical ventilation is attributable to the endotracheal tube, it would appear from the measurements of Sly et al. (100) that this increment is not sufficient to account for the magnitude of increase measured in patients with RDS.

Why R_L is increased in RDS has not received extensive attention. In their study demonstrating the association between increased R_L and the later development of BPD, Goldman et al. (54) suggested that increased resistance may result from airway damage secondary to endotracheal intubation, positive-pressure ventilation, or high inspired oxygen concentration, or that it may result from peribronchial edema caused by increased pulmonary blood flow or left heart failure secondary to a patent ductus arteriosus. It is also possible that increased resistance is related to the loss of lung volume in RDS. In this regard, further analysis of previously reported lung function measurements (46) reveals a highly significant correlation between G_{rs} and FRC ($R = 0.832$, $P < 0.0001$) measured during mechanical ventilation in premature infants with RDS. Interestingly, the regression coefficient of this relationship, 3.6×10^{-3} G_{rs}/ml FRC, is the same order of magnitude as the regression coefficient of G_{aw} as a function TGV reported in normal infants, $2.17–2.99 \times 10^{-3}$ G_{aw}/ml TGV (3). This similarity in change in conductance with change in lung volume between infants with RDS and normal infants would imply that the increased R_L in RDS is more the consequence of a decrease in the cross-sectional area of patent conducting airways leading to ventilated lung than the result of abnormal mechanical properties of conducting airways.

Lung resistance in RDS is usually measured as an average value for the total lung or respiratory system. In a compartmental analysis, Richardson et al. (101) demonstrated that the mechanics of passive exhalation in premature lambs with RDS were better described by two compartments with different time constants (RC) than by a single compartment. The difference in time constants between the two compartments was due to a marked difference in R, with $R_{rs} = 90\ cmH_2O \cdot ml^{-1} \cdot s$ in the fast compartment and $R_{rs} = 503\ cmH_2O \cdot ml^{-1} \cdot s$ in the slow compartment. These investigators proposed that the slow compartment was the result of a large increase in resistance in small airways surrounded by unstable surfactant deficient alveoli with decreased compliance.

VI. Conclusions

The abnormal mechanical properties of the lung in RDS described in this chapter are the consequence of a variety of interacting pathophysiological events. The data and arguments presented in the preceding sections of this chapter which explain how these events relate to abnormalities in compliance and resistance can be summarized in the following working hypothesis.

Compliance is decreased in RDS because of a decreased number (derecruitment) of ventilated terminal air spaces and because of an increase in the recoil pressure of ventilated terminal airspaces.

Derecruitment occurs as a result of collapse of unstable air spaces, displacement of air space gas volume by protein rich edema fluid, and frank obstruction of terminal airways by hyaline membrane formation. Instability of terminal air spaces is a direct consequence of surfactant deficiency. The difficulty to inflate unstable terminal air spaces and their tendency to collapse during expiration is made worse by the inherently unstable chest walls of premature infants. The lining of alveolar ducts in RDS is injured as a result of epithelial disruption when high transpulmonary pressures are required to inflate air spaces. Epithelial damage may also occur as a primary ischemic event in association with intrapartum asphyxia. With the resulting loss of epithelial integrity from either injury, and with a hydrostatic gradient augmented by high surface forces accompanying surfactant deficiency, ventilated terminal airways are flooded by protein-rich liquid. Hyaline membranes forming from the coagulum of sloughed epithelial cell debris may obstruct terminal air spaces from recruitment by interventions such as distending airway pressure or surfactant replacement.

Those air spaces which remain recruited present an increased recoil pressure because of increased surface forces and increased tissue elastic forces. Surface forces are increased as a result of inadequate surfactant function due to its lack of production and release, due to abnormalities of other factors in the surfactant system such as the surfactant associated proteins, or due to its inactivation by protein-containing edema fluid. Increased elastic recoil owing both to surface forces and to tissue forces will be presented by the reduced compartment of air spaces which remain recruited, since adequate gas exchange cannot be provided by this compartment unless it is ventilated to an overdistended volume where surfactant, even when present, has minimal effect and where tissue recoil is determined more by collagen than elastin. Left-to-right ductus shunting, either as part of the acute pathophysiology of RDS or when complicating its recovery, contributes to a further decrease in compliance as a result of pulmonary vascular engorgement and aggravation of pulmonary edema, conditions which may increase elastic recoil owing to surface and tissue forces. The presence of the hyaline membrane in the acute phase of RDS and the deposition of collagen and other structural constituents in the repair process following this lung injury may also add to the tissue component of increased elastic recoil.

Some of the increased resistance to airflow in RDS can be accounted for by the endotracheal tube. Much of the increase in resistance derives from a reduction in the cross-sectional area of conducting airways leading to ventilated terminal air spaces. The resistance offered by these conducting airways may be increased further by iatrogenic airway injury (endotracheal tube, pressure, oxygen) and by peribronchial edema. There may also be an additional contribution by tissue resistive forces, but this possible source of increased R_L is not well characterized in RDS.

Acknowledgment

Supported by National Institutes of Health Pediatric Pulmonary SCOR HL-14214.

References

1. Hoppin FG Jr, Stothert JC Jr, Greaves IA, et al. (1986). Lung recoil: Elastic and rheological properties. In: Macklem PT, Mead J, Fishman AP, Geiger SR, eds. Handbook of Physiology, Section 3: The Respiratory System, Vol. III. Bethesda: American Physiological Society, pp 195–215.
2. Rodarte JR, Rehder K. (1986). Dynamics of respiration. In Macklem PT, Mead J, Fishman AP, Geiger SR, eds. Handbook of Physiology, Section 3: The Respiratory System, Vol. III. Bethesda: American Physiological Society, pp 131–144.

3. Stocks J, Godfrey S. (1977). Specific airway conductance in relation to postconceptional age during infancy. J Appl Physiol 43:144–154.
4. Hogg JC, Williams J, Richardson JB, et al. (1970). Age as a factor in the distribution of lower-airway conductance and in the pathologic anatomy of obstructive lung disease. N Engl J Med 282:1283–1287.
5. Marshall R, DuBois AB. (1956). The measurement of the viscous resistance of the lung tissues in normal man. Clin Sci 15:161–170.
6. Polgar G, String ST. (1966). The viscous resistance of the lung tissues in newborn infants. J Pediatr 69:787–792.
7. Gerhardt T, Bancalari E. (1980). Chestwall compliance in full-term and premature infants. Acta Pœdiatr Scand 69:359–364.
8. Davis GM, Coates AL, Papageorgiou A, Bureau MA. (1988a). Direct measurement of static chest wall compliance in animal and human neonates. J Appl Physiol 65:1093–1098.
9. Mortola JP. (1987). Dynamics of Breathing in Newborn Mammals. Physiol Rev 67:187–243.
10. Thomson A, Elliott J, Silverman M. (1983). Pulmonary compliance in sick low birthweight infants. Arch Dis Child 58:891–896.
11. Bryan AC, Wohl MB. (1986). Respiratory mechanics in children. In: Macklem PT, Mead J, Fishman AP, Geiger SR, eds. Handbook of Physiology, Section 3: The Respiratory System, Vol. III. Bethesda: American Physiological Society, pp 179–191.
12. Sullivan KJ, Mortola JP. (1986). Dynamic lung compliance in newborn and adult cats. J Appl Physiol 60:743–750.
13. Mortola JP. (1992). Measurements of respiratory mechanics. In: Polin RA, Fox WW, eds. Fetal and Neonatal Physiology. Vol. 1. Mexico City: Saunders, pp 813–822.
14. LeSouëf PN, England SJ, Bryan AC. (1984). Passive respiratory mechanics in newborns and children. Am Rev Respir Dis 129:552–556.
15. Olinsky A, Bryan AC, Bryan MH. (1976). A simple method of measuring total respiratory system compliance in newborn infants. S Afr Med J 50:128–130.
16. Kelly E, Bryan H, Possmayer F, et al. (1993). Compliance of the respiratory system in newborn infants pre- and postsurfactant replacement therapy. Pediatr Pulmonol 15:225–230.
17. Sullivan KJ, Mortola JP. (1987). Age related changes in the rate of stress relaxation within the rat respiratory system. Respir Physiol 67:295–309.
18. Peslin R, Marchal F, Choné C. (1991). Viscoelastic properties of rabbit lung during growth. Respir Physiol 86:189–198.
19. Otis AB, McKerrow CB, Bartlett RA, et al. (1956). Mechanical factors in distribution of pulmonary ventilation. J Appl Physiol 8:427–443.
20. Hanson JS, Shinozaki T. (1970). Hybrid computer studies of ventilatory distribution and lung volume. Pediatrics 46:900–914.
21. Richardson CP, Jung AL. (1978). Effects of continuous positive airway pressure on pulmonary function and blood gases of infants with respiratory distress syndrome. Pediatr Res 12:771–774.
22. Sandberg K, Sjöqvist BA, Parker RA, et al. (1994). Surfactant therapy improves

ventilation inhomogeneity in infants with respiratory distress syndrome (RDS). Pediatr Res 35:351A (abstract).
23. Uhl RR, Lewis FJ. (1974). Digital computer calculation of human pulmonary mechanics using a least squares fit technique. Comput Biomed Res 7:489–495.
24. Bhutani VK, Sivieri EM, Abbasi S, Shaffer TH. (1988a). Evaluation of neonatal pulmonary mechanics and energetics: A two factor least mean square analysis. Pediatr Pulmonol 4:150–158.
25. Silberberg AR, Edberg KE, Sandberg K, Hjalmarson O. (1991). Respiratory system mechanics in ventilated newborn infants: Evaluation of single-compartment models. Technical Report 6:91, Research Laboratory of Medical Electronics, Chalmers University of Technology, Göteberg, Sweden, pp 1–25.
26. Mortola JP, Fisher JT, Smith B, et al. (1982). Dynamics of breathing in infants. J Appl Physiol 52:1209–1215.
27. Stocks J, Nöthen U, Sutherland P, et al. (1987). Improved accuracy of the occlusion technique for assessing total respiratory compliance in infants. Pediatr Pulmonol 3:71–77.
28. Guslits BG, Wilkie RA, England SJ, Bryan AC. (1987). Comparison of methods of measurement of compliance of the respiratory system in children. Am Rev Respir Dis 136:727–729.
29. Cook CD, Sutherland JM, Segal S, Cherry RB, et al. (1957). Studies of respiratory physiology in the newborn infant. III. Measurements of mechanics of respiration. J Clin Invest 36:440–448.
30. Swyer PR, Reiman RC, Wright JJ. (1960). Ventilation and ventilatory mechanics in the newborn. J Pediatr 56:612–622.
31. Chu J, Clements JA, Cotton EK, et al. (1967). Neonatal Pulmonary Ischemia: Part I: Clinical and Physiological Studies. Pediatrics 40:709–782.
32. Hjalmarson O, Olsson T, Riha M. (1974). Mechanics of breathing in newborn infants with pulmonary disease. Acta Pœdiatr Scand 247(suppl):26–48.
33. Sandberg K, Sjöqvist BA, Hjalmarson O, Olsson T. (1987). Lung function in newborn infants with tachypnea of unknown cause. Pediatr Res 22:581–586.
34. Mortola JP, Milic-Emili J, Noworaj A, et al. (1984). Muscle pressure and flow during expiration in infants. Am Rev Respir Dis 129:49–53.
35. Migdal M, Dreizzen E, Praud JP, et al. (1987). Compliance of the total respiratory system in healthy preterm and fuil-term newborns. Pediatr Pulmonol 3:214–218.
36. Karlberg P, Cook CD, O'Brien D, et al. (1954). Studies of respiratory physiology in the newborn infant. II. Observations during and after respiratory distress. Acta Pœdiatr Scand 43(suppl 100):397–411.
37. Auld PAM, Nelson NM, Cherry RB, et al. (1963). Measurement of the thoracic gas volume in the newborn infant. J Clin Invest 42:476–483.
38. Swyer RR, Levison H. (1965). The current status of the respiratory distress syndrome of the newly born. Can Med Assoc J 93:335–342.
39. Prod'hom LS, Levison H, Cherry RB, Smith CA. (1965). Adjustment of ventilation, intrapulmonary gas exchange, and acid-base balance during the first day of life. Pediatrics 35:662–676.
40. Davis JM, Veness-Meehan K, Notter RH, et al. (1988b). Changes in pulmonary

mechanics after the administration of surfactant to infants with respiratory distress syndrome. N Engl J Med 319:476–479.

41. Couser RJ, Ferrara TB, Ebert J, et al. (1990). Effects of exogenous surfactant therapy on dynamic compliance during mechanical breathing in preterm infants with hyaline membrane disease. J Pediatr 116:119–124.
42. Bhat R, Dziedzic K, Bhutani VK, Vidyasagar D. (1990). Effect of single dose surfactant on pulmonary function. Crit Care Med 18:590–595.
43. Edberg KE, Sandberg K, Silberberg A, et al. (1991). Lung volume, gas mixing, and mechanics of breathing in mechanically ventilated very low birth weight infants with idiopathic respiratory distress syndrome. Pediatr Res 30:496–500.
44. Goldsmith LS, Greenspan JS, Rubenstein D, et al. (1991). Immediate improvement in lung volume after exogenous surfactant: Alveolar recruitment versus increased distention. J Pediatr 119:424–428.
45. Bhutani VK, Abbasi S, Long WA, Gerdes JS. (1992). Pulmonary mechanics and energetics in preterm infants who had respiratory distress syndrome treated with synthetic surfactant. J Pediatr 120:S18–S24.
46. Cotton RB, Olsson T, Law AB, et al. (1993). The physiologic effects of surfactant treatment on gas exchange in newborn premature infants with hyaline membrane disease. Pediatr Res 34:495–501.
47. Miller J, Law AB, Parker RA, et al. (1994). Effects of morphine and pancuronium on lung volume and oxygenation in premature infants with hyaline membrane disease. J Pediatr 125:97–103.
48. Dreizzen E, Migdal M, Praud JP, et al. (1989). Passive total respiratory system compliance and gas exchange in newborns with hyaline membrane disease. Pediatr Pulmonol 6:2–7.
49. Tamura M, Kawano T. (1989). The effect of reconstituted bovine surfactant on pulmonary mechanics in infants with respiratory distress syndrome. Acta Pœdiatr Jpn 31:734–741.
50. Pfenninger J, Aebi C, Bachmann D, Wagner BP. (1992). Lung mechanics and gas exchange in ventilated preterm infants during treatment of hyaline membrane disease with multiple doses of artificial surfactant (Exosurf). Pediatr Pulmonol 14:10–15.
51. Baraldi E, Pettenazzo A, Filippone M, et al. (1993). Rapid improvement of static compliance after surfactant treatment in preterm infants with respiratory distress syndrome. Pediatr Pulmonol 15:157–162.
52. Vilstrup CT, Björklund LJ, Larsson A, Werner O. (1993). Lung function impairment in RDS (abstr). Pediatr Res 33:348A.
53. Edberg KE, Ekström-Jodal B, Hallman M, et al. (1990). Immediate effects on lung function of instilled human surfactant in mechanically ventilated newborn infants with IRDS. Acta Pœdiatr Scand 79:750–755.
54. Goldman SL, Gerhardt T, Sonni R, et al. (1983). Early prediction of chronic lung disease by pulmonary function testing. J Pediatr 102:613–617.
55. Bhutani VK, Abbasi S, Sivieri EM. (1988b). Continuous skeletal muscle paralysis: Effect on neonatal pulmonary mechanics. Pediatrics 81:419–422.
56. Gregory GA, Kitterman JA, Phibbs RH, et al. (1971). Treatment of the idiopathic respiratory-distress syndrome with continuous positive airway pressure. N Engl J Med 284:1333–1340.

57. Yu VYH, Rolfe P. (1977). Effect of continuous positive airway pressure breathing on cardiorespiratory function in infants with respiratory distress syndrome. Acta Pœdiatr Scand 66:59–64.
58. Bancalari E, Garcia OL, Jesse MJ. (1973). Effects of continuous negative pressure on lung mechanics in idiopathic respiratory distress syndrome. Pediatrics 51:485–493.
59. Shaffer TH, Koen PA, Moskowitz GD, et al. (1978). Positive end expiratory pressure: Effects on lung mechanics of premature lambs. Biol Neonate 34:1–10.
60. Philips JB III, Beale EF, Howard JE, et al. (1980). Effect of positive end-expiratory pressure on dynamic respiratory compliance in neonates. Biol Neonate 38: 270–275.
61. Cook CD, Mead J, Schreiner GL, et al. (1959). Pulmonary mechanics during induced pulmonary edema in anesthetized dogs. J Appl Physiol 14:177–186.
62. Sundell HW, Harris TR, Cannon JR, et al. (1987). Lung water and vascular permeability-surface area in premature newborn lambs with hyaline membrane disease. Circ Res 60:923–932.
63. Heaf DP, Belik J, Spitzer AR, et al. (1982). Changes in pulmonary function during the diuretic phase of respiratory distress syndrome. J Pediatr 101:103–107.
64. Yeh TF, Shibli A, Leu ST, et al. (1984). Early furosemide therapy in premature infants (≤2000 gm) with respiratory distress syndrome: A randomized controlled trial. J Pediatr 105:603–609.
65. Belik J, Spitzer AR, Clark BJ, et al. (1987). Effect of early furosemide administration in neonates with respiratory distress syndrome. Pediatr Pulmonol 3:219–225.
66. Najak ZD, Harris EM, Lazzara Jr A, Pruitt AW. (1983). Pulmonary effects of furosemide in preterm infants with lung disease. J Pediatr 102:758–763.
67. Balsan MJ, Jones JG, Guthrie RD. (1991). Effects of a clinically detectable PDA on pulmonary mechanics measures in VLBW infants with RDS. Pediatr Pulmonol 11:161–165.
68. Naulty CM, Horn S, Conry J, Avery GB. (1978). Improved lung compliance after liga- tion of patent ductus arteriosus in hyaline membrane disease. J Pediatr 93:682–684.
69. Stefano JL, Abbasi S, Pearlman SA, et al. (1991). Closure of the ductus arteriosus with indomethacin in ventilated neonates with respiratory distress syndrome. Am Rev Respir Dis 143:236–239.
70. Clyman RI, Mauray F, Heymann MA, Roman C. (1987). Cardiovascular effects of patent ductus arteriosus in preterm lambs with respiratory distress. J Pediatr 111:579–87.
71. Pérez Fontan JJ, Clyman RI, Mauray F, et al. (1987). Respiratory effects of a patent ductus arteriosus in premature newborn lambs. J Appl Physiol 63:2315–2324.
72. Graff MA, Novo RP, Diaz M, et al. (1986). Compliance measurement in respiratory distress syndrome: The prediction of outcome. Pediatr Pulmonol 2:332–336.
73. Cunningham MD. (1989). Intensive care monitoring of pulmonary mechanics for preterm infants undergoing mechanical ventilation. J Perinatol 9:56–59.
74. Freezer NJ, Sly PD. (1993). Predictive value of measurements of respiratory mechanics in preterm infants with HMD. Pediatr Pulmonol 16:116–123.
75. Bhutani VK, Abbasi S. (1992). Relative likelihood of bronchopulmonary dysplasia

based on pulmonary mechanics measured in preterm neonates during the first week of life. J Pediatr 120:605–613.

76. Kirpalani H, Schmidt B, Gaston S, et al. (1991). Birthweight, early passive respiratory system mechanics, and ventilator requirements as predictors of outcome in premature infants with respiratory failure. Pediatr Pulmonol 10:195–198.
77. Wallenbrock MA, Sekar KC, Toubas PL. (1992). Prediction of the acute response to surfactant therapy by pulmonary function testing. Pediatr Pulmonol 13:11–15.
78. Berglund G, Karlberg P. (1956). Determination of the functional residual capacity in newborn infants. Acta Pœdiatr 45:541–544.
79. Krauss AN, Auld PAM. (1970). Measurement of functional residual capacity in distressed neonates by helium rebreathing. J Pediatr 77:228–232.
80. Jackson JC, Standaert TA, Truog WE, et al. (1985). Changes in lung volume and deflation stability in hyaline membrane disease. J Appl Physiol 59:1783–1789.
81. Sandberg K, Edberg K, Benton W, et al. (1991). Surfactant improves gas mixing and alveolar ventilation in preterm lambs. Pediatr Res 30:181–189.
82. Bose CL, Lawson EE, Greene A, et al. (1986). Measurement of cardiopulmonary function in ventilated neonates with respiratory distress syndrome using rebreathing methodology. Pediatr Res 20:316–320.
83. Jackson JC, Mackenzie AP, Chi EY, et al. (1990). Mechanisms for reduced total lung capacity at birth and during hyaline membrane disease in premature newborn monkeys. Am Rev Respir Dis 142:413–419.
84. Clements JA, Hustead RF, Johnson RP, Gribetz I. (1961). Pulmonary surface tension and alveolar stability. J Appl Physiol 16:444–450.
85. Greaves IA, Hildebrandt J, Hoppin FG Jr. (1986). Micromechanics of the lung. In: Macklem PT, Mead J, Fishman AP, Geiger SR, eds. Handbook of Physiology, Section 3: The Respiratory System, Vol. III. Bethesda: American Physiological Society, pp 217–231.
86. Cotton RB. (1994). A model of the effect of surfactant treatment on gas exchange in hyaline membrane disease. Semin Perinatol 18:19–22.
87. Stahlman MT, LeQuire VS, Young WC, et al. (1964). Pathophysiology of respiratory distress in newborn lambs. Am J Dis Child 108:375–393.
88. Stahlman MT. (1977). Respiratory disorders in the newborn. In: Kendig EL, Chernick V, eds. Disorders of the Respiratory Tract in Children. Philadelphia: Saunders, pp 271–290.
89. Ikegami M, Jobe A, Jacobs H, Lam R. (1984). A protein from airways of premature lambs that inhibits surfactant function. J Appl Physiol 51:1134–1142.
90. Fuchimakai T, Fujiwara T, Takahashi A, Enhorning G. (1987). Artificial pulmonary surfactant inhibited by proteins. J Appl Physiol 62:429–437.
91. Kobayaski T, Nitta K, Ganzuka M, et al. (1991). Inactivation of exogenous surfactant by pulmonary edema fluid. Pediatr Res 29:353–356.
92. Amirkhanian JD, Taeusch HW. (1993). Reversible and irreversible inactivation of preformed pulmonary surfactant surface films by changes in subphase constituents. Biochim Biophys Acta 1165:321–326.
93. Amirkhanian JD, Bruni R, Waring AJ, Taeusch HW. (1991). Inhibition of mixtures of surfactant lipids and synthetic sequences of surfactant proteins SP-B and SP-C. Biochim Biophys Acta 1096:355–360.

94. Robertson B, Kobayashi T, Ganzuka M, et al. (1991). Experimental neonatal respiratory failure induced by a monoclonal antibody to the hydrophobic surfactant-associated protein SP-B. Pediatr Res 30:239–243.
95. Nogee LM, DeMello DE, Dehner LP, Colten HR. (1993). Brief report: Deficiency of pulmonary surfactant protein B in congenital alveolar proteinosis. N Engl J Med 328:406–410.
96. O'Brodovich H, Hannam V. (1993). Exogenous surfactant rapidly increases Pa_{O_2} in mature rabbits with lungs that contain large amounts of saline. Am Rev Respir Dis 147:1087–1090.
97. Corbet AJS, Ross JA, Beaudry PH, Stern L. (1974). Ventilation-perfusion relationships as assessed by aADN2 in hyaline membrane disease. J Appl Physiol 36:74–81.
98. Hansen TN, Corbet AJS, Kenny JD, et al. (1979). Effects of oxygen and constant positive pressure breathing on aADCO2 in hyaline membrane disease. Pediatr Res 13:1167–1171.
99. Hauge A, Bø G, Waaler BA (1975). Interrelations between pulmonary liquid volumes and lung compliance. J Appl Physiol 38:608–614.
100. Sly PD, Brown KA, Bates JHT, et al. (1988). Noninvasive determination of respiratory mechanics during mechanical ventilation of neonates: A review of current and future techniques. Pediatr Pulmonol 4:39–47.
101. Richardson P, Jarriel S, Hansen TN. (1989). Mechanics of the respiratory system during passive exhalation in preterm lambs. Pediatr Res 26:425–428.

8

Radiological Diagnosis of Neonatal Respiratory Distress Syndrome and Related Disorders

WILLIAM H. NORTHWAY, JR.
Stanford University School of Medicine
Stanford
and Lucile Packard Children's Hospital
Palo Alto, California

I. Introduction

A remarkable decline in mortality rate in infancy has taken place in this century. In the early 1900s, before the development of antibiotics, two thirds of all infant deaths occurred after the first 4 weeks of life primarily from infectious disease (1). By the mid 1950s, two thirds of infant deaths occurred during the first 4 weeks of life, with most occurring during the first week of life. Most of the deaths were secondary to pulmonary disorders, immaturity, birth injuries, and congenital malformations. The leading cause of death was the respiratory distress syndrome (RDS), or hyaline membrane disease, which occurs in 25% of all liveborn premature infants. With improvements in intensive care nursing, including the use of exogenous surfactants, mortality from RDS is no longer the leading cause of death, having been replaced by deaths from congenital malformations (2). Since 1953 when Donald and Steiner (3) described and documented the characteristic radiographic picture of RDS, chest radiography has played an important role in diagnosing specific pulmonary diseases in the neonatal period. The improved reliability of diagnosis that chest radiography provided facilitated the study of these diseases which led to specific treatments for them, including RDS. Chest radiography has also been helpful in identifying the acute and chronic complications associated with the treatment of neonatal RDS syndrome and related disorders.

II. Respiratory Distress Syndrome

Although the initial description of hyaline membranes in the lungs of newborns dying of respiratory disease was made in 1903 (4), as late as 1957 hyaline membrane disease was not included in the standard nomenclature of disease (5). Prior to 1953, the various causes of respiratory distress in the newborn infant were not easily separable by history and physical examination. The radiographic description in 1953 of the fine miliary mottling or granular pattern of density with air bronchograms seen in infants with proven RDS (Fig. 1) allowed the clinical diagnosis to be firmly established (3). Peterson and Pendleton in 1955 (6), in a controlled study, with postmortem correlation, differentiated the radiographic picture of RDS from that of aspiration pneumonia (Fig. 2). In RDS, the segmental bronchi are distended with air and are visible because of the density of the surrounding atelectatic and transudate-filled alveoli. In the first 4 hr following birth or in mild cases, the air bronchogram may be absent and the fine granularity inconspicuous. By 12 hr of age, approximately 50% of the premature infants with RDS will have the classic radiographic picture of air bronchogram

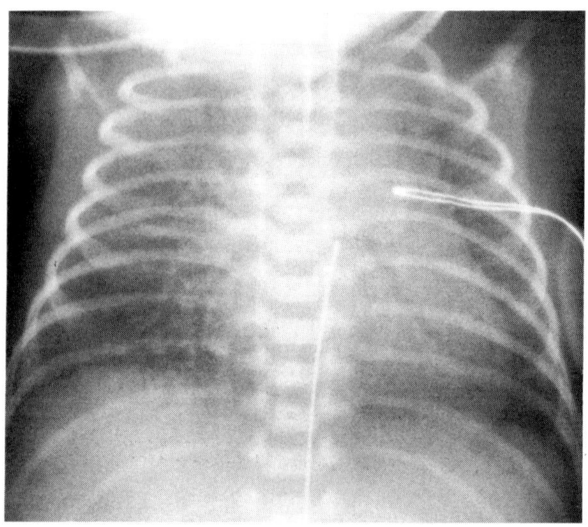

Figure 1 Prematurely born infant with respiratory distress. An initial chest radiograph shows bilateral fine granularity in the lungs with peripheral air bronchogram characteristic of RDS.

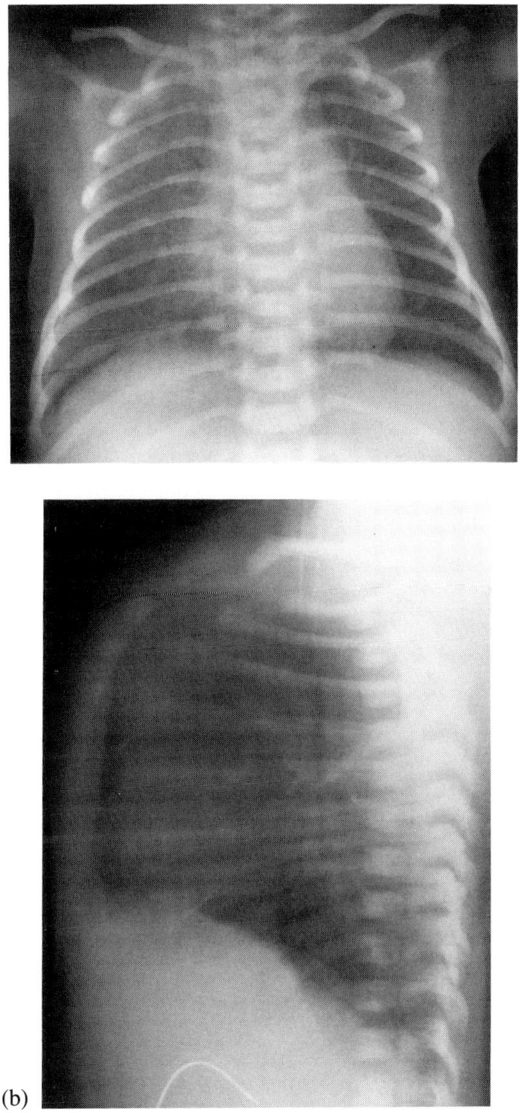

(a)

(b)

Figure 2 Full-term infant with respiratory distress and meconium staining of amniotic fluid. An initial anteroposterior (a) and lateral (b) chest radiograph shows bilateral hyperexpansion and nonuniform increase in pulmonary density most prominent on the right consistent with meconium aspiration pneumonia.

with bilateral fine granularity. If the radiographic findings are in question, a repeat chest radiograph can confirm the diagnosis by revealing the development of the characteristic pattern by 24 to 36 hr of age. The granularity of the lungs is present bilaterally and is homogeneously distributed throughout both lungs. The appearance in either lung of a patch of radiographic density and/or the presence of a pleural effusion raises the possibility of a superimposed bacterial pulmonary infection. The lungs in infants with RDS appear either normally expanded or underexpanded prior to endotracheal intubation. The radiographic appearance of the heart varies from normal to slightly increased in size. The heart size depends to some extent on the degree of lung inflation.

The severity of the pulmonary disease during the first 1–3 days of life roughly parallels the degree of granular opacification seen in the lungs. The course of radiographic change in mild RDS is one of progressive resolution of abnormal findings by 1 week of age. Prior to the use of mechanical ventilation, progressive radiographic opacification of the lungs was seen in severe disease, and, if therapy was unsuccessful, death occurred by 4 days of age. The radiographic and clinical course of severe RDS has been prolonged and modified by mechanical ventilation, supplemental oxygen therapy, and, most recently, by surfactant therapy.

Several diseases clinically resembling RDS can be differentiated from it radiographically in the immediate newborn period. These include:

1. Central nervous system hemorrhage, which presents radiographically with clear lungs
2. Meconium aspiration pneumonia, which presents in mature or postmature infants with coarse, irregular, nonuniform increase in radiographic pulmonary density, focal irregularities in aeration, and hyperexpanded lungs
3. Left-to-right shunting with congenital heart disease, which presents with an enlarged heart and large central pulmonary vessels

Diffuse pulmonary hemorrhage and viral interstitial pneumonia, although unusual at birth, may be indistinguishable from RDS radiographically (7).

III. Pulmonary Immaturity

RDS occurs primarily in prematurely born infants. By World Health Organization definition, these infants are live born before 37 weeks from the first day of the last menstrual period. Infants of extremely low birth weight, less than 750 g, have been referred to as immature neonates (1). As a result of improved mechanical ventilation techniques, extremely low birth weight prematurely born infants of 23–26 weeks' gestational age with respiratory distress are being managed in intensive care nurseries. Between 17 and 26 weeks' gestational age, the lung goes through a canalicular phase of development. The terminal units of the lung become lined by high cuboidal epithelium and the close relationship of the pulmonary capillaries to the gas-exchanging surfaces is developed at the end of this phase. Gas exchange becomes possible at 22 weeks' gestational age (8). Prematurely born infants below 900 g birth weight (26 weeks) who expire rapidly may not show evidence of hyaline membranes, so they technically do not have hyaline membrane disease even though the rest of the pathology of hyaline membrane disease or RDS may be present. The ability of these 23- to 26-week gestational age infants to maintain spontaneous ventilation and to oxygenate their blood is marginal. Almost all require mechanical ventilation and oxygen supplementation. The radiographic appearance of the lungs in these immature infants may initially be normal or show mild diffuse granularity without air bronchogram or a mild degree of interstitial edema (9) (Fig. 3).

IV. Bronchopulmonary Dysplasia

The decrease in mortality and prolongation of life seen with intensive care treatment of prematurely born infants with RDS has been associated with the

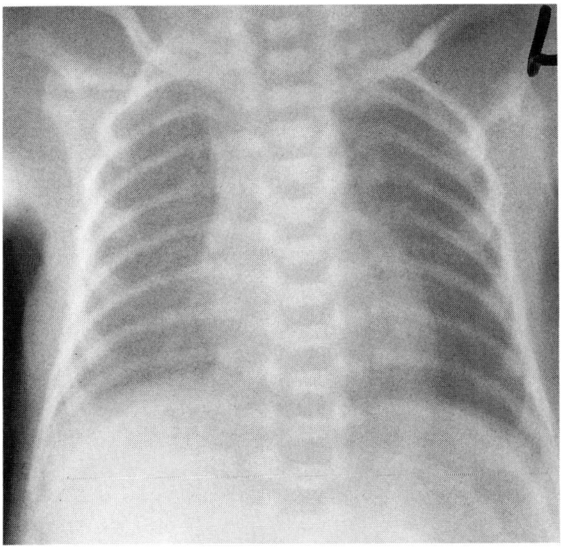

Figure 3 Extremely low birth weight prematurely born infant with apnea. Initial chest radiograph shows fine hazy pulmonary density without air bronchogram typical of immature lungs.

appearance of a chronic lung disease, bronchopulmonary dysplasia (BPD). BPD was first described by Northway, et al. in 1967 (10). They reported 32 infants with severe RDS who were treated with high concentrations of oxygen (80–100%) and mechanical ventilation. Prior to this type of therapy, infants with RDS either died by 4 days of age or recovered by 7 days of age without persistent respiratory difficulty (6). The initial report of BPD described a four-stage clinical-radiographic progression of disease which culminated at 30 days of age with stage IV disease which was chronic. At 30 days of age, the chest radiograph showed lungs which were hyperexpanded with a reticular pattern of alternating areas of linear density and cyst-like lucencies. The descriptive name of the disease process was chosen because of the pathological demonstration of injury and repair to the lung parenchyma and the airways which appeared to alter normal lung growth and development.

Analysis of the oxygen therapy of the original patient population with and without BPD suggested that the etiology was related to pulmonary oxygen toxicity (11). Research in animal models reported by several authors (12–15) has suggested that both pulmonary oxygen toxicity and barotrauma play a role in development of a BPD-like pathological picture in the newborn mammalian lung.

The major factors in the pathogenesis of BPD are now believed to be (1) premature birth, (2) respiratory failure, (3) supplemental oxygen therapy, and (4) mechanical ventilation. The respiratory failure is usually secondary to RDS. Respiratory failure caused by meconium aspiration pneumonia (16), other aspiration pneumonias (17–19), congestive heart failure (17–23), neonatal tetanus (24), congenital muscular disease (25), Wilson-Mikity syndrome (18), and marked prematurity (20,26–29) has also been associated with the development of BPD. Any factor that prolongs mechanical ventilation and supplemental oxygen therapy can contribute to the development of BPD. These include (1) interstitial emphysema, pneumothorax, and pneumomediastinum (30); (2) pulmonary edema from congestive heart failure or fluid overload (31); and (3) secondary pulmonary infection (32).

Since the original description of BPD, the four-stage radiographic progression to chronic disease has been modified as improvements in mechanical ventilation techniques have lowered the duration and concentration of supplemental oxygen exposure and peak inspiratory pressure. Originally, the four stages were:

Stage I (1–3 days of age): The chest radiograph was indistinguishable from uncomplicated RDS, but histologically early mucosal necrosis could be seen.

Stage II (4–10 days of age): The lungs became increasingly opaque on chest radiography and there was necrosis and alveolar epithelial repair with marked fluid exudation into the alveolar and airway lumen.

Stage III (10–20 days of age): The lungs became clearer on the chest radiograph but developed a cystic, bubbly pattern which reflected the underlying widespread alveolar emphysema and alveolar atelectasis with mucosal squamous metaplasia.

Stage IV (30 days of age and older): Beyond 1 month of age, the chest radiograph typically showed hyperexpansion, linear streaks of abnormal density, and areas of cystic lucency, with variable cardiomegaly (Fig. 4).

Although BPD represents a continuum of lung injury and repair that is recognized histologically after 1 week of artificial ventilation and supplemental oxygen therapy, the clinical diagnosis of BPD is difficult to document radiographically before 21–30 days of age. It is stage IV of this injury and repair process that currently is considered BPD. In 1989, the Bureau of Maternal and Child Health and Resources Development put forward the following diagnostic criteria for BPD (33):

1. Positive-pressure ventilation during the first 2 weeks of life for a minimum of 3 days
2. Clinical signs of respiratory compromise persisting longer than 28 days of age

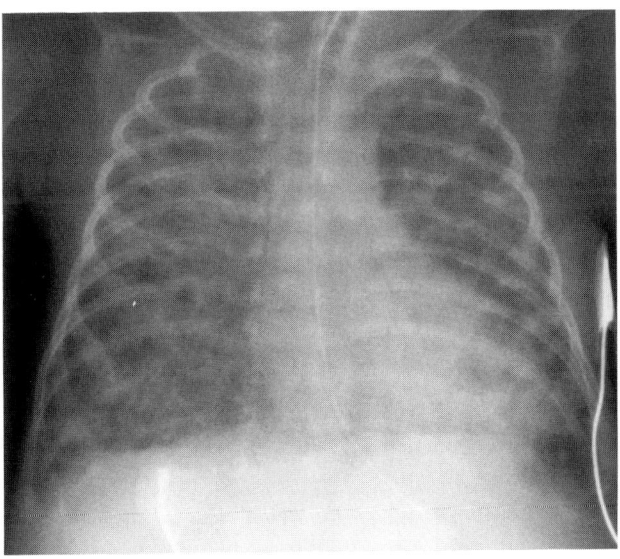

Figure 4 The same infant as in Fig. 1 with RDS following 1 month of treatment with mechanical ventilation and oxygen supplementation. The chest radiograph shows hyperexpansion, mottled density, and a cystic appearance of both lungs characteristic of severe BPD.

3. Requirement for supplemental oxygen longer than 28 days of age to maintain a $Pa_{O_2} > 50$ mmHg (>6.7 kPa)
4. Chest radiograph with findings characteristic of BPD

The radiographic criteria for BPD have been purposely left vague since the original radiographic four-stage progression has been modified by subsequent changes in supplemental oxygen and mechanical ventilation therapy. An additional clinical change has been the treatment of increasingly smaller, less mature infants for respiratory failure. Although the original four-stage radiographic development of BPD still occurs, it is less common. The chest radiographic changes are now usually less severe, and the progression to fine linear interstitial densities in the lungs may be more prolonged. The radiological progression of BPD may be obscured by intercurrent complications such as heart failure from a patent ductus arteriosus, pulmonary interstitial emphysema, pneumomediastinum, and pneumothorax, or infection. It is, therefore, difficult to diagnose BPD before 3 weeks of postnatal age. Bronchopulmonary dysplasia may gradually become apparent as a diffuse reticular interstitial pattern of increased density and alternating lucency that persists after the complicating factors have disappeared.

Very low birth weight infants with repeated apnea may present with an initial chest radiograph that is essentially normal. With mechanical ventilation and supplemental low concentration oxygen therapy, they slowly develop the radiographic picture of BPD with the appearance of a diffuse, fine increase in interstitial markings which may be most easily recognized after 30 days of age (26) (Fig. 5).

Northway and Edwards (11) have listed six radiographic features that are useful in diagnosing BPD: (1) Interstitial predominance, in which the radiographic changes are those of fine, linear densities rather than patchy densities suggesting alveolar disease; (2) lungs tend to be hyperexpanded; (3) abnormalities are diffuse throughout both lungs; (4) the pleura is not recognizably involved; (5) the onset of radiographic changes is gradual; (6) late appearance; the changes of BPD are rarely apparent before 3 weeks of life; and (7) chronicity; the changes of BPD persist from chest radiograph to chest radiograph and are not evanescent. Although atelectasis is a feature of chronic BPD, pleural effusions, adenopathy, and air bronchograms are not features of uncomplicated BPD and their presence should suggest infection or pulmonary edema.

Chest radiography has been demonstrated to underestimate the extent of BPD. When radiographic and pathological staging of BPD was compared (25,34,35), there was agreement in less than half of the cases, and radiographic staging lagged pathological staging in over half.

The differential diagnosis of BPD at 3–4 weeks of postnatal age includes persistent pulmonary interstitial emphysema, certain perinatal acquired viral pneumonitides, and Wilson-Mikity syndrome (7). Radiographically, the late

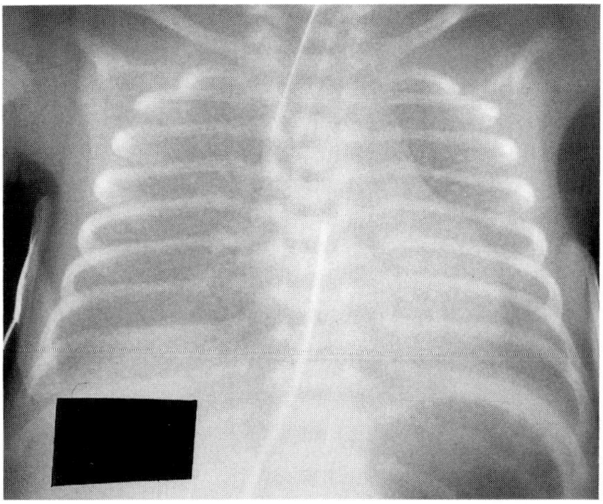

(a)

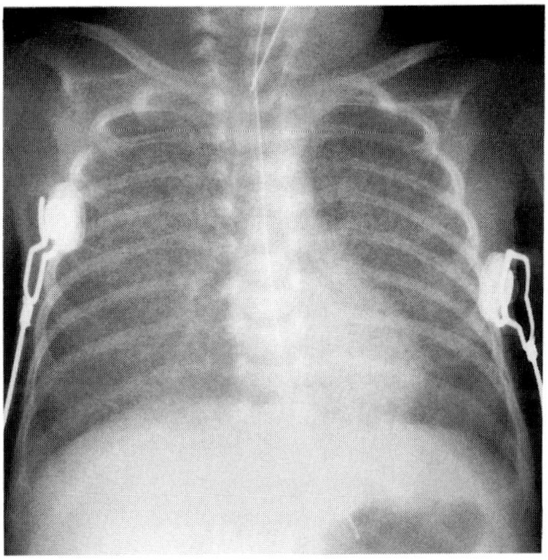

(b)

Figure 5 Very low birth weight prematurely born infant with RDS. (a) The initial chest radiograph shows bilateral granularity and air bronchogram. (b) Same infant on postnatal day 28, following mechanical ventilation and oxygen supplementation. The chest radiograph shows hyperexpansion and hazy pulmonary densities consistent with BPD. (c) Same infant on postnatal day 57, with continuing low concentration oxygen supplementation and more easily recognized fine linear densities in both lungs characteristic of BPD.

(c) 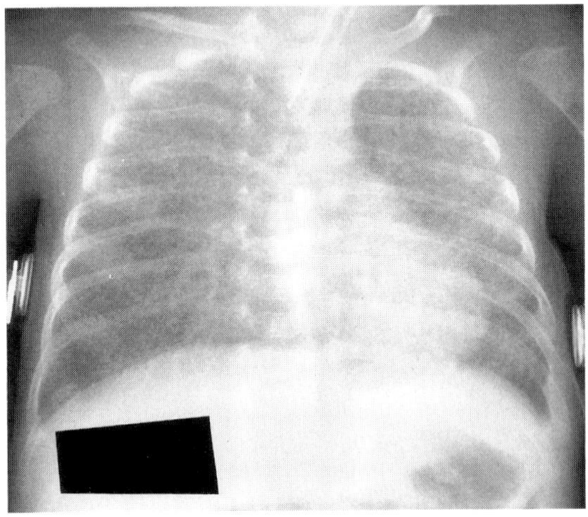

Figure 5 *(Continued)*

appearance of both pulmonary interstitial emphysema and BPD may be indistinguishable. Typically, pulmonary interstitial emphysema occurs early in the course of mechanical ventilation, is usually initially focal, is clearly present within 2 days, and is often associated with a pneumothorax. Any continuously ventilated infant with persistent pulmonary interstitial emphysema at 3 weeks of life undoubtedly also has BPD.

Complications of BPD include segmental and subsegmental areas of atelectasis, episodes of congestive heart failure, pulmonary arterial hypertension, left and right ventricular hypertrophy, systemic hypertension, subglottic stenosis, acquired tracheobronchial malacia, severe osteoporosis and rickets, and rib cage deformity (11).

V. Wilson-Mikity Syndrome

Although the Wilson-Mikity syndrome is much rarer than BPD, the chest radiographic appearance resembles that seen in BPD. The early clinical course and the histopathological findings in Wilson-Mikity syndrome (36,37) and BPD (10,38) are distinctly different. Wilson-Mikity syndrome was originally described in prematurely born infants who required supplemental oxygen support without mechanical ventilation for a few days, following which the infant was clinically normal (36). Respiratory distress ensued from 1 to 5 weeks of age and the chest radiograph revealed a bilateral increase in linear interstitial markings with a cystic-like appearance to the lungs (Fig. 6). In the original report, three of the

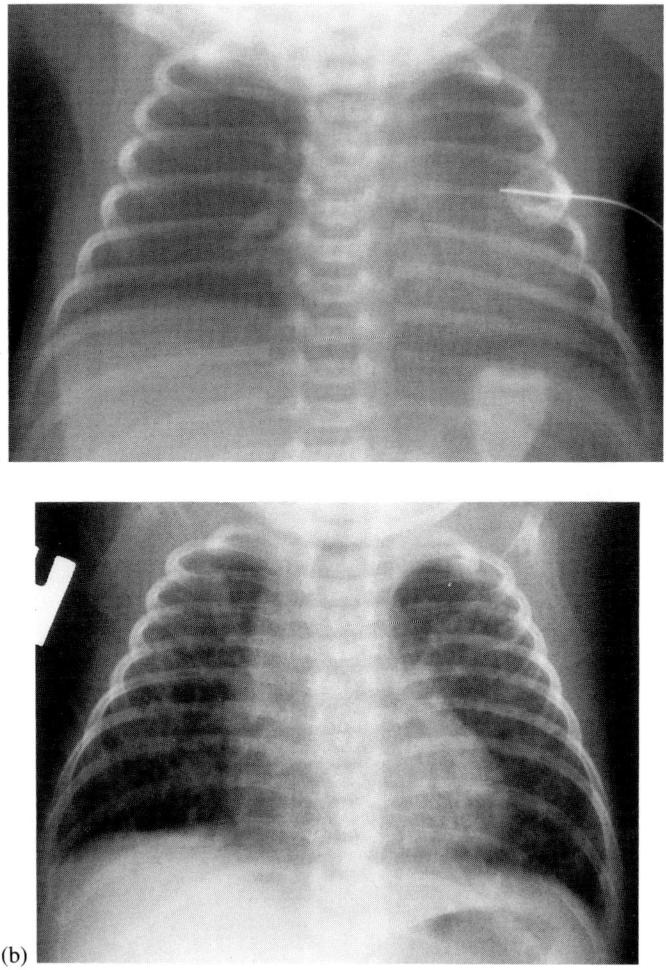

(a)

(b)

Figure 6 Very low birth weight prematurely born infant with neonatal respiratory distress treated with supplemental oxygen by nasal canula. (a) The initial chest radiograph is normal. (b) The infant continued to require supplemental oxygen by nasal canula, but received no mechanical ventilation. At 30 days of age, the chest radiograph shows a bilateral increase in linear markings with a cyst-like appearance to the lungs. The radiographic picture and the clinical setting are consistent with a diagnosis of the Wilson-Mikity syndrome. Because of the prolonged supplemental oxygen therapy, BPD can not be excluded.

five infants with this syndrome died. In a later report, 30% of 34 infants with the syndrome died during the period of severe respiratory distress (37). The lungs of infants with Wilson-Mikity syndrome who were biopsied or expired showed immature parenchyma with areas of atelectasis alternating with regions of overexpansion with few showing any fibrosis (37). These pathological findings contrast significantly with those seen in infants dying with BPD.

Originally, the clinical diagnosis of Wilson-Mikity syndrome was based on the fact that the infant had received little or no mechanical ventilation or supplemental oxygen treatment at birth. This contrasted with the typical patient with BPD, who received prolonged mechanical ventilation and supplemental oxygen therapy. Currently, Wilson-Mikity syndrome is less readily recognized, because many very low birth weight prematurely born infants are treated initially with mechanical ventilation with room air or low concentrations of oxygen for apnea or thoracic and diaphragmatic muscle fatigue. In this setting, the delayed appearance of respiratory distress characteristic of Wilson-Mikity syndrome will not be recognized and the chest radiographic picture of Wilson-Mikity syndrome may be misdiagnosed as BPD. If infants with the Wilson-Mikity syndrome require prolonged mechanical ventilation with increased concentrations of supplemental oxygen for increasing respiratory difficulty, they will eventually develop the pathology and radiographic picture of BPD. The etiology of Wilson-Mikity syndrome has not been identified and, because of the increased utilization of endotracheal intubation, mechanical ventilation, and oxygen supplementation at low levels for infants prone to develop Wilson-Mikity syndrome, further study of this syndrome will be difficult.

VI. Pulmonary Sequelae of BPD

Clinical worsening of the course of infants beyond 30 days of age with established BPD generally occurs in the setting of substantial continuing respiratory insufficiency requiring prolonged endotracheal intubation, oxygenation, and mechanical ventilation. The clinical course is often complicated by acute bouts of respiratory failure and pulmonary infections. Worsening of the chest radiograph reflects the underlying respiratory failure and its complications. Most patients with BPD, however, will show continued slow improvement which eventually leads to discontinuation of mechanical ventilation and supplemental oxygen therapy. The chest radiograph tends to improve slowly over time and has been said to be normal by 2–3 years of age (39). Chronic changes in the chest radiograph which can be seen as late as young adulthood are typically subtle and consist primarily of peribronchial cuffing, focal and diffuse fine linear densities, hyperexpansion, pleural scarring, and occasional pectus carinatum or pectus excavatum deformities (40). Infants with established BPD appear to have more severe and more frequent pneumonias than those survivors of RDS who do not have BPD (41). Infants and children with BPD have an increased risk of respiratory syncytial virus pneumonia (42) and greater severity of infection (43). Infants with established BPD also appear to have an increased frequency of sudden infant death syndrome (44). Infants with BPD and children and young adults with prior BPD are similar to asthmatics in their response to methacholine (40,45) and to bronchodilators (40,46,47) and commonly wheeze with lower respiratory tract infections. Adolescents and young adults with prior BPD may have an increased incidence of pulmonary dysfunction, as measured by pulmonary function testing, when compared with matched prematurely born and normal control populations (40). This dysfunction includes increased airway resistance, airway hyperreactivity, and air trapping. Usually, this pulmonary dysfunction is not severe or symptomatic.

VII. Adult Respiratory Distress Syndrome

A condition that occurs in children which leads to a setting similar to that which predisposes an infant to develop BPD is adult respiratory distress syndrome (ARDS). ARDS may occur in children ranging in age from several weeks to years. Proposed criteria for the diagnosis of this condition are: (1) previously normal lungs; (2) presence of an acute triggering injury or illness; (3) the need for mechanical ventilation with a minimum positive end-expiratory pressure of 6 cmH_2O within 3 days of the triggering event; (4) requirement of continuous positive-pressure ventilation for at least 48 hr, with a fraction of oxygen in the inspired gas of 0.5 for at least 12 hr; and (5) diffuse bilateral air space opacities on chest radiographs during the acute illness (48). This syndrome has occurred in pediatric patients as early as 2 weeks of age (49). Some of the acute diseases associated with ARDS include sepsis, viral pneumonia, smoke inhalation, near drowning, pulmonary contusion, or multiple trauma (50) (see also Chapter 29). Although ARDS is considered a single entity by some investigators (50), it clearly arises from a variety of insults to the lung which produce respiratory failure in the older infant and child. Regardless of the initial insult, the clinical course of ARDS in children follows a typical pattern with four stages: (1) acute injury, (2) latent period, (3) acute respiratory failure, and (4) severe physiological abnormalities, including intractable respiratory failure, metabolic and respiratory acidosis, death, or chronic lung disease requiring prolonged respiratory support (49). Important factors in the outcome of children with ARDS, in addition to the nature of the initial insult, include the late occurrence of multiple organ system failure, secondary infection, and progressive pulmonary dysfunction. Adult survivors of ARDS have a good prognosis for recovery of pulmonary

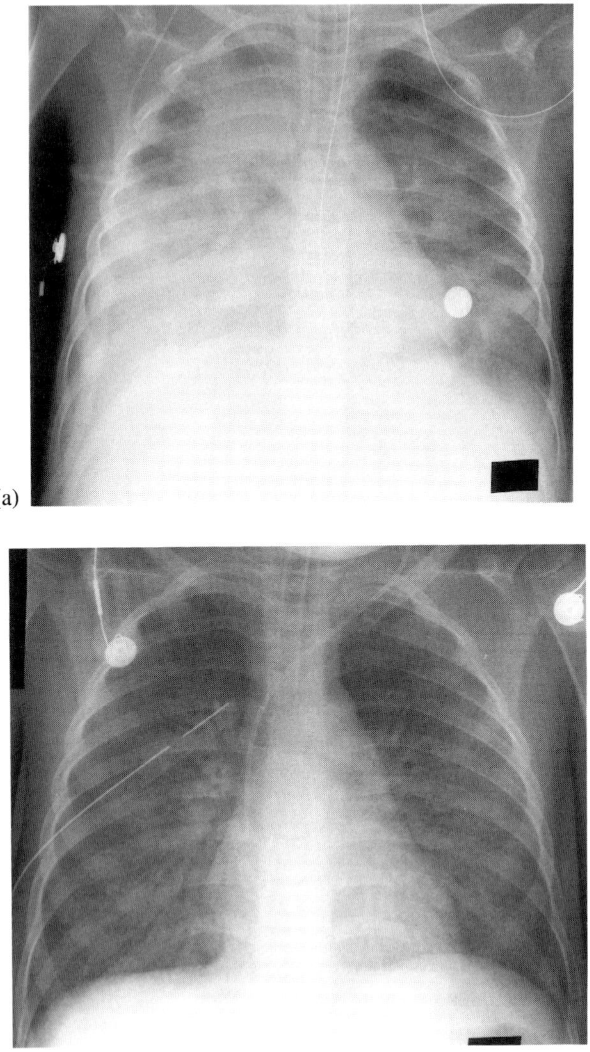

(a)

(b)

Figure 7 Five-year-old girl with nephrosis who developed *Klebsiella pneumoniae* pneumonia. (a) The initial chest radiograph shows bilateral consolidative partial lung opacification greater on the right than on the left. (b) After 5 days of treatment with antibiotics, mechanical ventilation, and supplemental oxygen, the lung consolidation has changed to a fine bilateral granularity with air bronchogram consistent with the diagnosis of ARDS.

function, but it is unclear whether children have a better or worse prognosis than adults in terms of long-term pulmonary sequelae (49).

The pulmonary pathological changes of ARDS are divided into three stages, the early exudative phase seen during the first 96 hr, followed by a cellular proliferative phase during the third to tenth day of illness, and a subsequent fibroproliferative phase (49). The chest radiographic changes mirror the histopathological changes and are modified by the initial illness precipitating the respiratory failure. Diffuse bilateral patchy air space increase in density is usually noted within 24–48 hr of the initiating illness (51). The initial bilateral increase in pulmonary density becomes increasingly diffuse and homogeneously distributed over the first 4 days and frequently resembles the appearance of diffuse granularity and air bronchogram seen in RDS in infants (Fig. 7). The diffuse increase in pulmonary density may partially clear, but the lungs may also become increasingly dense or show a gradual increase in interstitial markings later in the course of the disease (48). Pulmonary interstitial emphysema, pneumothorax, or pneumomediastinum is frequently detected (48,51).

Pulmonary function and radiologic follow-up of children surviving ARDS is limited. In one set of nine children surviving ARDS examined 0.9 to 4.2 years after the acute illness, all patients had pulmonary dysfunction measured by pulmonary function testing (52). Other reports summarizing pulmonary function studies in 58 adult patients surviving ARDS, indicated that approximately 40% had abnormal pulmonary function (53). The pulmonary function changes included mild restrictive impairment, diminished gas transfer, and decreases in arterial oxygenation as well as reactive airways disease which improved following bronchodilator administration. Although late radiological changes that resemble the changes of BPD have been described in adults with ARDS, such late changes have not yet been described in children (54).

VIII. Conclusions

Radiographic examination of the chest has been and will remain an important technique for diagnosing respiratory diseases which may be amenable to treatment by surfactant. Radiographic examination of the chest, including high-resolution computed tomographic scanning, should play an important role in evaluating the short and long-term results of surfactant therapy on the lungs of patients with these diseases (see Chapter 24).

References

1. Behrman RE. The field of neonatal—perinatal medicine and neonatal risks. In: Fanaroff AA, Martin RJ, eds. Neonatal Perinatal Medicine: Disease of the Fetus and Infant. St. Louis: Mosby, 1987:1–7.

2. Avery ME, Merritt TA. Surfactant-replacement therapy. N Engl J Med 1991; 324:910–911.
3. Donald T, Steiner RE. Radiography in the diagnosis of hyaline membrane. Lancet 1953; 2:846–849.
4. Hochheim, K. Über einige Befunde in den Lungen von Neugeborenen und die Beziehung derselben zur Aspiration von Fruchtwasser. Centralbl Pathol 1903; 14:537–538.
5. Curtis P. Hyaline membrane disease. J Pediatr 1957; 51:726–741.
6. Peterson HG Jr, Pendleton ME. Contrasting roentgenographic pulmonary patterns of the hyaline membrane and fetal aspiration syndromes. Am J Roentgenol 1955; 4:800–817.
7. Edwards, DK III. The radiology of bronchopulmonary dysplasia and its complications. In: Merritt TA, Northway WH Jr, Boynton BR, eds. Bronchopulmonary Dysplasia. Boston: Blackwell Scientific, 1988:185–234.
8. Thurlbeck WM. Prematurity and the developing lung. Clin Perinatol 1992; 19:497–519.
9. Wood BP, Davitt MA, Metlay LA. Lung disease in the very immature neonate: Radiographic and microscopic correlation. Pediatr Radiol 1989; 20:33–40.
10. Northway WH Jr, Rosan RC, Porter DY. Pulmonary disease following respiratory therapy of hyaline membrane disease: bronchopulmonary dysplasia. N Engl J Med 1967; 276:357–368.
11. Northway WH Jr, Edwards DK. Bronchopulmonary dysplasia: modern concepts and radiology. Postgrad Radiol 1992; 12:1–24.
12. Northway WH Jr, Petriceks R, Shahinian L Jr. Quantitative aspects of oxygen toxicity in the newborn: inhibition of lung DNA synthesis in the mouse. Pediatrics 1977; 50:67–72.
13. Frank L. Developmental aspects of experimental pulmonary oxygen toxicity. Free Radic Biol Med 1991; 11:463–494.
14. Franks L, Bucher JR, Roberts JR. Oxygen toxicity in neonatal and adult animals of various species. J Appl Physiol 1978; 45:699–704.
15. Nilsson R, Grossmann G, Robertson B. Bronchiolar epithelial lesions induced in the premature rabbit neonate by short periods of artificial ventilation. Acta Pathol Microbiol Scand [A] 1980; 88:359–367.
16. Rhodes PG, Hall TR, Leonidas JC. Chronic pulmonary disease in neonates with assisted ventilation. Pediatrics 1975; 55:788–796.
17. Bomsel F, Couchard M, Polje J, Larroche JC. Pulmonary sequelae of the hyaline membrane disease: iatrogenic factors? Radiological and anatomical study. Ann Radiol 1973; 16:70–74.
18. Pusey VA, MacPherson RI, Chernick V. Pulmonary fibroplasia following prolonged artificial ventilation of newborn infants. Can Med Assoc J 1969; 100:451–457.
19. Barnes ND, Glover WJ, Hull D, Milner AD. Effects of prolonged positive-pressure ventilation in infancy. Lancet 1969; 2:1096–1099.
20. Mayes L, Perkett E, Stahlman MT. Severe bronchopulmonary dysplasia: A retrospective review. Acta Paediatr Scand 1983; 72:225–229.
21. Jentzen J, Rockswold G, Anderson WR. Pulmonary oxygen toxic effect. Occurrence

in a newborn infant despite low PaO_2 due to an intracranial arteriovenous malformation. Arch Pathol Lab Med 1984; 108:334–337.
22. Campognone P, Singer DB. Neonatal sepsis due to nontypable haemophilus influenzae. Am J Dis Child 1986; 140:117–121.
23. Edwards DK. Radiographic aspects of bronchopulmonary dysplasia. J Pediatr 1979; 95:823–829.
24. Chew DTA, Yin ALS. Oxygen therapy and pulmonary fibroplasia: A review and case reports. Med J Malaya 1971; 26:122–128.
25. Oppermann HC, Wille L, Bleyl U, Obladen M. Bronchopulmonary dysplasia in premature infants. A radiological and pathological correlation. Pediatr Radiol 1977; 5:137–141.
26. Edwards DK, Jacob J, Gluck L. The immature lung: Radiographic appearance, course, and complications. Am J Roentgenol 1980; 135:659–666.
27. Loeber NV, Morray JP, Kettrick RG, Downes JJ. Pulmonary function in chronic respiratory failure of infancy. Crit Care Med 1980; 8:596–601.
28. Philip AGS. Oxygen plus pressure plus time: The etiology of bronchopulmonary dysplasia. Pediatrics 1975: 55:44–50.
29. Truog WE, Jackson JC, Badura RJ, et al. Bronchopulmonary dysplasia and pulmonary insufficiency of prematurity. Lack of correlation of outcome with gas exchange abnormalities at one month of life. Am J Dis Child 1985; 139:351–354.
30. Moylan FMB, Walker AM, Krammer SS, et al. Alveolar rupture as an independent predictor of bronchopulmonary dysplasia. Crit Care Med 1978; 6:10–13.
31. Brown ER, Stark A, Sosenki IRS, et al. Bronchopulmonary dysplasia: Possible relationship to pulmonary edema. J Pediatr 1978; 92:982–984.
32. Sawyer MH, Edwards DK, Spector SA. Cytomegalovirus infection and bronchopulmonary dysplasia in premature infants. Am J Dis Child 1987; 141:303–305.
33. Bureau of Maternal and Child Health and Resources Development. Bronchopulmonary dysplasia (BPD). Guidelines for the care of children with chronic lung disease. Pediatr Pulmonol 1989; Suppl 3: 3.
34. Edwards DK, Colby TV, Northway WH Jr. Radiographic-pathologic correlation in bronchopulmonary dysplasia. J Pediatr 1979; 95:834–836.
35. Kwok-Liu JP, Zylak CJ, deSa DJ. Bronchopulmonary dysplasia. A radiologic-pathologic correlation. J Can Assoc Radiol 1980; 31:238–241.
36. Wilson MG, Mikity VG. A new form of respiratory disease in premature infants. Am J Dis Child 1960; 99:489–499.
37. Hodgman JE, Mikity VG, Tatter D, Cleland RS. Chronic respiratory distress in the premature infant. Wilson-Mikity syndrome. Pediatrics 1969; 44:179–195.
38. Bonikos DS, Bensch KG, Northway WH Jr, Edwards DK. Bronchopulmonary dysplasia: the pulmonary pathologic sequel of necrotizing bronchiolitis and pulmonary fibrosis. Hum Pathol 1976; 7:643–666.
39. Mortensson W, Lindroth M. The course of bronchopulmonary dysplasia. A radiographic follow-up. Acta Radiol [Diagn] 1986; 27:19–22.
40. Northway WH Jr, Moss RB, Carlisle KB, et al. Late pulmonary sequelae of bronchopulmonary dysplasia. N Engl J Med 1990; 323:1793–1799.
41. Myers MG, McGuinness GA, Lachenbruch PA, et al. Respiratory illnesses in

survivors of infant respiratory distress syndrome. Am Rev Respir Dis 1986; 133:1011–1018.

42. Groothuis JR, Salbenblatt CK, Lauer BA. Severe respiratory syncytial virus infection in older children. Am J Dis Child 1990 144:346–348.
43. Meert K, Heideman S, Lieh-Lai M. Sarnaik AP. Clinical characteristics of respiratory syncytial virus infections in healthy versus previously compromised host. Pediatr Pulmonol 1989; 7:167–170.
44. Werthammer J, Brown ER, Neff RK, Taeusch HW Jr. Sudden infant death syndrome in infants with bronchopulmonary dysplasia. Pediatrics 1982: 69:301–304.
45. Smythe JA, Tabachnik E, Duncan WJ, et al. Pulmonary function and bronchial hyperreactivity in long-term survivors of bronchopulmonary dysplasia. Pediatrics 1981; 68:336–340.
46. Rooklin AR, Moomjian AS, Shutack JG, et al. Theophylline therapy in bronchopulmonary dysplasia. J Pediatr 1979; 95:882–885.
47. Kao LC, Warburton D, Platzker ACG, Keens TG. Effect of isoproterenol inhalation on airway resistance in chronic bronchopulmonary dysplasia. Pediatrics 1984; 73:509–514.
48. Pfenninger I, Gerber A, Tschäppler H, Zimmerman A. Adult respiratory distress syndrome in children. J Pediatr 1982; 101:352–357.
49. Royall JA, Levin DL. Adult respiratory distress syndrome in pediatric patients: Clinical aspects, pathophysiology, pathology, and mechanisms of lung injury. J Pediatr 1988; 112:169–180.
50. Davis SL, Furman DP, Costarino AT. Adult respiratory distress syndrome in children: associated disease, clinical course, and predictors of death. J Pediatr 1993; 123:35–45.
51. Effmann EL, Merten DF, Kirks DR, et al. Adult respiratory distress syndrome in children. Radiology 1985; 157:69–74.
52. Fanconi S, Kraemer R, Weber J, et al. Long-term sequelae in children surviving adult respiratory distress syndrome. J Pediatr 1985; 106:218–222.
53. Lakshmmarayan S, Hudson LD. Pulmonary function following adult respiratory distress syndrome. Semin Respir Med 1981; 11:160–164.
54. Churg A, Golden J, Fligiel S, Hogg JC. Bronchopulmonary dysplasia in the adult. Am Rev Respir Dis 1983; 127:117–120.

9

The Adult Respiratory Distress Syndrome: Pathophysiological Concepts Related to the Pulmonary Surfactant System

ULRICH PISON, JOHANNES C. BÖCK, SYLVIA PIETSCHMANN, SIEGFRIED VEIT, and KLAUS SLAMA
Universitätsklinikum Rudolf Virchow
Berlin, Germany

I. Introduction

The adult respiratory distress syndrome (ARDS) was first described as a clinical entity by Ashbaugh and colleagues in 1967 (1). ARDS is associated with, or caused by, many risk factors. These factors promote diffuse lung injury either directly (aspiration, toxic inhalation, pulmonary infection, near drowning, lung contusion) or via systemic mechanisms (severe trauma, sepsis, multiple transfusion, fat embolism). Despite the many etiologies, the clinical, pathophysiological, roentgenographic, and histopathological abnormalities in ARDS are quite uniform and resemble those seen in the neonatal respiratory distress syndrome (RDS) that often accompanies preterm birth prior to the maturation of the surfactant system.

The clinical importance of an intact surfactant system was first demonstrated in babies with RDS (2). The surfactant system of these infants is not fully developed, and many of them respond favorably to exogenous surfactants (see Chapters 19 and 20). Alterations of pulmonary surfactant may account also for some of the pathological characteristics in ARDS, including gas exchange disturbance refractory to oxygen therapy, decreased respiratory system compliance, ventilation-perfusion mismatching, lung fluid imbalance, and alveolar host defense deficiencies.

It is striking that advances in intensive care monitoring, ventilator management, and other support systems have not improved the ultimate outcome in patients with ARDS but have frequently increased the time of treatment, perpetuating a series of complications that usually culminate in sepsis and multiple organ failure. In this chapter, we will give a perspective of various concepts regarding the onset and evolution of ARDS, focusing on the available data concerning alterations of the pulmonary surfactant system.

II. Onset and Evolution of ARDS: Surfactant Abnormalities, Lung Edema, Inflammation, Panendothelial Injury and Sepsis, Lung Injury and Repair

A concise definition of ARDS is difficult, since ARDS, although a clinical entity, is not a specific disease. The criteria for diagnosis have been reevaluated recently by the American-European Consensus Conference on ARDS (3) and are summarized in Table 1. According to these criteria, ARDS is acute in onset and characterized by a constellation of clinical, roentgenographic, and physiological abnormalities that cannot be explained by, but may coexist with, left atrial or pulmonary capillary hypertension.

What explains the lung abnormalities in ARDS patients? Today, we believe that ARDS represents a pathophysiological sequence caused by diffuse lung injury and affecting parenchymal, intersititial, vascular, and airway components. However, the concepts explaining the onset and evolution of ARDS have changed over the years. Initial theories emphasized the similarities with neonatal RDS and cardiogenic pulmonary edema (4). A current theory focuses on inflammation, precipitating tissue injury with the lung as primary target (5,6). This theory was extended recently to include panendothelial injury mediated by humoral-cellular interactions at multiple vascular target sites (7), fitting clinical experience of the often multisystemic nature of ARDS with infection, sepsis, and multiple organ failure as the major cause of death (8–11). Finally, new theories about lung injury and repair were developed to explain the pathogenesis of ARDS (12–15). Such theories emphasize the ambivalent, i.e., both beneficial and harmful, nature

Table 1 Criteria for Diagnosis of ARDS

Timing: Acute onset
Oxygenation: $PaO_2/FiO_2 \leq 200$ mmHg (regardless of PEEP)
Chest radiograph: Bilateral infiltrates on frontal chest radiograph
Exclusion of left heart failure: Pulmonary artery occlusion pressure $\leq$18 mmHg when measured or no clinical evidence of left atrial hypertension

of host reactions to ARDS. Pathogenetic inferences from better understood processes, e.g., wound healing, may be applied to the acute and explosive nature so characteristic for ARDS and to the sequences that lead to chronic interstitial lung diseases and to apoptosis in general. Analogy between these processes may point to similarities of the transition between acute and chronic conditions of various organ failures, and to a common intrinsic genetic program that leads to cell death or repair. At present, neither the factors causing transformation from acute to chronic lung injury nor the intensity of the stimuli determining cell death are known.

A. Pulmonary Surfactant Deficiency

Initial theories on the pathogenesis of ARDS emphasized the similarities to neonatal RDS (1). It was speculated that the pulmonary surfactant system may be altered in ARDS as in acute lung failure due to prematurity (2). Indeed, postmortem analysis of lung specimens from ARDS patients revealed some evidence of functional surfactant deficiency (16,17). Difficulties in obtaining surfactant from these patients in vivo made available data incomplete for a long time. Only after bronchoalveolar lavage procedures became more accessible in intensive care units, Hallman et al. (18) demonstrated that surfactant is altered in lung lavage samples that were obtained from ARDS patients in vivo. Studies from our group confirmed their findings (19–21) and were extended recently for some of the surfactant-associated proteins by Gregory et al. (22) and by us (23). The surfactant abnormalities, however, are probably not a primary pathogenic factor in ARDS but another, and very specific, marker of lung injury. Nevertheless, the only therapeutic strategy that undoubtedly improves survival in ARDS at present is mechanical ventilation with a positive end-expiratory pressure (PEEP). Such intervention could be described as a "mechanical" surfactant substitution and points to the relevance of a functioning surfactant system for lung function. Since mechanical ventilation could cause its own complications through hyperoxia and rigid alveolar inflation, appropriate direct forms of surfactant substitution may diminish the hazardous potential of mechanical ventilation and serve as a reasonable strategy for treatment of ARDS, as discussed later in this book (Chapter 28).

B. Pathophysiology of Pulmonary Edema Formation

Acute respiratory failure associated with lung injury was previously known by a variety of names (e.g., traumatic wet lung, shock lung, congestive atelectasis, postperfusion lung, capillary leak syndrome) before it was termed ARDS. Brewer and colleagues (24) described one of the principal symptoms which characterizes ARDS following battlefield trauma as a "wet lung." They speculated that "in the late stages of shock the capillary permeability is increased in nontraumatic regions of the body so that blood plasma escapes into the tissue spaces. That which escapes into the pulmonary alveoli results in the clinical findings of pulmonary edema." Pulmonary edema results from lung liquid imbalances. What causes these imbalances? Starling in 1886 (25) proposed the physiological basis for liquid balance across any semipermeable barrier. Starling's equation predicts that the net flow of liquid across a semipermeable barrier is the product of the driving pressure (net intravascular minus interstitial hydrostatic and osmotic pressure differences, the latter influenced by the osmotic reflection coefficient) and the hydraulic conductance of the barrier. It should be noted that the forces and constants contained in the equation change in both horizontal and vertical directions within the lung and that the constants (reflection coefficient and hydraulic conductance) cannot easily be translated into a physiological system (26). In addition, two important factors that influence lung liquid balance are not or not directly included in the Starling equation: lymphatic function and the intrinsic surface pressure of the alveolar lining fluid (27). Staub and colleagues (28,29) studied lymph flow as a measure for the sequence of pulmonary edema formation. They attempted to simulate ARDS in an animal model in which the caudal mediastinal lymph duct of the sheep was cannulated to obtain lung lymph (30). They described alterations in lymph flow rate and in the concentration and molecular size of its constituent proteins as specific changes in driving pressure or membrane permeability for various experimental situations, assuming that in the steady state the composition of lung lymph is identical to that of the net fluxes of water, electrolytes, and proteins traversing the pulmonary endothelium. In their experimental models of ARDS, pulmonary edema resulted from increased alveolar capillary permeability. However, since the hydraulic conductivity of the capillary membrane includes both permeability as well as surface area over which filtration occurs, changes in lymph flow may not necessarily reflect changes in microvascular permeability. They also demonstrated, in excised dog lungs, a pressure gradient from the lung periphery to the hilum in the loose connective tissue space, which drains fluid from the alveolar wall interstitium (31).

Pulmonary blood flow is not affected by interstitial edema, but is markedly reduced when alveolar flooding occurs, suggesting that alteration of the alveolar epithelial barrier is more relevant for the development of respiratory distress than alteration of the endothelial barrier (32). Taylor and colleagues (26) proposed that ARDS is caused by an initial incidence of alveolar edema along with the formation of ischemic lung areas resulting from the alveolar hypoxic response, followed by subsequent reperfusion of the ischemic areas with ventilation therapy. If repeat cycles of these events occur, the lung will become more and more damaged by the increasing efforts needed to maintain adequate ventilation.

Many of the results from animal studies concerning the formation of pulmonary edema have been used to explain findings in patients with ARDS. Although ARDS can complicate hydrostatic edema and vice versa, pulmonary edema in these patients is not due to volume overload or congestive heart failure but is caused by the disturbance of alveolar capillary permeability (33–39).

In addition to the experimental analysis of factors contributing to pulmonary edema formation, two technologies have been introduced in intensive care medicine for studying critically ill patients at bedside. The introduction of flow-directed pulmonary artery catheters by Swan and colleagues in 1970 (40) allowed bedside monitoring of the hemodynamic status. The thermal-dye dilution technique was adopted for the measurement of extravascular lung water by Lewis and colleagues in 1979 (41) and allowed assessment of pulmonary edema by quantitative means in vivo (42). Measurements of the pulmonary capillary occlusion pressure confirmed that lung edema could be caused by permeability defects or by hydrostatic pressure increase; the latter characterizes congestive heart failure, the former usually accompanies ARDS (43). Measurements of extravascular lung water revealed that the degree of increased lung water content is not directly correlated with the degree of shunt in ARDS as is the case in cardiogenic edema (44,45). It could be misleading, however, if lung perfusion is nonhomogeneous (46) and may be influenced by ventilation distribution. Bedside measurements of hemodynamics and lung water have helped to document the sequence of pulmonary edema formation in ARDS patients and to monitor their therapeutic management during substitution of the intravascular volume and titration of inotropic drugs to maintain appropriate organ perfusion (47–50). In addition, it also became clear that the excess lung water, predominantly caused by altered permeability in ARDS, is not the sole factor responsible for respiratory failure (51).

C. Lung Inflammation and Tissue Injury

Pulmonary edema results from lung liquid imbalance, which is secondary to increased alveolar capillary permeability in ARDS. This, in turn, is part of an inflammatory process which also is the main cause of lung tissue injury. Three basic lines of evidence support this concept: (1) accumulation of inflammatory cells has been demonstrated in lung tissue from patients who dying from ARDS (52,53), and in brochoalveolar lavage fluid from such patients (54,55); (2) inflammatory mediators that are known to attract, or to be released from, inflammatory cells, and cause permeability defects are present in lung wash (56,57) and/or serum obtained from ARDS patients (58,59); and (3) respiratory distress could be produced in animal models mimicking ARDS by intravascular complement activation (60), or by intravenous infusion or intratracheal instillation of a broad spectrum of inflammatory mediators and bacterial toxins (61,62).

We believe that the process of inflammation that leads to lung injury consists of several important events characterized by complex humoral cellular interactions. Initial alterations in plasma or lung fluids may be independent of cells and affect the complement, coagulation/fibrinolysis, and kinin systems. The subsequent cellular responses may involve peripheral (neutrophils, monocytes, platelets) as well as lung resident populations of inflammatory cells (macrophages, lymphocytes), and pulmonary endothelial along with alveolar epithelial cells and interstitial fibroblasts. Cellular events which may play a role in the process that leads to lung injury include the delivery of inflammatory cells to the lung and their retention and migration into the alveolar space and the intra-alveolar release of mediators. Neutrophils have a preeminent, but not exclusive, role in the former (61) and resident macrophages in the latter events (63,64). In this regard, it is important to know that ARDS may be triggered by neutrophil-independent pathways, as in neutropenic patients (65). A conceptual framework of the regulation of the inflammatory process that leads to lung injury has been derived from experimental in vitro data and animal systems and presented recently (5). For a brief overview of this process, see Fig. 1.

Studies were performed in patients who suffered from ARDS and/or sepsis to test whether or not respiratory distress could be influenced by substances that were directed to modulate the inflammatory response. These substances include corticosteroids (68–70), prostaglandin E1 (71), nonsteroidal anti-inflammatory drugs (72–74), and antibodies directed against endotoxin (75,76) or tumor necrosis factor (77–79). None of the studies performed so far conclusively documented improved survival.

The precise sequence of events in the inflammatory response that leads to lung injury is not fully understood and may be different for various ARDS etiologies. It seems clear that ARDS is not caused by a single mediator and that no specific therapeutic drug is available for the disease (80).

D. Panendothelial Injury, Multiple Organ Failure, and Sepsis Syndrome

Advancements in ventilator therapy, extracorporeal lung support systems, fluid management, and the inhalation of nitric oxide effectively reduce the level of intrapulmonary shunting and maintains acceptable pulmonary gas exchange in ARDS but have not been shown in prospective studies to improve survival. Once ARDS develops, patient survival largely depends on whether the clinical course is complicated by extrapulmonary events such as systemic infection with sepsis syndrome and multiple organ failure (8–11,81). The risk of developing these complications increases with time spent on a mechanical ventilator. When ARDS is preceded by sepsis, the abdomen is the predominant site of primary infection, but when sepsis occurs after the onset of ARDS there is usually a pulmonary source (9). These and many other studies document a close interrelation between ARDS, multiple organ failure, and sepsis syndrome.

Since the lung receives the entire cardiac output and provides the first capillary system after the systemic circulation, it may serve as a kind of biological filter for mediators and activated or primed inflammatory cells (e.g., during severe trauma or peritonitis). This predisposes the lung to be the first failing organ following systemic insults. However, when the injurious potential persists, usually caused by uncontrolled infection, then other organs may follow. Especially in trauma patients, the associated multiple organ failure is sequential, starting with respiratory failure in the form of ARDS and continuing with the liver, gastrointestinal tract, and kidney (82). The sequential characteristic of multiple organ failure cannot be detected with certainty in medical patients, since the clinical recognition of ARDS is often considerably delayed in relation to the initial insult. In most of such cases, ARDS follows sepsis and then causes the progressive failure of multiple organs as a result of impaired gas exchange and tissue oxygen delivery. Or ARDS is simply the pulmonary component of a generalized panendothelial response to systemic sepsis, and this response leads to injury not only of the lungs, but also of the gastrointestinal tract, liver, kidneys, central nervous system, and heart (83). In addition, during the late stage of ARDS, metabolic functions of the lung fail and the lung itself releases inflammatory mediators into the systemic circulation, which contribute to multiple organ failure (84). In ARDS, the lungs cannot metabolize biogenic amines, prostaglandins, and vasoactive peptides (85). Such metabolic lung dysfunctions in ARDS can be detected using multiple-indicator dilution techniques and by concentration measurements of selected mediators in blood samples collected at precapillary and postcapillary sites of the lung. Serotonin and prostaglandin E1 have been assessed by the former method (86–88) and angiotensin-1 converting enzyme and endothelin-1 by the latter technique (89,90).

There is good evidence that both lung injury and nonpulmonary organ injury in ARDS are caused by similar mechanisms that often became clinically visible as sepsis syndrome. The clinical term *sepsis syndrome* could be translated at the cellular level as systemic inflammation that causes panendothelial injury, very similar to local lung inflammation that causes alveolar capillary leakage. Although this concept seems to explain the close interrelation between ARDS and multiple organ failure, the flaws of the inflammation theory persist: Because of the ambivalent character of the inflammatory response and the complexity of the networks regulating inflammation, it is not known whether selected events are pathological or homeostatic and directed toward increased injury or toward repair. Thus, beneficial pharmacological modifications of the inflammatory response are not available today. Whether inhaling nitric oxide for the treatment of ARDS (91) or compartmental modifications of the endogenous nitric oxide system during sepsis will reduce mortality remains to be investigated in clinical trials.

E. Mechanisms of Lung Tissue Injury and Repair

Over the last decade, the clinical risk factors for the development of ARDS have been identified (81) and a broad spectrum of mediators shown to be associated

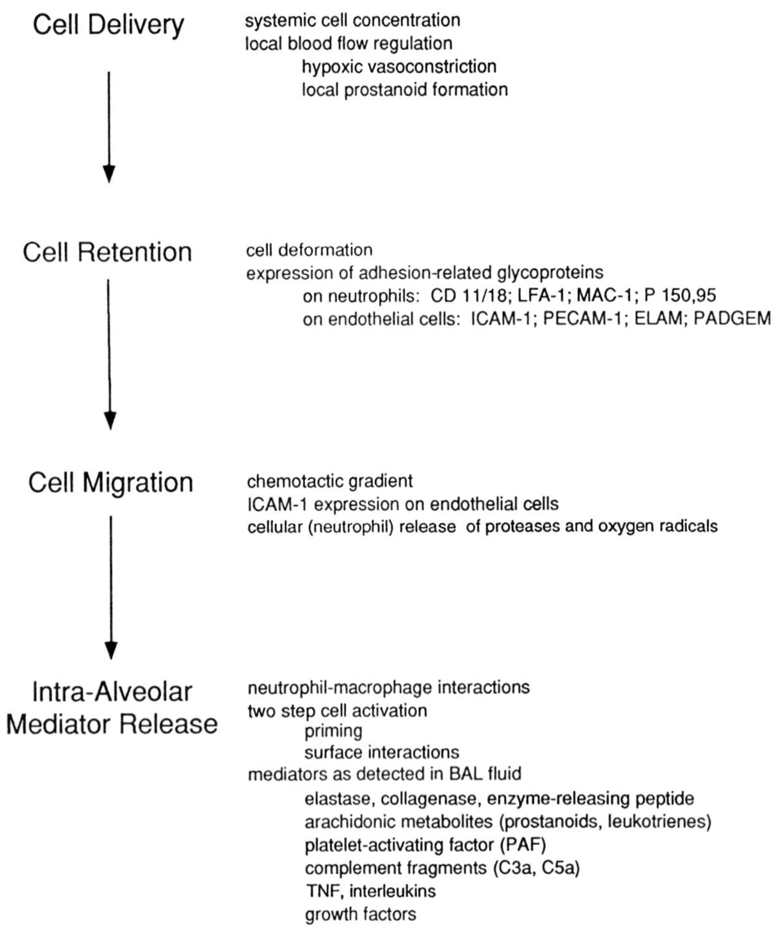

Figure 1

with lung injury (80,84). In contrast, relatively little is known about the lung's reparative mechanisms, although the clinical outcome of acute lung injury is closely related to the ability of the lung to heal. In theory, the speed of lung repair and the prevention of further alveolar damage are likely to contribute to outcome in a given patient. Lung repair depends on the integrity of the alveolar epithelial basement membrane in humans and animals (92–94). Extracorporeal lung support systems (95), new ventilatory strategies (96), and exogenous surfactant substitution for the treatment of ARDS (97) are medical interventions with the potential to optimize gas exchange while minimizing alveolar stretch and pressure that would cause further alveolar damage.

Figure 1 Regulation of peripheral cell (neutrophil) accumulation in the lung and of the injurious potential and mediator secretion in alveoli (according to Parsons et al. [5]). Regulation of neutrophil delivery to the lung depends on the concentration of inflammatory cells in the circulating blood and on local blood flow to the inflammatory site. The lung uses hypoxic vasoconstriction and generates local prostanoid derivatives to control regional blood flow. Regulation of neutrophil retention in lung capillaries includes two basic control mechanisms: The neutrophil must deform in order to transit any capillary and the cell must adhere in order to retain at preferred sites within the lung. Alteration in mechanical properties of the cell to retain in the lung is necessary because the neutrophil has an average diameter of 8 μm, and capillaries an average diameter of only 5.5 μm. The force for neutrophil deformation in lung is the local capillary pressure. Neutrophils deform easily under normal conditions, but became considerably more stiff in response to complement split products like C5a and C5a des arg, tumor necrosis factor (TNF), interleukin-1, and bacterial lipopolysaccarides. Cell adherence is controlled through the expression of adhesion-related glycoproteins in stimulated inflammatory and endothelial cells. Several different adherence glycoproteins have been identified on both the neutrophil and endothelial cell. The major neutrophil complexes include integrins like MAC-1, LFA-1, P150,95, and CD11/18, all of which share a common beta chain. The families of adhesion molecules on the endothelial cell include the cellular adhesion molecule (CAM) members of the immunoglobulin superfamily (intercellular adhesion molecule 1 [ICAM-1] and platelet endothelial cell adhesion molecule 1 [PECAM-1]), and the members of the endothelial-leukocyte adhesion molecule (ELAM) related family (ELAM-1 and platelet activation–dependent granule to external membrane protein [PADGEM]) (66). The regulation of neutrophil migration is different for the different anatomical structures to be passed on the way from the vascular to the alveolar space: Cells must migrate through the vascular endothelium and its basement membrane, the interstitial matrix, and the alveolar epithelium with its basement membrane. Traveling through the vascular endothelium is basically controlled by a gradient of chemoattractants and the upregulation of ICAM-1 in endothelial cells. Migration through the basement membrane and interstitial matrix may require the release of proteases by neutrophils to destroy these anatomic structures. Migration through the alveolar epithelium occurs through intercellular junctions, and this process can apparently occur without any associated epithelial injury. For the regulation of the injurious potential of inflammatory cells it is important to know that enhanced neutrophil retention within the pulmonary capillary bed is not necessarily associated with lung injury (67) and that resident macrophages are usually downregulated to avoid an inflammatory response in the delicate gas exchange region (64). For both cells, however, a multistep activation process through responsive, primed, and fully activated stages have been described. Responsive cells are primed with a distinct first stimulus inducing certain cell capacities, which are executed by a second stimulus leaving the cell fully activated; e.g., to release injurious material. Cell surface interactions modulate secretory events as well. The materials released by inflammatory cells that may be injurious include toxic oxygen metabolites, proteases, lipid mediators such as platelet-activating factor (PAF), prostaglandins and leukotrienes, nitric oxide, growth factors and cytokines, neuropeptides, and cationic proteins. Besides active cell secretion as the process to release this material, passive cell lysis could also contribute to the injurious concentration in alveoli during the course of ARDS.

From morphological studies we know that the high-permeability edema that accompanies ARDS is not simply a capillary leakage, but it more accurately reflects damage to both epithelial and endothelial cells, their respective basement membranes, and the connective tissue (52,98). Damage to the alveolar epithelial barrier and its basement membrane is probably much more relevant for the evolution of respiratory distress than damage to the endothelium, since the integrity of the epithelium (13) and the resolution of alveolar edema (99) are major determinants of lung tissue repair, and alveolar edema and collapse (microatelectasis) more problematic for restoration of lung tissue than interstitial edema alone (32,100).

It is interesting that the basement membrane disruption and the collagen deposition seen in severe ARDS and interstitial pulmonary fibrosis are indistinguishable (94), and the response of the lung to severe injury is very similar to that of other organs. In general: Orderly repair involves the migration and proliferation of viable cells along the preexisting connective tissue scaffolding. As a result, the normal architecture can often be restored when the connective tissue scaffolding is intact, but replacement with disorganized connective tissue elements occurs when the scaffolding is destroyed (101). In addition, rapid healing requires efficient clearance of cellular debris and inflammatory exudate, as well as reepithelialization. Small defects with minimal exudate usually heal rapidly, whereas large tissue defects accumulate abundant exudate, heal slowly, and often result in scarring (13).

Fibroproliferation is a key process after initial lung injury that could lead to either effective or unsuccessful repair. The regulation of the fibroproliferative response has been reviewed recently by Burkhardt (100), Crouch (13), and Marinelli and colleagues (102). We would like to attract the reader's attention to the following hypotheses guiding future research in these area: (1) Fibrosis is, at least at its inception, a repair reaction. (2) The initiation of a distinct genetic program (like in apoptosis), not just the regulation of a solitary gene, determines whether the repair process is effective or unsuccessful. (3) Oncogenes that regulate tumor growth or push cells into a suicidal track may gain importance not only for the biology of cancer but for the pathophysiological sequence underlying ARDS and acute failure of other organs.

III. Pulmonary Surfactant During the Course of ARDS

A. Biochemical Abnormalities of Surfactant in ARDS

Much of the surfactant research has been motivated by the finding of Avery and Mead in 1959 (2) that a deficiency of pulmonary surfactant is the primary cause of neonatal RDS. Evidence is now growing that surfactant is also altered in adult patients with acute respiratory failure.

Early studies addressing this issue showed a decreased total pulmonary phospholipid content (103) and altered surface properties (17) of lung lavage fluid from patients dying from ARDS. One of the most consistent findings in three recent studies using bronchoalveolar lavage (BAL) to obtain alevolar liquid samples during the course of ARDS is the modification of phospholipid composition with decreased relative amounts of phosphatidylcholine (PC) and phosphatidylglycerol (PG) (18,20,22) (Table 2). These biochemical abnormalities correlate with the severity of respiratory failure, suggesting that type II cell metabolic functions are altered in ARDS.

In contrast to the similarities concerning the relative distribution of various phospholipids in these studies, the absolute phospholipid concentrations that may reflect surfactant phospholipid pool size are different. These differences may be in part due to the limitations of the BAL technique and in part to the various isolation and analyzing procedures. As known from other studies using BAL, absolute values for a given substance, e.g., phospholipids, are characterized by a large variability. At least three factors contribute to this variability: (1) variable recovery of lavage fluid; (2) variable total lung area lavaged; and (3) variable contact time between lavage fluid and the lung area lavaged. Some of these problems might be overcome by using a marker substance whose concentration is not influenced by clinical conditions as a denominator in the lavage fluid, or by using ratios of absolute values of different variables (104). In addition, although it seems likely that type II cell alteration accounts for changes of surfactant components in the alveolar compartment, one needs to keep in mind that BAL fluid may be diluted by alveolar edema fluid and be contaminated by phospholipids and proteins from plasma or cells other than type II cells. Differences in absolute amounts of phospholipids may also be due to the variability of isolation procedures used to obtain the surfactant for quantitative measurements. Surfactant exists in many different forms in the alveoli, and these forms have different sedimentation characteristics. Hence, surfactant prepared from whole lung tissue or lung lavage, employing techniques such as centrifugation in aqueous media and extraction using organic solvents, may not reflect the actual alveolar lining material. Various components might be lost, gained, or modified during the preparation procedure. In the studies by Hallman, Pison, and coworkers (18,20,21), lipids were analyzed in the cell-free BAL supernatant, whereas Gregory et al. (22) studied surfactant composition in a BAL pellet obtained after centrifugation at 48,000*g*. The differences in the applied isolation techniques may explain differences in the reported results: unchanged phospholipid concentration in ARDS in the former studies, decreased phospholipid concentration in the latter.

Accurate quantitative measurements of surfactant phospholipid pool sizes in patients are not feasible. The best estimates in this regard come from animal studies using extensive lung lavage procedures, and are about 10–15 mg lipid/kg

Table 2 Phospholipids in ARDS Measured in Three Clinical Studies

	Hallman et al. (18)		Pison et al. (20)			Gregory et al. (22)		
Parameter[a]	normal	ARDS	normal	low ARDS score[b]	high ARDS score[b]	normal	at risk	ARDS
Total PL	0.6 μM	0.6 μM	84 μg/ml	66 μg/ml	65 μg/ml	8.0 μM/ml	3.5 mM/ml	2.5 μM/ml
PC (%)	73	60	63	56	48	76	73	63
PG (%)	12	0.3	10	1.6	1.9	12	7.3	6.5
PI (%)	2.7	3.1	8.3	14	14	3.9	4.7	6.9
PE (%)	2.6	4.3	4.8	14	19	3.3	4.9	5.9
SPH (%)	3.7	17	7.4	12	14	1.5	1.6	5.5

[a]PL, phospholipid; PC, phosphatidylcholine; PG, phosphatidylglycerol; PI, phosphatidylinositol; PE, phosphatidylethanolamine; SPH, sphingomyelin.
[b]The ARDS score used in this study combined separate evaluations of chest radiographs, oxygenation index, pulmonary artery pressures, and respiratory system compliance.

body weight under normal conditions (97). In some animal lung injury models, such as oleic acid infusion (105), bilateral vagotomy (106), N-nitroso-N-methylurethane (107), and 100% oxygen exposure (108), there are either no changes or decreased surfactant pool sizes at peak injury. Other models such as 85% oxygen exposure (109), administration of bleomycin (110), and silica instillation (111) can result in increased pool sizes. The type of injury may influence surfactant phospholipid pool size, although the injury itself may affect the efficiency of lavage.

Quantitative values for the surfactant-associated proteins as measured in BAL are compromised because pulmonary edema may dilute sample volume, but the absolute amounts of these proteins are not influenced by contamination with proteins from other sources, since surfactant proteins are specific for the alveolar epithelium. Therefore, quantitative data concerning the surfactant associated proteins in ARDS might reflect surfactant pool sizes more accurately, and type II cell alterations more specifically, than corresponding data for phospholipids. Gregory and colleagues (22) determined SP-A and SP-B in BAL fluid and found significantly lower concentrations in ARDS patients and patients at risk to develop ARDS as compared with normal individuals. In a study by Pison et al. (23), the SP-A concentrations were significantly different in patients with moderate lung injury compared with patients with severe lung injury and both were lower than normal.

Surfactant alterations depend not only on the severity of respiratory failure, but on the stage of ARDS. Little is known, however, about the sequential changes of surfactant components during the course of ARDS. In a prospective study, surfactant abnormalities were evaluated in lung washes from severely injured patients during the course of posttraumatic pulmonary dysfunction and compared with corresponding data from normal probands (20). Trauma patients were selected because of the homogeneity of the underlying disease and the consistency in time relationship between the insult and the development of respiratory failure in several of these patients. Phospholipid composition was changed dramatically very early after the initial insult. By 6 hr after trauma, mean PG was already decreased from 10 to 3.8% and there was a slight concomitant increase in phosphatidylinositol. By 24 hr after trauma, average PC had decreased from 63 to 58%. During the three stages of respiratory failure, PC and PG varied according to the severity of the disease. In the early stage of respiratory failure (first 2 days after trauma), PC was decreased significantly in patients who had severe, moderate, and mild respiratory failure. In the intermediate stage of respiratory failure (3–6 days after trauma), levels of PC normalized in patients with mild disease but dropped further in patients with severe and moderate respiratory failure. In the late stage of respiratory failure (7–18 days after trauma), PC tended to normalize in patients with moderate respiratory failure, but decreased further in patients with severe respiratory failure (Fig. 2A). PG was decreased in all

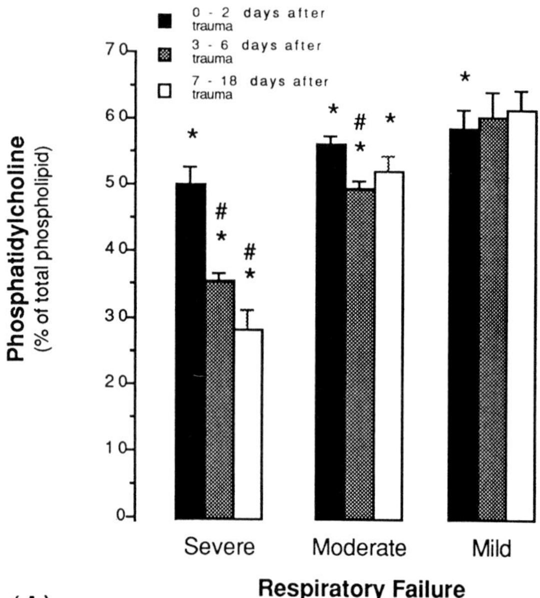
0 - 2 days after trauma
3 - 6 days after trauma
7 - 18 days after trauma
Phosphatidylcholine (% of total phospholipid)
70
60
50
40
30
20
10
0
Severe
Moderate
Mild
Respiratory Failure

(A)

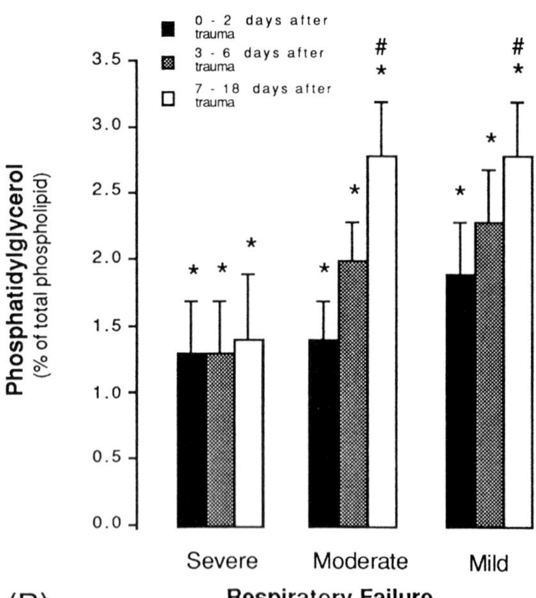
0 - 2 days after trauma
3 - 6 days after trauma
7 - 18 days after trauma
Phosphatidylglycerol (% of total phospholipid)
3.5
3.0
2.5
2.0
1.5
1.0
0.5
0.0
Severe
Moderate
Mild
Respiratory Failure

(B)

patients over the whole observation period, but tended to normalize 7–18 days after trauma in patients who had moderate or mild respiratory failure (Fig. 2B). When septicemia complicated the clinical course of multiple severe trauma patients with acute respiratory failure, the relative amount of alveolar phosphatidylethanolamine (PE) (normally 4.8% of total phospholipids) and alveolar PC (normally 63%) both approached the proportions found in the trachea (PE 33%, PC 36%), suggesting a specific pattern of surfactant alterations during septicemia and probably a decreased surfactant phospholipid pool size (21).

Sequential measurements of SP-A concentration in BAL fluid revealed a normalization for moderate but not for severe lung injury during the transition from early to later stages of the disease (23). However, values for SP-A in BAL fluid do not correlate with changes in phospholipid composition. These data indicate that the metabolic regulation of individual surfactant components might differ during lung injury and repair, as was suggested for bleomycin-induced lung injury in the rat (112). Additional support for this view comes from the observation that, during perinatal lung development and in type II cell in vitro culture systems, surfactant proteins and phospholipids are each influenced by distinct regulatory mechanisms (113). Surfactant protein synthesis is closely linked to the type II cell phenotype (114). Type II cells rapidly lose their phenotypic characteristics during lung injury and repair in vivo (115), and when isolated and cultured in vitro they change their phenotypic characteristics and their ability to synthesize surfactant proteins (116). Proteolysis of surfactant proteins might occur during lung injury (117) and that might also change the immunoreactive concentrations of surfactant proteins in the alveolar space.

In our own studies, the concentration of SP-A was not correlated with lung injury scores calculated for the time point when the individual lung lavage specimens were obtained. This is in contrast to changes in phospholipid composition, especially changes in the relative amount of PC in lung lavage samples, which were inversely correlated to the lung injury scores calculated for the same time point (20,21). This discrepancy is largely due to the tremendous increase of SP-A during the intermediate stage in patients with moderate lung injury (Fig. 3). SP-A measurements in BAL fluid may nevertheless serve as specific marker for the process of lung injury and repair.

Despite the limitations of BAL procedures, the liquid sampled by such

---

Figure 2 Changes in relative amounts of phosphatidylcholine (A) and phosphatidylglycerol (B) in lung lavage samples in relation to time after trauma and severity of lung injury in 30 polytraumatized patients. The control value for phosphatidylcholine in lung lavage sample from 10 healthy subjects was 63 ± 1.1% of total phospholipids. The control value for phosphatidylglycerol was 10 ± 0.7% of total phospholipids. *, significantly different from control ($P < 0.05$); #, significantly different from previous stage ($P < 0.05$) (From ref. 21; used with permission.)

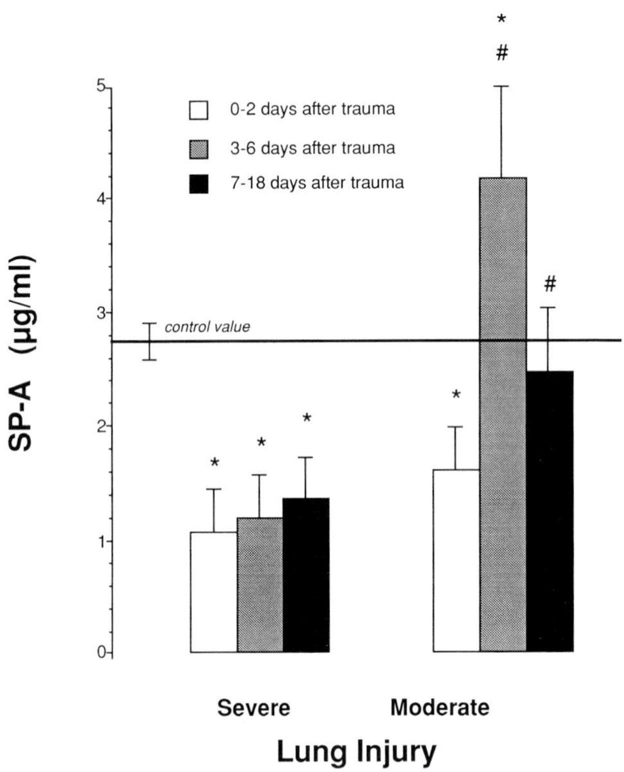

Figure 3 Changes in SP-A concentrations in lung lavage samples in relation to time after trauma and severity of lung injury in 19 polytraumatized patients. The control value for SP-A in lung lavage samples from 10 healthy subjects was 2.7 ± 0.3 μg/ml lavage fluid (dotted line). *, significantly different from control ($P < 0.05$); #, significantly different from previous stage ($P < 0.05$). (From ref. 23; used with permission.)

methods contains the various surfactant components, and its composition in different species is surprisingly similar, varying only during development and parenchymal lung injury. From the reported human data, surfactant compositional abnormalities clearly exist in patients with ARDS and these alterations reflect the severity of respiratory failure and the stage of the disease. Surfactant pool size changes during the course of ARDS have not been demonstrated conclusively.

B. Biophysical Surfactant Abnormalities in ARDS

Pulmonary surfactant exists in many different forms in the alveolar space and the heterogeneity of surfactant structure is clearly relevant to the interpretation of the results of surfactant compositional analysis as outlined above but even more for the explanation of biophysical activity measurements. Massaro and colleagues (118) showed that low volume ventilation without periodic large inflations in rats leads to diminished alveolar stability and to the accumulation of increased amounts of airway disaturated PC in large aggregates that sediment at 1000g; surfactant in this form lowers surface tension less rapidly than surfactant present in the 1000-g supernatant fraction. These findings demonstrate that the mode of ventilation may lead to decreased alveolar stability despite the presence of normal amounts of airway surfactant, and, by inference, indicate that the extracellular form or state of surfactant has an important effect on alveolar stability. These initial findings were extended in rabbits, where lung injury was induced with N-nitroso-N-methylurethane (119,120), and in mice with radiation pneumonitis (121). In the former type of lung injury, the conversion of large to small surfactant aggregate forms is abnormal, and the small and large surfactant aggregates isolated from injured lungs had decreased function compared with aggregates from normal animals. In the latter form of lung injury, the surfactant subtypes are qualitatively normal but their surface activity is impaired, presumably by extraneous material in the alveoli, and proportions of surfactant subtypes are radically altered by a combination of increased synthesis and decreased metabolism of the heavier subtypes.

Petty and coworkers (16) reported alterations in surface activity (expressed as film compressibility) and the density profile of surfactant isolated from one ARDS patient and alterations of surfactant film compressibility in five ARDS patients in a follow-up study (17). In patients with ARDS, surfactant activity has also been assessed in BAL samples obtained during the course of the disease. Hallman and colleagues (18) purified surfactant from BAL samples by sucrose density gradient centrifugation and dissolved the obtained lipid-protein complex in organic solvents before applying it to a surface balance. Pison and coworkers (20,21) used cell-free BAL supernatant, obtained after centrifugation at 180*g* and subsequently concentrated approximately four- to fivefold using positive-pressure ultrafiltration, for surface balance studies. Gregory et al. (22) used a surfactant pellet obtained at 48,000*g*, which was resuspended in saline for pulsating bubble measurements. All studies demonstrated alterations in the biophysical characteristics of surfactant in ARDS, although the parameters assessed were not equally changed (Table 3). These differences are most likely due to variations in the preparation of the surfactant material used for surface tension measurements.

The alteration of surfactant funcion in ARDS may be due to the compositional changes in surfactant as described in the previous section, alterations of the intra-alveolar conversion of surfactant aggregate forms, or by functional inactivation via various inhibitors (Fig. 4). Leakage of plasma proteins into the alveolar space may substantially contribute to the latter mechanism of surfactant

Table 3 Surfactant Activity in ARDS Measured in Four Clinical Studies

Reference	Material	Method	Variable[a]	Change[b]	n[c]
Petty et al. (17)	Lipid-protein complex obtained from postmortem BALF[d]	Surface balance	γ_{min}	Not significant	5
			Film compressibility	↑	
Hallman et al. (18)	Lipid-protein complex obtained from BALF	Surface balance	γ_{min}	↑	26
Pison et al. (20)	Cell-free BALF	Surface balance	γ_{min}	Not significant	17
			Hysteresis	↓	
Gregory et al. (22)	High-speed pellet obtained from BALF	Pulsating bubble surfactometer	γ_{min}	↑	66
			γ_{max}	↑	

[a] γ_{min}, minimum surface tension; γ_{max}, maximum surface tension; hysteresis, area bordered by the compression and the expansion limb in a Wilhelmy balance recording.
[b] Compared with normal.
[c] Number of ARDS patients studied.
[d] BALF, bronchoalveolar lavage fluid.

alteration in ARDS. Among different proteins that are usually elevated in BAL fluid obtained from ARDS patients, albumin (122), hemoglobin (123), and in particular fibrinogen or fibrin monomer (124–126) have strong surfactant inhibitory properties in vitro. The addition of surfactant-associated proteins to various surfactant lipid preparations in vitro increased the resistance of these preparations to plasma protein inhibition, and these findings may have important implications for the formulation of an exogenous surfactant for substitution therapy (127–129). Surfactant can be inhibited not only by plasma derived inhibitors, but also by cell-derived mediators: proteolytic enzymes (117,130), reactive oxygen metabolites (108,131,132), nitrogen radicals (133), and phospholipases (134). Furthermore, incorporation of surfactant phospholipids in fibrin strands has been recently demonstrated in vitro and this phenomenon may cause severe loss of functionally important surfactant in areas with hyaline membrane formation (135). (For a more detailed discussion of various mechanisms involved in surfactant inactivation, see Chapter 13.)

C. Metabolic and Genetic Aspects of the Surfactant System in ARDS

As predicted and confirmed by several studies, the chemical composition and functional activity of endogenous surfactant sampled by BAL is impaired in ARDS. Some studies reported time-dependent changes for phospholipids and for SP-A. From animal studies we know that the intra-alveolar conversion of surfactant forms is altered. Data from clinical and experimental studies furthermore indicate that metabolic functions of alveolar type II cells are changed in acute lung injury. To determine if such changes occur already on the pretranslational level, we measured mRNA for the surfactant-associated proteins in sheep wih unilateral lung injury (136). We induced lung injury with vaporized HCl (0.15 M) inhaled for 4 hr into one lung using a double-lumen tube. In the control group, 0.9% NaCl was used instead of hydrochloric acid. We obtained biopsies from both lungs of several sheep, isolated total RNA, and measured mRNA levels for surfactant proteins by Northern blot analysis using cDNA probes for human SP-A, SP-B and SP-C. All hybridization data were normalized to signals found with cDNA probes for β-actin and glyceraldehyde-3-phosphate dehydrogenase (G3PDH) which are constitutively expressed. We found in all animals after 4 hr of HCl inhalation decreased levels of mRNA encoding SP-A, SP-B, and SP-C on the injured lung side. No side differences were observed in the control group. Transcript abundance for β-actin and G3PDH was identical on both injured and normal lungs, indicating that the decrease of surfactant protein mRNA in injured lungs was not due to acid-related mRNA instability. Our results show alterations for surfactant proteins on the pretranslational level and are consistent with data of previous studies, in which

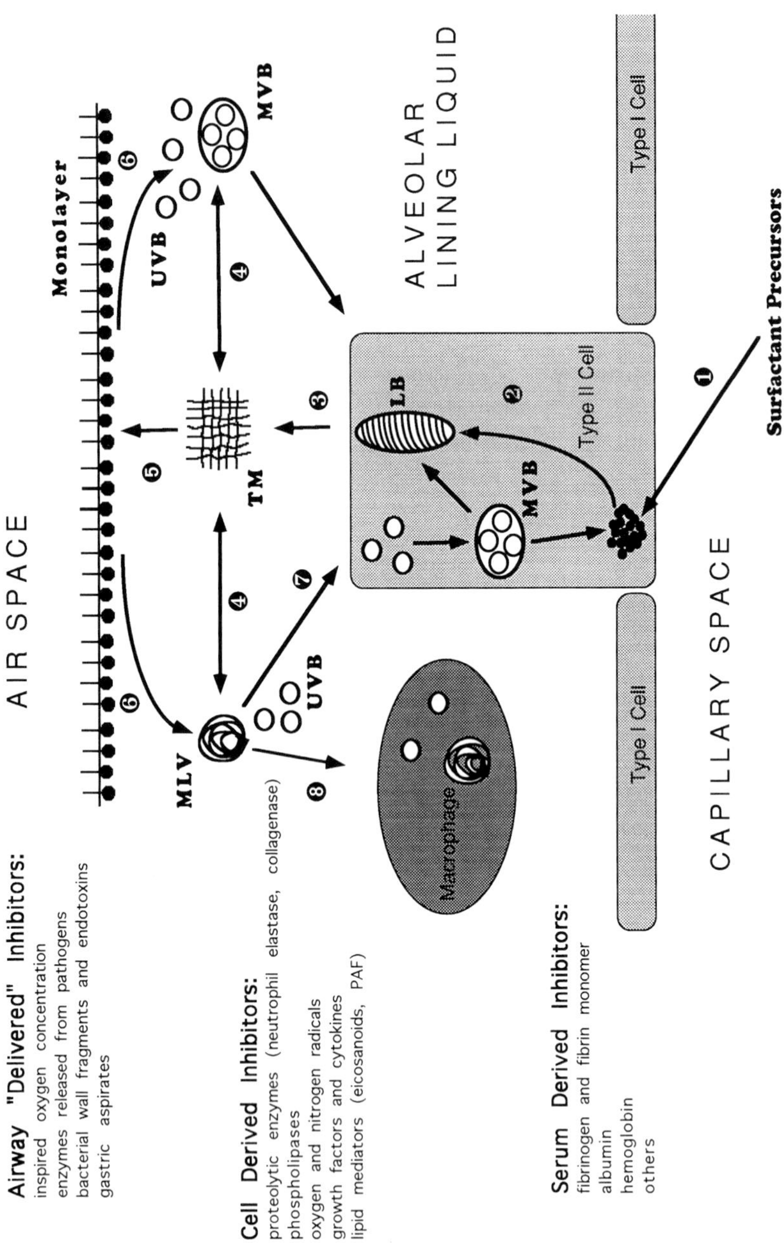

AIR SPACE
Monolayer
MLV
UVB
TM
MVB
LB
Type II Cell
Type I Cell
Macrophage
ALVEOLAR LINING LIQUID
CAPILLARY SPACE
Surfactant Precursors
Airway "Delivered" Inhibitors:
inspired oxygen concentration
enzymes released from pathogens
bacterial wall fragments and endotoxins
gastric aspirates
Cell Derived Inhibitors:
proteolytic enzymes (neutrophil elastase, collagenase)
phospholipases
oxygen and nitrogen radicals
growth factors and cytokines
lipid mediators (eicosanoids, PAF)
Serum Derived Inhibitors:
fibrinogen and fibrin monomer
albumin
hemoglobin
others

Figure 4

decreased amounts of SP-A and SP-B were found in BAL fluid from ARDS patients (22,23). As type II cells rapidly lose their phenotypic characteristics during lung injury and repair in vivo, we suggest that such phenotypic change is associated with decreased surfactant protein expression occurring already 4 hr after the initial insult.

Little is known about the influence of cytokines, generated during lung injury, on surfactant metabolism. Interferon-γ has a selective stimulatory effect on the synthesis of SP-A in fetal lung epithelial explants (137).

We know virtually nothing about the distribution of allelic variants of the genes encoding surfactant proteins in populations of ARDS patients. The heterogeneity of allelic variants of the 6A gene locus for human surfactant protein A was recently analyzed among white adults and infants with RDS and in black adults. Although the data did not reach statistical significance, the 6A/6A genotype tended to appear with higher frequency in blacks (138) (see also Chapter 5).

IV. Conclusions

ARDS is a multifaceted disease with high mortality. It can be initiated through various causes and the pathophysiological sequence of ARDS has been partially elucidated using different concepts.

Many markers of lung injury exist but it does not seem reasonable to search for a single pathogenic factor in ARDS. Alterations of the surfactant system as determined in BAL samples occur very early after the initial insult and changes in the amount of surfactant-associated proteins are probably the most specific

Figure 4 Cartoon of the life cycle of surfactant and various inhibitors of surfactant function. Abbreviations: LB, lamellar bodies; MLV, multi-lamellar vesicles; MVB, multi-vesicular bodies; TM, tubular myelin; UVB, univesicular bodies. (**1**) Surfactant precursors (amino acids, carbohydrates, fatty acids) move from the vasculature into type II cells, which synthesize the various surfactant components. (**2**) Newly synthesized or recycled surfactant is stored in LB. (**3**) Type II cells secrete surfactant as LB. Conversion of LB to TM may be triggered by calcium. (**4**) In the alveolar lining fluid TM can convert to MLV and vice versa. (**5**) From TM phospholipids adsorb to the air-liquid interface, generating a monolayer. (**6**) Surfactant squeezed out of the surface monolayer during expiration can be stored as MLV or UVB. (**7**) Reuptake of MLV and UVB surfactant structures by type II cells, a process which is mediated through SP-A. About 80% of the secreted surfactant will follow this pathway. (**8**) Phagocytosis of MLV and UVB surfactant structures by macrophages. Aboout 15% of the secreted surfactant will follow this pathway, the rest is cleared by the airways. Surfactant inhibitors can be "delivered" through the airways, or derived from inflammatory cells or serum. They can affect various steps of the life-cycle of surfactant, ultimately destroying the biological function of surfactant.

markers for lung injury today. Allelic variations exist for the genes coding for surfactant proteins and may determine outcome after lung injury. This hypothesis is presently under investigation.

Host responses after initial lung injury are ambivalent and may trigger both increased lung injury and repair. We do not know what causes the transformation from acute to chronic lung injury, but sequential SP-A measurements in BAL may serve as a specific marker to monitor the process of lung injury and repair. Whether distinct genetic programs determine the effectiveness of the repair process remains to be shown.

New therapeutic approaches for ARDS should aim at minimizing the hazardous potential of present medical interventions. Successful therapeutic strategies for ARDS should accelerate lung repair and prevent further alveolar damage. Surfactant therapy for ARDS has the potential to reduce lung lesions induced by mechanical ventilation. Whether specific therapies are applicable to different lung compartments, ARDS states, and etiologies awaits future studies.

References

1. Ashbaugh DG, Bigelow DB, Petty TL, Levine BE. Acute respiratory distress in adults. Lancet 1967; 2:319–323.
2. Avery ME, Mead J. Surface properties in relation to atelectasis and hyaline membrane disease. Am J Dis Child 1959; 97:517–523.
3. Bernard GR, Artigas A, Brigham KL, et al. The American-European consensus conference on ARDS. Definitions, mechanisms, relevant outcome, and clinical trial coordination. Am J Respir Crit Care Med 1994; 149:818–824.
4. Petty TL, Ashbaugh DG. The adult respiratory distress syndrome. Clinical features, factors influencing prognosis and principles of management. Chest 1971; 60:233–239.
5. Parsons PE, Worthen GS, Henson PM. Injury from inflammatory cells. In: Crystal RG, West JB, eds. The Lung, Scientific Foundation. New York: Raven Press, 1991:1981–1992.
6. Reynolds HY. Lung inflammation: normal host defense or a complication of some diseases? Annu Rev Med 1987; 38:295–323.
7. Heyman SJ, Rinaldo JE. Multiple system organ failure in the adult respiratory distress syndrome. J Int Care Med 1989; 4:192–200.
8. Bell RC, Coalson JJ, Smith JD, Johanson W Jr. Multiple organ system failure and infection in adult respiratory distress syndrome. Ann Intern Med 1983; 99:293–298.
9. Montgomery AB, Stager MA, Carrico CJ, Hudson LD. Causes of mortality in patients with the adult respiratory distress syndrome. Am Rev Respir Dis 1985; 132:485–489.
10. Seidenfeld JJ, Pohl DF, Bell RC, et al. Incidence, site, and outcome of infections in patients with the adult respiratory distress syndrome. Am Rev Respir Dis 1986; 134:12–16.

11. Bone RC, Balk R, Slotman G, et al. Adult respiratory distress syndrome. Sequence and importance of development of multiple organ failure. Chest 1992; 101:320–326.
12. Bitterman PB. Pathogenesis of fibrosis in acute lung injury. Am J Med 1992; 92:39S–43S.
13. Crouch E. Pathobiology of pulmonary fibrosis. Am. J. Physiol 1990; 259:L159–L184.
14. Cerra FB. Multiple organ failure syndrome. Disease of the Month 1992; 38:843–847.
15. Rinaldo JE, Rogers RM. Adult respiratory-distress syndrome: Changing concepts of lung injury and repair. N Engl J Med 1982; 306:900–909.
16. Petty TL, Reiss OK, Paul GW, et al. Characteristics of pulmonary surfactant in adult respiratory distress syndrome associated with trauma and shock. Am Rev Respir Dis 1977; 115:531–536.
17. Petty TL, Silvers GW, Paul GW, Stanford RE. Abnormalities in lung elastic properties and surfactant function in adult respiratory distress syndrome. Chest 1979; 75:571–574.
18. Hallman M, Spragg R, Harrell JH, et al. Evidence of lung surfactant abnormality in respiratory failure. Study of bronchoalveolar lavage phospholipids, surface activity, phospholipase activity, and plasma myoinositol. J Clin Invest 1982; 70:673–683.
19. Pison U, Gono E, Joka T, Obertacke U. Phospholipid lung profile in adult respiratory distress syndrome—Evidence for surfactant abnormality. Prog Clin Biol Res 1987; 236A:517–523.
20. Pison U, Seeger W, Buchhorn R, et al. Surfactant abnormalities in patients with respiratory failure after multiple trauma. Am Rev Respir Dis 1989; 140:1033–1039.
21. Pison U, Obertacke U, Brand M, et al. Altered pulmonary surfactant in uncomplicated and septicemia-complicated courses of acute respiratory failure. J Trauma 1990; 30:19–26.
22. Gregory TJ, Longmore WJ, Moxley MA, et al. Surfactant chemical composition and biophysical activity in acute respiratory distress syndrome. J Clin Invest 1991; 88:1976–1981.
23. Pison U, Obertacke U, Seeger W, Hawgood S. Surfactant protein A (SP-A) is decreased in acute parenchymal lung injury associated with polytrauma. Eur J Clin Invest 1992; 22:712–718.
24. Brewer LA, Burbank B, Samson PC, Schiff CA. The "wet lung" in war casualties. Ann Surg 1946; 123:343–362.
25. Starling EH. On the absorption of fluids from the connective tissue spaces. J Physiol 1886; 19:312–326.
26. Taylor AE, Barnard JW, Barman SA, Adkins WK. Fluid balance. In: Crystal RG, West JB, eds. The Lung, Scientific Foundation. New York: Raven Press, 1991:1147–1161.
27. Clements JA. Pulmonary edema and permeability of alveolar membranes. Arch Environ Health 1961; 2:280–283.
28. Staub NC. The pathogenesis of pulmonary edema. In: Staub NC, and Taylor AE, eds. Edema. New York: Raven Press, 1984:719–786.
29. Staub NC. New concepts about the pathophysiology of pulmonary edema. J Thorac Imaging 1988; 3:8–14.

30. Staub NC, Bland RD, Brigham KL, et al. Preparation of chronic lung lymph fistulas in sheep. J Surg Res 1975; 19:315–320.
31. Bhattacharya J, Staub NC. Direct measurement of microvascular pressures in the isolated perfused dog lung. Science 1980; 210:327–328.
32. Bhattacharya J, Nakahara K, Staub NC. Effect of edema on pulmonary blood flow in the isolated perfused dog lung lobe. J Appl Physiol 1980; 48:444–449.
33. Anderson RR, Holliday RL, Driedger AA, et al. Documentation of pulmonary capillary permeability in the adult respiratory distress syndrome accompanying human sepsis. Am Rev Respir Dis 1979; 119:869–877.
34. Braude S, Nolop KB, Hughes JM, et al. Comparison of lung vascular and epithelial permeability indices in the adult respiratory distress syndrome. Am Rev Respir Dis 1986; 133:1002–1005.
35. Calandrino F Jr, Anderson DJ, Mintun MA, Schuster DP. Pulmonary vascular permeability during the adult respiratory distress syndrome: A positron emission tomographic study. Am Rev Respir Dis 1988; 138:421–428.
36. Fein A, Wiener-Kronish JP, Niederman M, Matthay MA. Pathophysiology of the adult respiratory distress syndrome. What have we learned from human studies? Crit Care Clin 1986; 2:429–453.
37. Holter JF, Weiland JE, Pacht ER, et al. Protein permeability in the adult respiratory distress syndrome. Loss of size selectivity of the alveolar epithelium. J Clin Invest 1986; 78:1513–1522.
38. Rinaldo JE, Borovetz HS, Mancini MC, et al. Assessment of lung injury in the adult respiratory distress syndrome using multiple indicator dilution curves. Am Rev Respir Dis 1986; 133:1006–1010.
39. Sprung CL, Long WM, Marcial EH, et al. Distribution of proteins in pulmonary edema. The value of fractional concentrations. Am Rev Respir Dis 1987; 136:957–963.
40. Swan HJC, Ganz W, Forrester J, et al. Catheterization of the heart in man with use of a flow-directed balloon-tipped catheter. N Engl J Med 1970; 283:447–451.
41. Lewis FR, Elings VB, Sturm JA. Bedside measurement of extravascular lung water. J Surg Res 1979; 27:250–261.
42. Böck JC, Lewis FR. Clinical relevance of lung water measurement with the thermal-dye dilution technique. J Surg Res 1990; 48:254–265.
43. Unger KM, Shibel EM, Moser KM. Detection of left ventricular failure in patients with adult respiratory distress syndrome. Chest 1975; 67:8–13.
44. Breen PH, Schumacker PT, Sandoval J, et al. Increased cardiac output increases shunt: Role of pulmonary edema and perfusion. J Appl Physiol 1985; 59:1313–1321.
45. Lava J, Rice CL, Moss GS, et al. Pulmonary dysfunction in sepsis: Is pulmonary edema the culprit? J Trauma 1982; 22:280–284.
46. Allison RC, Carlile PJ, Gray BA. Thermodilution measurement of lung water. Clin Chest Med 1985; 6:439–457.
47. Dantzker DR, Lynch JP, Weg JG. Depression of cardiac output is a mechanism of shunt reduction in the therapy of acute respiratory failure. Chest 1980; 77:636–642.
48. Prewitt RM. Hemodynamic management in pulmonary embolism and acute hypoxemic respiratory failure. Crit Care Med 1990; 18:S61–S69.
49. Eisenberg PR, Hansbrough JR, Anderson D, Schuster DP. A prospective study of

lung water measurements during patient management in an intensive care unit. Am Rev Respir Dis 1987; 136:662–668.

50. Mitchell JP, Schuller D, Calandrino FS, Schuster DP. Improved outcome based on fluid management in critically ill patients requiring pulmonary artery catheterization. Am Rev Respir Dis 1992; 145:990–998.
51. Esbenshade AM, Newman JH, Lams PM, et al. Respiratory failure after endotoxin infusion in sheep: Lung mechanics and lung fluid balance. J Appl Physiol 1982; 53:967–976.
52. Bachofen A, Weibel ER. Alterations of the gas exchange apparatus in adult respiratory insufficiency associated with septicemia. Am Rev Respir Dis 1977; 116:589–615.
53. Tomashefski J Jr. Pulmonary pathology of the adult respiratory distress syndrome. Clin Chest Med 1990; 11:593–619.
54. Pison U, Brand M, Joka T. et al. Distribution and function of alveolar cells in multiply injured patients with trauma-induced ARDS. Intensive Care Med 1988; 14:602–609.
55. Weiland JE, Davis WB, Holter JF, et al. Lung neutrophils in the adult respiratory distress syndrome. Clinical and pathophysiologic significance. Am Rev Respir Dis 1986; 133:218–225.
56. Lee CT, Fein AM, Lippmann M, et al. Elastolytic activity in pulmonary lavage fluid from patients with adult respiratory-distress syndrome. N Engl J Med 1981; 304:192–196.
57. Fowler AA, Hyers TM, Fisher BJ, et al. The adult respiratory distress syndrome. Cell populations and soluble mediators in the air spaces of patients at high risk. Am Rev Respir Dis 1987; 136:1225–1231.
58. Duchateau J, Haas M, Schreyen H, et al. Complement activation in patients at risk of developing the adult respiratory distress syndrome. Am Rev Respir Dis 1984; 130:1058–1064.
59. Parsons PE, Worthen GS, Moore EE, et al. The association of circulating endotoxin with the development of the adult respiratory distress syndrome. Am Rev Respir Dis 1989; 140:294–301.
60. Ward PA, Johnson KJ, Till GO. Complement and experimental respiratory failure. Intensive Care Med 1986; 12:17–21.
61. Tate RM, Repine JE. Neutrophils and the adult respiratory distress syndrome. Am Rev Respir Dis 1983; 128:552–559.
62. Spragg RG, Smith RM. Biology of acute lung injury. In: Crystal RG, West JB, eds. The Lung, Scientific Foundation. New York: Raven Press, 1991; 2003–2017.
63. Jacobs RF, Kiel DP, Balk RA. Alveolar macrophage function in a canine model of endotoxin-induced lung injury. Am Rev Respir Dis 1986; 134:745–751.
64. Nathan C. Mechanisms and modulation of macrophage activation. Behring Inst Mitt 1991; 88:200–207.
65. Braude S, Apperley J, Krausz T, et al. Adult respiratory distress syndrome after allogeneic bone-marrow transplantation: Evidence for a neutrophil-independent mechanism. Lancet 1985; 1:1239–1242.
66. Pilewski, JM, Albelda SM. Adhesion molecules in the lung. An overview. Am Rev Respir Dis 1993; 148:S31–S37.

67. Webster RO, Larsen GL, Mitchell BC, et al. Absence of inflammatory lung injury in rabbits challenged intravascularly with complement-derived chemotactic factors. Am Rev Respir Dis 1982; 125:335–340.
68. Bernard GR, Luce JM, Sprung CL, et al. High-dose corticosteroids in patients with the adult respiratory distress syndrome. N Engl J Med 1987; 317:1565–1570.
69. Bone RC, Fisher CJ, Clemmer TP, et al. A controlled clinical trial of high-dose methylprednisolone in the treatment of severe sepsis and septic shock. N Engl J Med 1987; 317:653–658.
70. Luce JM, Montgomery AB, Marks JD, et al. Ineffectiveness of high-dose methylprednisolone in preventing parenchymal lung injury and improving mortality in patients with septic shock. Am Rev Respir Dis 1988; 138:62–68.
71. Bone RC, Slotman G, Maunder R, et al. Randomized double-blind, multicenter study of prostaglandin E1 in patients with the adult respiratory distress syndrome. Chest 1989; 96:114–119.
72. Steinberg SM, Rodriguez JL, Bitzer LG, et al. Indomethacin treatment of human adult respiratory distress syndrome. Circ Shock 1990; 30:375–384.
73. Bernard GR. N-acetylcysteine in experimental and clinical acute lung injury. Am J Med 1991; 91:54S–59S.
74. Bernard GR, Reines HD, Halushka PV, et al. Prostacyclin and thromboxane A2 formation is increased in human sepsis syndrome. Effects of cyclooxygenase inhibition. Am Rev Respir Dis 1991; 144:1095–1101.
75. Luce JM. Introduction of new technology into critical care practice: a history of HA-1A human monoclonal antibody against endotoxin. Crit Care Med 1993; 21:1233–1241.
76. Ziegler EJ, Fisher CJ, Sprung CL, et al. Treatment of gram-negative bacteremia and septic shock with HA-1A human monoclonal antibody against endotoxin. A randomized, double-blind, placebo-controlled trial. N Engl J Med 1991; 324:429–436.
77. Martin RA, Silva AT, Cohen J. Effect of anti–TNF-alpha treatment in an antibiotic treated murine model of shock due to Streptococcus pyogenes. FEMS Microbiol Lett 1993; 110:175–178.
78. Fisher CJ, Opal SM, Dhainaut JF, et al. Influence of an anti-tumor necrosis factor monoclonal antibody on cytokine levels in patients with sepsis. Crit Care Med 1993; 21:318–327.
79. Hinshaw LB, Emerson TJ, Taylor FJ, et al. Lethal Staphylococcus aureus–induced shock in primates: Prevention of death with anti-TNF antibody. J Trauma 1992; 33:568–573.
80. Rinaldo JE, Christman JW. Mechanisms and mediators of the adult respiratory distress syndrome. Clin Chest Med 1990; 11:621–632.
81. Fowler AA, Hamman RF, Good JT, et al. Adult respiratory distress syndrome: Risk with common predispositions. Ann Intern Med 1983; 98:593–597.
82. Fry DE, Pearlstein L, Fulton RL, Polk HJ. Multiple system organ failure. The role of uncontrolled infection. Arch Surg 1980; 115:136–140.
83. Niederman MS, Fein AM. Sepsis syndrome, the adult respiratory distress syndrome, and nosocomial pneumonia. A common clinical sequence. Clin Chest Med 1990; 11:633–656.
84. Demling RH. The role of mediators in human ARDS. J Crit Care 1989; 3:56–72.

85. Wiedemann HP, Matthay MA, Gillis CN. Pulmonary endothelial cell injury and altered lung metabolic function. Early detection of the adult respiratory distress syndrome and possible functional significance. Clin Chest Med 1990; 11:723–736.
86. Cox JW, Andreadis NA, Bone RC, et al. Pulmonary extraction and pharmacokinetics of prostaglandin E1 during continuous intravenous infusion in patients with adult respiratory distress syndrome. Am Rev Respir Dis 1988; 137:5–12.
87. Gillis CN, Pitt BR, Wiedemann HP, Hammond GL. Depressed prostaglandin E1 and 5-hydroxytryptamine removal in patients with adult respiratory distress syndrome. Am Rev Respir Dis 1986; 134:739–744.
88. Morel DR, Dargent F, Bachmann M, et al. Pulmonary extraction of serotonin and propranolol in patients with adult respiratory distress syndrome. Am Rev Respir Dis 1985; 132:479–484.
89. Johnson AR, Coalson JJ, Ashton J, et al. Neutral endopeptidase in serum samples from patients with adult respiratory distress syndrome. Comparison with angiotensin-converting enzyme. Am Rev Respir Dis 1985; 132:1262–1267.
90. Druml W, Stelzer H, Waldhäusl W, et al. Endothelin-1 in adult respiratory distress syndrome. Am Rev Respir Dis 1993; 148:1169–1173.
91. Rossaint R, Falke KJ, Lopez F, et al. Inhaled nitric oxide for the adult respiratory distress syndrome. N Engl J Med 1993; 328:399–405.
92. Fukuda Y, Ishizaki M, Masuda Y, et al. The role of intraalveolar fibrosis in the process of pulmonary structural remodeling in patients with diffuse alveolar damage. Am J Pathol 1987; 126:171–182.
93. Rennard SI, Bitterman PB, Crystal RG. Response of the lower respiratory tract to injury. Mechanisms of repair of the parenchymal cells of the alveolar wall. Chest 1983; 84:735–739.
94. Raghu G, Striker LJ, Hudson LD, Striker GE. Extracellular matrix in normal and fibrotic human lungs. Am Rev Respir Dis 1985; 131:281–289.
95. Gattinoni L, Pesenti A, Kolobow T, Damia G. A new look at therapy of the adult respiratory distress syndrome: motionless lungs. Int Anesthesiol Clin 1983; 21:97–117.
96. Marini JJ, Kelsen SG. Re-targeting ventilatory objectives in adult respiratory distress syndrome. New treatment prospects—Persistent questions. Am Rev Respir Dis 1992; 146:2–3.
97. Lewis JF, Jobe AH. Surfactant and the adult respiratory distress syndrome. Am Rev Respir Dis 1993; 147:218–233.
98. Bachofen M, Weibel ER. Structural alterations of lung parenchyma in the adult respiratory distress syndrome. Clin Chest Med 1982; 3:35–56.
99. Matthay MA, Wiener-Kronish JP. Intact epithelial barrier function is critical for the resolution of alveolar edema in humans. Am Rev Respir Dis 1990; 142:1250–1257.
100. Burkhardt A. Alveolitis and collapse in the pathogenesis of pulmonary fibrosis. Am Rev Respir Dis 1989; 140:513–524.
101. Vracko R. Basal lamina scaffold-anatomy and significance for maintenance of orderly tissue structure. Am J Pathol 1974; 77:314–346.
102. Marinelli WA, Henke CA, Harmon KR, et al. Mechanisms of alveolar fibrosis after acute lung injury. Clin Chest Med 1990; 11:657–672.
103. von Wichert P, Kohl FV. Decreased dipalmitoyllecithin content found in lung

specimens from patients with so-called shock-lung. Intensive Care Med 1977; 3:27–30.
104. Reynolds HY. Bronchoalveolar lavage. Am Rev Respir Dis 1987; 135:250–263.
105. Casals C, Herrera L, Miguel E, et al. Comparison between intra- and extracellular surfactant in respiratory distress induced by oleic acid. Biochim Biophys Acta 1989; 1003:201–203.
106. Berry D, Ikegami M, Jobe A. Respiratory distress and surfactant inhibition following vagotomy in rabbits. J Appl Physiol 1986; 61:1741–1748.
107. Liau DF, Barrett CR, Bell AL, Ryan SF. Functional abnormalities of lung surfactant in experimental acute alveolar injury in the dog. Am Rev Respir Dis 1987; 136:395–401.
108. Holm BA, Notter RH, Siegle J, Matalon S. Pulmonary physiological and surfactant changes during injury and recovery from hyperoxia. J Appl Physiol 1985; 59:1402–1409.
109. Young SL, Crapo JD, Kremers SA, Brumley GW. Pulmonary surfactant lipid production in oxygen-exposed rat lungs. Lab Invest 1982; 46:570–576.
110. Low RB, Adler KB, Woodcock-Mitchell J, et al. Bronchoalveolar lavage lipids during development of bleomycin-induced fibrosis in rats. Relationship to altered epithelial cell morphology. Am Rev Respir Dis 1988; 138:709–713.
111. Dethloff LA, Gilmore LB, Hook GE. The relationship between intra- and extra-cellular surfactant phospholipids in the lungs of rabbits and the effects of silica-induced lung injury. Biochem J 1986; 239:59–67.
112. Horiuchi T, Mason RJ, Kuroki Y, Cherniack RM. Surface and tissue forces, surfactant protein A, and the phospholipid components of pulmonary surfactant in bleomycin-induced pulmonary fibrosis in the rat. Am Rev Respir Dis 1990; 141:1006–1013.
113. Ballard PL. Hormonal regulation of pulmonary surfactant. Endocrinol Rev 1989; 10:165–181.
114. Walker SR, Williams MC, Benson B. Immunocytochemical localization of the major surfactant apoproteins in type II cells, Clara cells, and alveolar macrophages of rat lungs. J Histochem Cytochem 1986; 34:1137–1148.
115. King RJ, Jones MB, Minoo P. Regulation of lung cell proliferation by polypeptide growth factors. Am J Physiol 1989; 257:L23–L38.
116. Edelson JD, Shannon JM, Mason RJ. Alkaline phosphatase: A marker of alveolar type II cell differentiation. Am Rev Respir Dis 1988; 138:1268–1275.
117. Pison U, Tam EK, Caughey GH, Hawgood S. Proteolytic inactivation of dog lung surfactant-associated proteins by neutrophil elastase. Biochim Biophys Acta 1989; 992:251–257.
118. Massaro D, Clerch L, Temple D, Baier H. Surfactant deficiency in rats without a decreased amount of extracellular surfactant. J Clin Invest 1983; 71:1536–1543.
119. Higuchi R, Lewis J, Ikegami M. In vitro conversion of surfactant subtypes is altered in alveolar surfactant isolated from injured lungs. Am Rev Respir Dis 1992; 145:1416–1420.
120. Lewis JF, Ikegami M, Jobe AH. Altered surfactant function and metabolism in rabbits with acute lung injury. J Appl Physiol 1990; 69:2303–2310.
121. Gross NJ. Surfactant subtypes in experimental lung damage: Radiation pneumonitis. Am J Physiol 1991; 260:L302–L310.

122. Holm BA, Notter RH, Finkelstein JN. Surface property changes from interactions of albumin with natural lung surfactant and extracted lung lipids. Chem Phys. Lipids 1985; 38:287–298.
123. Holm BA, Notter RH. Effects of hemoglobin and cell membrane lipids on pulmonary surfactant activity. J Appl Physiol 1987; 63:1434–1442.
124. Taylor FB Jr, Abrams ME. Effect of surface active lipoprotein on clotting and fibrinolysis, and of fibrinogen on surface tension of surface active lipoprotein. Am J Med 1966; 40:346–350.
125. Seeger W, Stohr G, Wolf HR, Neuhof H. Alteration of surfactant function due to protein leakage: special interaction with fibrin monomer. J Appl Physiol 1985; 58:326–338.
126. Fuchimukai T, Fujiwara T, Takahashi A, Enhorning G. Artificial pulmonary surfactant inhibited by proteins. J Appl Physiol 1987; 62:429–437.
127. Venkitaraman AR, Hall SB, Whitsett JA, Notter RH. Enhancement of biophysical activity of lung surfactant extracts and phospholipid-apoprotein mixtures by surfactant protein A. Chem Phys Lipids 1990; 56:185–94.
128. Venkitaraman AR, Baatz JE, Whitsett JA, et al. Biophysical inhibition of synthetic phospholipid-lung surfactant apoprotein admixtures by plasma proteins. Chem Phys Lipids 1991; 57:49–57.
129. Cockshutt AM, Weitz J, Possmayer F. Pulmonary surfactant-associated protein A enhances the surface activity of lipid extract surfactant and reverses inhibition by blood proteins in vitro. Biochemistry 1990; 29:8424–8429.
130. Ryan SF, Ghassibi Y, Liau DF. Effects of activated polymorphonuclear leukocytes upon pulmonary surfactant in vitro. Am J Respir Cell Mol Biol 1991; 4:33–41.
131. Seeger W, Lepper H, Wolf HR, Neuhof H. Alteration of alveolar surfactant function after exposure to oxidative stress and to oxygenated and native arachidonic acid in vitro. Biochim Biophys Acta 1985; 835:58–67.
132. Oosting RS, Van IJ, Van BL, et al. Exposure of surfactant protein A to ozone in vitro and in vivo impairs its interactions with alveolar cells. Am J Physiol 1992; 262:L63–L68.
133. Haddad IY, Ischiropoulos H, Holm BA, et al. Mechanisms of peroxynitrite-induced injury to pulmonary surfactants. Am J Physiol 1993; 265:L555–L564.
134. Holm BA, Keicher L, Liu MY, et al. Inhibition of pulmonary surfactant function by phospholipases. J Appl Physiol 1991; 71:317–321.
135. Seeger W, Elssner A, Günther A, et al. Lung surfactant phospholipids associate with polymerizing fibrin: loss of surface activity. Am J Respir Cell Mol Biol 1993; 9:213–220.
136. Pietschmann S, Wrede C, Pison U. Lung injury in sheep decreases mRNA levels of surfactant associated proteins SP-A, SP-B, and SP-C. Am J Respir Crit Care Med 1994; 149:A126.
137. Ballard PL, Liley HG, Gonzales LW, et al. Interferon-gamma and synthesis of surfactant components by cultured human fetal lung. Am J Respir Cell Mol Biol 1990; 2:137–143.
138. Rishi A, Hatzis D, McAlmon K, Floros J. An allelic variant of the 6A gene for human surfactant protein A. Am J Physiol 1992; 262:L566–L573.

10

Evaluation of Lung Permeability in Neonatal and Adult Respiratory Distress Syndrome

PER WOLLMER and BJÖRN JONSON
University of Lund
Lund, Sweden

BURKHARD LACHMANN
Erasmus University
Rotterdam, The Netherlands

I. The Alveolocapillary Barrier

A prerequisite for effective gas exchange in the alveolocapillary unit of the lung is that alveolar air is brought into close contact with capillary gas. The thickness of the barrier separating alveolar gas from capillary blood varies somewhat in different parts of the alveolus (1). The thinnest parts are less than 1 μm thick, and consist of the alveolar surfactant layer with its aqueous hypophase, the alveolar epithelial type I cell, a fused basement membrane, and the capillary endothelial cell. Other parts of the alveolocapillary barrier are thicker, the basement membranes of the epithelial and endothelial cells being separated by a thin interstitial space. In the interstitial space surrounding somewhat larger vessels and bronchioles, there is a rich lymphatic network (2).

Exchange of hydrophilic solutes in the pulmonary microcirculation is considered to take place through intercellular junctions. In the normal situation, the barrier effectively limits the exchange of water and solutes to a small net filtration, which is balanced by lymphatic drainage.

The main force driving fluid filtration in the pulmonary microcirculation is the difference in hydrostatic pressure across the walls of the microvessels. Even in the normal situation, the pulmonary capillary pressure is highly variable, since it is profoundly influenced by gravitational effects on the lung. The perimicrovascular pressure in the lung is the interstitial pressure or the pericapillary pressure in the alveoli. Although the interstitial pressure in the lungs has proven difficult to measure precisely, it is generally held to be subatmospheric (3–5). The hydrostatic pressure around the capillaries not surrounded by interstitium, but rather by the thin fluid film in the alveoli, is dependent on the surface tension of the film. The relationship between surface tension and perimicrovascular pressure is further complicated by the fact that alveoli are not spheres but rather irregular. The contribution of surface forces to this pressure can be expressed according to the law of Laplace, which tells that the pressure is inversely proportional to the radius of the curvature of the surface. At least in theory, three situations can be distinguished: (1) The curvature of the gas-liquid interface in "alveolar corners" has a radius much smaller than the average radius. (2) The curvature of the free nearly flat alveolar wall has a radius approaching infinity. (3) Where and when capillaries may bulge into the alveolar space the radius of the interface becomes negative. Surface tension would then (1) lower, (2) leave unaffected, or (3) increase perimicrovascular pressure. We know that alveolar corner vessels remain open when capillaries in interalveolar septa are closed in lung zones with low precapillary pressure (6). This may reflect the importance of local geometry. Our knowledge about alveolar geometry in vivo is limited particularly for lungs with surfactant dysfunction. Therefore, theory leaves us with limited support as concerns the relationship between surface forces and alveolar liquid exchange. A review on the matter has been presented by Guyton et al. (7) (see also Chapter 2).

Fluid filtration in the pulmonary microvasculature is resisted by the transmural difference in colloid osmotic pressure. Maintainance of the osmotic pressure gradient relies on a low permeability to protein in the alveolocapillary barrier. The relative permeability of the endothelial and epithelial cells to proteins as well as to small solutes has been extensively studied, and there is general agreement that the permeability of the endothelium is considerably larger than that of the epithelium (8,9). The alveolar epithelial cells are thus considered to form the major structural component of the alveolocapillary barrier.

Lymph flow constitutes an important safety factor against the development of pulmonary edema. The pumping action of the lymphatics effectively drains the interstitium under normal conditions and contributes to the negative interstitial pressure in the lungs. The capacity of the lymphatics to increase flow is very large; when filtration pressure is increased, lymph flow may increase more than 10 times.

Pulmonary edema is traditionally considered as hydrostatic edema if the primary abnormality is increased intravascular pressure and the barrier permeability to protein is intact, and as high permeability edema if the integrity of the barrier is compromised. There is no absolute distinction between the two forms of edema, since increased permeability makes the lungs more susceptible to high intravascular pressures (10), and, on the other hand, high pressures eventually lead to permeability changes.

II. Surfactant and the Alveolocapillary Barrier

It has long been recognized that the alveolar surfactant system on theoretical grounds is very important for the alveolar liquid balance (11,12). There have, however, been rather few experimental studies of surfactant function in relation to the integrity of the alveolocapillary barrier. This is partly the consequence of methodological difficulties; the properties of the alveolocapillary barrier is often studied in fluid filled lungs, in which there is, of course, no alveolar air-liquid interface and no physiologically functioning alveolar surfactant.

A. Surfactant Dysfunction, Ventilation, and Blood Flow

Reduction of alveolar surface tension by surfactant is essential for the normal aeration of the lungs. Severe impairment of the integrity of the alveolar surfactant system inevitably leads to atelectasis in a spontaneously breathing animal and mechanical ventilation is generally required. Application of mechanical ventilation may, however, have unwanted consequences. Ventilation with large tidal volumes may lead to surfactant dysfunction, presumably due to elimination of surfactant from the alveoli into the terminal airways (13,14). Ventilation of a lung with surfactant dysfunction often requires high insufflation pressures. If traditional patterns of ventilation are used, there is often total collapse and reopening of whole lung regions within each insufflation (Levy P et al., personal communication). This soon results in structural damage to the terminal airways and alveoli (15), presumably due to high shear forces on opening of closed lung units (16,17). By application of appropriate mechanical ventilation, e.g., pressure-generated insufflation with short expiration, repeated closure and reopening of lung regions can largely be avoided (16). Even so, however, some damage to the structural elements of the alveolocapillary barrier is likely to occur in states of severe surfactant dysfunction.

The mechanical and structural effects of severe surfactant dysfunction also have secondary effects on hemodynamics. An increase in surface tension causing a reduction in perivascular pressure implies that the distending pressure of the vessel is increased. Nieman et al. (18) thus showed that the number of alveoli with continuous blood flow increased after lung lavage with a detergent solution elevating surface tension. The reverse has also been shown; i.e., when the lung is filled with saline to abolish surface tension, vascular resistance is increased (19). When alveolar edema develops, blood flow to the edematous lung region is severely reduced (20).

Several plasma proteins are known to inactivate surfactant (21) (see Chapter 13). Leakage of plasma into the alveolus may result from bronchiolar or alveolar damage. Irrespective of the primary cause, this will lead to surfactant dysfunction. The complex relationships between the structure of the small airways, alveolocapillary unit, pulmonary mechanics, hemodynamics, and surfactant function make it difficult to design experiments to investigate specifically the role of the surfactant system in maintaining liquid homeostasis in the lung.

B. Experimental Models of Surfactant Dysfunction

The most obvious pathophysiological model of surfactant dysfunction is, of course, the lungs of premature animals (see Chapter 12). A model with some similar features is total lung lavage in adult animals. A large proportion of the intra-alveolar phospholipids can be removed by repeated lung lavage with isotonic saline (22), resulting in drastically increased lung recoil and impaired gas exchange (23,24). The initial effects of lung lavage are presumably limited to surfactant removal, but very soon after lavage, ventilation of the poorly compliant lung results in structural damage to the epithelium (15). The pathophysiological and morphological characteristics of this model closely resemble those of adult respiratory distress syndrome (ARDS) (23). Lung lavage has also been performed with detergent solutions (18,25). Detergents interact with surfactant phospholipids to reduce surface activity which can be demonstrated by in vitro measurements of the surface activity of lung washings or extracts in the presence and absence of detergent (26). With detergent present in the lavage fluid, substantially greater effects on lung mechanics and gas exchange are obtained for a given lavage volume (18,26).

There are several disadvantages with the lavage techniques as models for investigation of the role of the surfactant system in the liquid homeostasis in the lungs. It is difficult to ensure that the lungs are affected uniformly by the lavage. The possibilities to obtain graded damage to the surfactant system are limited, and the result of lavage is frequently that of fully developed respiratory failure. The introduction of large volumes of liquid into the airspaces of the lung will in itself have adverse effects on lung mechanics and gas exchange and precludes; e.g., measurement of fluid accumulation in the lung as a consequence of surfactant dysfunction. An alternative model of surfactant dysfunction, based on administration of a synthetic detergent in aerosol form, was introduced by Nieman and Bredenberg (27). With this technique, the lungs are affected more uniformly, the damage can be graded by administration of different amounts of detergent, and the volume of liquid administered is sufficiently small not to interfere to any appreciable extent with measurements of fluid accumulation in the lungs. Surfactant dysfunction can be induced without any substantial cellular damage to the alveolocapillary unit (27), and there is no increase in the permeability of the barrier to protein (28).

C. Surfactant Dysfunction and Lung Water Content

The variables best reflecting the importance of the surfactant system for maintaining the alveolocapillary barrier function are measurement of water accumulation in the lungs and transfer of tracer molecules across the barrier. Parameters of overall lung function such as lung compliance and gas exchange mainly reflect the consequences of alveolar liquid filling and/or alveolar collapse. In states of such gross pathology, there may also be structural damage to the barrier, and the abnormalities measured may not predominantly reflect alveolar surfactant dysfunction.

Albert et al. (29) studied the effect of surfactant dysfunction on fluid filtration in dog lungs. Surfactant dysfunction was induced by cooling the lung and ventilating it with large tidal volume. The isogravimetric pressure, i.e., the intravascular pressure required to balance perimicrovascular pressure so that lung weight was constant, was measured (while oncotic pressure was kept constant). Isogravimetric pressure was reduced after induction of surfactant dysfunction, compatible with a reduced perimicrovascular pressure. In a morphological study, Bachofen et al. (30) performed perfusion fixation of isolated rabbit lungs expanded by negative pleural pressure. They noted that alveolar edema was more pronounced in lungs lavaged with a detergent solution than in untreated control lungs. The finding is compatible with reduced perimicrovascular pressure and increased filtration pressure in the lavaged lungs. The effect of surfactant dysfunction on the wet/dry weight ratio of the lung has been studied by Bredenberg et al. (26) after lung lavage with a detergent solution and by Nieman and Bredenberg (27) after administration of detergent in aerosol form. Both studies showed detergent treatment to increase the wet/dry weight ratio, compatible with increased transudation of fluid in the alveolocapillary unit.

D. Surfactant Dysfunction and Solute Exchange

Fluid-Filled Lungs

Exchange of solutes between the alveolar space, the pulmonary tissue, and the alveoli has often been studied in fluid-filled lungs. Although no information about the surfactant system is obtained, the importance of surfactant for the solute exchange in the neonatal lung during the phase of inflation may be studied with this technique. Measurement of the alveolocapillary transfer has been accomplished by instillation of radiolabeled tracers into the lungs of fetuses before the first breath. The leakage of solutes has similarly been measured after injection of radiolabeled tracers and measurement in alveolar lavage fluid. Egan et al. (31) measured the rate of absorption of tracers from the lungs of premature ventilated goats of varying gestational age. Lung maturity was assessed by measurement of surface activity of amniotic fluid. The rate of absorption of solutes was much greater in fetuses with low surface activity of amniotic fluid than in more mature fetuses.

The transfer of albumin in both directions across the alveolocapillary barrier in premature lambs has been studied by Jobe et al. (32). These authors also measured the effect of surfactant instillation before the first breath. The transfer of albumin during the first 3 hr of mechanical ventilation was substantially reduced by surfactant treatment. In a similar study of immature rabbit fetuses, Robertson et al. (33) measured the rate of transfer of albumin in both directions across the alveolocapillary barrier during the first hour of mechanical ventilation with and without surfactant instillation before the first breath. Surfactant treatment substantially reduced the albumin transfer (Fig. 1). On histological

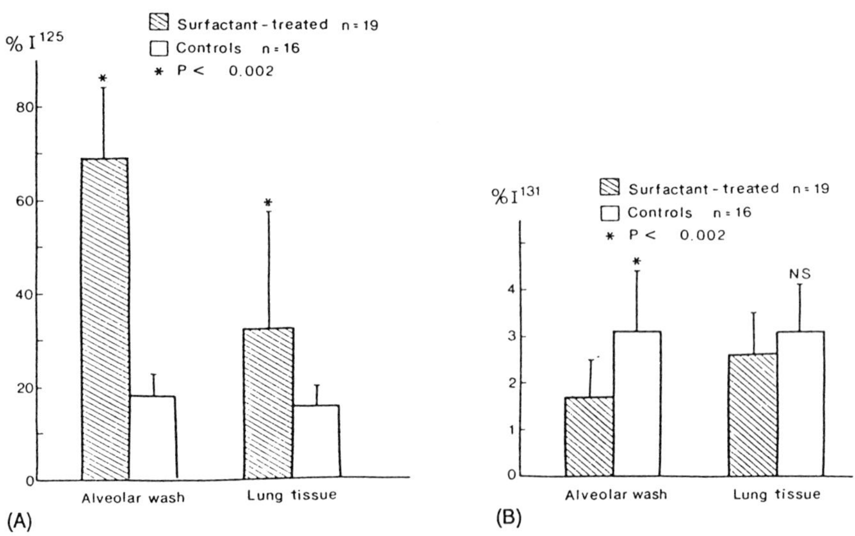

Figure 1 Transfer of radiolabeled albumin across the alveolocapillary barrier in premature rabbits. (A) ^{125}I-albumin in saline solution (open columns) or mixed with natural surfactant (hatched columns) was instilled into the airways before the first breath. (B) ^{131}I-albumin was injected intravenously. The animals were mechanically ventilated for 60 min and the lungs were then lavaged with saline. The recovery of ^{125}I-albumin in lavage fluid was higher in surfactant treated animals than in controls, indicating that surfactant treatment reduced the rate of absorption of the tracer. The recovery of ^{131}I-albumin in lavage fluid was lower in surfactant treated animals than in controls, indicating that surfactant reduced the leakage of protein from the circulation into the alveoli. (From ref. 33; used with permission.)

examination, the lungs of animals treated with surfactant showed considerably less abnormalities than control animals, but were not quite normal. These studies show that alveolar surfactant is essential for a normal alveolocapillary barrier after birth. From the studies, it is, however, impossible to determine if this is a direct action of surfactant on the alveolocapillary barrier or if surfactant merely reduced the structural damage caused by mechanical ventilation of the surfactant-deficient lung.

Inflated Lungs

Aerosol Tracer Technique

Evaluation of the functional integrity of the alveolocapillary barrier in the inflated lung is greatly facilitated by administration of radiolabeled tracer substances in aerosol form. In order to reach the alveoli, aerosol particles should have a diameter less than 2 μm. Several commercially available air jet nebulizers produce particles in this size range. Appropriate amounts of radiolabeled tracer substances may thus be administered in a volume less than 1 ml (34). After inhalation, the rate of absorption of radioactive tracers from the lungs is measured by external recording of the radioactivity over the chest with a single detector or a gamma camera. An attractive feature of the technique is that it can be applied in the same way in animal experiments and in clinical studies. The most widely used tracer is the water-soluble complex ^{99m}Tc-diethylene triamine pentaacetate (^{99m}Tc-DTPA, Mw 492 Da), but several other radiolabeled compounds have been used, including proteins (35–38). ^{99m}Tc-DTPA is generally considered to traverse the alveolocapillary barrier by simple diffusion via the paracellular route from the alveolar space into the blood. Very little tracer is cleared by the lymphatics in normal lungs (39), but lymphatic clearance may increase in disease states (40). Clearance of the tracer from the lungs is also largely independent of blood flow. Ritzk et al. (41) found that clearance was reduced, but not absent, after unilateral pulmonary artery occlusion. There was no effect of the increase in flow on the contralateral side. Bronchial artery occlusion did not affect the pulmonary clearance of ^{99m}Tc-DTPA. Measurement of the clearance of the tracer from the lungs thus mainly reflects its rate of transfer across the alveolocapillary barrier.

Experimental Studies

Experimental as well as clinical studies of the pulmonary clearance of ^{99m}Tc-DTPA have indicated that the permeability of the alveolocapillary barrier is considerably more variable than previously appreciated. The rate of clearance increases substantially with increases in lung volume (41–46), whether caused by voluntary hyperinflation or application of positive expiratory pressure, and with ventilation with large tidal volume (47). The mechanism is often considered to be stretching of the alveolar wall with widening of intercellular junctions. The increased clearance during high tidal volume ventilation has been suggested to result from increased elimination of surfactant from the alveoli into the airways (47).

Pulmonary clearance of ^{99m}Tc-DTPA has been studied in a number of experimental models of acute lung injury, e.g., hydrochloric acid aspiration (48) total lung lavage (49,50), oleic acid injection (37,48,51–55), and injection of α-naphthylthiourea (56). These studies all show dramatically increased clearance rate, in contrast to studies of hydrostatic pulmonary edema, which do not show any increase in clearance rate (52,53). The rate of clearance of ^{99m}Tc-DTPA increases promptly after the various provocations, indicating that it reflects an early event in the pathogenesis of acute lung injury. In view of the complexity of the situation, it is, of course, difficult to determine the exact mechanism for the increased clearance of ^{99m}Tc-DTPA. Evander et al. (49) performed surfactant replacement in rabbits after total lung lavage with saline, and found that this to some extent attenuated the effect on clearance of ^{99m}Tc-DTPA. It could not be determined if this was a direct effect of surfactant on the alveolocapillary barrier or an effect of reduced lung injury during mechanical ventilation of the lavaged lung.

The relation between surfactant function and the clearance of ^{99m}Tc-DTPA has been studied more specifically with the provocation technique based on aerosolized detergent. Administration of detergent aerosol causes a dramatic increase in the rate of clearance of ^{99m}Tc-DTPA (37,38,57–59). Clearance increases within 1 min after detergent administration (Fig. 2) (37) in a dose-related manner (60). Although low doses of detergent increase clearance without causing any substantial change in dynamic compliance of the respiratory system or gas exchange impairment (37,38,57), high doses increase clearance in conjunction with the development of frank pulmonary edema accompanied by abnormal lung mechanics and gas exchange (58,59). Clearance of ^{99m}Tc-DTPA has also been studied in experimental models of increased alveolar surfactant content. Bos et al. (61) treated rabbits with ambroxol to stimulate surfactant synthesis and release, and also instilled natural surfactant into the lungs of rabbits. In both conditions, the clearance of ^{99m}Tc-DTPA was reduced compared with untreated control animals (Fig. 3). Surfactant dysfunction thus increases the permeability of the alveolocapillary barrier to ^{99m}Tc-DTPA in the absence of other substantial changes in the function of the alveolocapillary unit, and increased alveolar surfactant content similarly reduces the permeability. These experimental observations indicate that surfactant may have a primary role in the regulation of the permeability of the alveolocapillary barrier.

Clinical Studies

The most striking clinical finding in studies of the pulmonary clearance of ^{99m}Tc-DTPA has been that of greatly increased clearance in otherwise normal

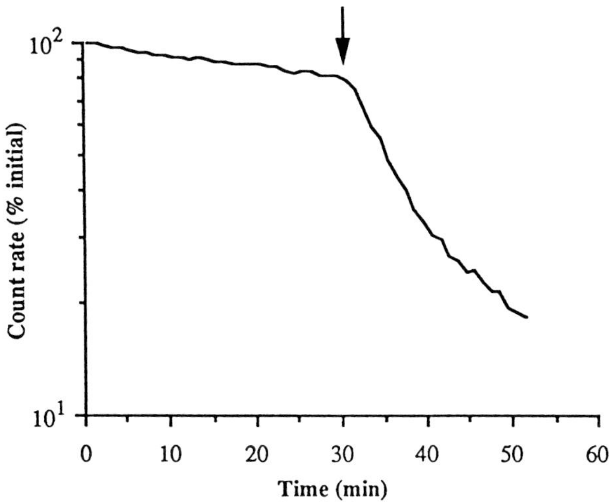

Figure 2 Pulmonary clearance of ^{99m}Tc-DTPA before and after administration of a synthetic detergent in aerosol form. The graph shows the count rate over the lungs corrected for physical decay and recirculation of tracer. During the first 30 min of measurement the count rate slowly declines, reflecting the normal clearance rate. Detergent administration at 30 min (arrow) immediately results in a dramatic increase in clearance rate. (From ref. 37; used with permission.)

smokers (62–66). The mechanism has generally been assumed to be adverse effects of smoking on the pulmonary epithelium, but this has been difficult to substantiate. Smoking is, on the other hand, known to reduce the amount of phospholipids recoverable by bronchoalveolar lavage (67–69), an abnormality which precedes ultrastructural damage to the cells (68). Schmekel et al. (65) recently showed that the rate of clearance of ^{99m}Tc-DTPA correlated with the amount of phosphatidylcholine recovered by lung lavage in smokers and nonsmokers, supporting the notion that surfactant dysfunction may partly explain the increased permeability of the alveolocapillary barrier in smokers.

The pulmonary clearance of ^{99m}Tc-DTPA has also been studied in patients with acute lung injury, notably in babies with respiratory distress syndrome (RDS) (70). All infants studied within the first 72 hr of life had an increased rate of clearance of ^{99m}Tc-DTPA. In 11 of 14 patients, improvement was seen in a follow-up study just prior to extubation on the fourth to eighth day of life. In a subsequent study, O'Brodovich and Coates (71) studied babies with RDS who subsequently developed bronchopulmonary dysplasia (BPD). Although some of these infants had abnormal clearance of ^{99m}Tc-DTPA after 1 week of age, others had normalized the clearance. These studies indicate that in the acute stage of RDS, dominated by surfactant deficiency and pulmonary edema, the

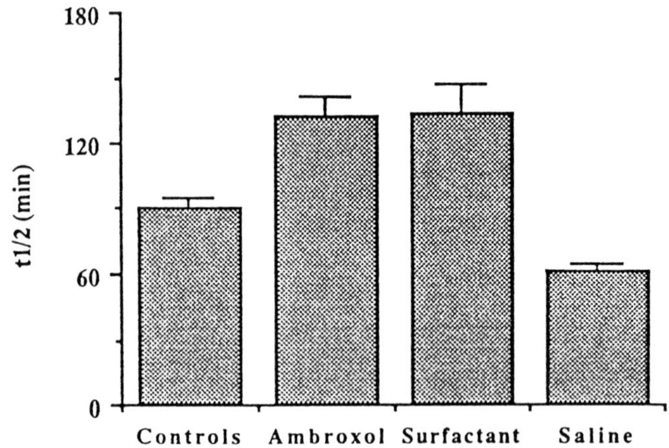

Figure 3 Rate of pulmonary clearance of ^{99m}Tc-DTPA in rabbits with increased alveolar surfactant content. Normal rabbits were treated by intravenous injection of ambroxol (ambroxol, five doses of 50 mg/kg) or tracheal instillation of natural surfactant (surfactant, 100 mg/kg). Control animals were untreated (controls) or given physiological saline by tracheal instillation (saline, 5 ml). The rate of clearance of ^{99m}Tc-DTPA is reduced (longer half-life) in animals with increased alveolar surfactant content relative to controls. In animals treated with tracheal instillation of saline, the rate of clearance is increased relative to untreated controls. (From ref. 61; used with permission.)

alveolocapillary barrier function is abnormal. In babies recovering from RDS, i.e., in babies with increasing surfactant production, the barrier to absorption of small solutes tends to improve. Improvement may be seen even in infants who subsequently develop BPD; i.e., patients in whom the integrity of the pulmonary tissue is certainly compromised. No studies of the effect of surfactant instillation on the clearance of ^{99m}Tc-DTPA in premature infants are, as yet, available.

Pulmonary clearance of ^{99m}Tc-DTPA is increased in patients with adult respiratory distress syndrome (ARDS), in contrast to patients with cardiogenic pulmonary edema, who are mostly normal (54,72,73). The rate of clearance in patients with ARDS is often in the same range as that in smokers (54,74), which limits the clinical usefulness of the technique with respect to differential diagnostics. Measurement of the clearance of ^{99m}Tc-DTPA in patients at risk for developing ARDS identified all patients who subsequently developed respiratory failure in the study by Tennenberg et al. (75). A considerable number of patients who did not develop ARDS also had abnormal clearance, indicating that the clearance measurement reflects early pathophysiological abnormalities which can still be reversed. Once ARDS is established in a patient, the abnormal clearance often persists for a long time compared with radiographic abnormalities (54), and it has little or no prognostic value (76).

III. Conclusions

The alveolar surfactant system is of fundamental importance for reducing the alveolar surface tension and reducing the pressure needed to inflate the lungs. It has long been recognized that surfactant also reduces the transmural hydrostatic pressure gradient in the alveolar microvasculature and thereby constitutes a safety factor against pulmonary edema. Evidence is now accumulating that alveolar surfactant may also affect the permeability of the alveolocapillary barrier to solutes. The alveolar epithelial cell is undoubtedly the major structural barrier separating air from blood and interstitial fluid, but it appears possible that surfactant may modify the permeability of the epithelium. The precise mechanisms involved can only be speculated on, but may involve adsorption of phospholipids to cell membranes in the alveolocapillary barrier (77).

References

1. Weibel ER. Morphometry of the Human Lung. Berlin: Springer-Verlag, 1963.
2. Lauweryns JM. The juxta-alveolar lymphatics in the human adult lung. Histologic studies in 15 cases of drowning. Am Rev Respir Dis 1970; 102:877–885.
3. Meyer BJ, Meyer A, Guyton AC. Interstitial fluid pressure. V. Negative pressure in the lungs. Circ Res 1968; 22:263–271.
4. Parker JD, Guyton AC, Taylor AE. Pulmonary interstitial and capillary pressures estimated from intra-alveolar fluid pressures. J Appl Physiol 1978; 44:267–276.
5. Bhattacharya J, Gropper MA, Staub NC. Interstitial fluid pressure gradient measured by micropuncture in excised dog lung. J Appl Physiol 1984; 56:271–277.
6. Warrel DA, Evans JW, Clarke RO, et al. Pattern of filling in the pulmonary capillary bed. J Appl Physiol 1972; 32:346–356.
7. Guyton AC, Moffatt DS, Adair TH. Role of alveolar surface tension in transepithelial movement of fluid. In: Robertson B, van Golde LMG, Batenburg JJ, eds. Pulmonary Surfactant. Amsterdam: Elsevier Science, 1984:171–185.
8. Gorin AB, Stewart PA. Differential permeability of endothelial and epithelial barriers to albumin flux. J Appl Physiol 1979; 47:1315–1324.
9. Effros RM, Mason GR, Silverman P, et al. Movement of ions and small solutes across endothelium and epithelium of perfused rabbit lungs. J Appl Physiol 1986; 60:100–107.
10. Huchon GJ, Hopewell PC, Murray JF. Interactions between permeability and hydrostatic pressure in perfused dogs' lungs. J Appl Physiol 1981; 50:905–911.
11. Pattle RE. Surface lining of lung alveoli. Physiol Rev 1965; 45:48–79.
12. Clements JA. Pulmonary edema and permeability of alveolar membranes. Arch Environ Health 1961; 2:104–107.
13. Faridy EE. Effect of distension on release of surfactant in excised dogs' lungs. Respir Physiol 1976; 27:99–114.
14. Wyszogrodski I, Kyei-Aboagye K, Taeusch HW Jr, Avery ME. Surfactant

inactivation by hyperventilation: Conservation by end-expiratory pressure. J Appl Physiol 1975; 38:461–466.
15. Nilsson R, Grossmann G, Robertson B. Bronchiolar epithelial lesions induced in the premature rabbit neonate by short periods of artificial ventilation. Acta Pathol Microbiol Scand [A] 1980; 88:359–367.
16. Lachmann B, Jonson B, Lindroth M, Robertson B. Modes of artificial ventilation in severe respiratory distress syndrome. Crit Care Med 1982; 10:724–732.
17. Mead J, Takashima T, Leith D. Stress distribution in lungs: A model of pulmonary elasticity. J Appl Physiol 1970; 28:596–608.
18. Nieman GF, Bredenberg CE, Clark WR, West NR. Alveolar function following surfactant deactivation. J Appl Physiol 1981; 51:895–904.
19. Bruderman I, Somers K, Hamilton WK, et al. Effect of surface tension on circulation in the excised lungs of dogs. J Appl Physiol 1964; 19:707–712.
20. Bhattacharya J, Nakahara K, Staub NC. Effect of edema on pulmonary blood flow in the isolated perfused dog lung lobe. J Appl Physiol 1980; 48:444–449.
21. Seeger W, Stöhr G, Wolf HRD, Neuhof H. Alteration of surfactant function due to protein leakage: Special interaction with fibrin monomer. J Appl Physiol 1985; 58:326–338.
22. Fujiwara T, Adams FH, El-Salawy A, Sipos S. "Alveolar" and whole lung phospholipids of newborn lambs. Proc Soc Exp Biol Med 1968; 127:962–969.
23. Lachmann B, Robertson B, Vogel J. In vivo lung lavage as an experimental model of the respiratory distress syndrome. Acta Anaesthesiol Scand 1980; 24:231–236.
24. Huber GL, Edmunds LH Jr, Finley TN. Acute effect of saline lung washing on pulmonary mechanics and morphology. Surg Forum 1966; 17:113–114.
25. Yoshida S. Effects of surfactants or fat solvent on static pressure-volume hysteresis of excised dog lung. Am J Physiol 1962; 203:725–730.
26. Bredenberg CE, Paskanik AM, Nieman GF. High surface tension pulmonary edema. J Surg Res 1983; 34:515–523.
27. Nieman GF, Bredenberg CE. High surface tension pulmonary edema induced by detergent aerosol. J Appl Physiol 1985; 58:129–136.
28. Bredenberg CE, Nieman GF, Paskanik AM, Hart KE. Microvascular membrane permeability in high surface tension pulmonary edema. J Appl Physiol 1986; 60:253–259.
29. Albert RK, Lakshminarayan S, Hildebrandt J, et al. Increased surface tension favors pulmonary edema formation in anesthetized dogs' lungs. J Clin Invest 1979; 63:1015–1018.
30. Bachofen H, Gehr P, Weibel ER. Alterations of mechanical properties and morphology in excised rabbit lungs rinsed with a detergent. J Appl Physiol 1979; 47:1002–1010.
31. Egan EA, Nelson RM, Beale EF. Lung solute permeability and lung liquid absorption in premature ventilated fetal goats. Pediatr Res 1980; 14:314–318.
32. Jobe A, Ikegami M, Jacobs H, et al. Permeability of premature lamb lungs to protein and the effect of surfactant on that permeability. J Appl Physiol 1983; 55:169–176.
33. Robertson B, Berry D, Curstedt T, et al. Leakage of protein in the immature rabbit lung; effect of surfactant replacement. Respir Physiol 1985; 61:265–276.

34. Dahlbäck M, Wollmer P, Drefeldt B, Jonson B. Controlled aerosol delivery during mechanical ventilation. J Aerosol Med 1989; 2:339–347.
35. Barrowcliffe MP, Zanelli GD, Jones JG. Pulmonary clearance of radiotracers after positive end-expiratory pressure or acute lung injury. J Appl Physiol 1989; 66:288–294.
36. Huchon GJ, Montgomery AB, Lipavsky A, et al. Respiratory clearance of aerosolized radioactive solutes of varying molecular weight. J Nucl Med 1987; 28:894–902.
37. Nilsson K, Wollmer P. Pulmonary clearance of ^{99m}Tc-DTPA and ^{99m}Tc-albumin in rabbits with surfactant dysfunction and lung injury. Clin Physiol 1992; 12:587–594.
38. Nilsson K, Wollmer P. Pulmonary clearance of tracers with different lipid and water solubility in experimental surfactant dysfunction. Eur Respir J 1993; 6:505–508.
39. Coates G, O'Brodovich HM. The contribution of lymphatic drainage to the clearance of inhaled ^{99m}Tc-DTPA from the lungs. Clin Invest Med 1986; 9:15–20.
40. Peterson BT, Gray LD. Pulmonary lymphatic clearance of ^{99m}Tc-DTPA from air spaces during lung inflation and lung injury. J Appl Physiol 1987; 63:1136–1141.
41. Rizk NW, Luce JM, Hoeffel JM, et al. Site of deposition and factors affecting clearance of aerosolized solute from canine lungs. J Appl Physiol 1984; 56:723–729.
42. Marks JD, Luce JM, Lazar NM, et al. Effect of increases in lung volume on clearance of aerosolized solute from human lungs. J Appl Physiol 1985; 59:1242–1248.
43. O'Brodovich H, Coates G, Marrin M. Effect of inspiratory resistance and PEEP on ^{99m}Tc-DTPA clearance. J Appl Physiol 1986; 60:1461–1465.
44. Nolop KB, Maxwell DL, Royston D, Hughes JMB. Effect of raised thoracic pressure and volume on ^{99m}Tc-DTPA clearance in humans. J Appl Physiol 1986; 60:1493–1497.
45. Cooper JA, van der Zee H, Line BR, Malik AB. Relationship of end-expiratory pressure, lung volume, and ^{99m}Tc-DTPA clearance. J Appl Physiol 1987; 63:1586–1590.
46. Peterson BT, James HL, McLarty JW. Effects of lung volume on clearance of solutes from the air spaces of lungs. J Appl Physiol 1988; 64:1068–1075.
47. Evander E, Wollmer P, Jonson B. Pulmonary clearance of inhaled ^{99}Tc^{m} DTPA: effects of ventilation pattern. Clin Physiol 1990; 10:189–199.
48. Huchon GJ, Little JW, Murray JF. Assessment of alveolar-capillary membrane permeability of dogs by aerosolization. J Appl Physiol 1981; 51:955–962.
49. Evander E, Wollmer P, Jonson B, Lachmann B. Pulmonary clearance of inhaled ^{99m}Tc-DTPA: Effects of surfactant depletion by lung lavage. J Appl Physiol 1987; 62:1611–1614.
50. Bos JAH, Erdmann W, Lachmann B. ^{99m}Tc-DTPA clearance: A sensitive method for early detection of an impending disturbance in gas exchange. In: Goldstick TK, McCabe M, Maguire DJ, eds. Oxygen Transport to Tissue XIII. New York: Plenum Press, 1992:311–317.
51. Jones JG, Minty BD, Beeley JM, et al. Pulmonary epithelial permeability is immediately increased after embolisation with oleic acid but not with neutral fat. Thorax 1982; 37:169–174.

52. Huchon GJ, Montgomery AB, Lipavsky A, et al. Pulmonary clearance of three aerosolized solutes in oleic acid-induced lung injury. J Appl Physiol 1988; 64:1171–1178.
53. Peterson BT, Dickerson KD, James HL, et al. Comparison of three tracers for detecting lung epithelial injury in anesthetized sheep. J Appl Physiol 1989; 66:2374–2383.
54. Barrowcliffe MP, Jones JG. Pulmonary clearance of ^{99m}Tc-DTPA in the diagnosis and evolution of increased permeability pulmonary oedema. Anaesth Intensive Care 1989; 17:422–432.
55. O'Brodovich H, Coates G, Kay J, Muysson D. Simultaneous measurement of lung clearance rates for Tc- and In-DTPA in normal and damaged lungs. J Appl Physiol 1989; 66:2293–2297.
56. Minty BD, Scudder CM, Grantham CJ, et al. Sequential changes in lung metabolism, permeability, and edema after ANTU. J Appl Physiol 1987; 62:491–496.
57. Evander E, Wollmer P, Jonson B. Pulmonary clearance of inhaled ^{99m}Tc-DTPA: Effect of the detergent dioctyl sodium sulfosuccinate in aerosol. Clin Physiol 1988; 8:105–111.
58. Jefferies AL, Kawano T, Mori S, Burger R. Effect of increased surface tension and assisted ventilation on ^{99m}Tc-DTPA clearance. J Appl Physiol 1988; 64:562–568.
59. Nieman G, Ritter-Hrncirik C, Grossman Z, et al. High alveolar surface tension increases clearance of technetium 99m diethylenetriamine-pentaacetic acid. J Thorac Cardiovasc Surg 1990; 100:129–133.
60. Evander E, Wollmer P, Valind S, et al. Bi-exponential pulmonary clearance of ^{99m}Tc-DTPA induced by detergent aerosol. J Appl Physiol 1994; 77:190–196.
61. Bos JAH, Wollmer P, Bakker W, et al. Clearance of ^{99m}Tc-DTPA and experimentally increased alveolar surfactant content. J Appl Physiol 1992; 72:1413–1417.
62. Jones JG, Minty BD, Lawler P, et al. Increased alveolar epithelial permeability in cigarette smokers. Lancet 1980; 1:66–68.
63. Huchon GJ, Russel JA, Barritault LG, et al. Chronic air-flow limitation does not increase respiratory epithelial permeability assessed by aerosolized solute, but smoking does. Am Rev Respir Dis 1984; 130:457–460.
64. Kennedy SM, Elwood RK, Wiggs BJR, et al. Increased airway mucosal permeability of smokers. Am Rev Respir Dis 1984; 129:143–148.
65. Schmekel B, Bos JAH, Khan AR, et al. Integrity of the alveolar-capillary barrier and alveolar surfactant system in smokers. Thorax 1992; 47:603–608.
66. Wollmer P, Evander E. Biphasic pulmonary clearance of ^{99m}Tc-DTPA in smokers. Clin Physiol 1994; 14:547–559.
67. Finley TN, Ladman AJ. Low yield of pulmonary surfactant in cigarette smokers. N Engl J Med 1972; 286:223–227.
68. Le Mesurier SM, Stewart BW, Lykke AW. Injury to type-2 pneumocytes in rats exposed to cigarette smoke. Environ Res 1981; 24:207–217.
69. Schmekel B, Khan AR, Linden M, Wollmer P. Recoveries of phosphatidylcholine and alveolar macrophages in lung lavage from healthy light smokers. Clin Physiol 1991; 11:431–438.

70. Jefferies AL, Coates G, O'Brodovich H. Pulmonary epithelial permeability in hyaline-membrane disease. N Engl J Med 1984; 311:1075–1080.
71. O'Brodovich H, Coates G. Pulmonary clearance of ^{99m}Tc-DTPA in infants who subsequently develop bronchopulmonary dysplasia. Am Rev Respir Dis 1988; 137:210–212.
72. Mason GR, Effros RM, Uszler JM, Mena I. Small solute clearance from the lungs of patients with cardiogenic and noncardiogenic pulmonary edema. Chest 1985; 88:327–334.
73. Todisco T, Dottorini M, Rossi F, et al. Pulmonary epithelial permeability in ARDS and cardiogenic pulmonary oedema. Eur Respir J 1988; 1:918–922.
74. Braude S, Nolop KB, Hughes JMB, et al. Comparison of lung vascular and epithelial permeability indices in the adult respiratory distress syndrome. Am Rev Respir Dis 1986; 133:1002–1005.
75. Tennenberg SD, Jacobs MP, Solomkin JS, et al. Increased pulmonary alveolar-capillary permeability in patients at risk for adult respiratory distress syndrome. Crit Care Med 1987; 15:289–293.
76. Royston D, Braude S, Nolop KB. Failure of aerosolized ^{99m}TcDTPA clearance to predict outcome in patients with adult respiratory distress syndrome. Thorax 1987; 42:494–499.
77. Hills BA. The Biology of Surfactant. Cambridge, England: Cambridge University Press, 1988.

Part Three

PHARMACOLOGY OF EXOGENOUS SURFACTANT

11

Essential and Nonessential Constituents of Exogenous Surfactants

PINAR BONCUK-DAYANIKLI
University of California, San Francisco
San Francisco, California

H. WILLIAM TAEUSCH
University of California, San Francisco
and San Francisco General Hospital
San Francisco, California

I. Introduction

Like insulin, pulmonary surfactant is essential for life, its absence and/or inactivation is associated with disease, the cure for which in some cases is replacement of the essential substance. Unlike insulin, pulmonary surfactant is a complex mixture of constituents, the stoichiometry of which, first defined 20 years ago (1), is still not completely understood.

II. Composition of Surfactant

The composition of surfactant may vary with such factors as species, age, lung compartment, its point in its metabolic cycle, disease states, diet, exercise, lung volume history, toxin exposure, temperature, and its method of isolation. Various natural and various synthetic constituents can substitute for each other in surfactant. Therefore, even a nonrigorous definition of what is surfactant and what should be included in a therapeutic surfactant is situationally dependent. Surfactant isolated from lung lavage of healthy mammals contains about 10% protein (half of which is surfactant specific), and 90% lipids; of which 80% is phospholipid and 20% neutral lipid, including 10% unesterified cholesterol. The phospholipid fraction contains mostly (76%) phosphatidylcholine (PC); about two thirds is dipalmitoyl phosphatidylcholine (DPPC), and the rest is unsaturated. Eleven percent of the phospholipids are made up of phosphatidylglycerol (PG), 4% phosphatidylinositol, 3% phosphatidylethanolamine, 2% phosphatidylserine, 1.5% sphingomyelin, and 0.2% lysophosphatidylcholine (2). Surfactant protein (SP-A) represents 4% of surfactant and SP-B and SP-C each make up less than 1% according to current estimates (see also Chapter 3).

The form in which alveolar surfactant exists is of importance, but has not been studied much with regard to forms of surfactant used for therapy. In animals, at birth, alveolar surfactant is mostly in a large aggregate form (3). The small (catabolic) forms of surfactant increase to become 30–50% of the alveolar surfactant pool within a few hours of term birth (4). Not much difference exists between small and large aggregate forms of surfactant in terms of phospholipid composition, despite nearly all of the functional activity being vested in the large aggregate forms (3,5), a phenomenon probably due to the presence of surfactant proteins in the large aggregate (newly secreted) forms (6).

A. Elements of Ideal Surfactant for Therapy

The ideal therapeutic surfactant should share many of the attributes of any ideal therapy. It should be stable, readily available, easy to make, inexpensive and have an easy route of administration, a half-life consonant with the disease process, and fully understood mechanisms of action, metabolism, and catabolism. It should have maximum efficacy for the disease without toxicity, intolerance, immunogenicity, or side effects (Table 1). Its use should completely reverse the primary disease process and repair or allow the body to repair secondary damage from the primary disease.

After Avery and Mead (7) described surfactant insufficiency in infants dying with respiratory distress syndrome (RDS), a number of clinical approaches

Table 1 Attributes of Optimal Therapeutic Surfactants

Mimic effects of pulmonary surfactant in vitro
Nonimmunogenic
Improve gas exchange
Improve lung mechanics
Improve functional residual capacity
Resist inactivation
Optimal distribution characteristics
Known clearance mechanisms
Minimal toxicity

were taken to overcome this problem. Initial attempts at improving RDS with surfactant replacement during the 1960s (8) failed largely because of a lack of knowledge about surfactant composition, surfactant delivery, and optimal ways of positive-pressure ventilation with positive end-expiratory pressure. Liggins and colleagues (9), in the early 1970s, were the first to utilize corticosteroids for the enhancement of fetal lung maturation (including surfactant production), thereby reducing the risk and complications of RDS after birth. It is probable that combining prenatal corticosteroids with thyroid-releasing hormone will enhance prenatal prophylaxis for RDS (10) (see also Chapter 18). Hallman and coworkers (11) have suggested giving inositol as a substrate for surfactant production to infants early in the course of RDS, a therapy that has been as successful as administration of surfactant (in the single clinical trial of this approach).

A number of approaches for the design and the use of surfactant replacement for RDS have also been tried. The most straightforward approach is to replace with whole human surfactant. Hallman and coworkers (12) isolated whole human surfactant containing SP-A, SP-B, SP-C from human amniotic fluid that was obtained from volunteers who were undergoing elective cesarean sections at term. This preparation was successful in clinical trials, but because of difficulties in obtaining large quantities of surfactant, it is not in commercial production.

A second approach is to learn the function of various surfactant constituents and then construct surfactants from substitutes that might be more easily obtained or less expensive than the isolation of natural products. Clements devised Exosurf in this manner, a preparation containing DPPC, hexadecanol, and tyloxapol. Hexadecanol and tyloxapol mimic the functions to some degree of surfactant proteins, PG, and other lipids in natural surfactant. Several groups have added surfactant proteins to lipids, designing the proteins to mimic structure and function of native surfactant proteins (13,14). Strategies that add surfactant proteins to lipid mixtures include formulating proteins using de novo peptide synthesis or recombinant DNA techniques (15).

Surfactant recipes based on estimates of minimal essential ingredients of natural surfactant have been used clinically. Morley and coworkers (16) developed a surfactant that they named Artificial Lung Expanding Compound (ALEC) which contains only DPPC and PG.

It is conceivable that delivery of surfactant constituents, or "incomplete" surfactants may be useful in certain diseases involving surfactant dysfunction (Table 2). By analyzing tracheal aspirates taken serially from infants with RDS, Shelley and coworkers (17) found changes in the composition presumably of alveolar surfactant as the infants improved and also noted a gradual increase in palmitic acid with recovery. Chida and coworkers (18) made similar observations over time with regard to surfactant proteins. One can imagine the goal of treatment in some infants might be to enrich their alveolar concentration for a

Table 2 Diseases for Which Surfactants Are Now Being Used Clinically

Condition	Rationale for surfactant therapy
Respiratory distress syndrome	Deficiency, inactivation
Adult respiratory distress syndrome	Inactivation, deficiency
Congenital diaphragmatic hernia	Surfactant deficiency in remaining lung
Infants treated with ECMO	Surfactant production impaired?
Meconium aspiration pneumonia	Inactivation

specific lipid or protein. Perhaps the clearest current indication for this approach would be protein or gene therapy treatment of infants having damaged genetic control specifically for the synthesis of SP-B (19).

B. Types of Surfactant Now Available for Clinical Use

Available therapeutic surfactants are of two types: those that are prepared from mammalian lungs and those made from synthetic compounds (Table 3). Bovine and porcine surfactants contain SP-B and SP-C associated with phospholipids. SP-A and SP-D are only present in the whole natural surfactant derived from the amniotic fluid which was used only in efficacy trials and is not available commercially. The synthetic surfactants are Exosurf and a 7:3 mixture of DPPC and PG (ALEC).

Surfactant TA

Surfactant TA (Surfacten, Tokyo Tanabe, Tokyo, Japan) was developed by Fujiwara and coworkers (20), and it was the first clearly efficacious surfactant used in human beings. The TA stands for Tokyo and Akita, the two cities in Japan where the surfactant was developed. Surfactant TA is prepared by organic solvent extractions of bovine lung mince, with the final surfactant composed of 1% SP-B, SP-C, 8% palmitic acid, 7% tripalmitin, and 84% phospholipids. It is delivered as 25 mg/ml of phospholipid at a dose of 100 mg (4 ml)/kg body weight. In Japan as in the United States, when beef is slaughtered for human consumption, the surface of the lung must be cut for inspection for evidence of infection. Therefore, lung mince is easier to obtain than lung lavage. Surfactant TA is supplied as a lyophilized powder that is reconstituted with saline. Electron microscopy of pellets of Surfactant TA shows marked heterogeneity of forms, including lamellae, variably sized vesicles, and amorphous material resembling protein (21).

Survanta

Survanta (Beractant, Abbott, North Chicago, IL is a natural bovine lung extract containing phospholipids, neutral lipids, fatty acids, and surfactant-associated

Table 3 Surfactants for Human Use

Surfactant	Possible advantages	Possible disadvantages
Human	Contains SP-A, which may decrease risk of infection	Not currently available SP-A may affect surfactant secretion and catabolism Possible unwanted constituents, e.g., infectious agents
Surfactant TA	Powder	Not available outside Japan
Exosurf	Inexpensive ingredients No protein Completely defined formulation	Incompletely defined metablism of tyloxapol Lower resistance to inactivation Less rapid improvement in gas exchange
Survanta	Has SP-B, SP-C No mixing	Cow lung mince Unwanted constituents
Alveofact	Bovine lung lavage	Not widely available Unwanted constituents
Infasurf	Lavage not mince Young calves vs. older cows	Not FDA approved Unwanted constituents
Curosurf	Higher concentration and dose	Pig lung mince Unwanted constituents
CLSE	Calf lung lavage	Unwanted constituents
ALEC	No protein Completely defined formulation	Not widely availablc Lacks SP-B and SP-C

proteins to which DPPC, palmitic acid, and tripalmitin are added to improve surface tension–lowering properties. This product is similar to Surfactant TA. Ross/Abbott Labs. (Columbus, OH) bought distribution rights for Surfactant TA outside parts of Asia. Unlike Surfactant TA, Survanta is distributed as a liquid. It is not clear whether there are other substantive differences in its manufacture. The composition of Survanta is 25 mg/ml phospholipids (including 11.0–15.5 mg/ml DPPC), 0.5–1.75 mg/ml triglycerides, 1.4–3.5 mg/ml free fatty acids, no cholesterol, and less than 1 mg/ml protein in the form of SP-B and SP-C. Survanta is one of the clinically useful surfactants with a lower SP-B content than Calf Lung Surfactant Extract (CLSE) or Alveofact (see below) (22).

Each dose of Survanta is 4 ml/kg = 100 ml/kg phospholipids (~44–62 mg/ml DPPC) that is administered intratracheally through a 5 French end-hole catheter inserted into the endotracheal tube. There have now been several randomized trials with one or multiple doses of Survanta used either prophylactically or as rescue therapy. Results are in favor of immediate improvements in gas exchange after a single or multiple doses (23,24) (see Chapter 19).

Calf Lung Surfactant Extract

Calf Lung Surfactant Extract (CLSE, Rochester, NY) is prepared from calf lung lavage from which lipids and lipophilic proteins are extracted. It was developed in a collaboration of groups from Rochester and Buffalo, New York and London, Ontario, Canada, by Shapiro, Notter, Egan, and Possmayer, and coworkers (25,26,92). CLSE is made privately in Canada. In the United States CLSE, or a similar compound, has been developed as Infasurf (see below). It contains 63% saturated PC, 32% other phospholipids, 4% cholesterol and cholesterol esters, and 1% hydrophobic protein (SP-B, SP-C) (25). Controlled trials of prophylactic use of CLSE have been done in infants of 24–28 weeks' and 25–29 weeks' gestation (26). Mortality and morbidity decreased significantly (27).

Infasurf

Infasurf (Forrest Labs, St. Louis, MO) is a surfactant is a chloroform-methanol extract of neonatal calf lung lavage without supplements. It is undergoing final clinical trials before anticipated release in the United States after approval by the Federal Drug Administration. It contains SP-B and SP-C, but it does not contain SP-A. Clinical trials comparing it with Exosurf or Survanta are in progress. Because Infasurf is prepared from lung lavage rather than lung mince, it may contain less unwanted ingredients. In vitro testing by Seeger et al. (22) indicates that Infasurf and CLSE may be the clinically available surfactants that are most refractory to inactivation. Infasurf contains 35 mg/ml phospholipids, 55–70% of which is saturated PC. The usual dose is 3 ml/kg = 105 mg phospholipids/kg. Infasurf has been the only surfactant used in infants with congenital diaphragmatic hernia (28). In a recent review, Infrasurf was found to reduce the incidence of retinopathy of prematurity along with a significant improvement in survival in infants with birth weights <1000 g (29). Auten and coworkers (30) used Infasurf in the treatment of respiratory failure secondary to meconium aspiration syn- drome/pneumonia with improvement in oxygenation.

Alveofact

Alveofact (Thomae GmbH, Biberach, Germany) is a compound obtained from bovine lung lavage and made up of 1% SP-B, SP-C, 88% phospholipids, 4% cholesterol, and 8% other lipids. According to results of in vitro studies (22), Alveofact contains relatively higher amounts of SP-B. Alveofact has been used in some clinical trials mainly in Germany. The dosing is 1.2 ml/kg; approximately 50 mg phospholipid/kg, and because of this lower dose it may be considered superior to the other surfactants in terms of risks with transient airway obstruction in neonates. In a multicenter trial, Alveofact given in the first hour following birth to infants of 25–30 weeks' gestation was shown to increase the incidence of survival without bronchopulmonary dysplasia with no effect on the incidence of air leaks, patent ductus arteriosus, or intracranial hemorrhage (31).

Curosurf

Curosurf (Chiesi Farmaceutici, Parma, Italy) is a surfactant that is made from minced pig lung by chloroform-methanol extraction and liquid-gel chromatography. The name of this surfactant derives from the names of the inventors: *Cu*stedt and *Ro*bertson. It contains 41–48% saturated PC, 51–58% other phospholipids, and ~1% SP-B, SP-C, without triglycerides, cholesterol, or free fatty acids (32). Like Survanta, Curosurf has been shown to contain a smaller amount of SP-B (22). It is used at a higher dose, 200 mg/kg = 2.5 ml/kg, and administered via a feeding tube (FS 5) inserted into the endotracheal tube. Curosurf has been used as prophylaxis and rescue therapy in several European multicenter trials with subsequent decrease in the incidence and severity of RDS (33–36).

Exosurf

Exosurf (Exogenous surfactant; Exosurf Neonatal, Burroughs Wellcome, Research Triangle Park, NC) is a synthetic, protein-free surfactant composed of 85% DPPC, 9% hexadecanol (cetyl alcohol), and 6% tyloxapol by weight, all in the form of lyophilized powder. When admixed with water, its concentration is 13.5 mg DPPC per milliliter. A single dose of 5 ml/kg body weight delivers 67 mg DPPC/kg. The cetyl alcohol and tyloxapol facilitate adsorption and spreading of DPPC. Exosurf is injected via the side port of an endotracheal tube adapter (see Chapter 15). In a multicenter, double-blind, placebo-controlled trial conducted at 23 hospitals in the United States, death from RDS was reduced with a single prophylactic dose (37). Short-term changes such as decreased ventilatory requirement and a drop in the incidence of air leaks have been the major findings in a variety of controlled trials done to date (38,39).

Artificial Lung Expanding Compound

Artificial Lung Expanding Compound (ALEC) (Pumactant, Britannia, Pharmaceuticals, Redhill, Surrey, UK) is composed of DPPC and unsaturated PG in a weight ratio of 7:3 and no protein (40). It is used as a suspension in cold saline and is administered two to four times as 100 mg in 1.0–1.2 ml, a relatively small volume compared with other surfactants. Clinical trials with ALEC showed improvement in lung compliance at 6 and 24 hr (41) and a decrease in mortality related to RDS.

III. Comparison of Surfactants In Vitro

The in vitro surface properties thought to be essential for good in vivo function are rapid adsorption of the surfactant from the subphase to the air-water interface, low minimum surface tension on dynamic compression, low compressibility, lack of degradation on repeated expansion and compression, and resistance to inhibition (see Chapters 1 and 12). These attributes vary when clinically useful surfactants are tested in vitro (Table 4). For example, in adsorption experiments, CLSE (containing SP-B and SP-C) achieves significantly lower surface tension than Survanta (containing SP-B and SP-C and palmitic acid). Addition of SP-B and SP-C to Exosurf improves its surface tension–lowering ability to a level comparable with CLSE (42).

Recently, marked differences among surfactants have been observed in vitro in the presence of putative surfactant inactivators (see Chapter 13). Inactivation in the presence of fibrinogen, albumin, and hemoglobin was studied with CLSE, Alveofact, Curosurf, Survanta, and an apoprotein-based synthetic phospholipid mixture supplemented with human recombinant SP-C and natural SP-B. Only Curosurf and Survanta were inhibited by all three proteins, whereas Alveofact and the synthetic surfactant were not. Susceptibility to inactivation was least in the two surfactants with the highest concentrations of SP-B (22). Using synthetic peptides modeled on SP-B and SP-C, Amirkhanian and coworkers found similar results (49). Venkitaraman and coworkers (50) have found that SP-A added to mixtures of lipids and low molecular weight surfactant proteins also prevents inactivation by serum inhibitors.

IV. Comparison of Surfactants In Vivo

In vivo responses can vary also in ways not necessarily predictable from in vitro results (Table 5). Ikegami and coworkers (51) compared four different surfactants (Surfactant TA, human surfactant, natural rabbit surfactant, natural sheep surfactant). Of the four surfactants studied, Surfactant TA required the least concentration to lower surface tension optimally. However, in studies with preterm lambs (120–122 days' gestation), initial oxygenation and ventilatory requirements were most improved with sheep surfactant. Human surfactant caused a transient improvement in gas exchange. Although differences in gas exchange and ventilatory settings existed among the four surfactants, reduction of protein leak into alveolar spaces was similar for the four.

Durand and colleagues (52) studied the effect of Exosurf and natural surfactant in slightly more mature preterm lambs of 132 days' gestation and found that survival rates in each group to be 80 and 100%, respectively. Similar experiments were done on preterm rabbits with natural surfactant and Exosurf.

Table 4 Important In Vitro Characteristics of Various Surfactants

Surfactant	Minimum surface tension	Lipid concentration (mg/ml) necessary to achieve surface tension <10 mN/m	Equilibrium surface tension at 0.5–3.0 mg/ml (mN/m)	Relative resistance to inactivation (arbitrary scale 0–5)	Approx. SP-B content
Exosurf	25–40 (42,46,48) 0 (43)	–[a]	38 (42)	1 (42)	0
Surfactant TA	7 (45)	2–3 (21)	–	–	–
Survanta	5–16 (22,42,46,48)	>2 (22)	28–36 (22,42,48)	3 (22,42)	<0.1% (22)
Alveofact	0 (22)	1 (22)	20–25 (22)	5(22)	1.7% (22)
Curosurf	0 (22)	1 (22)	20–25 (22)	3 (22)	0.2% (22)
CLSE	0 (22,42)	1 (22)	20–25 (22,42)	5 (22,42)	1.7% (22)
Lipid+SP-B,C	0–9 (22,42,45)	0.5 (22)	20–25 (22)	4 (42)	–
Bovine	0–3 (47)	–	–	–	–
Human	3 (12)	–	–	–	–
Sheep	0 (48)	–	<1 (44)	–	–
Infasurf	0–11 (46)	–	22 (48)	–	–

[a]Dashes indication no information available.

Source: Based on pulsating bubble measurements of 20 cycles/min (22,42,45–48) and captive bubble experiments (43).

Table 5 Important In Vivo Characteristics of Surfactants

Surfactant	Relative increase in oxygenation at the first hour after therapy (arbitrary scale 0–5)	Relative restoration of total lung capacity	Phospholipid content of lavage fluid after treatment (total recovery; mg)
Control	0 (45,48)	0% (48)	4.5–5.0 (48,51)
Exosurf	1–3 (48,52)	6–10% (42,45) 50% (53)	65 (48)
Surfactant TA	5 (45)	–	28 (51)
Survanta	4 (48)	40–50% (42,48)	50 (48)
Natural sheep	5 (48)	65–70% (48)	40–47 (48,51)
Human	–[a]	–	20 (51)
Lipid + SP-B	4 (45)	–	–
CLSE	–	100% (42)	–
Infasurf	5 (48)	100% (48)	75 (48)
Curosurf	5 (58,59)	–	–

[a]Dashes indicate no information available.
Source: Based on data from experiments on preterm (48,51,52), rats (42,45), in rabbits (53,59), and guinea pigs (58).

Tooley and colleagues (53) were able to show significant improvement in the lung mechanics of preterm rabbits that were given natural surfactant or Exosurf. Inspiratory pressures during the first hour of ventilation were significantly lower and the lung compliance was higher than the saline-treated control group. Natural surfactant was more effective than Exosurf in improving both of the parameters mentioned above.

Different results were found in a recent study that compared natural sheep surfactant, Infasurf, Survanta, and Exosurf in preterm lambs with a gestational age of 126 days (48). Although initial responses were good with the first three, sustained oxygenation and reduced need for ventilator support were only seen in animals treated with Infasurf. Average arterial to alveolar oxygen ratios showed significant initial improvements that declined over the first 12 hr of treatment with Survanta and natural sheep surfactant, whereas sustained oxygenation was maintained with Infasurf. Beneficial effects of natural sheep surfactant on oxygenation were not sustained possibly because SP-A may enhance alveolar uptake of this surfactant as well as decreasing type II cell secretion of surfactant (53,54). Therefore, if studies with adult type II cells are relevant to the in vivo metabolism of surfactant in immature animals, then surfactants containing SP-A may have enhanced uptake from the alveolar spaces and may decrease endogenous surfactant secretion when compared with surfactants that lack SP-A.

Ineffectiveness of Exosurf in this study could be explained by the way the study was conducted. Exosurf, but not the other surfactants, was administered after ventilation was begun. The dose of Exosurf was about half the dose of the other surfactants. Exosurf was given in multiple aliquots, whereas the other surfactants were given as a single-dose bolus.

The presence or absence of SP-A would not explain differences in activity between, say, Infasurf and Survanta, because both lack SP-A. Survanta is enriched in palmitic acid, a constituent that may enhance surface adsorption and distribution of DPPC (56). However, Survanta loses its efficacy in parallel with the disappearance of palmitic acid from the airways (48,57). Infasurf may have more efficacy, because it is derived from lung lavage rather than lung mince, and thus may have less unwanted constituents; e.g., infectious agents, or prostaglandin, lipid, and protein metabolites.

V. Direct Comparisons of Clinical Surfactants in Human Studies

Clinical trials with bovine, human, or pig surfactants compared with trials with Exosurf also give some indication that surfactant proteins may be important constituents of therapeutic surfactants in some infants. In meta-analyses of published and unpublished data, the Oxford Perinatal Group found differences of about 15% in air leak, death, and bronchopulmonary dysplasia (BPD) in the groups treated with surfactants containing surfactant proteins versus Exosurf-treated groups (60).

In a large multicenter randomized trial comparing Survanta and Exosurf, infants weighing 501 to 1500 g with RDS were given four intratracheal doses of either Survanta or Exosurf and outcome was compared in terms of death and chronic lung disease at 28 days (23). Although Survanta recipients required less oxygen and mean airway pressures during the first 72 hr following the initial dose, at the end of 28 days, there was no significant difference between the groups in the incidence of death or chronic lung disease. A nearly identical but much smaller study has come to the same conclusion and added the observation that nonresponders were more frequent in the Exosurf group. These studies indicate that results from in vitro and in vivo experiments with regard to the effects of surfactant proteins on the degree of surfactant inactivation may be clinically relevant (24).

VI. Major Constituents of Therapeutic Surfactants

A. DPPC

The key element in all pulmonary surfactants is DPPC, a compound known to be extremely effective at reducing surface tension. DPPC cannot be administered by itself into the lung because it adsorbs from subphase to the air-liquid interfaces slowly (61,62). Hall and coworkers (42) ranked the surface tension–lowering ability of various surfactants and surfactant mixtures using the pulsating bubble surfactometer and found an order of DPPC $<$ Exosurf $=$ tyloxapol $<$ Survanta $<$ CLSE. Addition of tyloxapol to DPPC improved performance significantly.

B. PG

PG, which makes up about 10% of total phospholipids of human surfactant, is generally essential for surface activity of pulmonary surfactant. The unique attribute of PG that is probably responsible for its activity in surfactant is its negative charge. King and coworkers (63) found that PG, in the presence of surfactant lipids and calcium, interacts with SP-A to form a complex that more readily adsorbs and spreads at an air-liquid interface than do the lipids alone. Another negatively charged phospholipid, phosphatidylinositol, can substitute for PG (64). PG can stimulate uptake of liposomal PC by type II cells (65), which might indicate that PG is associated with surfactant lipid turnover.

C. Fatty Acids

Palmitic acid is the primary free fatty acid in surfactants isolated from mammalian lung. It interacts with DPPC and/or SP-B to enhance the movement of surfactant from the subphase and to stabilize the surfactant complex at the air-water interface (56,62,66,67). Survanta and Surfactant TA both contain 7% palmitic acid and 7% tripalmitin. In vivo, palmitic acid disappears within an hour from the airways, a finding that may account for short-lived responses to these surfactants (48,57).

D. Hexadecanol

This substance is metabolized to palmitic acid, which is later utilized in the synthesis of phospholipids. It may serve the same function in Exosurf as palmitic acid does in Survanta and Surfactant TA. Elimination is more through expired air than through fecal or kidney route (68). In surface tension experiments, hexadecanol and DPPC have the same effect as DPPC alone (42).

E. Tyloxapol

Tyloxapol is a detergent that is used in Exosurf to disperse DPPC. Metabolites of tyloxapol are released into the blood from the lungs and excreted through the kidneys and intestinal tract (69). Tyloxapol alone is as effective as Exosurf or a DPPC-tyloxapol mixture, and it is significantly more so than DPPC-hexadecanol in decreasing surface tension in oscillating bubble experiments (42).

F. SP-A

During the past few years, a wealth of information on the composition and sequence of the pulmonary surfactant proteins has been published (70–76). In the presence of surfactant proteins SP-B and SP-C, SP-A enhances the surface activity of the phospholipids (77). SP-A may play a key role in the regulation of the surfactant turnover by facilitating the uptake and by inhibiting the secretion of phospholipids by type II pneumocytes (54,78). When CLSE was compared with CLSE + SP-A in the presence of albumin, the CLSE + SP-A was more resistant to inactivation (42). Cockshutt and coworkers (78) also observed an increase in resistance to inactivation in presence of SP-A. SP-A has also been shown to stimulate macrophage migration in a concentration-dependent manner by enhancing chemotaxis (79). SP-A collaborates with SP-B in transforming surfactant from the intracellular storage form to tubular myelin (80). Granted the effects of SP-A on phenomena that might affect risk of infection, and SP-A regulation of the intra-alveolar surfactant pool, it is not yet clear whether SP-A would be helpful or detrimental as a constituent of therapeutic surfactants.

G. SP-B

That SP-B is essential for natural surfactant function has been shown by a number of lines of evidence. By inducing tumors that secrete monoclonal antibodies to SP-B in mice, Suzuki and coworkers (81) have found that severe respiratory failure ensues. This group has also demonstrated the importance of SP-B by eliminating the efficacy of SP-B-containing surfactants by premixing them with anti-SP-B antibody (82). SP-B has been shown in vitro to be important in the cycling of PG from the monolayer to the subphase during the compression and expansion of the film (83). Two groups have imitated SP-B by making synthetic peptides that are similar to the amino acid sequence of native SP-B or that have secondary structures (helical) similar to that of SP-B (45,84). For the most part, results show that these mock peptides can demonstrate the function of SP-B in surfactant mixtures.

H. SP-C

The specific function of SP-C in surfactant is not known. SP-C has much less surface activity when added to surfactant lipids than SP-B (47). SP-B and SP-C, added together to surfactant lipids, improve not only the surface activity, but also the ability to resist inactivation to an extent greater than found with either protein alone (49). Similar findings were observed when these two hydrophobic proteins were added to DPPC alone or Exosurf (42).

I. SP-D

SP-D still remains to be the least known among the components of surfactant. It possesses some structural similarities to SP-A (see Chapter 3). It does not appear to be surface active. Smith and coworkers (85) found that surfactant lipids without proteins were ineffective in restoring pulmonary mechanics in rats made surfactant deficient. Rider and coworkers (86) had similar findings in 27-day gestation preterm rabbits. Results in terms of ventilatory pressures and lung compliance favored lipids combined with SP-B or lipids combined with SP-A and SP-B, over lipids alone or lipid SP-A and SP-C combinations (Fig. 1). Recovery of albumin in the alveolar washes, used as an index of protein leak into alveolar spaces, was the greatest in the lipid alone group.

VII. Obvious Remaining Questions Pertaining to Composition of Surfactants for Clinical Use

1. *Does the composition of surfactant have implications for dosage, means of delivery, or technique for posttreatment ventilation*? The question of how much to use for treatment depends to some degree on estimates of the pool size of endogenous surfactant. In infants with

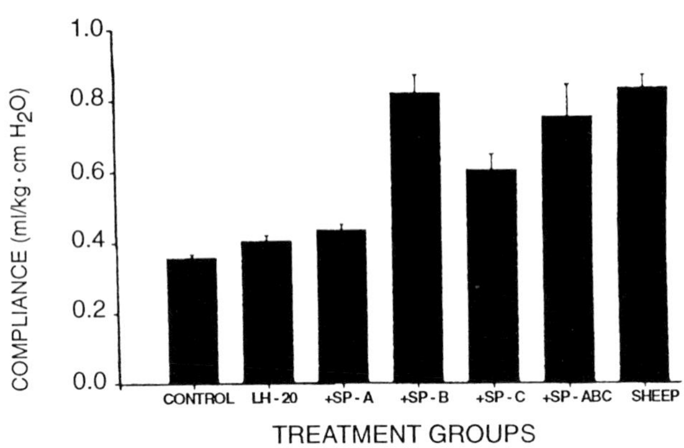

Figure 1 Dynamic compliance responses in rabbits ventilated with 3 cmH_2O PEEP and low tidal volume strategy. Addition of SP-A to the natural surfactant lipids did not significantly increase dynamic compliance, whereas addition of the hydrophobic proteins alone and in combination resulted in marked improvement in the response ($P < 0.05$ + SP-B, +SP-ABC, > +SP-C > +SP-A, LH-20 > Control). Addition of SP-B alone increased dynamic compliance to levels achieved after sheep surfactant treatment, whereas SP-C had an intermediate effect. (From ref. 86; used with permission) (*Sheep*; natural sheep surfactant recovered from saline alveolar washes of adult sheep lungs, *SP-A*, *SP-B*; isolated from sheep surfactant, *SP-C*; extracted from natural bovine surfactant, *LH-20*; protein free natural surfactant lipids isolated from natural sheep surfactant, *Control*; 0.45% NaCl).

RDS, the concentration of surfactant lipids and proteins increases over the first 4 days of age (17,18). Amounts of surfactant in the alveolar spaces approximate 100 mg/kg in healthy term animals (87,88). Preterm animals have pool sizes of 7–20 mg/kg of body weight. Preterm infants who have died soon after birth or who have severe disease may have 1–10 mg/kg (89). Jobe and coworkers (88) found 1.5–15.5 mg/kg body weight (2–20 μmol/kg) of saturated phosphatidylcholine in preterm lambs with RDS. These dosage considerations are predicated on the assumption that surfactant is a single compound, with all constiutents being deficient in proportion in cases of RDS. It is possible, especially during recovery from RDS or when surfactant inactivation predominates over surfactant deficiency that treatments wherein specific surfactant constituents are optimized may be indicated. Do we want therapeutic surfactants to affect the life cycle of surfactant by enhancing endogenous surfactant secretion or by decreasing metabolism or uptake? SP-A is a known factor that would affect these attributes of alveolar surfactant (54). As discussed in Chapter 17, it is probable that different infants will require different doses depending on disease severity, postnatal age, degree of surfactant inactivation, and relative lung maturity, yet rational guidelines for individualizing therapy do not yet exist. Similarly, surfactants with different attributes may require different styles of ventilator treatment (see Chapter 23).

2. *How do surfactant proteins, charged phospholipids, and DPPC interact at the molecular level to explain the biophysical behavior of surfactant in the alveoli*? This question has been revisited many times over past decades with increasing sensitivity and sophistication of techniques used to address it. Nonetheless, the molecular anatomy of surfactant lipids and proteins during their complex alveolar life cycles are not yet understood (90).
3. *Can surfactants serve as carriers or as vehicles for delivery of additional therapeutic agents*? Table 6 indicates the sorts of drugs that might be delivered to the lung using surfactant. Drugs encapsulated with surfactant liposomes would exploit the capability of surfactant to disperse rapidly on aqueous surfaces throughout the lung (91). Alternatively, therapeutic proteins could be covalently bound to surfactant proteins or lipids and thereby distributed into the lung. As yet there are no combined surfactant-drug treatments available for human use.
4. *Can some surfactants, or some surfactant constituents, under some conditions cause harm to patients*? The answer to this question must almost certainly be yes, but as yet these situations remain completely undefined. The most obvious condition where surfactant treatment

Table 6 Potential Uses of Surfactant in Pulmonary Drug Delivery

Disease	Possible drug delivery
Asthma	Bronchodilators
Bronchopulmonary dysplasia	Anti inflammatory agents
Lung infections	Immunotherapy
Persistent pulmonary hypertension	Vasodilators
Lung infections	Antibiotics
Lung hypoplasia	Growth factors
Bronchopulmonary dysplasia (Vit A)	Drugs enhancing epithelial integrity
Respiratory distress syndrome	Factors accelerating lung maturation
Cancer	Anti-neoplastic drugs
Cystic fibrosis, alveolar proteinosis	Lung lavage with surfactant replacement and drugs
Congenital SP-B deficiency	Gene therapy

would not be helpful would be in patients who fail to respond. This group of infants has not been well defined in clinical studies, although they appear to be the most immature and the sickest infants and/or those with surfactant inactivation as a predominant feature of their disease. Whether this group of patients accrues adverse effects from surfactant treatment is not yet known.

Acknowledgment

We thank John A. Clements for a very thorough review of the manuscript.

References

1. King RJ, Clements JA. Surface active materials from dog lung II. Composition and physiological correlations. Am J Physiol 1972; 223:715–726.
2. King RJ. Isolation and chemical composition of pulmonary surfactant. In: Robertson B, van Golde LMG, Batenburg JJ, eds. Pulmonary Surfactant. Amsterdam: Elsevier, 1984:1–15.
3. Magoon MW, Wright JR. Baritussio A, et al. Subfraction of lung surfactant. Implications for metabolism and surface activity. Biochim Biophys Acta 1983; 958:255–267.
4. Stevens PA, Wright JR, Clements JA. Changes in quantity, composition, and surface activity of alvolar surfactant at birth. J Appl Physiol 1987; 63:1049–1057.
5. Yamada T, Ikegami M, Jobe A. Effect of large and small aggregate surfactant subfractions on preterm rabbit lungs. Clin Res 1989; 37:211A.

6. Wright JR, Wager RE, Hamilton RL, et al. Uptake of lung surfactant subfractions into lamellar bodies of adult rabbit lungs. J Appl Physiol 1986; 60:817–825.
7. Avery ME, Mead J. Surface properties in relation to atelectasis and hyaline membrane disease. Am J Dis Child 1959; 97:517–523.
8. Chu J, Clements JA, Cotton EK, et al. Neonatal pulmonary ischemia: Clinical and physiological studies. Pediatrics 1967; 40:709–782.
9. Liggins GC, Howie RN. A controlled trial of antepartum glucocorticoid treatment for prevention of the respiratory distress syndrome in premature infants. Pediatrics 1972; 50:515–520.
10. Althabe F, Fustinana C, Althabe O, Cernadas C., Controlled trial of prenatal betamethasone plus TRH vs. betamethasone plus placebo for prevention of RDS in preterm infants. Pediatr Res 1991; 29:200A.
11. Hallman M, Bry K, Hoppu K, et al. Inositol supplementation in premature infants with respiratory distress syndrome. N Engl J Med 1992; 326:1233–1239.
12. Hallman M, Merritt TA, Schneider H, et al. Isolation of human surfactant from amniotic fluid and a pilot study of its efficacy in respiratory distress syndrome. Pediatrics 1983; 71:473–482.
13. Cochrane CG, Revak SD. Pulmonary surfactant protein (SP-B): Structure-function relationships. Science 1991; 254:566–568.
14. Bruni R, Taeusch HW, Waring AJ. Surfactant protein B: Lipid interactions of synthetic peptides representing the amino-terminal amphiphathic domain. Proc Natl Acad Sci USA 1991; 88:7451–7455.
15. Yao L-J, Richardson C, Ford C. Expression of mature pulmonary surfactant-associated protein B in Escherichia coli, using truncated human SP-B cDNA's. Biochem Cell Biol 1990; 68:559–566.
16. Morley CJ, Bangham AD, Miller N, Davis JA. Dry artificial surfactant and its effects on very premature babies. Lancet 1981; 1:64–68.
17. Shelley S, Kovacevic M, Paciga JE, Balis JU. Sequential changes of surfactant phosphatidylcholine in hyaline membrane disease. N Engl J Med 1979; 300:112–116.
18. Chida S, Phelps DS, Cordle C, et al. Surfactant-associated proteins in tracheal aspirates of infants with respiratory distress syndrome after exogenous surfactant therapy. Am Rev Respir Dis 1988; 137:943–947.
19. Nogee LM, deMello DE, Dehner LP, Colten HR. Brief report: Deficiency of pulmonary surfactant protein B in congenital alveolar proteinosis. N Engl J Med 1993; 328:406–410.
20. Fujiwara T, Maeta H, Chida S, et al. Artificial surfactant therapy in hyaline membrane disease. Lancet 1980; 1:55–59.
21. Taeusch HW, Keough KMW, Williams M, et al. Characterization of bovine surfactant for infants with respiratory distress syndrome. Pediatrics 1986; 77:572–581.
22. Seeger W, Grube C, Günther A, Schmidt R. Surfactant inhibition by plasma proteins: differential sensitivity of various surfactant preparations. Eur Respir J 1993; 6:971–977.
23. Horbar JD, Wright L, Soll R. A multicenter randomized trial comparing two surfactants for the treatment of neonatal RDS. Pediatrics 1993; 123:757–765.

24. Sehgal S, Ewing C, Richards T, Taeusch HW. Modified bovine surfactant (Survanta) versus a protein free surfactant (Exosurf) in the treatment of respiratory distress syndrome in preterm infants: A pilot study. J Natl Med Assoc 1994; 86:46–52.
25. Shapiro DL, Notter RH, Morin IIIFC, et al. Double-blind, randomized trial of a calf lung surfactant extract administered at birth to very premature infants for prevention of respiratory distress syndrome. Pediatrics 1985; 76:593–599.
26. Kwong MS, Egan EA, Notter RH, Shapiro DI. Double blind clinical trial of calf lung surfactant extract for the prevention of hyaline membrane disease in extremely premature infants. Pediatrics 1985; 76:585–592.
27. Kendig JW, Notter RH, Cox C. Surfactant replacement therapy at birth: final analysis of a clinical trial and comparison with similar trials. Pediatrics 1988; 82:756–762.
28. Glick PL, Leach CL, Besner GE, et al. Exogenous surfactant therapy for the high-risk neonate with CDH. J Pediatr Surg 1992; 27:866–869.
29. Repka MX, Hudak ML, Parsa CF, Tielsch JM. Calf lung surfactant extract prophylaxis and retinopathy of prematurity. Ophthalmology 1992; 99:531–536.
30. Auten RL, Notter RH, Kendig JW, et al. Surfactant treatment of full-term newborns with respiratory failure. Pediatrics 1991; 87:101–107.
31. Gortner L, Bartmann P, Pohlandt F, et al. Early treatment of respiratory distress syndrome with bovine surfactant in very preterm infants: a multicenter controlled clinical trial. Pediatr Pulmonol 1992; 14:4–9.
32. Curstedt T, Jörnvall H, Berggren P, Robertson B. Artificial surfactants based on different hydrophobic low-molecular-weight proteins. In: Lachmann B, ed. Surfactant Replacement Therapy in Neonatal and Adult Respiratory Distress Syndrome. Berlin: Springer-Verlag, 1988:332–337.
33. Egberts J, de Winter P, Sedin G, et al. Comparison of prophylaxis and rescue treatment with Curosurf in neonates less than 30 weeks' gestation: A randomized trial. Pediatrics 1993; 92:768–774.
34. Collaborative European Multicenter Study Group. Surfactant replacement therapy for severe neonatal respiratory distress syndrome: An international randomized clinical trial. Pediatrics 1988; 82:683–691.
35. Speer CP, Robertson B, Curstedt T, et al. Randomized European multicenter trial of surfactant replacement therapy for severe neonatal respiratory distress syndrome: single versus multiple doses of Curosurf. Pediatrics 1991; 89:13–20.
36. Bevilacqua G, Halliday H, Parmigiani S, Robertson B. Randomized multicentre trial of treatment with porcine natural surfactant for moderately severe neonatal respiratory distress syndrome. J Perinat Med 1993; 21:329–340.
37. Stevenson D, Walther F, Long W, et al. Controlled trial of a single dose of synthetic surfactant at birth in premature infants weighing 500 to 699 grams. The American Exosurf Neonatal Study Group. J Pediatr 1992; 120:S3–12.
38. Corbet A, Bucciarelli R, Goldman S. Decreased mortality rate among small premature infants treated at birth with a single dose of synthetic surfactant: a multicenter controlled trial. J Pediatr 1991; 118:277–284.
39. Information from The Wellcome Foundation. Effects of two 5 ml/kg doses of Exosurf in established respiratory distress syndrome.

40. Bangham AD, Morley CJ, Phillips MC. The physical properties of an effective lung surfactant. Biochim Biophys Acta 1979; 573:552–556.
41. Morley CJ, Greenough A. Respiratory compliance in premature babies treated with artificial surfactant (ALEC). Arch Dis Child 1991; 66:467–471.
42. Hall SB, Venkitaraman AR, Whitsett JA, Notter RH. Importance of hydrophobic apoproteins as constituents of clinical exogenous surfactants. Am Rev Respir Dis 1992; 145:24–30.
43. Schürch FS. Surface tension properties of surfactant. Clin Perinatol 1993; 20:669–682.
44. Holm BA, Enhorning G, Notter RN. A biophysical mechanism by which plasma proteins inhibit lung surfactant activity. Chem Phys Lipids 1988; 49:49–55.
45. Waring A, Taeusch HW, Bruni R, et al. Synthetic amphipathic sequences of surfactant protein-B mimic several physicochemical and in vivo properties of native pulmonary surfactant proteins. Peptide Res 1989; 2:308–313.
46. Scarpelli EM, David E, Cordova M, Mautone AJ. Surface tension of therapeutic surfactants (Exosurf Neonatal, Infasurf, Survanta). Am J Perinatol 1992; 9:414–419.
47. Takahashi A, Waring A, Amirkhanian J, et al. Structure-function relationships of bovine pulmonary surfactant proteins: SP-B and SP-C. Biochim Biophys Acta 1990; 1044:43–49.
48. Cummings JJ, Holm BA, Hudak ML, et al. A controlled clinical comparison of four different surfactant preparations in surfactant deficient lambs. Am Rev Respir Dis 1992; 145:999–1004.
49. Amirkhanian JD, Bruni R, Waring AJ, et al. Full length synthetic surfactant proteins, SP-B and SP-C reduce surfactant inactivation by serum. Biochim Biophys Acta 1993; 1168:315–320.
50. Venkitaraman A, Hall S, Whitsett J, Notter R. Enhancement of biophysical activity of lung surfactant extracts and phospholipid-apoprotein mixtures by surfactant protein A. Chem Phys Lipids 1990; 56:185–194.
51. Ikegami M, Agata Y, Elkady T, et al. Comparison of four surfactants: In vitro surface properties and responses of preterm lambs to treatment at birth. Pediatrics 1987; 79:38–46.
52. Durand DJ, Clyman RI, Heymann HA et al. Effects of a protein-free, synthetic surfactant on survival and pulmonary function in preterm lambs. J Pediatr 1985; 107:775–780.
53. Tooley WH, Clements JA, Muramatsu K, et al. Lung function in prematurely delivered rabbits treated with a synthetic surfactant. Am Rev Respir Dis 1987; 136:651–656.
54. Corbet A, Bedi H, Owens M, Taeusch HW. Surfactant protein-A inhibits lavage-induced surfactant secretion in newborn rabbits. Am J Med Sci 1992; 304:246–251.
55. Wright JR, Wagner RE, Hawgood S, et al. Surfactant apoprotein Mr = 26000–36000 enhances uptake of liposomes by type 2 cells. J Biol Chem 1986; 262:2888–2894.
56. Longo ML, Bisango AM, Zasadzinski JAN, et al. A function of lung surfactant protein SP-B. Science 1993; 261:453–456.
57. Tabor B, Ikegami M, Yamada T, Jobe A. Rapid clearance of surfactant-associated palmitic acid from the lungs of developing and adult animals. Pediatr Res 1990; 27:268–273.

58. Berggren P, Lachmann B, Curstedt T, et al. Gas exchange and lung morphology after surfactant replacement in experimental adult respiratory distress syndrome induced by repeated lung lavage. Acta Anaesthesiol Scand 1986; 30:321–328.
59. Bambang Oetomo S, de Ley L, Curstedt T, et al. Distribution of endotracheally instilled surfactant protein SP-C in lung lavaged rabbits. Pediatr Res 1991; 29:178–181.
60. The OSIRIS Collaborative Group (Open Study of Infants at high risk of or with Respiratory Insufficiency—The role of Surfactant). Early versus delayed neonatal administration of a synthetic surfactant—the judgement of OSIRIS. Lancet 1992; 340:1363–1369.
61. Longo ML, Waring A, Zasadzinski JAN. Lipid bilayer surface association of lung surfactant protein SP-B, amphipathic segment detected by flow immunofluorescence. J Biophysiol 1992; 63:760–773.
62. Cockshutt A, Absolom D, Possmayer F. The role of palmitic acid in pulmonary surfactant: Enhancement of surface activity and prevention of inhibition by blood proteins. Biochim Biophys Acta 1991; 1085:248–256.
63. King RJ, MacBeth MC. Interaction of the lipid and protein components of pulmonary surfactant. Role of phosphatidylglycerol and calcium. Biochim Biophys Acta 1981; 647:159–168.
64. Beppu OS, Clements JA, Goerke J. Phosphatidylglycerol-deficient lung surfactant has normal properties. J Appl Physiol 1983; 55:496–502.
65. Bates SR, Ibach PB, Fisher AB. Phospholipids co-isolated with rat surfactant protein C account for the apparent protein-enhanced uptake of liposomes into lung granular pneumocytes. Exp Lung Res 1989; 15:695–708.
66. Holm BA, Venkitaraman AR, Enhorning G, Notter R. Biophysical inhibition of synthetic lung surfactants. Chem Phys Lipids 1990; 52:243–250.
67. Tanaka Y, Takei T, Aiba T, et al. Development of synthetic lung surfactants. J Lipid Res 1986; 27:475–485.
68. Findlay JWA, Kearney MF, Barnes ER. Disposition of Exosurf components in the rabbit after intratracheal administration: I. Hexadecanol. J Pediatr. In press.
69. DeAngelis RL, Kearney MF, Barnes ER. Disposition of Exosurf components in the rabbit after intratracheal administration: III. Tyloxapol. J Pediatr. In press.
70. Floros J, Phelps DS, Kourembanas S, Taeusch HW. Primary translation products, biosynthesis, and tissue specificity of the major surfactant protein in rat. J Biol Chem 1986; 261:828–831.
71. Floros J, Steinbrink R, Jacobs K, et al. Isolation and characterization of cDNA clones for the 35 kDa pulmonary surfactant associated protein (PSP-A). J Biol Chem 1986; 261:9029–9033.
72. White RT, Damm D, Miller J, et al. Isolation and characterization of the human pulmonary surfactant apoprotein gene. Nature 1985; 317:361–363.
73. Sano K, Fisher J, Mason RJ, et al. Isolation and sequence of a cDNA clone for the rat pulmonary surfactant-associated protein (PSP-A). Biochem Biophys Res Commun 1987; 144:367–374.
74. Warr RG, Hawgood S, Buckley DI, et al. Low molecular weight human pulmonary surfactant protein (SP5): isolation, characterization and cDNA and amino acid sequences. Proc Natl Acad Sci USA 1987; 84:7915–7919.

75. Glasser SW, Korfhagen TR, Weaver TE, et al. cDNA, deduced polypeptide structure and chromosomal assignment of human pulmonary surfactant proteolipid, SPL(pVal). J Biol Chem 1988; 263:9–12.
76. Hawgood S, Benson BJ, Schilling J, et al. Nucletide and amino acid sequences of pulmonary surfactant protein SP 18 and evidence for cooperation between SP 18 and SP 28–36 in surfactant lipid adsorption. Proc Natl Acad Sci USA 1987; 84:66–70.
77. Hawgood S, Benson BJ, Hamilton RL Jr. Effects of a surface associated protein and calcium ions on the structure and surface activity of lung surfactant lipids. Biochemistry 1985; 24:184–190.
78. Cockshutt A, Weitz J, Possmayer F. Pulmonary surfactant-associated protein A enhances the surface activity of lipid extract surfactant and reverses inhibition by blood proteins in vitro. Biochem Biophys Res Commun 1990; 29:8424–8429.
79. Wright JR, Youmans DC. Pulmonary SP-A stimulates chemotaxis of alveolar macrophage. Am J Physiol 1993; 264:6338–6344.
80. Williams M, Hawgood S, Hamilton RL. Changes in lipid structure produced by surfactant proteins SP-A, SP-B, and SP-C. Am J Resp Cell Mol Biol 1991; 5:41–50.
81. Suzuki Y, Robertson B, Fujita Y, et al. Lung protein leakage in respiratory failure induced by a hybridoma making monoclonal antibody to the hydrophobic surfactant-associated polypeptide SP-B. Int J Exp Pathol 1992; 73:325–333.
82. Robertson B, Kobayashi T, Ganzuka M, et al. Experimental neonatal respiratory failure induced by a monoclonal antibody to the hydrophobic surfactant-associated protein SP-B. Pediatr Res 1991; 30:239–243.
83. Yu S, Possmayer F. Role of bovine pulmonary surfactant-associated proteins in the surface-active property of phospholipid mixtures. Biochim Biophys Acta 1990; 1046:233–241.
84. McLean LR, Lewis JE, Krstenansky JL, et al. An amphipathic alpha helical decapeptide in phosphatidylcholine is an effective synthetic lung surfactant. Am Rev Respir Dis 1993; 147:462–465.
85. Smith G, Taeusch HW, Phelps D, Keough K. Mixtures of low molecular weight surfactant proteins and dipalmitoyl phosphatidylcholine duplicate effects of pulmonary surfactant in vitro and in vivo. Pediatr Res 1988; 23:484–489.
86. Rider E, Ikegami M, Whitsett J, et al. Treatment responses to surfactants containing natural surfactant proteins in preterm rabbits. Am Rev Respir Dis 1993; 147:669–676.
87. Jackson JC, Palmer S, Standaert TA. Developmental changes of surface active material in newborn nonhuman primates. Am Rev Respir Dis 1984; 129:A204.
88. Jobe AH, Ikegami M, Jacobs HC, Jones SJ. Surfactant pool sizes and severity of respiratory distress syndrome in prematurely delivered lambs. Am Rev Respir Dis 1983; 127:751–755.
89. Adams FH, Fujiwara T, Emmanouilides G, Räihä N. Lung phospholipids of human fetuses and infants with and without hyaline membrane disease. J Pediatr 1970; 77:833–841.
90. Taeusch HW, Waring AJ. Surfactant proteins and surfactant therapy. In: Frantz ID, ed. Surfactant Replacement Therapy—A Clinical Symposium. Newtown, PA: Ross Laboratories/Associates in Medical Marketing, 1993; 5–17.

91. Kharasch VS, Sweeney TD, Fredberg J, et al. Pulmonary surfactant as a vehicle for intratracheal delivery of technetium sulfur colloid and pentamidine in hamster lungs. Am Rev Respir Dis 1991; 144:909–913.
92.. Enhorning G, Shennan A, Possmayer F, et al: Prevention of neonatal respiratory distress syndrome by tracheal instillation of surfactant: A randomized clinical trial. Pediatrics 1985; 76:145–153.

12

Experimental Models for Evaluation of Exogenous Surfactants

BENGT ROBERTSON
Karolinska Institute
Stockholm, Sweden

I. Introduction

The first successful experimental demonstration of improved lung function after surfactant replacement in animal models of surfactant deficiency (1,2) triggered a rapidly growing interest in the clinical potential of this new treatment for neonatal respiratory distress syndrome (RDS) and other forms of lung disease. As reviewed elsewhere in this this volume (Chapter 19), several thousand newborn babies have now been treated with various types of exogenous surfactants in controlled clinical trials. The results are generally concordant and corroborated by meta-analyses of pooled data from multiple randomized trials (3,4). Prophylactic treatment of surfactant reduces the incidence and severity of RDS and its complications in babies at risk, and treatment of established RDS reduces air leads and lowers mortality (see Chapters 18–20). Animal experiments are no longer needed to document these important effects of surfactant treatment, but they may still be useful for the detection of potentially important physical and physiological differences between surfactants in clinical use, as well as for preliminary evaluation of new surfactant substitutes.

This chapter will review experimental studies of various exogenous surfactants in in vitro systems and in animal models of surfactant dysfunction and pneumonia, with particular reference to differential effects on lung mechanics, protein leakage, morphology, and bacterial proliferation. Accumulated evidence from such studies indicates that the quality of an exogenous surfactant depends on both lipid composition and the presence of surfactant-associated proteins, especially the hydrophobic polypeptides. Also, the hydrophilic proteins may be important to increase resistance to inhibition and to stimulate alveolar macrophages in case of pulmonary infection. These latter aspects are discussed in detail in Chapters 4, 11, and 13.

II. Comparative Physicochemical Studies of Exogenous Surfactants

The physical properties of surfactant preparations are usually described in terms of surface adsorption from the hypophase, surface spreading and respreadability, film compressibility, and changes in surface tension during cyclic film compression (see Chapter 1). The biophysical requirements of an "optimal" exogenous surfactant may vary in different clinical situations. If exogenous surfactant is to influence lung mechanics during the first few breaths of a newborn baby, it must adsorb within a second to the rapidly expanding air-liquid interfaces of the lung. Similarly, in a patient with severe respiratory failure due to surfactant deficiency, rapid spreading is probably essential for the therapeutic effect by allowing the exogenous surfactant to reach its site of action in terminal air spaces with a minimum of delay. In a less critical clinical situation, rapid improvement of lung function may not be crucial, and the main mission of an exogenous surfactant may then be to enlarge the pool of intra-alveolar phospholipids available for recycling.

Effective respreadability, i.e., reentry of squeezed-out surfactant molecules into the surface film, is probably important for the economy of the surfactant system, as it reduces the consumption rate and thus the need for film replenishment from either newly secreted lamellar bodies or additional doses of exogenous surfactant. Low surface compressibility is believed to be important for alveolar stability, since low surface tension can then be attained with only minimal dimensional changes (5). These physical properties are temperature dependent and furthermore vary with the concentration of surfactant in the hypophase (6,7). Maximum and minimum surface tension during cyclic film compression in a Wilhelmy balance or pulsating-bubble system also depend on the cycling speed and the degree of area oscillation. In vitro comparison of different surfactants, therefore, calls for well-standardized experimental conditions.

Several in vitro model systems have been developed for testing of physical properties of exogenous surfactants. These include the automated Wilhelmy balance (a modern version of this instrument is marketed by Biegler Electronic,

Mauerbach, Austria), the Pulsating-Bubble Surfactometer (Electronetics, Amherst, NY) originally developed by Enhorning (8), and the captive bubble device recently described by Schürch et al. (9) (see Chapter 1). Each of these methods has its advantages and drawbacks. The commercially available Wilhelmy balance and pulsating-bubble systems are easy to handle, but film leakage during compression of surfactant films is a notorious problem with both methods. Barrow and Hills (10), in a critical assessment of the Wilhelmy balance method, also pointed out a contact angle problem that tends to render erroneously low minimum surface tension values for surfactant films unless appropriate corrections are made.

The advantages of the pulsating-bubble system includes small sample volume (20 μl), and access to dynamic surface tension measurements during rapid area oscillation simulating normal respiratory frequency. On the other hand, calculations of surface tension from the pressure gradient across the bubble wall become inexact when the pressure gradient approaches zero (which characteristically happens during compression of monolayers with a high content of dipalmitoyl phosphatidylcholine [DPPC]), because the bubble loses its spherical shape. However, the absolute error is small (<0.5 mN/m at minimum bubble size) and does not, therefore, affect the validity of the results (11). Several of these problems are avoided with the captive bubble system, in which there is no escape for the surface film during compression and surface tension is calculated from variations in bubble shape (9) (see Chapter 1).

A. Adsorption and Spreading Kinetics

Surfactant TA

Surfactant TA (Surfacten, Tokyo Tanabe, Tokyo, Japan), a modification of the preparation used in the first successful clinical study of replacement therapy for neonatal RDS (12–14), is an organic solvent extract of minced bovine lungs to which the synthetic lipids DPPC, triacylglycerol, and palmitic acid have been added to standardize composition and improve surface properties. This surfactant spreads within a few seconds when applied as a droplet onto a hypophase of saline and generates an equilibrium surface tension of about 30 mN/m (14). When dispersed in a hypophase of saline at a phospholipid concentration of 50 μg/ml, it adsorbs within less than 1 min to reach a surface tension of 27–30 mN/m (14). Similar adsorption kinetics have been reported for Survanta (Beractant, Abbot, North Chicago, IL), a modified bovine surfactant analogous to Surfactant TA (15). CLSE (Calf Lung Surfactant Extract) (16) adsorbs even more effectively in the same assay system and the equilibrium surface tension is below 25 mN/m (15).

Curosurf

Curosurf (Chiesi Farmaceutici, Parma, Italy), a modified natural surfactant isolated from pig lungs by extraction with organic solvents and further purified by liquid-gel chromatography (17), spreads within less than 1 sec from a droplet applied on a saline hypophase, and generates an equilibrium surface tension of about 25 mN/m (18). Studies with the captive bubble system have revealed that Curosurf adsorbs extremely rapidly from a hypophase of saline. When suspended at a concentration of 1 mg/ml in saline, less than 1 sec is required to lower surface tension to about 26 mN/m. As pointed out elsewhere in this volume (Chapter 1), the adsorption of Curosurf frequently seems to occur in "quantum jumps" corresponding to the simultaneous insertion of a large number of phospholipid molecules (about 10^{14} or about 120 ng of phospholipid) in the monolayer at the air-liquid interface (19). These adsorbing complexes must be highly enriched in DPPC, as only little film compression is required to lower surface tension to a level close to 0 mN/m (see Section II.D). The mechanism behind this selective adsorption is not known, but is probably related to the presence of hydrophobic proteins (20,21).

"Lipid Extract Surfactant"

Lipid extract surfactant, a preparation equivalent to Infasurf (ONY, Amherst, New York) or CLSE, also exhibits very rapid adsorption in the captive bubble system. When suspended at a concentration >0.8 mg/ml in 0.9% NaCl and 1.5 mM $CaCl_2$, it requires less than 1 sec to lower surface tension <30 mN/m, and less than 5 sec to establish an equilibrium surface tension of about 25 mN/m. Similar rates of adsorption can be observed at even lower surfactant concentrations if SP-A is added to the sample (22).

Artificial Surfactants

Artificial Lung Expanding Compound (ALEC) (Pumactant, Britannia Pharmaceuticals, Redhill, Surrey, UK), a protein-free surfactant prepared from DPPC and unsaturated glycerol (7:3) spreads as rapidly as modified natural surfactant provided that the material is applied as dry particles onto the hypophase (14,23). The same lipid mixture suspended in the hypophase exhibits very slow and ineffective surface adsorption, probably because the lipids aggregate as micelles or other "closed" complexes in the water phase (24). Exosurf (Burroughs Wellcome, Research Triangle Park, NC), a synthetic surfactant made from DPPC, hexadecanol, and tyloxapol (a detergent) (25) adsorbs slowly from a hypophase of saline; at a hypophase concentration of 0.5 mg/ml, it takes about 20 min to lower surface tension from 70 to 38 mN/m (15). Similar adsorption kinetics were noted for tyloxapol alone, whereas the adsorption isotherm for hexadecanol alone was characterized by a much more rapid initial fall in surface tension and an equilibrium surface tension of about 25 mN/m. On the other hand, hexadecanol alone did not accelerate adsorption of DPPC. These intriguing data suggest that the surface properties of Exosurf during adsorption are largely determined by the detergent present in the mixture (15). In a recent study using the captive bubble system, Exosurf at a concentration of 1 mg/ml required about 4 min to adsorb to a static surface tension of 38 mN/m (26).

B. Dynamic Surface Tension in Wilhelmy Balance

Films of Surfactant TA, generated from a droplet applied onto a hypophase of saline, have a minimum surface tension below 5 mN/m during 50% cyclic surface compression in a Wilhelmy balance system. These films have a low compressibility (<0.02 m/mN at surface tension 10 mN/m), reflecting the high content of "stiff" saturated fatty acid chains in the monolayer, and effective respreadability (14). Human amniotic fluid surfactant, isolated by sucrose gradient centrifugation, is characterized by a higher film compressibility (0.04 m/mN); such films require 90% compression to reduce surface tension to 3 mN/m (27). In contrast, films of CLSE spread from hexane:ethanol (9:1) solutions require only 20% compression to lower surface tension <5 mN/m (28). Minimum surface tension of Exosurf films approaches 0 mN/m during the first 90% compression cycle in a Wilhelmy balance system, but increases to 8 mN/m in subsequent cycles, indicating inadequate replenishment of the monolayer during film expansion (29). This is similar to the dynamic surface properties reported for DPPC plus high-density lipoprotein (10:1, w/w), an artificial surfactant developed by Meban (30) and used in a randomized clinical trial for prophylaxis of neonatal RDS without convincing effects (31). Films of DPPC plus unsaturated PG, spread from dry particles, lower surface tension <5 mN/m during 50% surface compression (23).

Sun et al. (32) recently studied the "economy" of surfactant films generated by various methods in a Wilhelmy balance system. Different amounts of modified porcine surfactant (Curosurf) were applied onto the surface as dry particles or droplets, or were suspended in the hypophase, and the films generated by this material were subjected to 50% cyclic compression at a rate of 1 cycle/min. Film spreading was faster from droplets than from dry particles of surfactant, but the period during which minimum surface tension of the compressed film remained <5 mN/m was significantly longer for the dry material than for a similar amount of material applied in droplet form. This suggests that the "wet" surfactant became dispersed more quickly in the (huge) hypophase of the system and, therefore, was less readily available for film replenishment during prolonged cycling. Nevertheless, modified porcine surfactant, suspended in the hypophase at a phospholipid concentration of 0.5 mg/ml, generated very stable films. Minimum surface tension dropped below 5 mN/m within a few cycles, and this low value usually persisted for several hours of cyclic film compression.

C. Pulsating Bubble Measurements

In the Pulsating-Bubble Surfactometer (8), modified natural surfactants characteristically exhibit rapid adsorption and low minimum surface tension at hypophase concentrations >5 mg/ml. However, at lower surfactant concentrations, biophysical differences between various surfactants become recognizable. Surfactant TA thus requires a hypophase concentration of only 1.25 mg/ml to generate a film with minimum surface tension <10 mN/m during 50% surface compression (33); with Curosurf, this critical concentration is significantly higher, about 5 mg/ml (17). Exosurf at a hypophase concentration of 10 mg/ml was originally reported to generate, in a pulsating-bubble system, a minimum surface tension close to 0 mN/m during 40% surface compression (29), but this observation has not been confirmed by others. Hall et al. (15) found a minimum surface tension of 29 mN/m for Exosurf at a concentration of 10 mg/ml. Recent measurements reported by Corcoran et al. (34) gave similar results. With CLSE and Survanta at 2.5 mg/ml, minimum surface tension values during pulsation were 1 and 2 mN/m, respectively (15).

D. Surface Tension Measurements in Captive Bubble

Films of lipid extract surfactant (equivalent to Infasurf and CLSE) or Curosurf, generated in a captive bubble, require only 20–30% compression to reduce quasi-static surface tension from about 25 mN/m to near 0 mN/m (19,22) (see also Chapter 1). As mentioned above, this indicates selective adsorption of DPPC to the air-liquid interface, probably mediated by hydrophobic proteins. Films of Exosurf studied under similar quasi-static conditions have to be compressed by 80% to achieve very low minimum surface tension; however, by increasing the cycling speed to 50/min, minimum surface tension near 0 mN/m could be obtained with only 40% surface compression (26).

E. Comments

Surfactant preparations currently used in clinical practice thus show a considerable variation in surface properties under standardized experimental conditions, with adsorption rates ranging from <1 sec to several minutes, equilibrium surface tension from <25 to about 40 mN/m, and the degree of surface compression required to lower surface tension <5 mN/m from 20 to 80%. Yet, all these exogenous surfactants are effective in clinical practice, albeit with different time course in the therapeutic response (see Chapters 19–21).

Nohara et al. (35) studied possible correlations between in vitro and in vivo physiological properties of various modified natural surfactants. A surfactant with rapid adsorption and comparatively high minimum surface tension in Wilhelmy balance (>15 mN/m) was isolated from minced bovine lungs by a combination of chloroform-methanol extraction and liquid-gel chromatography.

By adding synthetic DPPC, tripalmitin, and palmitic acid in proportions suggested by Tanaka et al. (36), minimum surface tension was lowered and the surface area versus surface tension isotherms recorded in Wilhelmy balance became similar to those of Surfactant TA. However, this was associated with a slightly retarded surface adsorption and did not improve the therapeutic effect of the same preparation in experiments in ventilated immature newborn rabbits.

There may be a certain "tolerance" in regard to the phospholipid composition of an exogenous surfactant, as a film of mixed surfactant phospholipids tends to refine spontaneously during cyclic film compression, gradually increasing the proportion of saturated species, especially DPPC (37). The presence or absence of the surfactant-specific proteins is probably more critical for surfactant function. Hall et al. (15) recently made the interesting observation that the physical and physiological properties of Exosurf can be improved by adding hydrophobic proteins (SP-B, SP-C). Other investigators have shown that adsorption kinetics and dynamic surface tension of a modified natural surfactant, prepared by extraction of lung lavage fluid with an organic solvent, can be further improved by addition of SP-A (22,38). The presence of SP-A also renders the surfactant more resistant to inactivation by leaking serum proteins (38) (see Chapter 13).

III. Animal Models

In general, in vitro surface properties of a surfactant preparation do not predict the physiological effects in experimental animals (39). A surfactant with rapid adsorption and low minimum surface tension under clean in vitro conditions may behave differently in immature alveoli flooded with proteinaceous edema fluid (40–42), interfering with surfactant function (43–45). Protein-free synthetic surfactants with seemingly satisfactory surface properties in a pulsating-bubble system may fail to improve lung function when instilled into the airways of surfactant-depleted animals, presumably because the material is very sensitive to inhibition by leaking serum proteins (46). Several studies have shown that the resistance to such inhibition depends on the presence of surfactant-specific proteins. A protein-free suspension of surfactant phospholipids is more easily inactivated by fibrinogen than a mixture of the same phospholipids and synthetic SP-C (47). The presence of both hydrophobic proteins makes the surfactant more resistant to inhibition (48,49), and the additional presence of SP-A further increases resistance to inactivation by fibrinogen (38). For reasons that are incompletely understood, the sensitivity to inhibition varies between surfactant preparations with a similar content of hydrophobic proteins, with Curosurf and Survanta being more sensitive than Alveofact and CLSE (50). Resistance to inhibition also depends on the lipid components of a surfactant preparation. In general, lysophosphatidylcholine sensitizes lipid extract surfactant to inhibition by serum proteins (51), and the presence of palmitic acid increases resistance to inhibition (52).

Using a microbubble stability test (53), we have confirmed that a surfactant containing only polar lipids and hydrophobic proteins is more easily inactivated by albumin than a "complete" natural surfactant isolated by sucrose gradient centrifugation and thus containing containing both hydrophilic and hydrophobic proteins (54). Presumably, differences in the supply of endogenous surfactant-associated proteins may influence the clinical response to surfactant preparations containing no or only some of these specific proteins. Preclinical evaluation of surfactant substitutes, therefore, requires well standardized animal experiments. (The problem of surfactant inactivation is further discussed in Chapter 13.)

A. Comparative Studies in Newborn Rabbits

Immature newborn rabbits, delivered at a gestational age of 26–27 days (term, 31 days), are commonly used for experimental evaluation of surfactant substitutes. These animals have very little endogenous surfactant and fail to establish functional residual capacity (FRC) at birth. When subjected to artificial ventilation (a prerequisite for survival), they develop widespread epithelial necrosis in peripheral airways and a profuse leakage of protein both from the vascular compartment into the alveoli and from the alveoli into the blood stream (41). Using human albumin as a marker injected intravenously at birth, Anceschi et al. (42) showed that approximately 5% of the pool of serum albumin leaks into the air spaces of immature newborn rabbits during a 15-min period of ventilation. When human recombinant SP-A was injected as a marker into the airways of these immature animals at birth, we demonstrated a substantial permeation of this surfactant-specific protein into the blood (55), confirming clinical observations by Chida et al. (56). This suggests that determination of serum levels of SP-A may serve as a diagnostic tool for early detection of increased alveolar permeability in various forms of lung disease.

Tracheal instillation of an adequate dose of an effective surfactant substitute improves static pressure-volume properties, as well as lung volumes and compliance under dynamic conditions. In a surfactant-deficient immature rabbit fetus with a gestational age of 27 days, static lung volumes >40 ml/kg at 5 cmH_2O deflation pressure indicate a satisfactory response. Such volumes have been reported for Surfactant TA (57), human surfactant (58), and Curosurf (18), but not with protein-free synthetic surfactants such as ALEC (57) or Exosurf (29).

Ventilated immature newborn rabbits are useful for in vivo evaluation of lung mechanics after surfactant replacement. Pertinent information can be obtained by ventilating the animals with a sequence of defined ventilator pressures

(59,60) or with a standardized tidal volume (61–63). The level of positive end-expiratory pressure (PEEP) must be standardized in comparative studies of different surfactants, since it influences several parameters of surfactant function and the effects may differ for different surfactants (64). By clamping the tube from the ventilator at end expiration, and determining lung volumes and wet weight, end-expiratory lung gas volume can be calculated (this is roughly equivalent to FRC) (60). Lung protein leakage can be determined by intravenous injection of markers such as radiolabeled albumin (41) or iron dextran (65) before the onset of ventilation and quantification of the markers in lung lavage fluid at the end of the experiment. Alternatively, the marker is instilled into the airways at birth and then quantified in blood after the period of ventilation. As mentioned above, recombinant human SP-A can be used as a lung permeability marker with this latter type of protocol (55). If the lungs of animals not subjected to lung lavage are fixed by vascular perfusion at a standardized transpulmonary deflation pressure of 10 cmH_2O (this is a sensitive region of the pressure-volume curve, where substantial differences in lung volume are to be expected between surfactant-deficient and normal lungs), alveolar volume density in histological sections correlates very well with compliance measurements obtained during ventilation (35).

In preterms rabbits with surfactant deficiency, treatment with an effective surfactant improves dynamic lung-thorax compliance and P_{CO_2} in heart blood to nearly mature levels (63) (Fig. 1). It also reduces the bidirectional leakage of protein in the lungs (41). Lungs of ventilated immature animals receiving an effective surfactant show, in addition, a significant increase in alveolar volume density (63) and well-preserved airway mucosa contrasting to the widespread necrosis and desquamation of bronchiolar epithelium characteristically found in control animals (66,67).

The first study comparing the effects of artificial and natural surfactant in preterm newborn rabbits was reported by Morley et al. (68). In these experiments, fetuses with a gestational age of 27 days (body weight about 30 g) were tracheotomized at birth and treated via the tracheal cannula with either 62 mg/kg of dry artificial surfactant made from DPPC and unsaturated PG, mixed in weight proportions 7:3 (this is identical to the composition of ALEC), or with 14 mg/kg of natural surfactant prepared by centrifugation of lung lavage fluid from adult rabbits; nontreated littermates served as controls. All animals were then ventilated for 30 min with a standardized insufflation pressure of 22 cmH_2O. After 60 min, both groups of surfactant-treated animals showed a more than threefold improvement in lung-thorax compliance in comparison with controls. The compliance level was similar in animals receiving artificial and natural surfactant (mean values 0.27 and 0.29 ml/cm $H_2O \cdot kg$, respectively), despite the huge difference in dose. However, the response to exogenous surfactant must be regarded as unsatisfactory in both groups of treated animals, as their compliance levels were

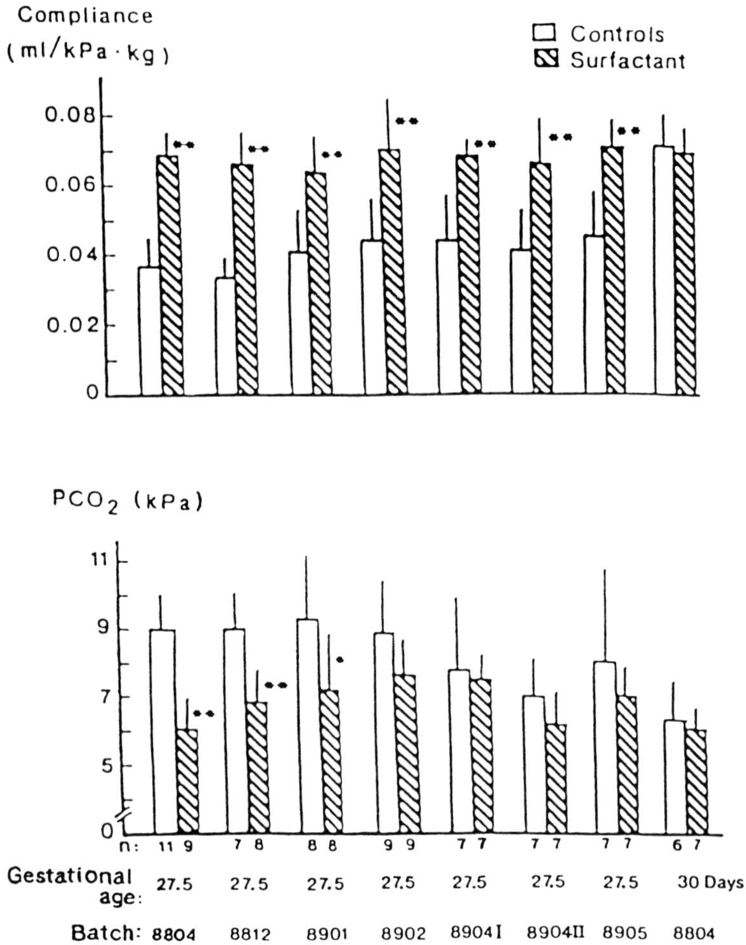

Figure 1 Data (mean, SD) from experiments testing the physiological effects of different batches of Curosurf in immature newborn rabbits with a gestational age of 27.5 days and in near-term animals with a gestational age of 30 days. The animals were ventilated for 30 min with 100% oxygen, pressure-constant ventilation, standardized tidal volume (approximately 10 ml/kg), frequency 40/min, and 50% inspiration time. No positive end-expiratory pressure was applied. Treatment with surfactant (160 mg/kg) before onset of ventilation improved lung-thorax compliance of immature animals to a level similar to that recorded in mature animals (upper panel, representing values recorded after 30 min). Surfactant treatment also lowered P_{CO_2} in heart blood sampled at the end of the experiment (lower panel). Instillation of surfactant had no adverse effect in mature animals. **P versus littermate controls <0.01; *P versus littermate controls <0.05. Conversion factors 1 kPa = 10.2 cmH_2O = 7.5 mmHg. (From ref. 63; used with permission.)

less than half the values recorded under similar conditions after treatment with modified natural surfactant (59). We also know from more recent studies that the dose of natural surfactant given in these experiments was much too low for an optimal response (69). In other words, this confrontation of two surfactants documented only a modest effect of the artificial product.

In experiments on premature newborn rabbits, Halliday et al. (70) compared artificial surfactant made from DPPC and high-density lipoprotein (10:1) (30) with a modified porcine surfactant equivalent to Curosurf. The artificial surfactant was administered at a dose of either 40 or 200 mg/kg and the modified natural surfactant at a dose of 160 mg/kg. After receiving surfactant, the animals were ventilated for 30 min with a standardized sequence of insufflation pressures. In comparison with untreated littermate controls, both groups of treated animals had increased tidal volumes at a peak pressure of 25 cmH_2O. However, tidal volumes were more than four times larger in animals treated with modified natural surfactant than in those receiving artificial surfactant. Lung-thorax compliance in this latter group was, in fact, similar to that of animals treated with dry artificial surfactant in the study cited above (68). Alveolar volume density, evaluated with automated image analysis, was more than doubled in animals receiving modified natural surfactant in comparison with the control group, but it was not improved in neonates treated with DPPC + high-density lipoprotein. In view of these disappointing experimental findings, the negative results obtained with this artificial surfactant in a clinical trial (31) are hardly surprising.

In a more recent study, Rider et al. (64) compared the physiological effects of two commercially available exogenous surfactants, Exosurf and Survanta, in ventilated preterm rabbits. These experiments also evaluated the influence of PEEP (3 cmH_2O) on the therapeutic response to surfactant. Exosurf and Survanta were administered at doses recommended by the manufacturers (67 and 100 mg/kg, respectively). A "negative" control group received saline (4 ml/kg) via the airways, and a "positive" control group was treated with complete natural sheep surfactant (100 mg/kg). Yet another group was treated with a protein-free lipid extract of natural sheep surfactant (100 mg/kg). The ventilatory pressure required to maintain a standardized tidal volume during ventilation without PEEP was lowered only in animals treated with natural sheep surfactant or Survanta, whereas animals receiving Exosurf did not differ from untreated controls (Fig. 2A). During ventilation with PEEP, however, the pressure needed to maintain a slightly lower standardized tidal volume was reduced in both Exosurf- and Survanta-treated animals. With both ventilator settings, natural sheep surfactant was superior to Survanta, and Survanta superior to Exosurf. A similar pattern was obtained for another important parameter of surfactant function, the vascular-to-alveolar leak of protein. Radiolabeled albumin, injected intravenously at birth, was used as a marker. The recovery of the label in alveolar wash

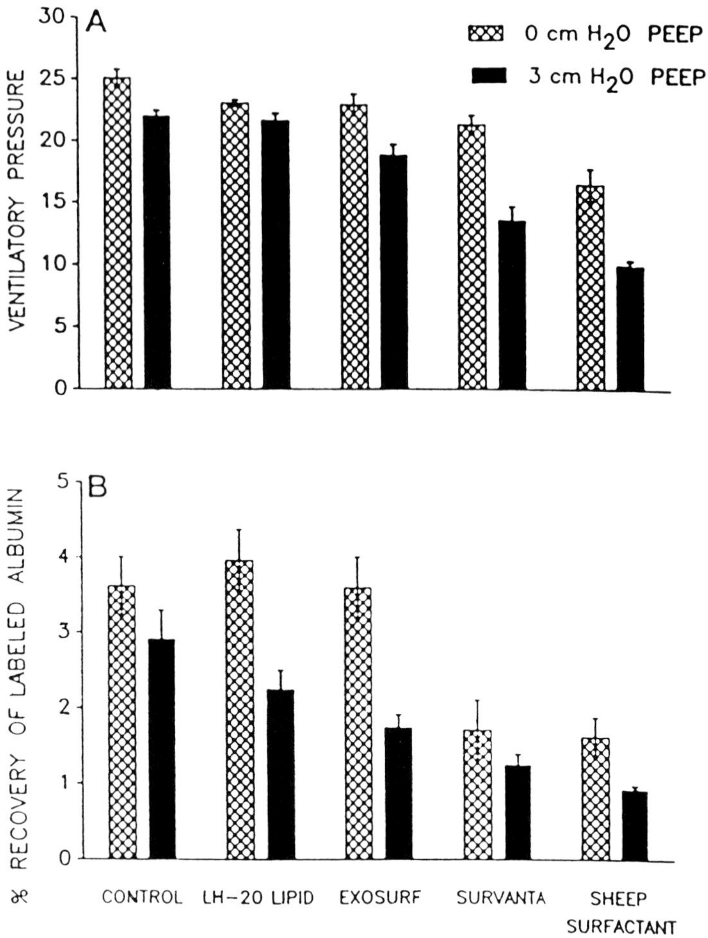

Figure 2 Ventilatory pressures and vascular-to-alveolar leak of albumin in immature newborn rabbits (gestational age 27 days) treated at birth with clinically recommended doses of Exosurf (67 mg lipid/kg) or Survanta (100 mg/kg). Littermates were treated with natural sheep surfactant (100 mg/kg), sheep surfactant lipids stripped of protein (LH-20 lipid, 100 mg/kg), or saline (Control). Animals were ventilated for 30 min without or with PEEP, using standardized tidal volumes of 10–11 ml/kg or 7–8 ml/kg, respectively. Ventilatory pressure is defined as peak inspiratory pressure minus PEEP. Leak of radiolabeled albumin, injected intravenously at birth, is expressed as percentage recovery in alveolar wash. Values are shown as mean and SEM. (A) With 0 cmH_2O PEEP, ventilatory pressures were decreased relative to controls by Survanta ($P < 0.05$) and by sheep surfactant relative to all other groups ($P < 0.01$). The use of 3 cmH_2O PEEP resulted in decreased pressures in the following sequence: control, LH-20 lipid > Exosurf > Survanta > sheep surfactant ($P < 0.05$). (B) Recoveries of labeled albumin in alveolar washes decreased in Survanta- and sheep surfactant-treated animals relative to all other groups in absence of PEEP ($P < 0.01$). With 3 cmH_2O PEEP, recoveries in control animals were higher than for sheep surfactant-treated rabbits, and treatment with LH-20 lipid resulted in higher recoveries than for Survanta- and sheep surfactant-treated rabbits ($P < 0.05$). (From ref. 64; used with permission.)

after 30 min of ventilation without PEEP was reduced only in animals receiving natural sheep surfactant or Survanta. With a PEEP level of 3 cmH_2O, a reduced leak was observed also in animals treated with Exosurf (Fig. 2B). These interesting data document significant differences in the acute physiological effects between Survanta and Exosurf, favoring the modified natural surfactant, and furthermore indicate that this difference can be to some extent masked by application of PEEP—most likely because PEEP compensates for the failure of alveolar stabilization in animals treated with the less effective surfactant.

In two recent studies, Curosurf and Exosurf were compared in experiments on ventilated preterm rabbits. Bongrani et al. (60) measured tidal volumes during ventilation with a standardized sequence of insufflation pressures, expiratory time constant (a parameter of lung stability), and end-expiratory lung gas volume (an equivalent to FRC) in animals treated with clinical doses of either surfactant and in animals receiving tyloxapol (the detergent component of Exosurf), Tween 20 (another detergent), or saline. Tidal volumes were improved in all groups of animals receiving surfactant or detergents. However, the expiratory time constant was significantly longer, and end-expiratory lung gas volume significantly larger in animals treated with Curosurf than in those receiving Exosurf or detergents (Fig. 3). Data from these experiments suggest that the acute physiological effects of Exosurf can largely be attributed to the detergent present in the product.

Corcoran et al. (34) reported lung-thorax compliance measurements and histological observations in preterm newborn rabbits ventilated for 60 min with a standardized tidal volume after treatment with clinical doses of Curosurf or Exosurf. Animals receiving Curosurf showed the expected improvement in compliance and alveolar volume density in comparison with nontreated controls, whereas intermediate values were noted for both parameters in animals treated with Exosurf. Necrosis of airway epithelium, a typical finding in ventilated surfactant-deficient animals (66), was more prominent in Exosurf-treated animals than in those receiving Curosurf. These data, together with the information generated by other experiments summarized above, indicate that the acute physiological effects of protein-free artificial surfactants are inferior to those of natural or modified natural surfactants (containing as a minimum requirement polar surfactant lipids, SP-B and SP-C). To some extent, this difference can be reduced by ventilation with PEEP. A strictly standardized ventilator setting is therefore mandatory in animal experiments aiming at comparing physiological effects of different surfactants.

B. Comparative Studies in Newborn Lambs

The ventilated preterm lamb is another useful experimental model of neonatal RDS (71) which has been applied by several workers for evaluation of various natural and synthetic surfactants. Significant and sustained improvements of gas

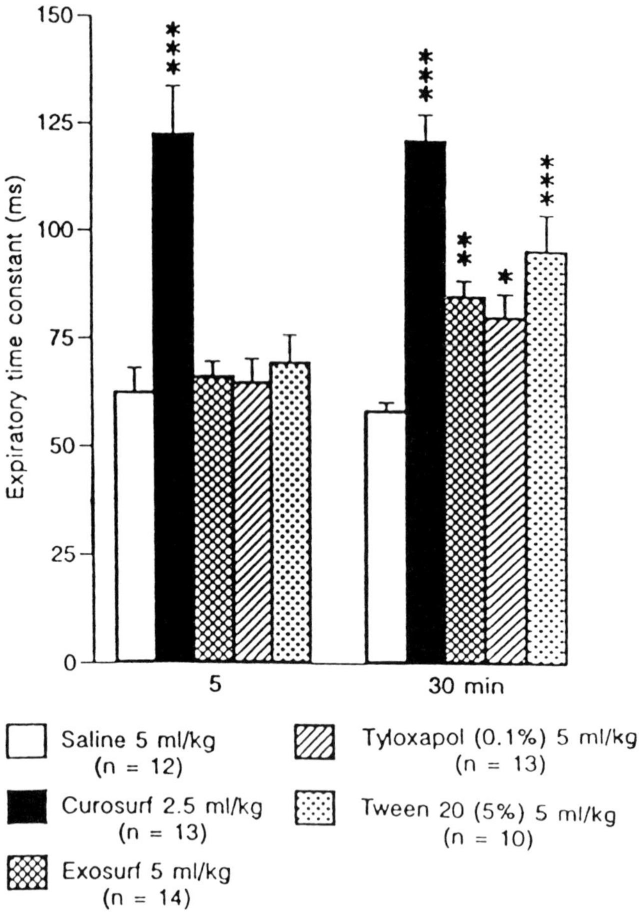

(A)

Figure 3 Expiratory time constants and end-expiratory lung gas volumes in immature newborn rabbits (gestational age 27 days) treated at birth with saline, Curosurf (80 mg/ml), Exosurf (13.5 mg lipid/ml), tyloxapol, or Tween 20. Animals were ventilated for a total time of 30 min with a standardized sequence of ventilation pressures. Each set of data in the diagrams was obtained after a 5-min period of ventilation with a peak pressure of 25 cmH_2O. Values are shown as mean and SEM. (A) Expiratory time constant is prolonged especially in animals receiving Curosurf, but after 30 min also in neonates receiving Exosurf, tyloxapol, or Tween 20. $*P \leq 0.05$; $**P \leq 0.01$; $***P \leq 0.001$ versus saline. (B) Lung gas volume is much larger in animals treated with Curosurf than in the other groups. $*P \leq 0.05$; $***P \leq 0.001$ versus saline. (From ref. 60; used with permission.)

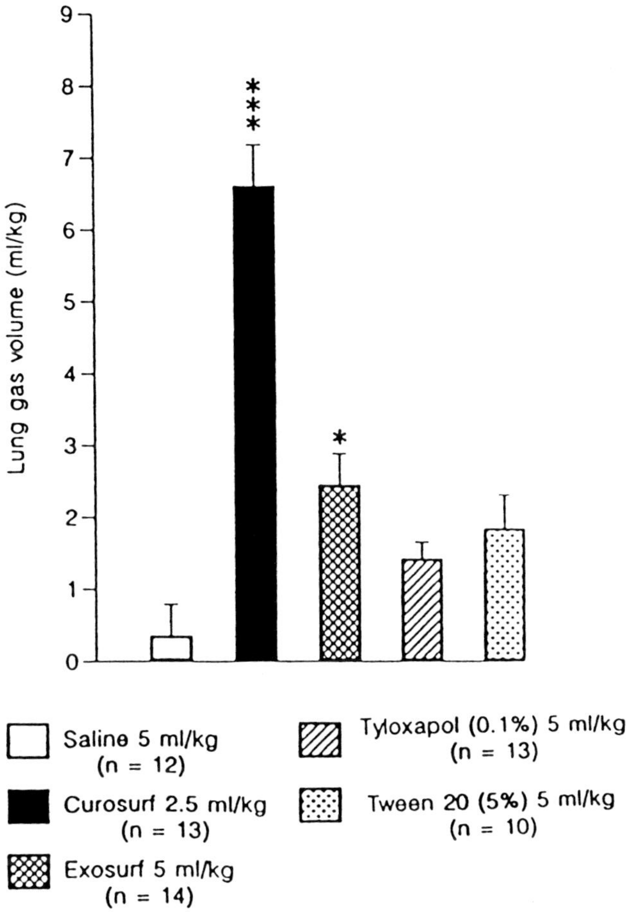

(B)

exchange and lung compliance have been documented after administration of comparatively low doses of CLSE (15–30 mg/kg) (28) or Alveofact (35 mg/kg) (72) to lambs with a gestational age of 124–130 days (term, 145 days). In contrast, a saline suspension of DPPC + unsaturated PG (7:3) did not improve lung function under these experimental conditions (28).

In experiments on very immature lambs with a gestational age of 120–122 days, Ikegami et al. (73) compared the physiological effects of four different exogenous surfactants: Surfactant TA, human surfactant isolated from amniotic fluid, natural rabbit surfactant, and natural sheep surfactant. All animals were treated with the same dose of surfactant (50 mg/kg) and ventilated for 4 hr. In this setting, the effect of Surfactant TA on gas exchange was inferior to that obtained with natural rabbit or sheep surfactant, and animals receiving human surfactant showed a more transient response that faded more rapidly than in the other treatment groups. The vascular-to-alveolar leak of albumin was larger in animals treated with Surfactant TA than in lambs receiving sheep or rabbit surfactant, but on the other hand, Surfactant TA was more resistant to inhibition by alveolar wash proteins than were the other surfactants. Surfactant TA and human surfactant were cleared more rapidly from the air spaces than the other two surfactants. This may explain the more prolonged response following treatment with natural rabbit or sheep surfactant. These experiments demonstrated several important physiological differences between the four surfactant preparations that could not be predicted on the basis of their biophysical properties under in vitro conditions. For example, the amount of film material required to reduce surface tension <10 mN/m in a Wilhelmy balance system was much lower for Surfactant TA than for the other preparations. Thus, enrichment of bovine surfactant extract with synthetic lipids "improves" in vitro surface properties without necessarily improving in vivo effects.

In more recent experiments Ikegami et al. (74) compared the physiological effects of Survanta, Exosurf, and a mixture of synthetic lipids (DPPC + palmitoyl-oleoylphosphatidylglycerol + palmitic acid; 69:22:9 by weight) in moderately premature lambs, delivered at a gestational age of 131–132 days. During a 5-hr period of mechanical ventilation, animals who received Survanta at the recommended clinical dose (100 mg/kg) responded with a significant improvement in dynamic lung compliance and "ventilation efficiency index" (75), whereas values for animals treated with Exosurf (67.5 mg/kg) were improved only slightly and were not significantly different from those of nontreated controls. Animals treated with the synthetic lipid mixture showed an intermediate response. A novel methodological approach was then chosen for the second part of the experiment. The lungs of the treated lambs were washed, the surfactant material in the lavage fluid was isolated and analyzed with particular reference to SP-A content, and the physiological effects of the reisolated material were tested in immature newborn rabbits as described above (Section III.A). Interestingly, the quality of the material recovered from the air spaces of the treated lambs was superior to the original surfactant. This improvement, which was more prominent for Survanta than for Exosurf, was associated with the appearance of SP-A in the recovered surfactant. Since SP-A was absent in the exogenous surfactants, it must have been derived from the lamb lungs. These intriguing data, which seem to open a "new level of understanding" (76), demonstrate that exogenous surfactant may become "activated" by associating with endogenous proteins or other components, either directly or by entering the metabolic pathways for recycling. This could explain why protein-free synthetic surfactants with poor physiological effects in short-term experiments on very immature animals may nevertheless improve long-term lung function and survival in preterm babies with some, albeit an insufficient, supply of endogenous surfactant.

Cummings et al. (77) recently compared efficacy of Exosurf, Infasurf (equivalent to CLSE), Survanta, and natural sheep surfactant in immature lambs delivered at a gestational age of 126 days. The first three preparations were given at the dose recommended by the manufacturers, and natural sheep surfactant surfactant was given at a dose of 100 mg/kg. Gas exchange, survival, and pulmonary pressure-volume characteristics were significantly improved after treatment with both the natural and modified natural surfactants, but this therapeutic response was sustained only in animals receiving Infasurf. Lambs treated with Exosurf did not differ from nontreated controls (Fig. 4). These data seem to contradict earlier observations on slightly more mature lambs with a gestational age of 131–133 days, in which Exosurf was reported to be nearly equivalent to natural surfactant (78). Perhaps the therapeutic effect of Exosurf depends on some endogenous surfactant component which was absent in the more immature animals studied by Cummings et al. (77). If so, these experimental observations suggest certain limitations to the clinical use of Exosurf and other protein-free synthetic surfactant substitutes especially in very low birth weight babies.

C. Comparative Studies in Other Animal Models

Adult experimental animals subjected to lung lavage have been used by several investigators as a model of surfactant depletion, suitable for evaluation of surfactant substitutes. Criteria for a satisfactory response to surfactant replacement in ventilated animals have been formulated (79). Following repeated lung lavage, there is a significant fall in arterial PO_2 due to intrapulmonary shunting, but this can be restored to prelavage levels by tracheal instillation of an adequate dose of surfactant (80), and the animal can subsequently be weaned from the ventilator (81). The therapeutic effect of surfactant replacement in this model depends on ventilation with PEEP (82). As in experiments on immature newborn animals, ventilator settings must therefore be standardized to allow meaningful comparison between different surfactants. The model has been used to document the physiological activity of Surfactant TA (83) and Curosurf (80,84). No dose-response studies and no comparative studies on live animals have been reported.

A protocol for surfactant depletion of excised rat lungs by repeated lavage was developed by Bermel et al. (85). Following the lavage procedure, the deflation limb of the pressure-volume loop becomes shifted to the right, indicating failure to stabilize the alveoli at low transpulmonary pressures. Instillation of natural surfactant via the airways restores normal lung stability during deflation. Hall et al. (15) used this model in the comparative studies of Exosurf, Survanta,

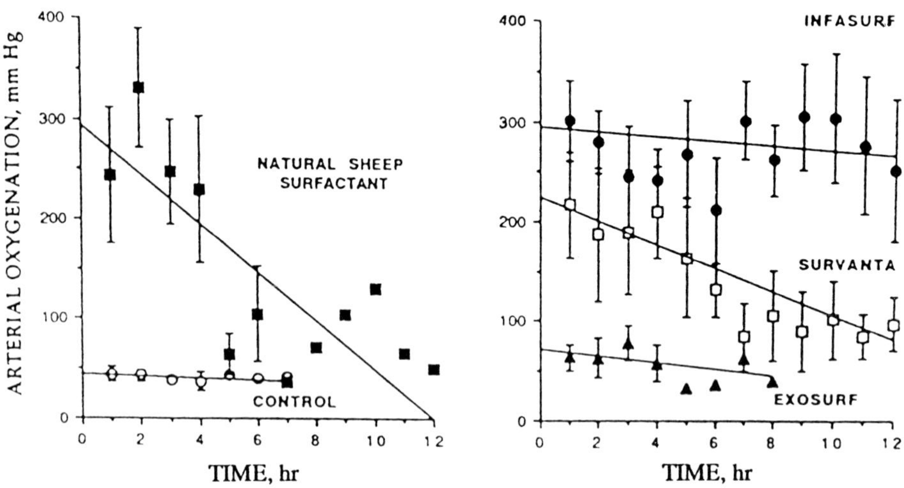

Surfactant Group	Intial Response (y-intercept), mm Hg	Rate of Change (slope) mm Hg/h
Control	44 ± 7	−1 ± 2
Natural sheep	292 ± 35*	−24 ± 6*
Exosurf	72 ± 15†	−4 ± 4†
Infasurf	290 ± 33*	−2 ± 5†
Survanta	223 ± 31*	−13 ± 5*

Figure 4 Arterial oxygenation in immature newborn lambs (gestational age 126 days) treated at birth with natural sheep surfactant (100 mg/kg), Infasurf (105 mg/kg), Survanta (100 mg/kg), Exosurf (67.5 mg/kg), or no surfactant (control group). The animals were ventilated with 100% oxygen until moribund from respiratory failure or until killed at 24 hr after delivery. Values are mean ± SEM. Left panel shows the control and natural sheep surfactant groups; right panel shows the three commercially available surfactant preparations. Open circles, controls; closed squares, natural sheep surfactant; closed circles, Infasurf; open squares, Survanta; closed triangles, Exosurf. Regression data in table are mean ± SD. **P* <0.02 compared with control group; †*P* <0.02 compared with natural sheep surfactant group. (From ref. 77; used with permission.)

and CLSE referred to above. Instillation of Exosurf caused slight improvement of lung stability, whereas administration of CLSE restored the pressure-volume characteristics to normal. With Survanta, there was an intermediate response. In accordance with the in vitro data reported in the same paper, the physiological properties of Exosurf in the surfactant-depleted excised lungs could be improved significantly by the addition of hydrophobic proteins (SP-B, SP-C), although the effect obtained with this modified synthetic preparation remained inferior to that obtained with CSLE (Fig. 5).

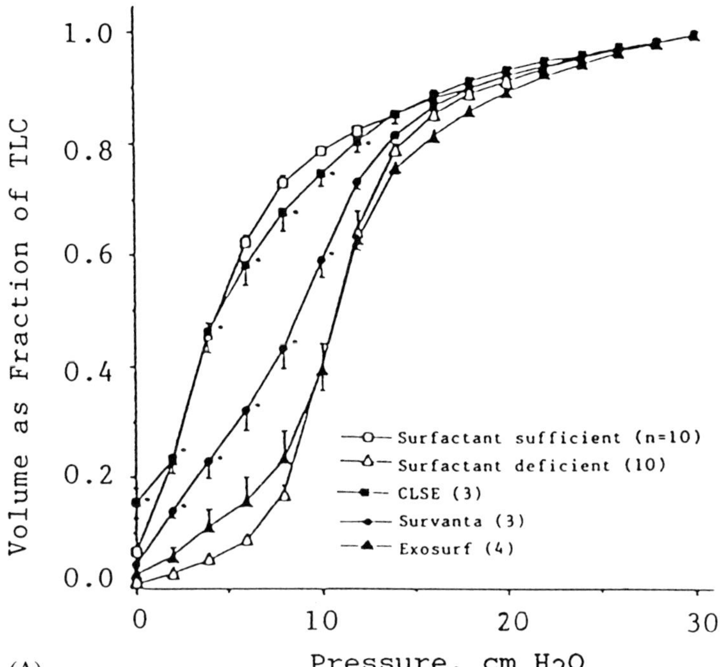

(A)

Figure 5 Pressure-volume properties of surfactant-depleted excised adult rat lungs after administration of CLSE, Survanta, Exosurf, or Exosurf + SP-B, SP-C (1% by weight). Measurements were obtained at 37°C during deflation from total lung capacity (TLC), before (surfactant-sufficient), and after (surfactant-deficient) the lungs were lavaged multiple times with normal saline, and following instillation of surfactant. CLSE and Survanta were instilled at a total dose of 20 mg and Exosurf at a total dose of 37.5 mg lipid in 2.5 ml of saline. Values are mean and SEM. (A) Clinically used surfactants. (B) Effect of SP-B, SP-C on Exosurf activity. Data for Exosurf are presented in both A and B to facilitate comparison. **P* versus surfactant-deficient lungs <0.05. (From ref. 15; used with permission.)

Surfactant depletion by repeated lung lavage is a fairly "clean" model in that it involves no other primary insult to the parenchyma. However, ventilation of these lungs leads to airway epithelial disruption, intra-alveolar edema, hyaline membranes, and recruitment of inflammatory cells to the air spaces (80). The dose of surfactant required to improve lung function may then vary with the time interval between the lavage procedure and surfactant treatment, as well as with the quality of the surfactant preparation, especially its resistance to inactivation by leaking serum proteins. As pointed out above, this resistance largely depends on the presence of surfactant-specific proteins.

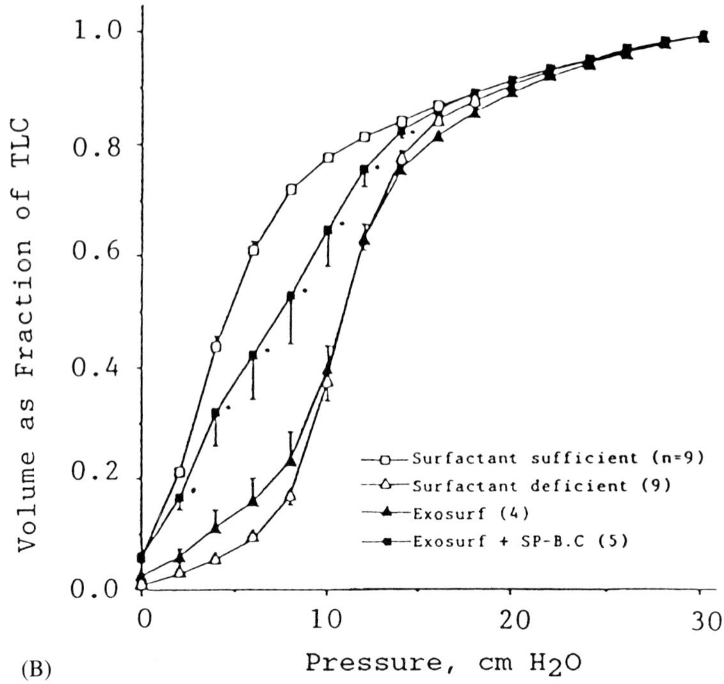

(B)

Figure 5 *(Continued)*

D. Surfactant Treatment in Experimental Meconium Aspiration

Meconium aspiration syndrome is a new potential clinical target for surfactant replacement therapy (see Chapter 21). Aspirated meconium interferes with lung function not only by mechanical obstruction of airways and by inducing a "chemical" pneumonitis, but also by disturbing surfactant function (86,87). Surfactant inhibitors are present in both the chloroform-soluble fraction of meconium (free fatty cids, cholesterol, triglycerides) and in the water-soluble fraction (proteins, bilirubin), but the specific inhibitory activity of the former fraction is much stronger (87).

In near-term newborn rabbits, respiratory failure characterized by decreased lung compliance, alveolar collapse, and fall in Pa_{O_2} was induced by tracheal instillation of a saline suspension of human meconium (87). The meconium used in these experiments was filtered (particle size ≤ 3 μm) and did not block the larger airways. Treatment with modified porcine surfactant (Curosurf, 200 mg/kg) led to a significant improvement of both compliance and Pa_{O_2} but did not restore normal lung function. Surfactant-treated animals also had improved alveolar volume density in histological sections, indicating stabilization of the terminal air spaces (88).

Sun et al. (89) recently evaluated the effects of surfactant treatment in an adult rat model of meconium aspiration. When respiratory failure was established after instillation of meconium into the airways, animals were treated with either natural porcine surfactant isolated by sucrose gradient centrifugation (100 mg/kg) or modified porcine surfactant (Curosurf, 100 or 200 mg/kg). Blood gases and compliance were recorded before treatment and at regular intervals during a 3-hr period of mechanical ventilation after surfactant instillation. As in the experiments on near-term rabbits cited above (88), treatment with a high dose of modified porcine surfactant (200 mg/kg) improved oxygenation, compliance, and alveolar volume density, but did not restore normal lung function. Treatment with the lower dose of modified porcine surfactant (100 mg/kg) had only a transient effect on oxygenation, whereas with natural surfactant given at the same dose there was an intermediate response. The presence of SP-A in the natural surfactant may have rendered this preparation more resistant to inactivation by meconium and serum proteins leaking into the air spaces during the period of artificial ventilation.

The combined evidence from the in vitro and in vivo experiments summarized above indicates that the pathophysiology of meconium aspiration syndrome includes an element of surfactant inactivation, and that this inactivation can be overcome by upgrading the pool of surfactant in the air spaces. The optimal dose and composition of exogenous surfactant for treatment of neonatal meconium aspiration remains to be defined in animal experiments and clinical trials.

E. Experimental Neonatal Pneumonia

Some babies with primary RDS have concomitant pulmonary infection, and some babies with primary infection (especially pneumonia caused by group B streptococci, GBS) have symptoms that can easily be mistaken for RDS. In either case, the baby is likely to be treated with exogenous surfactant. Pneumonia is also a common complication of adult respiratory distress syndrome, now recognized as a new potential target for surfactant therapy (see Chapter 28). In all these clinical situations, the possible influence of the exogenous surfactant on bacterial proliferation in the lungs is a matter of concern.

In principle, the stimulating acute effects of SP-A and SP-D on phagocytic cells (see Chapter 4) should be beneficial in a patient with bacterial or viral pneumonia. On the other hand, overloading of alveolar macrophages with surfactant lipids may be associated with decreased phagocytic and metabolic activity (90). It is also possible that exogenous surfactant could either stimulate or depress bacterial growth by direct interaction with the microorganisms.

Data from experiments on premature and fullterm newborn rabbits indicated that exogenous natural surfactant reduces the capacity of alveolar macrophages to kill GBS which are delivered into the lungs by aerosolization (91). This new observation led to a second set of experiments comparing the effect of clinically used surfactants in the same animal model. As illustrated in Fig. 6, only the synthetic surfactant Exosurf reduced growth of GBS in preterm rabbits. In animals treated with human amniotic fluid surfactant or modified natural surfactants (CLSE, Surfactant TA), bacterial proliferation did not differ from that in nontreated control animals. Similar results were obtained by direct in vitro exposure of GBS to the same surfactants: bacterial growth was not inhibited by natural or modified natural surfactants but was depressed by Exosurf (92). This suggests that the bacteriostatic effect was not mediated by interaction of the synthetic surfactant with alveolar macrophages. In term animals not receiving surfactant, the number of bacteria decreased after inoculation; i.e., bacteria were killed by an effective inflammatory reaction.

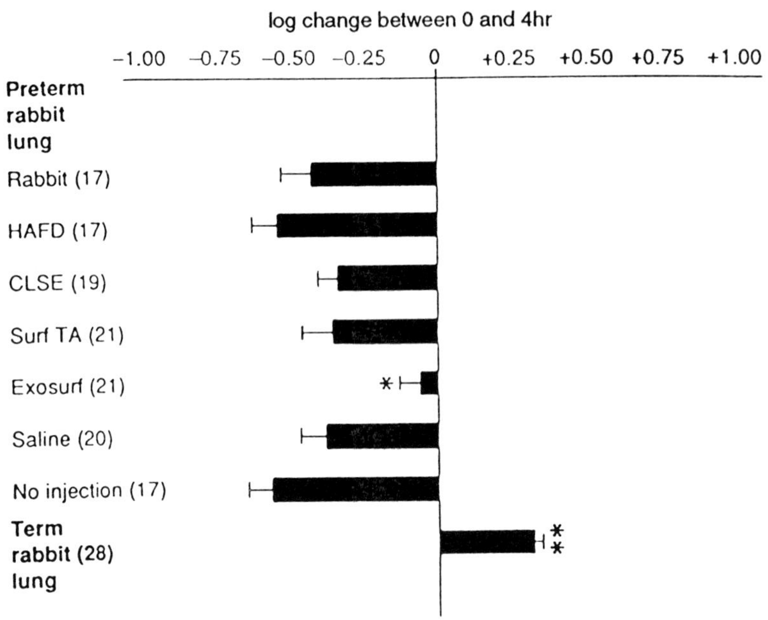

Figure 6 Effect of surfactant therapy on proliferation of GBS in premature newborn rabbits (gestational age 28 days) and in term newborn rabbits. The animals were infected with an aerosol of GBS, and then treated with natural rabbit surfactant (Rabbit), human amniotic fluid–derived surfactant (HAFD), CLSE, Surfactant TA (Surf TA), Exosurf, or saline. All surfactant preparations were administered at a dose of 60 mg/kg. The bars represent means and SEM; the numbers of animals studied at 0 and 4 hr are given in brackets. A negative log change to the left of zero means that bacterial proliferation took place in the lung and a positive log change to the right of zero indicates that bacterial killing occurred in the lung. *P <0.01 for Exosurf versus the other preterm groups; **P <0.001 for term rabbits versus the preterm groups. (From ref. 92; used with permission.)

Herting et al. (93) recently reported experiments on near-term newborn rabbits in which a standardized volume (5 ml/mg) of GBS suspended in saline (10^9 bacteria per milliliter) was instilled into the airways 15 min after birth. Fifteen minutes later, the animals were treated with Curosurf (200 mg/kg). Irrespective of this treatment, infected animals developed septicemia and histological evidence of pneumonia similar to GBS pneumonia in newborn babies. However, bacterial proliferation during a 5-hr period of artificial ventilation, evaluated from the number of colony-forming units in lung homogenate, was reduced by approximately 80% in Curosurf-treated animals in comparison with nontreated GBS-infected controls.

These slightly conflicting data from in vitro and in vivo experiments indicate that exogenous surfactant may influence bacterial proliferation in the lungs and that the effect may vary depending on lung maturity and surfactant composition. Systematic studies, confronting different surfactants with different bacteria, are required to further clarify possible interactions between exogenous surfactant, phagocytic cells, and invading microorganisms in various forms of infectious lung disease.

IV. Conclusions

The data reviewed in this chapter indicate significant differences in physical and physiological properties between surfactants currently used in clinical practice. These differences relate to surface adsorption rate, film compressibility, minimum surface tension during surface compression, time course and magnitude of therapeutic response, resistance to inhibition by serum proteins, and interaction with bacteria. Subtle differences in dose-response relationships may be masked by the administration of large doses of surfactant, and differences in lung-stabilizing properties may, in a ventilated patient, be compensated for by adjusting respiratory frequency and PEEP to match the expiratory time constant of the respiratory system.

In general, the significance of these differences depends on the clinical situation. A baby with moderately severe RDS and some endogenous supply of surfactant lipids and proteins may do well with a slow-acting surfactant preparation, especially as this surfactant may become "activated" by entering the metabolic pathways for recycling (74). An emergency situation may call for a rapidly acting surfactant containing, as a minimum requirement, polar lipids and hydrophobic proteins. In a clinical situation characterized by flooding of the air spaces with proteinaceous edema or other surfactant inhibitors, resistance to inactivation may be an important quality of the exogenous surfactant and this may require the presence of both SP-A and hydrophobic proteins. The presence of SP-A may also serve as an important stimulus of alveolar macrophages in patients with a combination of surfactant deficiency and pneumonia. Further basic studies are required to identify the optimal composition and dose regimen for exogenous surfactants in different clinical situations.

Acknowledgments

This work was supported by the Swedish Medical Research Council (Project No. 3351), Oscar II:s Jubileumsfond, the General Maternity Hospital Foundation, Axel Tielman's Minnesfond, and the Research Funds of the Karolinska Institute.

References

1. Rüfer R. Der Einfluss oberflächenaktiver Substanzen auf Entfaltung und Retraktion isolierter Lungen. Pflugers Arch 1967; 298:170–184.
2. Enhörning G, Robertson B. Lung expansion in the premature rabbit fetus after tracheal deposition of surfactant. Pediatrics 1972; 50:58–66.
3. Soll RF. Surfactant replacement therapy: overview of clinical trials. Int Proceed J 1991; 1:29–42.
4. Jobe AH. Pulmonary surfactant therapy. N Engl J Med 1993; 328:861–868.
5. King R, Clements JA. Surface active materials from dog lung. II. Composition and physiological correlations. Am J Physiol 1972; 223:715–726.
6. Kobayashi T, Shido A, Nitta K, et al. The critical concentration of surfactant in fetal lung liquid at birth. Respir Physiol 1990; 80:181–192.
7. Schürch S, Bachofen H, Goerke J, Green F. Surface properties of rat pulmonary surfactant studied with the captive bubble method: adsorption, hysteresis, stability. Biochim Biophys Acta 1992; 1103:127–136.
8. Enhorning G. Pulsating bubble technique for evaluating pulmonary surfactant. J Appl Physiol 1977; 43:198–203.
9. Schürch S, Bachofen H, Goerke J, Possmayer F. A captive bubble method reproduces the in situ behavior of lung surfactant monolayers. J Appl Physiol 1989; 67:2389–2396.
10. Barrow RE, Hills BA. A critical assessment of the Wilhelmy method in studying lung surfactants. J Physiol (Lond) 1979; 295:217–227.
11. Hall SB, Bermel MS, Ko YT, et al. Approximations in the measurement of surface tension on the oscillating bubble surfactometer. J Appl Physiol 1993; 75:468–477.
12. Fujiwara T, Maeta H, Chida S, et al. Artificial surfactant therapy in hyaline membrane disease. Lancet 1980; 1:55–59.
13. Fujiwara T, Adams FH. Surfactant for hyaline membrane disease. Pediatrics 1980; 66:795–798.
14. Fujiwara T. Surfactant replacement in neonatal RDS. In: Robertson B, van Golde LMG, Batenburg JJ, eds. Pulmonary Surfactant. Amsterdam: Elsevier, 1984:479–503.
15. Hall SB, Ventikaraman AR, Whitsett JA, et al. Importance of hydrophobic

apoproteins as constituents of clinical exogenous surfactants. Am Rev Respir Dis 1992; 145:24–30.
16. Shapiro DL, Notter RH, Morin FC III, et al. Double-blind, randomized trial of a calf lung surfactant extract administered at birth to very premature infants for prevention of respiratory distress syndrome. Pediatrics 1985; 76:593–599.
17. Robertson B, Curstedt T, Johansson J, et al. Structural and functional characterization of porcine surfactant isolated by liquid-gel chromatography. In: von Wichert P. Müller B, eds. Basic Research on Lung Surfactant. Progress in Respiration Research, Vol. 25. Basel: Karger, 1990:237–246.
18. Fujiwara T, Robertson B. Pharmacology of exogenous surfactant. In: Robertson B, van Golde LMG, Batenburg JJ, eds. Pulmonary Surfactant. From Molecular Biology to Clinical Practice. Amsterdam: Elsevier, 1992:561–592.
19. Schürch S, Schürch D, Curstedt T, Robertson B. Surface activity of lipid extract surfactant in relation to film area compression and collapse. J Appl Physiol 1994; 77:974–986.
20. Oosterlaken MA, Haagsman HP, van Golde LMG, Demel RA. Interaction of lipid vesicles with monomolecular layers containing lung surfactant proteins SP-B or SP-C. Biochemistry 1991; 30:8276–8281.
21. Oosterlaken MA, Haagsman HP, van Golde LMG, Demel RA. Characterization of lipid insertion into monomolecular layers mediated by lung surfactant proteins SP-B and SP-C. Biochemistry 1991; 30:10965–10971.
22. Schürch S, Possmayer F, Cheng S, Cockshutt AM. Pulmonary SP-A enhances adsorption and appears to induce surface sorting of lipid extract surfactant. Am J Physiol 1992; 263 (Lung Cell Mol Physiol 7):L210–L218.
23. Morley CJ, Bangham AD, Miller N, Davis JA. Dry artificial lung surfactant and its effect on very premature babies. Lancet 1981; 1:64–68.
24. Morley CJ, Bangham AD, Johnson P, et al. Physical and physiological properties of dry lung surfactant. Nature 1978; 271:162–163.
25. Dechant KL, Faulds D. Colfosceril palmitate. A review of the therapeutic efficacy and clinical tolerability of a synthetic surfactant preparation (Exosurf[R] Neonatal[TM]) in neonatal respiratory distress syndrome. Drugs 1991; 42:877–894.
26. Schürch S. Surface tension properties of surfactant. Clin Perinatol 1993; 20:669–682.
27. Hallman M, Merritt A, Schneider H, et al. Isolation of human surfactant from amniotic fluid and a pilot study of its efficacy in respiratory distress syndrome. Pediatrics 1983; 71:473–481.
28. Egan E, Notter RH, Kwong MS, Shapiro DL. Natural and artificial lung surfactant replacement therapy in premature lambs. J Appl Physiol 1983; 55:875–883.
29. Tooley WH, Clements JA, Muramatsu K, et al. Lung function in prematurely delivered rabbits treated with a synthetic surfactant. Am Rev Respir Dis 1987; 136:651–656.
30. Meban C. Effect of lipids and other substances on the adsorption of dipalmitoyl phosphatidylcholine. Pediatr Res 1981; 15:1029–1031.
31. Halliday HL, McClure G, Reid MMcC, Lappin TRJ, Meban C, Thomas PS. Controlled trial of artificial surfactant to prevent respiratory distress syndrome. Lancet 1984; 1:476–478.

32. Sun B, Curstedt T, Robertson B. Long-term cycling of surfactant films in Wilhelmy balance. J Dev Physiol. In press.
33. Sasaki M. Comparison of five pulmonary surfactants: In vitro surface properties and ultrastructures. J Iwate Med Assoc 1990; 42:883–896.
34. Corcoran JD, Berggren P, Sun B, et al. Comparison of surface properties and physiological effects in preterm rabbits of a synthetic and a natural surfactant. Arch Dis Child 1994; 71:F165–F169.
35. Nohara K, Berggren P, Curstedt T, et al. Correlations between physical and physiological properties of various preparations of lung surfactant. Eur J Respir Dis 1987; 69:321–335.
36. Tanaka Y, Takei T, Aiba T, et al. Development of synthetic lung surfactants. J Lipid Res 1986; 27:475–485.
37. Morley C, Bangham A. Physical properties of surfactant under compression. In: von Wichert P, ed. Clinical Importance of Surfactant Defects. Progress in Respiration Research, Vol 15. Basel: Karger, 1981:188–193.
38. Cockshutt AM, Weitz J, Possmayer F. Pulmonary surfactant-associated protein A enhances the surface activity of lipid extract surfactant and reverses inhibition by blood proteins in vitro. Biochemistry 1990; 29:8424–8429.
39. Lachmann B. In vivo tests for evaluation of pulmonary surfactant. In: Lachmann B, ed. Surfactant Replacement Therapy in Neonatal and Adult Respiratory Distress Syndrome. Berlin: Springer Verlag, 1988:28–36.
40. Jobe A, Ikegami M, Jacobs H, et al. Permeability of premature lamb lungs to protein and the effect of surfactant on that permeability. J Appl Physiol 1983; 55,169–176.
41. Robertson B, Berry D, Curstedt T, et al. Leakage of protein in the immature rabbit lung; effect of surfactant replacement. Respir Physiol 1985; 61:265–276.
42. Anceschi MM, Robertson B, Broccucci L, et al. Immunochemical and immunohistochemical evaluation of lung permeability in ventilated newborn rabbits. Exp Lung Res 1990; 16:593–605.
43. Seeger W, Stöhr G, Wolf HRD, Neuhof H. Alteration of surfactant function due to protein leakage: Special interaction with fibrin monomer. J Appl Physiol 1985; 58:326–338.
44. Fuchimukai T, Fujiwara T, Takahashi A, Enhorning G. Artificial pulmonary surfactant inhibited by proteins. J Appl Physiol 1987; 62:429–437.
45. Kobayashi T, Nitta K, Ganzuka M, et al. Inactivation of exogenous surfactant by pulmonary edema fluid. Pediatr Res 1991; 29:353–356.
46. Holm BA, Venkitaraman AR, Enhorning G, Notter RH. Biophysical inhibition of synthetic lung surfactant. Chem Phys Lipids 1990; 52:243–250.
47. Seeger W, Thede C, Günther A, Grube C. Surface properties and sensitivity to protein-inhibition of a recombinant apoprotein C–based phospholipid mixture in vitro—Comparison to natural surfactant. Biochim Biophys Acta 1991; 1081:45–52.
48. Amirkhanian JD, Bruni R, Waring AJ, Taeusch HW. Inhibition of mixtures of surfactant lipids and synthetic sequences of surfactant proteins SP-B and SP-C. Biochim Biophys Acta 1991; 1096:355–360.
49. Seeger W, Günther A, Thede C. Differential sensitivity to fibrinogen inhibition of SP-C- vs. SP-B-based surfactants. Am J Physiol 1992; 261 (Lung Cell Mol Physiol 5):L286–L291.

50. Seeger W, Grube C, Günther A, Schmidt R. Surfactant inhibition by plasma proteins: Different sensitivity of various surfactant preparations. Eur Respir J 1993; 6:971–977.
51. Cockshutt AM, Possmayer F. Lysophosphatidylcholine sensitizes lipid extracts of pulmonary surfactant to inhibition by serum proteins. Biochim Biophys Acta 1991; 1086:63–71.
52. Cockshutt AM, Absolom DR, Possmayer F. The role of palmitic acid in pulmonary surfactant: Enhancement of surface activity and prevention of inhibition by blood proteins. Biochim Biophys Acta 1991; 1085:248–256.
53. Berggren P, Eklind J, Linderholm B, Robertson B. Bubbles and computer aided image analysis for evaluation of surfactant inhibition. Biol Neonate 1992; 61(Suppl 1):15–20.
54. Robertson B. Surfactant deficiency and surfactant inactivation in experimental neonatal respiratory distress syndrome. In: Müller B, von Wichert P, eds. Lung Surfactant: Basic Research in the Pathogenesis of Lung Disorders. Progress in Respiration Research, Vol. 27. Basel: Karger, 1994:232–239.
55. Robertson B, Curstedt T, Herting E, et al. Alveolar-to-vascular leakage of surfactant protein A in ventilated immature newborn rabbits. Biol Neonate. In press.
56. Chida S, Phelps DS, Soll RF, Tauesch HW. Surfactant proteins and antisurfactant antibodies in sera from infants with respiratory distress syndrome with and without surfactant treatment. Pediatrics 1991; 88:84–89.
57. Maeta H, Asakura K, Konishi M, Fujiwara T. Effect of Surfactant-TA on alveolar stability of premature rabbit fetus: Comparison with term rabbit fetus and dry surfactant (70% DPPC and 30% PG). Acta Neonat Jpn 1983; 48:600.
58. Schneider HA, Hallman M, Benirschke K, Gluck L. Human surfactant: A therapeutic trial in premature rabbits. J Pediatr 1982; 100:619–622.
59. Berggren P, Curstedt T, Grossmann G, et al. Physiological activity of pulmonary surfactant with low protein content; effect of enrichment with synthetic phospholipids. Exp Lung Res 1985; 8:29–51.
60. Bongrani S, Fornasier M, Papotti M, et al. Lung gas volumes and expiratory time constant in immature newborn rabbits treated with natural or synthetic surfactant or detergents. Biol Neonate 1994; 65:406–415.
61. Ikegami M, Berry D, Elkady T, et al. Corticosteroids and surfactant change lung function and protein leaks in the lungs of ventilated premature rabbits. J Clin Invest 1987; 79:1371–1378.
62. Ikegami M, Jobe AH, Pettenazzo A, et al. Effects of maternal treatment with corticosteroids, T_3, TRH, and their combinations on lung function of ventilated preterm rabbits with and without surfactant treatments. Am Rev Respir Dis 1987; 136:892–898.
63. Sun B, Kobayashi T, Curstedt T, et al. Application of a new ventilator–multi-plethysmograph system for testing efficacy of surfactant replacement in newborn rabbits. Eur Respir J 1991; 4:364–370.
64. Rider E, Jobe A, Ikegami M, Sun B. Different ventilation strategies alter surfactant responses in preterm rabbits. J Appl Physiol 1992; 73:2089–2096.
65. Robertson B, Grossmann G, Jobe A, et al. Vascular to alveolar leak of iron dextran (120 kDa) in the immature ventilated rabbit lung. Pediatr Res 1989; 25:130–135.

66. Nilsson R, Grossmann G, Robertson B. Lung surfactant and the pathogenesis of neonatal bronchiolar lesions induced by artificial ventilation. Pediatr Res 1978; 12:249–255.
67. Grossmann G, Nilsson R, Robertson B. Scanning electron microscopy of epithelial lesions induced by artificial ventilation of the immature neonatal lung; the prophylactic effect of surfactant replacement. Eur J Pediatr 1986; 145:361–367.
68. Morley C, Robertson B, Lachmann B, et al. Artificial surfactant and natural surfactant. Comparative study of the effects on premature rabbit lungs. Arch Dis Child 1980; 55:758–765.
69. Nilsson R, Grossmann G, Berggren P, Robertson B. Surfactant treatment in experimental hyaline membrane disease. Eur J Respir Dis 1981; 62:441–449.
70. Halliday H, Robertson B, Nilsson R, et al. Automated image analysis of alveolar expansion patterns in immature newborn rabbits treated with natural or artificial surfactant. Br J Exp Pathol 1987; 68:727–732.
71. Jobe A, Ikegami M. The prematurely delivered lamb as a model for studies of neonatal adaptation. In: Nathanielsz PW, ed. Animal Models in Fetal Medicine. Ithaca, NY: Perinatology Press, 1984:1–30.
72. Gortner L, Pohlandt F, Weller E. Effects of bovine surfactant in premature lambs after intratracheal application. Eur J Pediatr 1990; 149:280–283.
73. Ikegami M, Agata Y, Elkady T, et al. Comparison of four surfactants: In vitro surface properties and responses of preterm lambs to treatment at birth. Pediatrics 1987; 79:38–46.
74. Ikegami M, Ueda T, Absolom D, et al. Changes in exogenous surfactant in ventilated preterm lamb lungs. Am Rev Respir Dis 1993; 148:837–844.
75. Notter RH, Egan EA, Kwong MS, et al. Lung surfactant replacement in premature lambs with extracted lipids from bovine lung lavage: effects of dose, dispersion technique, and gestational age. Pediatr Res 1985; 19:569–577.
76. Holm BA. Surfactant replacement therapy. Am Rev Respir Dis 1993; 148:834–836.
77. Cummings JJ, Holm BA, Hudak ML, et al. A controlled clinical comparison of four different surfactant preparations in surfactant-deficient preterm lambs. Am Rev Respir Dis 1992; 145:999–1004.
78. Durand D, Clyman RI, Heyman MA, et al. Effects of a protein-free, synthetic surfactant on survival and pulmonary function in preterm lambs. J Pediatr 1985; 107:775–780.
79. Robertson B, Lachmann B. Experimental evaluation of surfactants for replacement therapy. Exp Lung Res 1988; 14:279–310.
80. Berggren P, Lachmann B, Curstedt T, et al. Gas exchange and lung morphology after surfactant replacement in experimental adult respiratory distress syndrome induced by repeated lung lavage. Acta Anaesthesiol Scand 1986; 30:321–328.
81. Bambang Oetomo S, Reijngoud DJ, Ennema JJ, et al. Surfactant replacement therapy in surfactant-deficient rabbits: Early effects on lung function and biochemical aspects. Lung 1988; 166:65–73.
82. Kobayashi T, Kataoka H, Ueda T, et al. Effects of surfactant supplement and end-expiratory pressure in lung lavaged rabbits. J Appl Physiol 1984; 57:995–1001.
83. Taeusch HW, Keough KMW, Williams M, et al. Characterization of bovine surfactant for infants with respiratory distress syndrome. Pediatrics 1986; 77:572–581.

84. Bambang Oetomo S, de Ley L, Curstedt T, et al. Distribution of endotracheally instilled surfactant protein SP-C in lung-lavaged rabbits. Pediatr Res 1991; 29:178–181.
85. Bermel MS, McBride JT, Notter RH. Lavaged excised rat lungs as a model of surfactant deficiency. Lung 1984; 162:99–113.
86. Moses D, Holm BA, Spitale P, et al. Inhibition of pulmonary surfactant function by meconium. Am J Obstet Gynecol 1991; 164:477–481.
87. Sun B, Curstedt T, Robertson B. Surfactant inhibition in experimental meconium aspiration. Acta Paediatr 1993; 82:182–189.
88. Sun B, Curstedt T, Song GW, Robertson B. Surfactant improves lung function and morphology in newborn rabbits with meconium aspiration. Biol Neonate 1993; 63:96–104.
89. Sun B, Herting E, Curstedt T, Robertson B. Exogenous surfactant improves lung compliance and oxygenation in adult rats with meconium aspiration. J Appl Physiol 1994; 77:1961–1971.
90. Johansson A, Camner P, Jarstrand C, Wiernik A. Morphology and function of alveolar macrophages after long-term nickel exposure. Environ Res 1980; 23:170–180.
91. Sherman MP, D'Ambola JB, Aeberhard EE, Barrett CT. Surfactant therapy of newborn rabbits impairs lung macrophage bactericidal activity. J Appl Physiol 1988; 65:137–145.
92. Sherman MP, Campbell LA, Merritt TA, et al. The infected preterm rabbit lung. A model to test the effect of surfactant replacement on lung host defenses. In: von Wichert P, Müller B, eds. Basic Research on Lung Surfactant. Progress in Respiration Research, Vol. 25. Basel: Karger, 1990:204–208.
93. Herting E, Jarstrand C, Rasool O, et al. Experimental neonatal group B streptococcal pneumonia: Effect of a modified porcine surfactant on bacterial proliferation in ventilated near-term rabbits. Pediatr Res 1994; 36:784–791.

13

Resistance to Surfactant Inactivation

ANDREAS GÜNTHER and WERNER SEEGER
Justus-Liebig University
Giessen, Germany

I. Introduction

As detailed in Chapter 9, surfactant abnormalities represent a key event in the development of the adult respiratory distress syndrome (ARDS) (1,2). These abnormalities include lack of surface-active compounds and changes in surfactant composition (3–5) or metabolism (2), as well as inhibition of surface properties by inflammatory mediators (6–12) and plasma-derived proteins (3–5). Leakage of plasma proteins into the alveolar space due to increased endothelial and epithelial permeability is of major importance in the pathogenetic sequence of surfactant abnormalities in ARDS and is regularly noticed during the course of neonatal respiratory distress syndrome (RDS). This chapter will focus on the inactivation of sufactant function by plasma proteins, in particular fibrinogen and fibrin, and on the factors influencing the resistance of different surfactant preparations to this inhibitory stress.

II. Proteins Involved in Inhibition of Surfactant

Severe inhibition of natural surfactant function in vitro and in vivo was observed after addition of blood, serum, plasma, or alveolar washings obtained during severe states of plasma leakage (13–17). Among the different proteins involved, albumin (7,15,18–21), hemoglobin (22), immunoglobulin (21), C-reactive protein (23), and in particular fibrinogen or fibrinmonomer (7,15,18,24–28) possess defined surfactant-inhibitory properties in vitro. Figs. 1 and 2 display the inhibitory effect of albumin, hemoglobin, immunoglobulins, and fibrinogen on the surface activity of various natural surfactants, including Curosurf, Calf Lung Surfactant Extract (CLSE), Alveofact, and Survanta, as well as the synthetic surfactant preparation, PLM-C/B, a mixture of dipalmitoyl phosphatidylcholine (DPPC), phosphatidylglycerol (PG), and palmitic acid (PA) (68.5:22:5), supplemented with 1% natural bovine surfactant protein B (SP-B) and 2% recombinant human surfactant protein C (SP-C). All plasma proteins

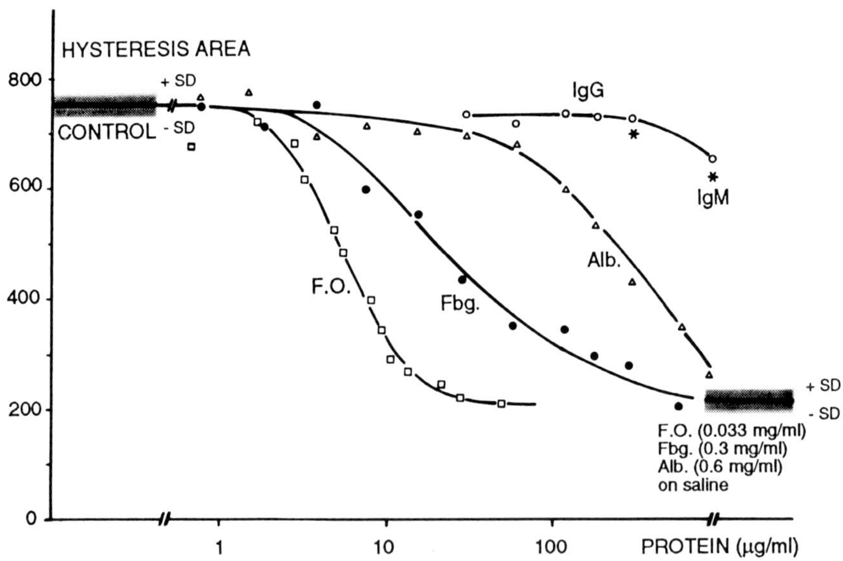

Figure 1 Dose-effect curves of immunoglobulins G and M (human), albumin (bovine; Alb.), fibrinogen (bovine; Fbg) and fibrin monomers/fibrin oligomers (bovine; F.O.) on surface tension characteristics of natural rabbit surfactant. Biophysical measurements were undertaken in diluted surfactant material in the Wilhelmy balance/Langmuir trough system (50 μg/ml phospholipids); the hysteresis of the surface tension–surface area relationship is given (arbitrary units). The shaded area indicates mean $\pm$ SD of hysteresis area of control surfactant without protein addition and of protein effects on pure saline. Fibrinmonomers were first dissolved in a small volume in urea-TRIS buffer and then admixed as a bolus to the surfactant material; arising large fibrin strands (but not small fibrin oligomers) were removed from the soluble phase by centrifugation before measuring surface tension. (From ref. 21; used with permission.)

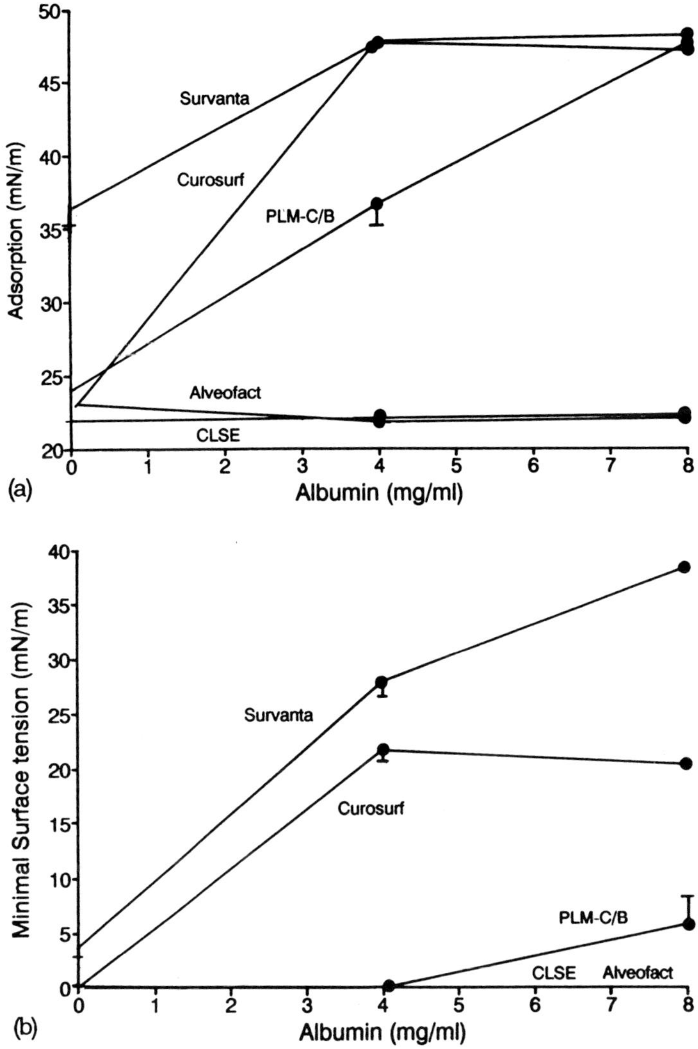

Figure 2 Dose-related influence of albumin (a & b), hemoglobin (c & d) and fibrinogen (e & f) on adsorption kinetics and dynamic surface tension–lowering properties of a synthetic surfactant (PLM-C/B, a mixture of DPPC:PG:PA [68.5:22.5:9], 2% human recombinant SP-C, and 1% natural bovine SP-B) and of several natural surfactant extracts (Calf Lung Surfactant Extract [CLSE], Survanta, Curosurf, and Alveofact). The experiments were performed in the Pulsating Bubble Surfactometer at a phospholipid concentration of 2 mg/ml. Surface tension after 12 sec of adsorption (top) and minimal surface tension after 5 min of film oscillation (bottom) are shown. Means ± SEM of at least five experiments are given. SEM bars are missing when falling within symbol. (From ref. 29; used with permission.)

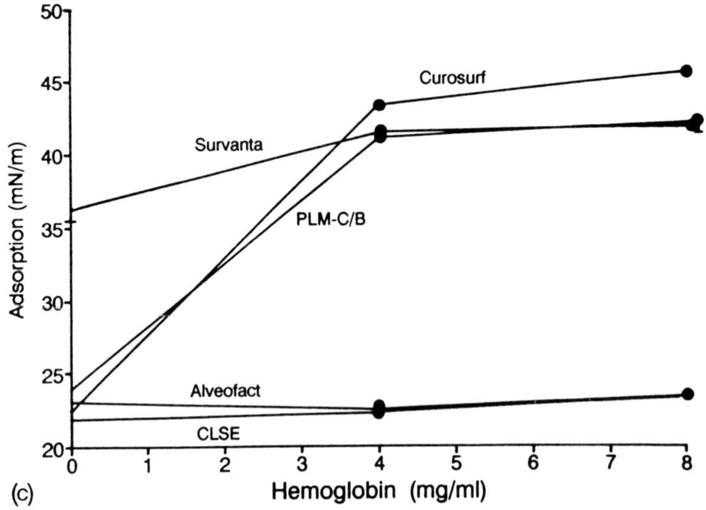

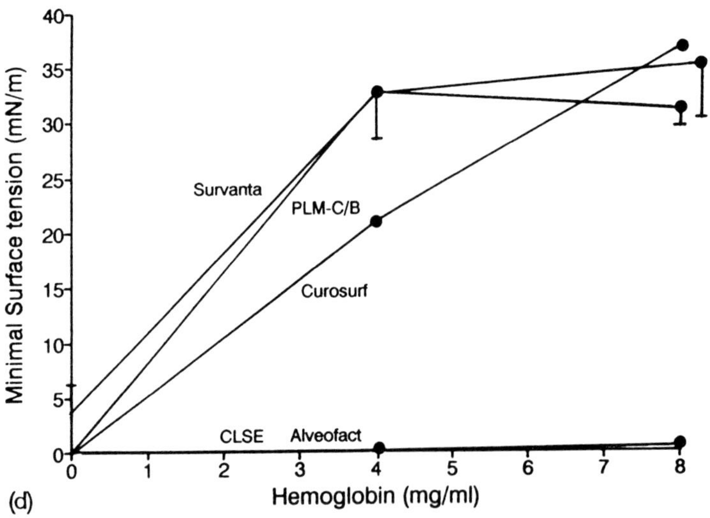

Figure 2 *(Continued)*

caused a dose-dependent inactivation of surfactant function in vitro, as judged from a decrease in the hysteresis area in the Wilhelmy balance system (Fig. 1), as well as a decrease in adsorption rate (reflected by the increased surface tension after 12 sec of adsorption; γads) and increased minimum surface tension (γmin) after 5 min of film oscillation in the pulsating bubble system (Fig. 2). Regardless of the surfactant material employed, the dose-effect curves of Figs. 1 and 2

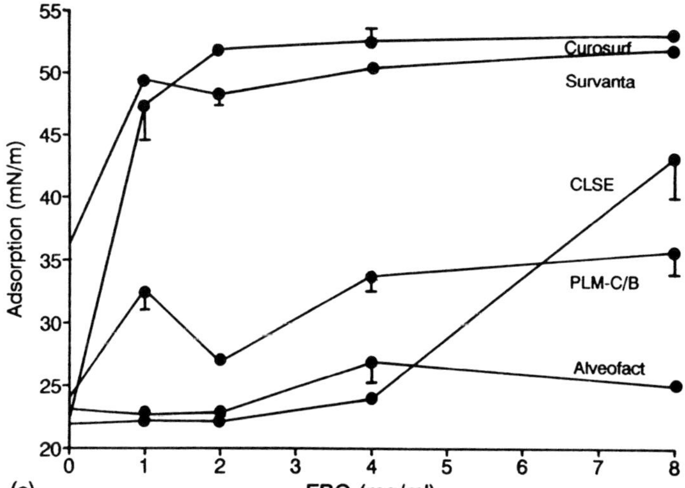

(e)

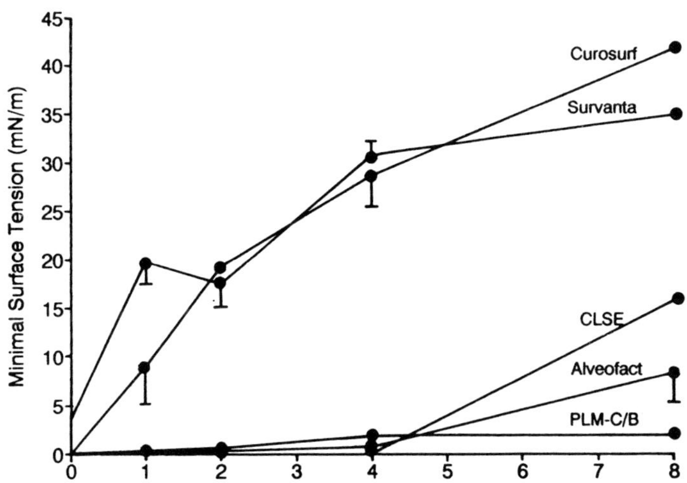

(f)

support the notion that fibrinogen has a markedly higher sufactant-inhibitory capacity in vitro compared with albumin, hemoglobin or immunoglobulins.

III. Differential Sensitivity of Various Surfactants to Protein Inhibition

Differential sensitivity toward protein inhibition of the various surfactant preparations has been noted, with higher susceptibility of Survanta and Curosurf, intermediate sensitivity of PLM-B/C, and low sensitivity of CLSE and Alveofact (29) (Fig. 2). With the exception of Survanta, these striking differences in protein sensitivity could not be explained by impaired surface activity in the absence of contaminating proteins (see starting points throughout Figs. 2A–C), since all surfactant preparations (except Survanta) displayed excellent baseline surface activity (γads = 20–25 mN/m; γmin = zero or near zero mN/m). Two main aspects may underlie these marked differences in protein sensitivity.

A. Variations in Lipid Composition

The relative phospholipid content is 84% for Survanta, 92% for CLSE, and 99% for Curosurf (30); in Alveofact, the phospholipids represent approximately 88% of the lipids. Triglycerides and free fatty acids are virtually absent in Curosurf (31) and percentages range up to 6% each in Survanta (32). Cholesterol is missing in Curosurf (31) Survanta (32), and the percentage ranges around 4% in CLSE (33) and Alveofact (34). As detailed in Table 1, marked differences in the phospholipid profiles were additionally noted, in particular with respect to the percentages of PG, sphingomyelin, and lysophosphatidylcholine. These variations in the lipid composition of the different surfactant preparations may influence the surface properties under inhibitory stress. Interestingly, addition of PA to a lipid extract surfactant reduces its sensitivity to inhibition by proteins

Table 1 Phospholipid Classes of Natural Surfactant Preparations[a]

	PC	LPC	SPH	PI	PE	PG	CL
Survanta	87.2 ±1.2	2.2 ±0.2	4.8 ±0.8	0.5 ±0.1	2.2 ±0.3	3.2 ±0.2	n.d.
Alveofact	82.0 ±1.4	4.0 ±0.2	1.4 ±0.3	0.5 ±0.2	3.0 ±0.4	9.0 ±1.3	n.d.
CLSE	89.3 ±1.1	n.d.	1.4 ±0.3	2.5 ±0.5	2.5 ±0.3	3.6 ±0.3	0.8 ±0.2
Curosurf	74.5 ±0.8	6.9 ±0.7	8.1 ±0.8	3.3 ±0.4	4.5 ±0.6	1.2 ±0.3	n.d.

[a]Phospholipids were separated by thin layer chromatography, using silica gel 60 plates. Samples were applied with a Linomat IV applicator. Chloroform:methanol:acetic acid:distilled water (50:37.5:3.5:2; by vol) was used as the mobile phase and the phospholipids were stained with molybdenum blue reagent and quantified by densitometric scanning at 700 nm with a TLC-Scanner II. Mean values SD ± (n = 5) of each phospholipid class are given in percentage of total phospholipid; PC, phosphatidylcholine; LPC, lysophosphatidylcholine; SPH, sphingomyelin; PI, phosphatidylinositol; PE, phosphatidylethanolamine; PG, phosphatidylglycerol; CL, cardiolipin; n.d., not detectable. (From ref. 29; used with permission.)

(35), and high contents of lysophosphatidylcholine increases the sensitivity to inhibition by fibrinogen (but not albumin) (7).

B. Variations in Apoprotein Composition

Since all natural surfactant preparations underwent organic solvent extraction, no substantial quantities of surfactant protein A (SP-A) are present. SP-B and SP-C are coextracted with the lipids. However, the molar ratio between these two hydrophobic proteins has hitherto only been reported for Curosurf (1:3, [31]). Quantification of the SP-B contents by ELISA technique revealed marked differences between the various surfactants, at least the batches investigated, with CLSE and Alveofact containing high amounts (>1.5% wt/wt related to the lipids) and Curosurf and Survanta containing low percentages (<0.2% wt/wt related to the lipids). Interestingly, these differences correspond to the differential sensitivities to inhibitory proteins as shown in Figs. 2a-f (high sensitivity of Curosurf and Survanta and low susceptibility of CLSE and Alveofact). Differential sensitivity toward inhibition by fibrinogen in spite of virtually identical base line activity has been shown also for the synthetic surfactant phospholipid mixture (PLM) defined above, reconstituted with either recombinant or natural SP-C or natural SP-B (Fig. 3). Low fibrinogen susceptibility was encountered for the SP-B–based PLM, higher sensitivity was found for the SP-C–based PLM, and the apoprotein-free PLM displayed the highest susceptibility (Fig. 3). Accordingly, the resistance to fibrinogen inhibition of a recombinant SP-C–based PLM was markedly increased by supplementation with small amounts of SP-B (Fig. 4). Vice versa, the low fibrinogen sensitivity of CLSE was found to be substantially increased by functional inhibition of its SP-B with a monoclonal antibody (Fig. 5). Thus, there is ample evidence that SP-B plays a major role in counteracting protein inhibition of natural and synthetic surfactants in vitro. Correspondingly, SP-B was recently found to enhance the in vivo efficacy of exogenously applied surfactant preparations in animal models of surfactant deficiency (36,37). In addition, supplementation of an organic extract of bovine surfactant (thus containing the hydrophobic apoproteins) with SP-A was recently noted to counteract the inhibitory effect of fibrinogen (38,39). Accordingly, SP-A enrichment of a solvent-extracted bovine lavage material improved its functional activity in a preterm ventilated rabbit model, in which alveolar protein leakage is known to occur rapidly (40). Thus, modification of surfactant apoprotein profiles appears to be of critical importance to achieve resistance for protein inhibition of the surface active material.

IV. Surfactant Function and the Influence of Clotting and Fibrin(ogen)olysis

Intra-alveolar accumulation of clot material, characterized as hyaline membranes, is commonly found in delayed or untreated neonatal RDS and in ARDS, as well

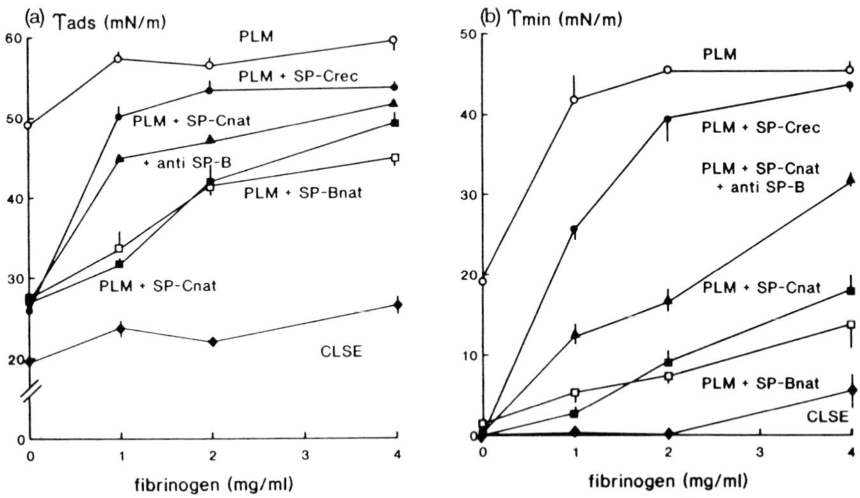

Figure 3 Dose-dependent influence of fibrinogen on adsorption kinetics and dynamic surface tension–lowering properties of Calf Lung Surfactant Extract (CLSE) and of a synthetic phospholipid mixture (PLM, containing DPPC:PG:PA, 68.5:22.5:9) in the absence of apoprotein or recombined with different hydrophobic apoproteins (natural bovine SP-B [SP-Bnat] natural bovine SP-C [SP-Cnat], recombinant human SP-C [SP-Crec] at a concentration of 2% relative to the lipids), assessed with the Pulsating Bubble Surfactometer. The phospholipid concentration was 2 mg/ml in all experiments, and the fibrinogen concentration ranged from 1–4 mg/ml. Surface tension after 12 sec of adsorption (γads, a) and minimum surface tension after 5 min of film oscillation (γmin, b) are shown. In separate experiments, PLM + SP-C_{nat} was incubated with 0.25 mg/ml monoclonal antibody against SP-B prior to exposure to fibrinogen (+ anti SP-B) in order to avoid any contamination of the natural SP-C with natural SP-B. Control experiments with 0.25 mg/ml nonspecific mouse immunoglobulin were additionally performed, but the results did not differ from those of PLM + SP-C_{nat} in the absence of antibody. Each point gives the mean ± SEM of five independent experiments. No error bars are shown if error fell within symbol. (Modified from ref. 26; used with permission.)

as in other acute or chronic inflammatory diseases of the lung (41–46). In the alveolar milieu, the extrinsic coagulation sequence (tissue factor in compound with factor VII) represents the predominant clotting pathway (47–52). This alveolar procoagulant activity was markedly increased in ARDS as well as in RDS patients (50,53–57) and in several experimental models of acute lung injury (58–61). In contrast, concentrations of urokinase-type plasminogen activator, representing the main fibrinolysis pathway within the alveolar spaces of adults (50,52,62,63), were decreased in alveolar lavage fluids from patients with ARDS; concomitantly, increased levels of plasminogen activator inhibitor 1 and α_2-antiplasmin were detected (50,51,56,62). Moreover, natural surfactant preparations

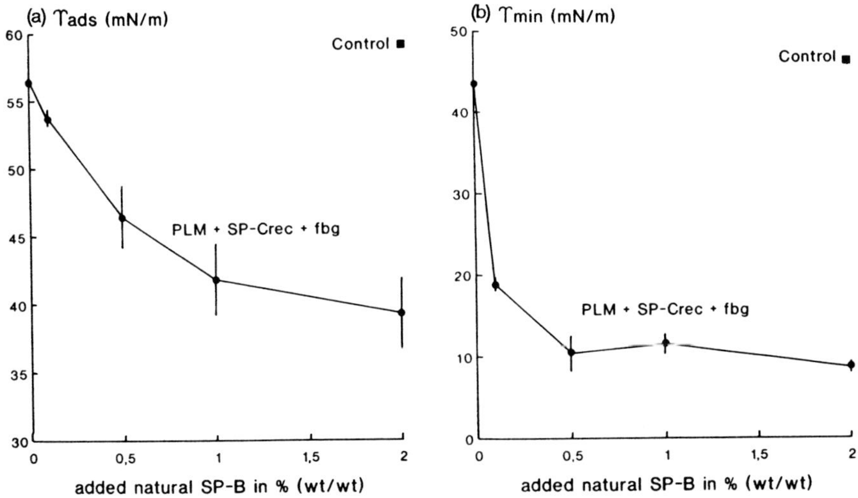

Figure 4 Effect of additional supplementation of a recombinant SP-C (SP-C_{rec}) based phospholipid mixture (PLM, containing DPPC:PG:PA [68.5:22.5:9] and 2% human SP-C_{rec}) with natural SP-B on its sensitivity to fibrinogen inhibition. The mixture was supplemented with increasing concentrations of natural bovine SP-B. All surfactant preparations were studied at a phospholipid concentration of 2 mg/ml in the presence of 4 mg/ml fibrinogen. Values for surface tension after 12 sec of adsorption (γads, a) and minimum surface tension after 5 min of film oscillation (γmin, b), recorded with the Pulsating Bubble Surfactometer, are shown. Each point indicates the mean ± SEM of five independent experiments. No error bars are shown if error fell within symbol. In separate experiments, SP-C_{rec}–based PLM was supplemented with additional 2% of SP-C_{rec} (amounting to in total 4% SP-C_{rec} in this mixture) and exposed to fibrinogen in corresponding manner (Control). (From ref. 26; used with permission.)

and synthetic phospholipid mixtures enriched with SP-C and SP-B were found to inhibit the plasmin-induced fibrino(geno)lysis (64,65). Thus, the hemostatic balance within the alveolar milieu appears to be shifted toward a predominance of procoagulant and antifibrinolytic activity in acutely or chronically inflamed lung regions.

Thrombin-induced coagulation of human fibrinogen (range 0.04–4.0 mg/ml) in the presence of CLSE (diluted to a phospholipid concentration of 2 mg/ml) resulted in a progressive loss of surface tension–lowering properties and adsorption facilities of this surfactant preparation; the CLSE-inhibitory capacity of desAABB-fibrin surpassed that of fibrinogen by more than two orders of magnitude (66) (Fig. 6). In parallel with the loss of surface activity, association of the predominant surfactant phospholipid DPPC (^{14}C-labeled, admixed to CLSE) with polymerizing desAABB-fibrin was observed (66) (Fig. 7). At a

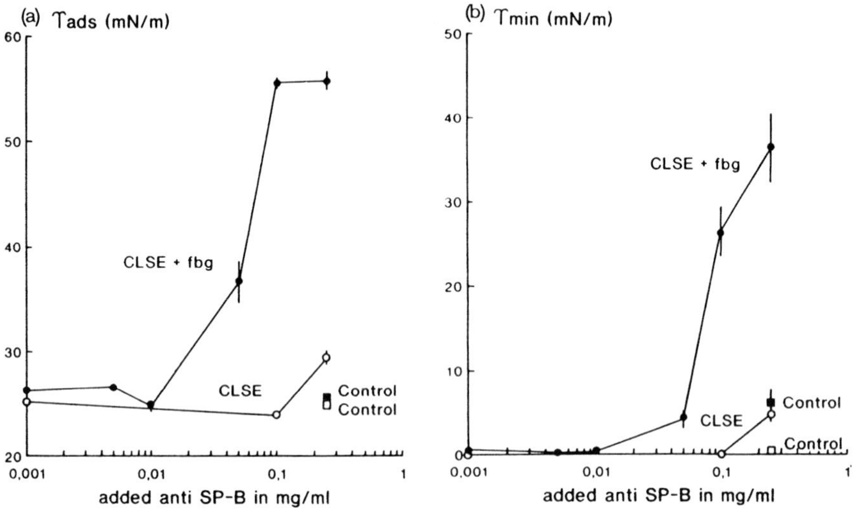

Figure 5 Dose-dependent effect of antibody against SP-B (anti–SP-B) on surface properties and fibrinogen sensitivity of Calf Lung Surfactant Extract (CLSE), assessed with the Pulsating Bubble Surfactometer. CLSE was incubated with increasing concentrations of anti–SP-B up to 0.25 mg/ml (log scale). It was used at a phospholipid concentration of 2 mg/ml in all experiments, in the absence or presence of 4 mg/ml of fibrinogen (fbg). Surface tension after 12 sec of adsorption (γads, left panel) and minimum surface tension after 5 min of film oscillation (γmin, right panel) are shown. Control experiments included those with admixture of 0.25 mg/ml of nonspecific mouse immunoglobulin to CLSE alone (open symbol) or to CLSE in the presence of fibrinogen (closed symbol). Each point gives the mean ± SEM of five independent experiments. No error bars are shown if error fell within symbol. (From ref. 26; used with permission.)

concentration of 0.3 mg/ml insoluble fibrin removed 50%, and at a concentration of 0.6 mg/ml it removed >90% of DPPC from the aqueous phase. Dioleoylphosphatidylcholine, dipalmitoylphosphatidic acid, stearic acid, PA, and arachidonic acid, admixed to CLSE as labeled compounds, as well as total CLSE phospholipids were retained in polymerizing desAABB-fibrin with dose-effect curves superimposable on that of DPPC; no fibrin association was noted for ^{14}C-glycerol-3-phosphate (66) (Fig. 8). Polymerizing desAA-fibrin, generated by incubation of CLSE-fibrinogen mixtures with arvin, captured DPPC and resulted in a loss of surface properties at even lower concentrations as compared with desAABB-fibrin. In contrast, CLSE incubation with preformed desAABB- and desAA-fibrin polymers did not effect substantial phospholipid coupling with the clot material or loss of surface properties. Microtiter plate-immobilized fibrinogen, desAABB-, and desAA-fibrinmonomers did not bind CLSE phospholipids mixed with ^{14}C-DPPC. Soluble desAABB- and desAA-fibrinmono-

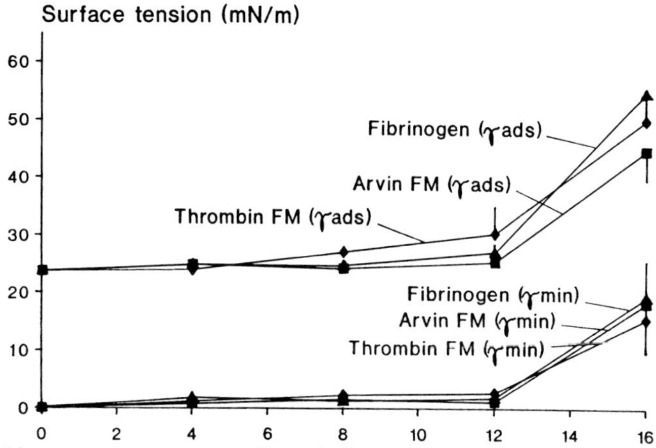

(a)

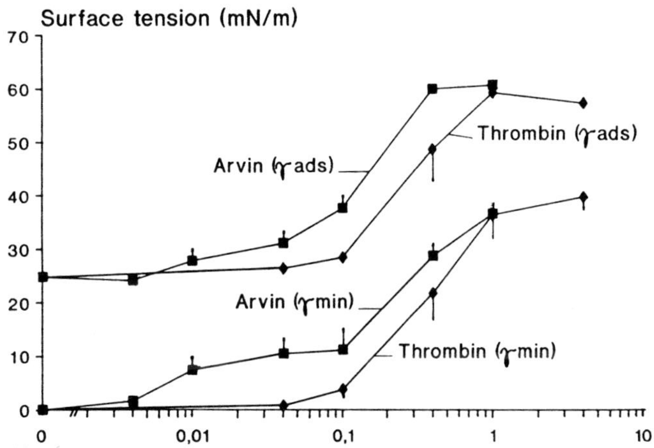

(b)

Figure 6 Dose-dependent inhibition of Calf Lung Surfactant Extract (CLSE) surface properties by fibrinogen, desAABBfibrinomnomer (Thrombin FM), and desAA-fibrin-monomer (Arvin FM; all (a) as well as desAABB- and desAAfibrin (b). The assays were performed according to the following protocols:

Influence of fibrinogen on CLSE function. CLSE was diluted to 2 mg/ml phospholipids in Ca^{2+} (3 mM)–containing saline, mixed with various fibrinogen concentrations (4–16 mg/ml), and time-matched incubation with gentle vortexing was performed in analogy to the subsequent protocols. Samples were directly transferred to the Pulsating Bubble Surfactometer. (Continued on p. 280.)

mers, generated in the presence of GLY-PRO-ARG-PRO, did not exhibit surfactant inhibitory properties different from those of fibrinogen (minimum inhibitory concentrations >12 mg/ml for 2 mg/ml of CLSE (66) (Fig. 6). Thus, these findings indicate the loss of surface active material into nascent fibrin clots with concomitant deterioration of surface tension properties. This mechanism may—in concert with protein-derived surfactant inhibition at the alveolar air-liquid interface and in the hypophase—contribute substantially to the surfactant inactivation and the decline of local phospholipid and apoprotein concentration in the alveolar space that occurs in neonatal RDS and ARDS.

Dissolution of alveolar deposits of fibrinogen and fibrin requires enzymatic degradation by plasmin or leukocyte-derived proteases. Plasmin-derived cleavage products of fibrinogen exhibited markedly increased inhibitory capacities on the natural and synthetic surfactant preparations in vitro (Fig. 9a,b) as compared with the native fibrinogen molecule (cf. Fig. 2e,f). Among the plasmic fragments, fibrinogen split product D (≈85 kDa), but not E (≈50 kDa), represented the predominant inhibitory compound (Figs. 9c-f). Only sequential cleavage of fibrinogen with trypsin and endoproteinase to low molecular weight split products (<25 kDa) resulted in a decrease of surfactant-inhibitory capacity (67) (Fig. 9g,h).

Plasmic cleavage of an insoluble clot with embedded natural surfactant material (CLSE) and subsequent characterization of surface properties resulted in an impressive reconstitution of surface properties (65) (Fig. 10). No significant

---

Influence of desAA- and desAABB-fibrinmonomers on CLSE function. CLSE (2 mg/ml)–fibrinogen (4–16 mg/ml) mixtures were incubated with 60 mM GLY-PRO-ARG-PRO for 30 min (37°C). Next, thrombin (5 mU/ml) or arvin (0.5 U/ml) was admixed for generation of desAABB-fibrin- and desAA-fibrinmonomers, respectively, and incubation was continued for another 1-hr period at 37°C before transferring samples to the Surfactometer. Control experiments with use of a fibrinopeptide-A ELISA documented >95% conversion of fibrinogen to fibrin(monomer) for both thrombin and arvin incubation procedures (data not given in detail). No clot formation was observed in the presence of of GLY-PRO-ARG-PRO. Control studies confirmed absence of direct inhibitory effect of the applied concentrations of GLY-PRO-ARG-PRO, thrombin and arvin on CLSE function; as well as lack of influence of this tetrapeptide on the surface properties of CLSE-fibrinogen mixtures in the absence thrombin and arvin.

Influence of fibrin clot formation on CLSE surface properties. CLSE (2mg/ml)–fibrinogen (0.004–4.0 mg/ml)–mixtures were incubated with thrombin (5 mU/ml) or arvin (0.5 U/ml) for 1 hr, aqueous phases were separated from clot material by filter passage as detailed in the legend to Fig. 7, and filtrate samples were transferred to the Pulsating Bubble Surfactometer. Control experiments (not given in detail) showed that the filter passage per se did not influence surface properties of CLSE-fibrinogen mixtures.

Surface tension after 12-sec of adsorption (γads, upper curves) and minimum surface tension after 5 min of film oscillation (γmin, lower curves) are given. Each point reflects the mean ± SEM of at least four independent experiments; no error bars are shown when error fell within symbol. (From ref. 66; used with permission.)

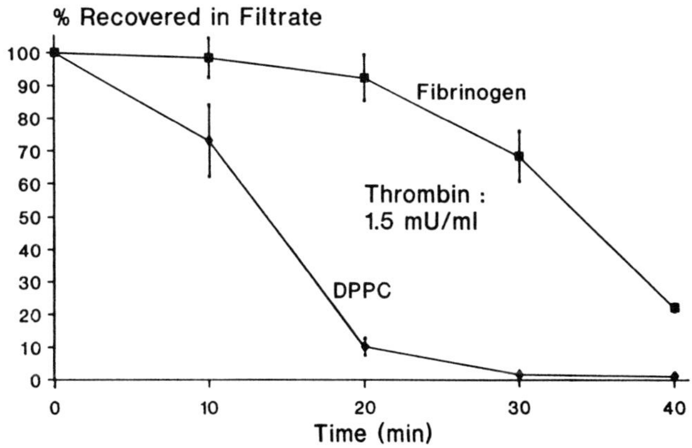

Figure 7 Time dependency of thrombin-induced fibrin formation and dipalmitoyl phosphatidylcholine (DPPC) clot association. In parallel experiments, Calf Lung Surfactant Extract (CLSE, 2 mg/ml, containing ^{14}C-DPPC or unlabeled)–fibrinogen (4 mg/ml, ^{125}I-labeled or unlabeled) mixtures were incubated with 1.5 mU/ml of thrombin for 10–40 min. Thrombin activity was stopped by heparin/antithrombin III admixture after the respective time periods and samples were centrifuged through a 100 μm nylon gauze and filtrate counts were measured in β- and γ-counters, respectively. Filtrate counts are given in % of initial total radioactivity. Note the gap between the fibrinogen and DPPC curves, being most evident after 20 min of incubation, where ≈10% polymerized fibrin retained ≈90% DPPC. In control experiments, direct quantification of phospholipids in the filtrate gave superimposable recovery curves. Each point reflects the mean ±SEM of at least four independent experiments; no error bars are shown when error fell within symbol. (From ref. 66; used with permission.)

differences between the dose-effect curves of plasmic fibrinogen or fibrin split products on the surface properties of CLSE were observed, suggesting release of surface active material with full functional integrity from preformed fibrin clots into the soluble phase.

V. Conclusions

The inhibition of surfactant function by soluble plasma proteins and—even more dramatically—by incorporation of hydrophobic surfactant components into a nascent fibrin clot must be assumed to contribute substantially to alveolar instability and collapse. Resistance to inhibitory stress thus represents a desirable criterion of artificial surfactants for use in acute respiratory failure. The degree of protein sensitivity of synthetic and natural surfactants depends on both the lipid and the apoprotein composition. In particular, the apoproteins SP-B and

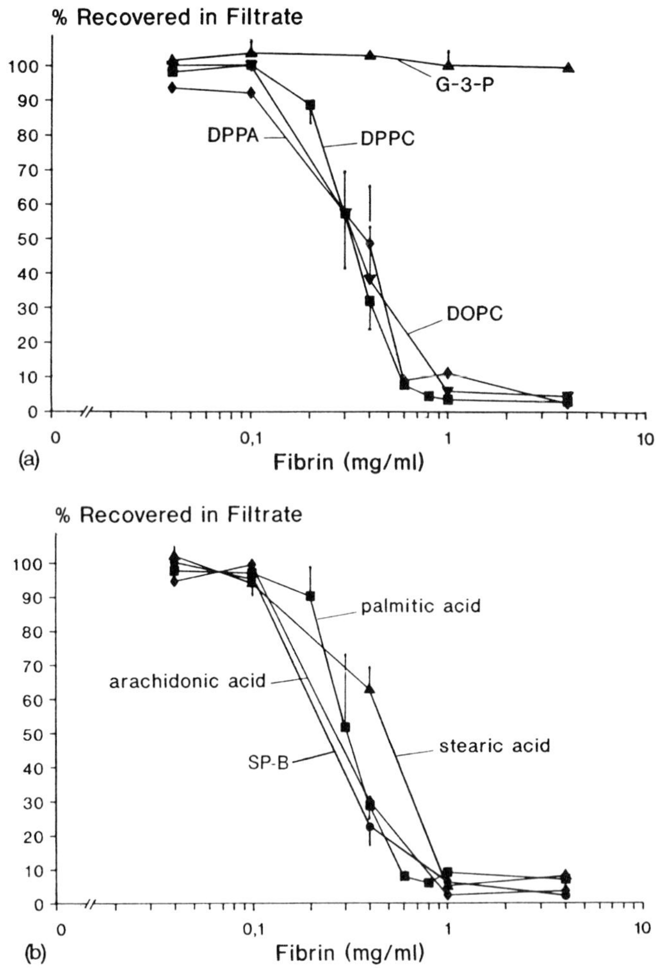

Figure 8 Association of different labeled lipids and SP-B with growing desAABB-fibrin clots. Calf Lung Surfactant Extract (CLSE; 2 mg/ml) was mixed with different radioactively labeled lipids and increasing concentrations of fibrinogen. Complete conversion into insoluble fibrin was achieved by subsequent incubation with 5 mU/ml thrombin for 1 h at 37°C. Samples were centrifuged through a 100 μm nylon gauze filter, and recovery of labeled lipid in the filtrate is given in % of the initial total quantity of tracer, in relation to the fibrin concentration (log scale). In addition, SP-B content of the filtrates was measured by use of the ELISA technique and is given in % of the initial total amount. Separate control experiments with admixture of ^{125}I-fibrinogen or quantification of nonlabeled fibrinogen by ultraviolet-detection at 280 nm documented that for all fibrinogen concentrations used, >95% of the protein was captured as insoluble clot material upon filter passage (data not shown). Each point reflects the mean ±SEM of at least 4 independent experiments; no error bars are shown when error fell within symbol. DPPC, dipalmitoylphosphatidylcholine; DOPC, dioleoylphosphatidylcholine; DPPA, dipalmitoylphosphatidic acid; G-3-P, glycerol-3-phosphate. (From ref. 66; used with permission.)

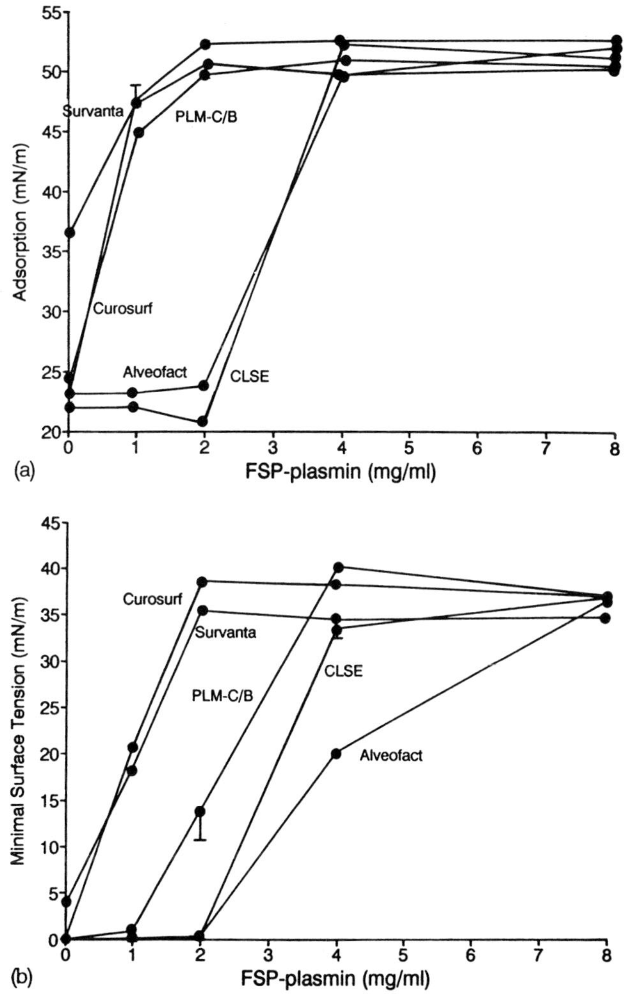

Figure 9 Dose-related influence of plasmic cleavage products of fibrinogen (FSP-plasmin; a and b), fibrinogen split product D (FS-D; c and d), fibrinogen split product E (FS-E; e and f) and trypsin and endoproteinase derived cleavage products of fibrinogen (FSP-endoproteinase + trypsin; g and h) on adsorption kinetics and dynamic surface tension lowering properties of several surfactant preparations. FSP-plasmin was previously obtained by incubation of 25 mg/ml of fibrinogen with 3.125 U/ml of plasmin for 3 hr at 37°C. FS-D and FS-E were purified from plasma- derived fibrinogen cleavage products. FSP-endoproteinase + trypsin was prepared by incubation of 25 mg/ml of fibrinogen with 1000 U/ml of trypsin for 48 hr and subsequent incubation of this mixture with 4 U/ml of *Staphylococcus aureus* endoproteinase Glu-C for 24 hr at 37°C. The final concentrations of the split products correspond to the indicated predigestion concentrations of fibrinogen. (Continued on p. 284.)

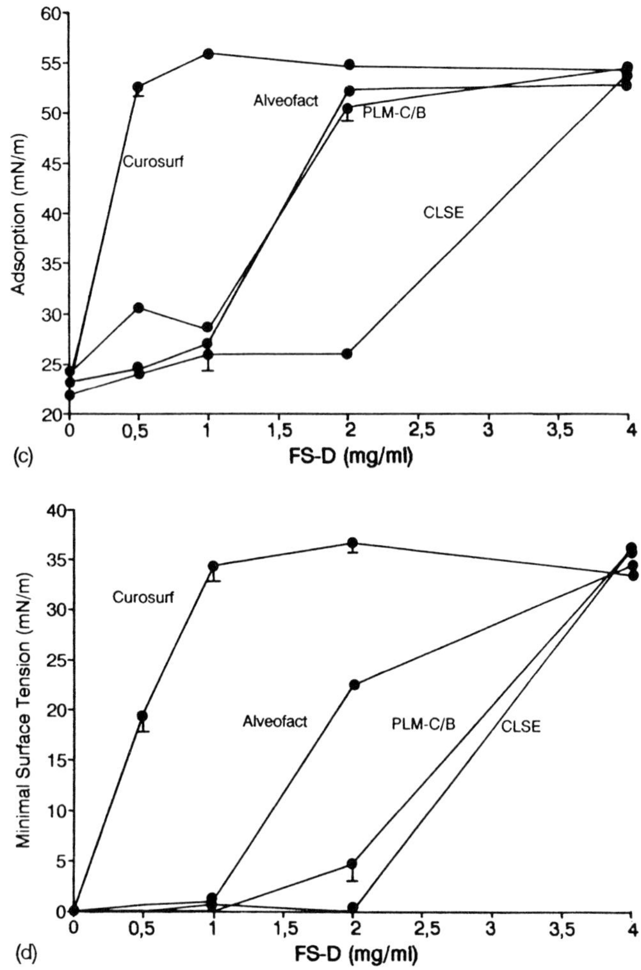

Figure 9 *(Continued)*

A synthetic surfactant (PLM-C/B containing DPPC:PG:PA [68.5:22.5:9], 2% human recombinant SP-C, and 1% natural bovine SP-B) and several natural surfactant extracts (Calf Lung Surfactant Extract [CLSE], Survanta, Curosurf, and Alveofact) were studied. Surfactant at a concentration of 2 mg/ml was mixed and incubated (37°C, 5 min) with increasing concentrations of FSP-plasmin (a,b), FS-D (c,d), FS-E (e,f), or FSP-endoproteinase + trypsin (g and h). The indicated FS-D or FS-E concentrations correspond to a dose range of the natural fibrinogen between 1 and 8 mg/ml, thus allowing direct comparison with the dose-effect curves in Figs. 2e and f and 9a and b. The experiments were performed in the Pulsating Bubble Surfactometer and surface tension after 12 sec of adsorption (top) and minimal surface tension after 5 min of film oscillation (bottom) are shown. Means ± SEM of at least five experiments are given. SEM bars are missing when falling within symbol. (From ref. 67; used with permission.)

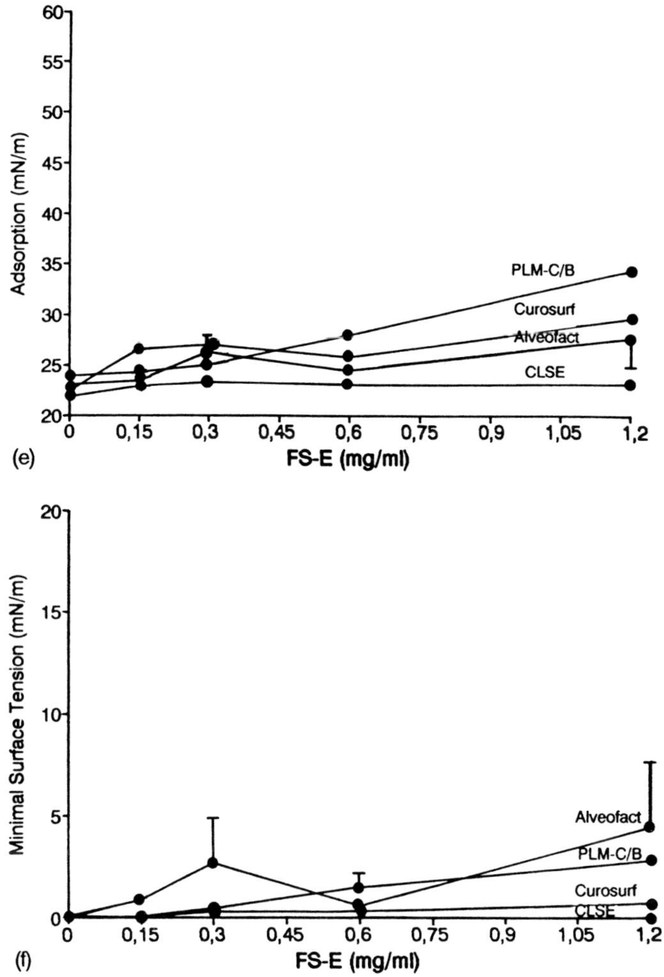

Figure 9 *(Continued)*

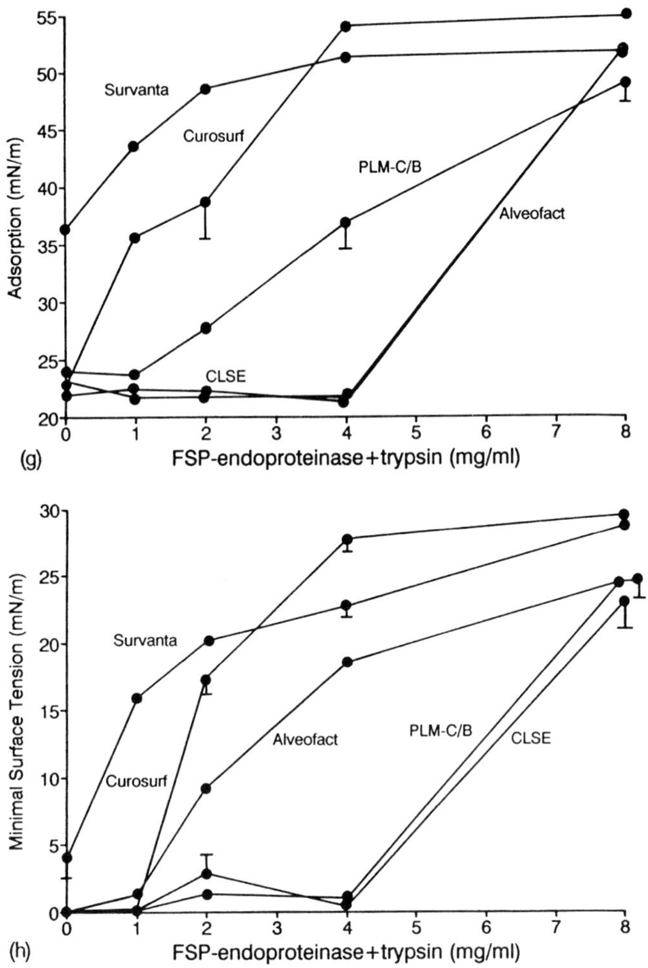

Figure 9 *(Continued)*

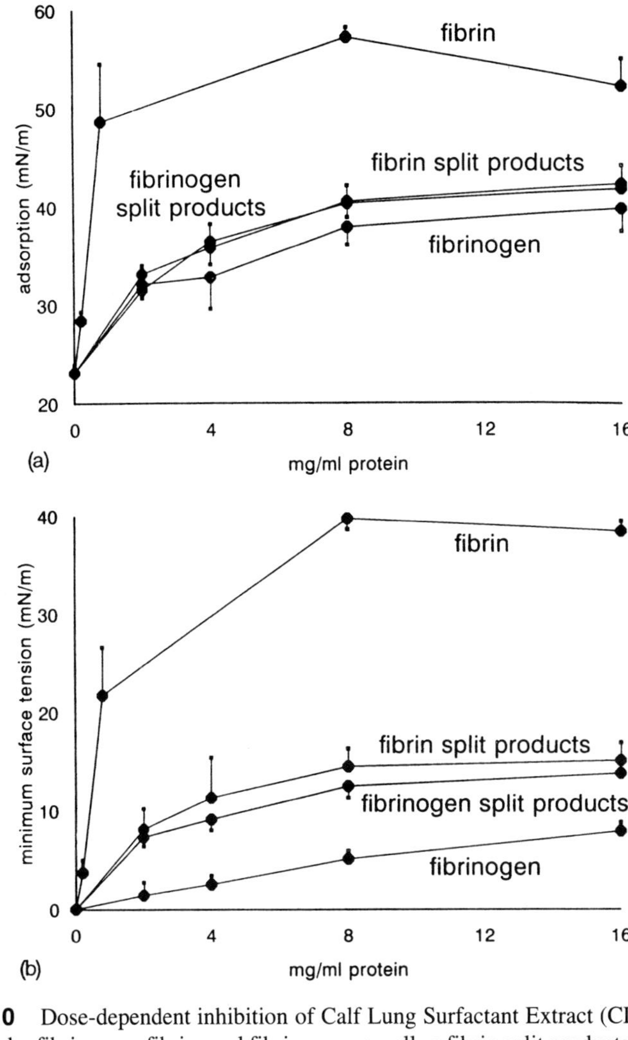

Figure 10 Dose-dependent inhibition of Calf Lung Surfactant Extract (CLSE) surface properties by fibrinogen, fibrin, and fibrinogen as well as fibrin split products, as assessed with the Pulsating Bubble Surfactometer. The assays were performed according to the following protocols:

Influence of fibrinogen on CLSE function. CLSE was diluted in 3 mM Ca^{2+} containing saline to a final concentration of 4 mg/ml phospholipids and was incubated for 25 min at 37°C. Fibrinogen (2, 4, 8, and 16 mg/ml) was admixed, the mixture was sonified for 1 min (50 W, 25 kHz), and incubated for another 5 min at 37°C.

Influence of fibrinogen split products on CLSE function. Fibrinogen (20 mg/ml) was incubated with plasmin (0.156 U/ml) for 24 hr at 37°C. The split products (2–16 mg/ml were admixed as described for fibrinogen. (Continued on p. 288.)

SP-A may protect against protein inhibition. The influence of these surfactant apoproteins on the incorporation of lipophilic surfactant material into growing fibrin networks has not yet been addressed, but it deserves to be investigated.

References

1. Seeger W, Günther A, Walmrath HD, et al. Alveolar surfactant and adult respiratory distress syndrome—pathogenetic role and therapeutic perspectives. Clin Invest 1993; 71:177–190.
2. Lewis JF, Jobe AH. Surfactant and the adult respiratory distress syndrome. Am Rev Respir Dis 1993; 147:218–233.
3. Hallman M, Spragg R, Harrell JH, Moser KM. Evidence of lung surfactant failure in respiratory distress syndrome. J Clin Invest 1982; 70:673–683.
4. Gregory TJ, Longmore WJ, Moxley MA, et al. Surfactant chemical composition and biophysical activity in acute respiratory distress syndrome. J Clin Invest 1991; 88:1976–1981.
5. Pison U, Seeger W, Buchhorn R, et al. Surfactant abnormalities in patients with respiratory failure after multiple trauma. Am Rev Respir Dis 1989; 140:1033–1039.
6. Holm BA, Keicher L, Liu MY, et al. Inhibition of pulmonary surfactant function by phospholipases. J Appl Physiol 1991; 71 317–321.
7. Cockshutt AM, Possmayer F. Lysophosphatidylcholine sensitizes lipid extracts of pulmonary surfactant to inhibition by serum proteins. Biochim Biophys Acta 1991; 1086:63–71.
8. Hallman M. Lung surfactant in respiratory distress syndrome. Acta Anaesthesiol Scand 1991; 35(suppl 95):15–21.
9. Wispe JR, Clark JC, Warner BB, et al. Tumor necrosis factor-alpha inhibits expression of pulmonary surfactant protein. J Clin Invest 1990; 86:1954–1960.
10. Pison U, Tam EK, Caughey GH, Hawgood S. Proteolytic inactivation of dog lung surfactant-associated proteins by neutrophil elastase. Biochim Biophys Acta 1989; 992:251–257.
11. Ryan SF, Ghassibi Y, Liau DF. Effects of activated polymorphonuclear leukocytes upon pulmonary surfactant in vitro. Am J Respir Cell Mol Physiol 1990, 4:33–41.

Influence of fibrin clot formation on CLSE function. Mixtures of CLSE (4 mg/ml) and increasing quantities of fibrin (1, 8, and 16 mg/ml) were filtered for separation of clot material from the soluble phase as described in the legend to Fig. 6.

Influence of fibrin scission products on CLSE function. CLSE (4 mg/ml) and 2, 4, 8, or 16 mg/ml of fibrinogen in saline/Ca^{2+} were mixed and clotting was induced by incubation with 5 mU/ml thrombin (12 hr at 37°C). Plasmin was added at a final concentration of 0.156 U/ml and the mixture was again incubated for another 18 hr at 37°C.

Values for surface tension after 12 sec of adsorption (top) and minimum surface tension after 5 min of film oscillation (bottom) are given. Each point reflects the mean ± SEM of at least four independent experiments; no SEM bars are shown when error fell within symbol. (From ref. 65; used with permission.)

12. Seeger W, Lepper H, Wolf HR, Neuhof H. Alteration of alveolar surfactant function after exposure to oxidative stress and to oxygenated and native arachidonic acid in vitro. Biochim Biophys Acta 1985; 835:58–67.
13. Kobayashi T, Nitta K, Ganzuka M, et al. Inactivation of exogenous surfactant by pulmonary edema fluid. Pediatr Res 1991; 29:353–356.
14. Berry D, Ikegami M, Jobe A. Respiratory distress and surfactant inhibition following vagotomy in rabbits. J Appl Physiol 1986; 61:1741–1748.
15. Fuchimukai T, Fujiwara T, Takahashi A, Enhorning G. Artificial pulmonary surfactant inhibited by proteins. J Appl Physiol 1987; 62:429–437.
16. Ikegami M, Agata Y, Elkady T, et al. Comparison of four surfactants: in vitro surface properties and responses of preterm lambs to treatment at birth. Pediatrics 1987; 79:38–46.
17. Tierney DF, Johnson RP. Altered surface tension of lung extracts and lung mechanics. J Appl Physiol 1965; 20:1253–1260.
18. Holm BA, Venkitaraman AR, Enhorning G, Notter RH. Biophysical inhibition of synthetic lung surfactants. Chem Phys Lipids 1990; 52:243–250.
19. Holm BA, Enhorning G, Notter RH. A biophysical mechanism by which plasma proteins inhibit lung surfactant activity. Chem Phys Lipids 1988; 49:49–55.
20. Holm BA, Notter RH, Finkelstein JN. Surface property changes from interactions of albumin with natural lung surfactant and extracted lung lipids. Chem Phys Lipids 1985; 38:287–298.
21. Seeger W, Stoehr G, Wolf HR, Neuhof H. Alteration of surfactant function due to protein leakage: special interaction with fibrin monomer. J Appl Physiol 1985; 58:326–338.
22. Holm BA, Notter RH. Effects of hemoglobin and cell membrane lipids on pulmonary surfactant activity. J Appl Physiol 1987; 63:1434–1442.
23. McEachren T, Keough KMW. Effects of C-reactive protein (CRP) and the complement component (C1Q) on the adsorption rate of pulmonary surface active material (SAM) to the air-water interface (abstr). Am Rev Respir Dis 1993; 147:A991.
24. O'Brodovich HM, Weitz JI, Possmayer F. Effect of fibrinogen degradation products and lung ground substance on surfactant function. Biol Neonate 1990; 57:325–333.
25. Rüfer R, Stolz C. Inaktivierung von alveolären Oberflächenfilmen durch Erniedrigung der Oberflächenspannung der Hypophase. Pflugers Arch 1969; 307:89–103.
26. Seeger W, Günther A, Thede C. Differential sensitivity to fibrinogen inhibition of SP-C- vs SP-B-based surfactants. Am J Physiol 1992; 262:L286–L291.
27. Seeger W, Thede C, Günther A, Grube C. Surface properties and sensitivity to protein-inhibition of a recombinant apoprotein C-based phospholipid mixture in vitro—comparison to natural surfactant. Biochim Biophys Acta 1991; 1081:45–52.
28. Taylor FB, Abrams ME. Effect of surface active lipoprotein on clotting and fibrinolysis, and of fibrinogen on surface tension of surface active lipoprotein. Am J Med 1966; 40:346–350.
29. Seeger W, Grube C, Günther A, Schmidt R. Surfactant inhibition by plasma proteins: differential sensitivity of various surfactant preparations. Eur Respir J 1993; 6:971–977.

30. Halliday HL. Clinical experience with exogenous natural surfactant. Dev Pharmacol Ther 1989; 13:173–181.
31. Robertson B, Curstedt T, Johansson J, et al. Structural and functional characterization of porcine surfactant isolated by liquid chromatography. In: von Wichert P, Müller B, eds. Basic Research on Lung Surfactant. Progress in Respiration Research. Vol. 25. Basel; Karger, 1990:237–246.
32. Taeusch HW, Keough KM, Williams M, et al. Characterization of bovine surfactant for infants with respiratory distress syndrome. Pediatrics 1986; 77:572–581.
33. Shapiro DL, Notter RH, Morin FC III, et al. Double-blind, randomized trial of a calf lung surfactant extract administered at birth to very premature infants for prevention of respiratory distress syndrome. Pediatrics 1985; 76:593–599.
34. Gortner L, Pohlandt F, Disse B, Weller E. Effects of bovine surfactant in premature lambs after intra-tracheal application. Eur J Pediatr 1990; 149:280–283.
35. Cockshutt AM, Absolom DR, Possmayer F. The role of palmitic acid in pulmonary surfactant: enhancement of surface activity and prevention of inhibition by blood proteins. Biochim Biophys Acta 1991; 1085:248–256.
36. Rider ED, Ikegami M, Whitsett JA, et al. Treatment responses to surfactants containing natural surfactant proteins in preterm rabbits. Am Rev Respir Dis 1993; 147:669–676.
37. Kobayashi T, Nitta K, Takahashi R, et al. Activity of pulmonary surfactant after blocking the associated proteins SP-A and SP-B. J Appl Physiol 1991; 71:530–536.
38. Cockshutt AM, Weitz J, Possmayer F. Pulmonary surfactant-associated protein A enhances the surface activity of lipid extract surfactant and reverses inhibition by blood proteins in vitro. Biochemistry 1990; 29:8424–8429.
39. Venkitaraman AR, Hall SB, Whitsett JA, Notter RH. Enhancement of biophysical activity of lung surfactant extracts and phospholipid-apoprotein mixtures by surfactant protein A. Chem Phys Lipids 1990; 56:185–194.
40. Yamada T, Ikegami M, Tabor BL, Jobe AH. Effects of surfactant protein-A on surfactant function in preterm ventilated rabbits. Am Rev Respir Dis 1990; 142:754–757.
41. Bachofen M, Weibel ER. Structural alterations of lung parenchyma in the adult respiratory distress syndrome. Clin Chest Med 1982; 3:35–56.
42. Jackson LK. Idiopathic pulmonary fibrosis. Clin Chest Med 1982; 3:579–592.
43. Spencer H. Pathology of the Lung. 3rd ed. Philadelphia: Saunders, 1977:235–240.
44. Pratt PC. Pathology of adult respiratory distress syndrome. In: Thurlbeck WM, Abell MR, eds. The Lung: Structure, Function, and Disease. Baltimore: Williams & Wilkins, 1978: 43–57.
45. Burkhardt A. Alveolitis and collapse in the pathogenesis of pulmonary fibrosis. Am Rev Respir Dis 1989; 140:513–524.
46. Hallman M, Maasilta P, Kivisaari L, Mattson K. Changes in surfactant in bronchoalveolar lavage fluid after hemithorax irradiation in patients with mesothelioma. Am Rev Respir Dis 1990; 141:998–1005.
47. Chapman HA, Allen CL, Stone L. Abnormalities in pathways of alveolar fibrin turnover among patients with interstitial lung disease. Am Rev Respir Dis 1986; 133:437–443.
48. Chapman HA, Stahl M, Allen CL, et al. Regulation of the procoagulant activity

within the bronchoalveolar compartment of normal human lung. Am Rev Respir Dis 1988; 137:1417–1425.

49. Gross TJ, Simon RH, Sitrin RG. Tissue factor procoagulant expression by rat alveolar epithelial cells. Am J Respir Cell Mol Biol 6:397–403.
50. Idell S, James KK, Levin EG, et al. Local abnormalities in coagulation and fibrinolytic pathways predispose to alveolar fibrin deposition in the adult respiratory distress syndrome. J Clin Invest 1989; 84:695–705.
51. Nakstad B, Lyberg T, Skjonsberg OH, Boye NP. Local activation of the coagulation and fibrinolysis systems in lung disease. Thromb Res 1990; 57:827–838.
52. Hasday JD, Bachwich PR, Lynch JP, Sitrin RG. Procoagulant and plasminogen activator activities of bronchoalveolar fluid in patients with pulmonary sarcoidosis. Exp Lung Res 1988; 14:261–278.
53. Idell S, James KK, Levin EG, et al. Local abnormalities in coagulation and fibrinolytic pathways predispose to alveolar fibrin deposition in the adult respiratory distress syndrome. J Clin Invest 1989; 84:695–705.
54. Viscardi RM, Broderick K, Sun C-CJ, et al. Disordered pathways of fibrin turnover in lung lavage of premature infants with respiratory distress syndrome. Am Rev Respir Dis 1992; 146:492–499.
55. Idell S, Gonzalez K, Bradford H, et al. Procoagulant activity in bronchoalveolar lavage in the adult respiratory distress syndrome. Contribution of tissue factor associated with factor VII. Am Rev Respir Dis 1987; 136:1466–1474.
56. Idell S, Koenig KB, Fair DS, et al. Serial abnormalities of fibrin turnover in evolving adult respiratory distress syndrome. Am J Physiol 1991; 261:L240–L248.
57. Seeger W, Hübel J, Klapettek K, et al. Procoagulant in bronchoalveolar lavage of severly traumatized patients—relation to the development of acute respiratory distress. Thromb Res 1991; 91:45–52.
58. Idell S, Gonzalez KK, MacArthur CK, et al. Bronchoalveolar lavage procoagulant activity in bleomycin-induced lung injury in marmosets. Characterization and relationship to fibrin deposition and fibrosis. Am Rev Respir Dis 1987; 136:124–133.
59. Idell S, Peters J, James KK, et al. Local abnormalities of coagulation and fibrinolytic pathways that promote alveolar fibrin deposition in the lungs of baboons with diffuse alveolar damage. J Clin Invest 1989; 84:181–193.
60. Idell S, James KK, Gillies C, et al. Abnormalities of pathways of fibrin turnover in lung lavage of rats with oleic acid and bleomycin-induced lung injury support alveolar fibrin deposition. Am J Pathol 1989; 135:387–399.
61. Idell S, Peterson BT, Gonzalez KK, et al. Local abnormalities of coagulation and fibrinolysis and alveolar fibrin deposition in sheep with oleic acid-induced lung injury. Am Rev Respir Dis 1988; 138:1282–1294.
62. Bertozzi P, Astedt B, Zenzius L, et al. Depressed bronchoalveolar urokinase activity in patients with adult respiratory distress syndrome. N Engl J Med 1990; 322:890–897.
63. Chapman HA, Bertozzi P, Sailor LZ, Nusrat AR. Alveolar macrophage urokinase receptors localize enzyme activity to the cell surface. Am J Physiol 1990; 259:L432–L438.
64. Günther A, Bleyl H, Seeger W. Apoprotein-based synthetic surfactants inhibit plasmic cleavage of fibrinogen in vitro. Am J Physiol 1993; 265:L186–L192.

65. Günther A, Kalinowski M, Elssner A, Seeger W. Clot-embedded surfactant: Kinetics of fibrinolysis and surface activity. Am J Physiol 267:L618–624, 1994.
66. Seeger W, Elssner A, Günther A, et al. Lung surfactant phospholipids associate with polymerizing fibrin-loss of surfactant activity. Am J Respir Cell Mol Physiol 1993; 9:213–220.
67. Seeger W, Grube C, Günther A. Proteolytic cleavage of fibrinogen: Amplification of its surfactant inhibitory capacity. Am J Respir Cell Mol Physiol 1993; 9:239–247.

14

Antigenicity of Surfactant Proteins A, B, and C

TIMOTHY E. WEAVER and JEFFREY A. WHITSETT
Children's Hospital Medical Center
Cincinnati, Ohio

I. Introduction

Surfactant proteins (SP) A, B, and C play an integral part in the organization, function, and metabolism of surfactant phospholipids that reduce surface tension at the air-liquid interface in the alveolus of the lung. Purification of the proteins associated with the surfactant complex and molecular cloning of the genes encoding them has now provided the reagents, including antibodies and cDNA probes, that have been highly useful in extending our knowledge of surfactant biology. Exogenous surfactant replacement is now standard in the treatment of respiratory distress syndrome (RDS) in neonates (see Chapters 19 and 20), and it is presently being tested for treatment of adult respiratory distress syndrome (ARDS) (see Chapter 28). Since nonhuman surfactant proteins are present in some of the surfactant preparations in clinical use, therapy may be associated with exposure to foreign antigens that may be immunogenic. This chapter describes some of the antigenic properties of SP-A, SP-B, and SP-C and their precursors. We will review biochemical, physiological, and clinical studies that have addressed the potential risks of antisurfactant protein antibodies in the clinical setting.

II. Antigenicity of Surfactant Proteins

A. SP-A

SP-A was first recognized as a lung-specific antigen comprising a group of related proteins migrating with Mr = 26,000–36,000 in the presence of a sulfhydryl-reducing agent. Peptide mapping, sequencing, and molecular cloning studies ultimately defined the primary structure of SP-A as a variably glycosylated polypeptide consisting of discrete domains that include an amphipathic-helical, an aminoterminal collagen-like region, and a globular, carboxylterminal domain that contains asparagine-linked oligosaccharide (1,2). There are two closely related SP-A genes in the human genome that encode SP-A I and SP-A II polypeptides (3,4). SP-A molecules oligomerize to form octodecamers that are associated by intermolecular sulfhydryl bonds and noncovalent intermolecular interactions (5,6). SP-A has close structural relationships to other peptides within a family of calcium-dependent lectins that include surfactant protein D (SP-D), the mannose-binding protein, and other collectins (7,8). SP-A is also subject to extensive posttranscriptional modifications, including sulfation, acetylation, hydroxylation (of proline residues), and glycosylation, with the latter consisting of both O-linked and asparagine-linked carbohydrates (2). These domains comprise distinct antigenic epitopes, and it is not surprising that some of these are highly antigenic (Fig. 1). A number of highly useful antibodies and antisera have been generated against SP-A from a variety of species. Since surfactant proteins accumulate in the lungs of patients with alveolar proteinosis, numerous laboratories have prepared antibodies against SP-A purified from alveolar lavage material from these patients.

SP-A is relatively antigenic and both polyclonal and monoclonal antibodies can be readily produced in animals. In our laboratory, antibodies or antisera have been produced against canine, human, rat, rabbit, and cow SP-A that recognize epitopes derived from both carbohydrate and polypeptide determinants. These reagents have been used for immunohistochemistry, immunocytochemistry, cDNA cloning, ELISA, immunoprecipitation, Western blot analysis, and functional assays.

Polypeptide Epitopes of SP-A

Polyclonal and monoclonal antibodies have been produced against the SP-A polypeptide that recognize both the aminoterminal (collagenous) and carboxylterminal (lectin-like) domains. Some of these reagents are also selective for oligomerized as opposed to monomeric SP-A, as assessed by Western blot analyses (9). Antibodies against SP-A cross react with type IV collagen, supporting the concept that the collagenous region offers a significant antigenic epitope (10); the collagenous domain is predicted to be relatively immunogenic

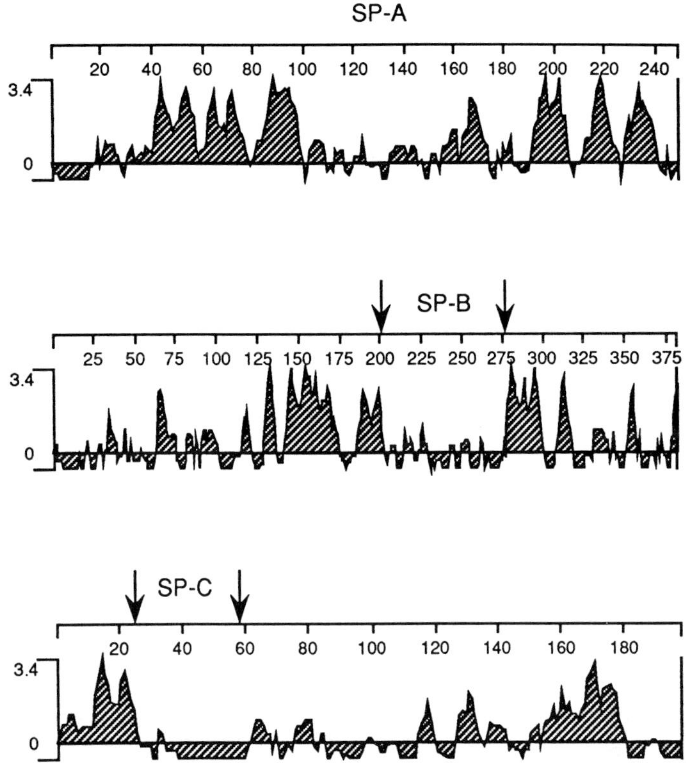

Figure 1 Surfactant protein antigenic indices. Potential antigenic determinants of surfactant proteins were predicted using an algorithm described by Jameson and Wolf (11). The algorithm incorporates hydrophilicity values, surface probabilities, chain flexibility, and secondary structure predictions to generate an antigenic index for a given polypeptide. The position of mature SP-B and SP-C peptides within their respective precursor proteins is marked by arrows.

on the basis of the antigenic index of Jameson and Wolf (11) (Fig. 1). It has also been possible to produce antibodies against the carboxylterminus of SP-A, as demonstrated by their reactivity against the Mr = 18–22 proteins remaining after collagenase digestion (9). Most polyclonal antibodies react with the primary translation products generated by in vitro translation of SP-A mRNA, demonstrating that these antibodies react against epitopes that are not dependent on posttranslational modification. Antibodies against the carboxylterminus of SP-A block lipid aggregation in the presence of calcium and block the inhibitory effects of SP-A on type II cell phospholipid secretion in vitro, supporting the importance of the carboxylterminal domain in signal transduction and in binding to type II epithelial cells (6,12,13). Deglycosylation of SP-A results in a protein which still inhibits phospholipid secretion by type II cells (6); however, the deglycosylated protein has a decreased ability to aggregate phospholipids in the presence of calcium (14), supporting the concept that the carbohydrate-dependent interactions play a role in the intermolecular organization of SP-A molecules. Antibodies against deglycosylated SP-A selectively stain epithelial cells within the respiratory tract, including serous cells in tracheobronchial glands, some bronchiolar cells, and alveolar type II cells (15). These antisera fail to stain nonpulmonary cells in human tissues either in fetal or postnatal specimens. Taken together, these studies demonstrate the presence of SP-A in cells of the proximal and distal respiratory epithelium. Present data demonstrate that SP-A expression is confined to the lung, although it remains possible SP-A may be present in other tissues at levels below the detectability of the present antisera or RNA probes.

Carbohydrate-Dependent Epitopes

Complex carbohydrate represents nearly one third of the mass of SP-A and consists of at least two distinct epitopes present in human SP-A (9,16–18) (Fig. 2). In our laboratory, we noted that polyclonal antisera and a number of monoclonal antibodies produced against highly purified human SP-A reacted strongly with epithelial cells in a variety of tissues, including salivary gland, pancreas, mammary glands, and the gastrointestinal tract in distribution similar to that of blood group antigenic determinants (9). A similar pattern of reactivity was seen in rat tissues with antirat SP-A antibodies. In human patients, these antibodies stain blood group A but not blood group O or B tissues as assessed by immunohistochemistry. Antihuman SP-A antibodies clumped blood group A cells and reacted strongly with glycosylated, but not with deglycosylated, SP-A, which is consistent with reactivity against blood group antigenic epitopes. Two distinct carbohydrate-dependent epitopes were subsequently mapped on human SP-A (9). Cleavage of the N-linked oligosaccharide from the carboxylterminal region of the human SP-A molecule removed the site on ^{187}Asn. A distinct antigenic epitope was not removed by endoglycosidase F treatment but was entirely removed by β-elimination which removes O-linked carbohydrate. Blood group A antigenic determinants in SP-A were strongly antigenic and required extensive absorption of the antisera with blood group A red cells or tissues to create an antisera that was selective for the polypeptide domains of SP-A. Polyclonal antisera against polypeptide was produced against endoglycosidase F, β-eliminated SP-A, with subsequent loss of reactivity against blood group A erythrocytes or blood group A antigenic sites in other epithelial tissues, as assessed by immunohistochemistry (9). The presence of strong blood group A–dependent antigenic sites presents important analytic issues in assessing

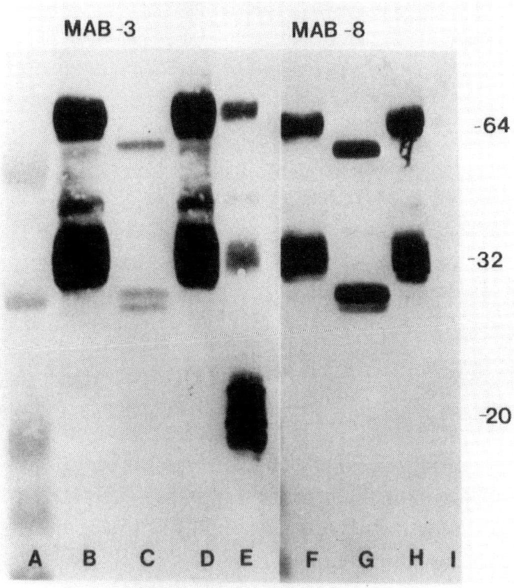

Figure 2 Human SP-A contains two distinct blood group A–dependent epitopes. Purified SP-A from a blood group A individual with alveolar proteinosis was separated by SDS-polyacrylamide gel electrophoresis and transferred to nitrocellulose for immunoblot reactions with murine monoclonal antibody (MAb). Approximate molecular weight ($\times 10^{-3}$) is indicated to the right of the figure. Lanes contain standard markers (lane a), SP-A (control) in endoglycosidase-F buffer (lanes b and f), endoglycosidase-F–treated SP-A (lanes c and g), SP-A (control) in collagenase buffers (lanes d and h), and collagenase-treated SP-A (lanes e and i). The proteins were reacted with MAb-3 (lanes a–e) or MAb-8 (lanes f–i). Both antibodies react with blood group A–dependent carbohydrates located in distinct portions of the SP-A molecule. MAb-3 reacts with asparagine-linked carbohydrate, removed by endoglycosidase-F, and present in the collagenase-resistant fragment (20 kDa). The MAb-8–binding site is removed in collagenase digestion demonstrating its presence on the NH_2-terminal collagenous domain of SP-A. Binding of MAb-8 to the NH_2-terminal peptide was resistant to endoglycosidase-F but sensitive to β-elimination, supporting the presence of and O-linked carbohydrate–dependent epitope.

anti–SP-A antibodies or antibody complexes that might circulate in patients with lung disease or after therapy with surfactant replacement preparation. Since isoimmune antibodies against blood group A are strongly reactive with human SP-A (9), it is not surprising that many individuals will bear antibodies against SP-A. Likewise, the interpretation of the localization of SP-A, as assessed by immunohistochemistry in other tissues, is complicated by the presence of potentially cross-reactive carbohydrate-dependent antigenic epitopes that are present in high concentrations in epithelial cells in a variety of organs. It is notable that human, rat, cow, sheep, and a variety of other mammalian species express blood group A antigens that may confound analyses utilizing SP-A antibodies.

Distribution of SP-A as Assessed by Immunohistochemistry and In Situ Hybridization

SP-A has been demonstrated in both bronchiolar and alveolar epithelium by both immunohistochemistry and in situ hybridization analyses in a variety of species. In the human, SP-A is present in high concentration in distinct cells of serous portions of tracheobronchial submucosal glands, as well as in discrete cells of the bronchiolar and alveolar epithelium (15). In the alveolar epithelium, SP-A is concentrated in type II cells, and it has been detected both in intracellular membranous organelles such as the rough endoplasmic reticulum and Golgi network and in association with lamellar bodies (19–21). Extracellular SP-A can be readily detected in the alveolar space associated with tubular myelin complex and closely associated with the cell surface (22,23). The distribution of SP-A in the respiratory tract is identical to that of SP-A mRNA as assessed by in situ hybridization analysis (15). As mentioned above, SP-A has not been found in tissues other than the respiratory tract, although it remains possible that SP-A may be present in tissues at levels below detectability by available reagents for in situ hybridization and immunohistochemistry.

B. SP-B

Human SP-B is synthesized by the alveolar type II cell as a preproprotein of 381 amino acids (2). The biophysically active mature peptide (residues 201–279) is generated by proteolytic processing of the SP-B precursor within the secretory pathway. Biochemical and morphological studies suggest that the multivesicular body is the site of processing and that the lamellar body contains only the mature form of SP-B (19,24,25). Therefore, under normal physiological conditions, it is likely that only mature SP-B is secreted with surfactant phospholipids into the airway. Although studies with primary cultures of type II cells suggest that the SP-B proprotein may also be constitutively secreted, the precursor form of SP-B is not detectable in alveolar lavage fluid (25). These results suggest that in vivo the SP-B proprotein is either not secreted or is rapidly processed to the mature peptide following release; in either event, the only detectable extracellular form of SP-B is the mature peptide and this is the only form present in surfactant replacement mixtures derived from animal lung extracts. The issue of whether multiple forms of SP-B are secreted under pathophysiological conditions remains unresolved.

Antigenic indices for the aminoterminal propeptide (residues 24–200) and the carboxylterminal peptide (residues 280–381) of the SP-B precursor indicate that these regions are likely to be immunogenic (Fig. 1). In keeping with this prediction, high titer polyclonal antibodies have been generated against full-length recombinant human SP-B proprotein, as well as the recombinant N- and C-terminal peptides (26). In contrast to the flanking peptides, the mature SP-B peptide (residues 201–279) is very hydrophobic and has a correspondingly low surface probability plot predicting low antigenicity. Despite an overall negative antigenic index, polyclonal antisera have been generated against native, mature SP-B and synthetic SP-B peptides, and monoclonal antibodies have been generated against the native peptide in several laboratories (27–31). Collectively, the results of these studies underscore the potential for immunological complications arising from airway instillation of surfactant replacement mixtures containing bovine or porcine SP-B.

C. SP-C

Human SP-C is synthesized by the alveolar type II cell as proprotein of 191 or 197 amino acids, depending on which alternatively spliced RNA is translated (2). As for the SP-B precursor protein, the biophysically active mature SP-C peptide (residues 24–58) is generated by proteolytic processing within the secretory pathway (32); however, unlike SP-B, very little is known about the kinetics of SP-C processing. Although the SP-C proprotein does not contain an NH_2-terminal signal peptide, there is evidence that the hydrophobic mature peptide mediates translocation into the endoplasmic reticulum resulting in an integral membrane protein (33,34). The SP-C proprotein is detected in multivesicular bodies but not in lamellar bodies, which is consistent with processing in the former compartment (32,35), whereas the mature peptide is detected in the lamellar body. It is, therefore, likely that mature SP-C is secreted with mature SP-B and surfactant phospholipids into the airway; it is not clear if the processed aminoterminal propeptide (residues 1–23) and the carboxylterminal peptide (residues 59–191/197) are secreted. A very recent study of infants born without any detectable SP-B (36) identified an aberrantly processed form of secreted SP-C containing a portion of the amino- and/or carboxylterminal peptide in amniotic fluid; therefore, under certain pathophysiological conditions, multiple forms of SP-C may be released into the airway (37). However, under normal physiological conditions, the mature peptide is the only form of SP-C associated with surfactant phospholipids and this is the only form present in surfactant replacement mixture derived from animal lung extracts.

The antigenic index for the SP-C proprotein indicates regions of potential antigenicity in the amino- and carboxylterminal peptides of the SP-C proprotein (Fig. 1). Antibodies have been successfully generated against these domains using either recombinant fusion proteins or synthetic peptides as antigens (33,38).

In contrast to these peptides, the mature SP-C peptide is a very poor immunogen. Although low-titer polyclonal antisera have been generated against mixtures of mature SP-B and SP-C peptides, a monospecific SP-C antiserum has not yet been described despite extensive efforts to develop this reagent (29). There is a single report of monoclonal SP-C antibody, but the specificity of this antiserum has not been confirmed (39). Given the low antigenicity of mature, native SP-C, the risk of immunological complications arising from SP-C containing surfactant replacement mixtures would appear to be minimal.

III. Clinical Relevance of Surfactant Antibodies

Ventilation of the surfactant-deficient lung leads to lesions in the distal respiratory epithelium resulting in increased epithelial permeability and flux of proteins into and out of the alveolus (40–42). The potential for circulating surfactant proteins raises the possibility of immunological consequences arising from the formation of antigen-antibody complexes. Surfactant protein antibodies have been shown to inhibit the biophysical activity of surfactant preparations in vitro (31,43,44), and direct instillation of SP-B monoclonal antibody into the airways of near-term newborn rabbits resulted in severe RDS (45). The finding that monoclonal antibodies generated against porcine surfactant protein B (the active peptide) caused respiratory failure after passive transfer to mice clearly demonstrated the potential toxicity of antisurfactant antibodies in vivo (46,47). Since exogenous surfactant preparations derived from bovine and porcine sources contain SP-B and SP-C, foreign antigens may be provided in the surfactant replacement regimens that have been widely used for the treatment of respiratory distress. The presence of endogenous antibodies against surfactant proteins as well as the possibility that antibodies might be produced in patients after surfactant replacement therapy raised important issues regarding the safety of such therapies.

There are a paucity of clinical studies that assess the presence of surfactant proteins or antisurfactant protein antibodies. Initial studies assessed the possibility that antibodies may be generated against whole human surfactant that was administered for therapy of RDS (48). Surfactant in these studies was obtained from pooled amniotic fluid from infants at birth and likely contained SP-A, SP-B, and SP-C, as well as smaller amounts of contaminating non–surfactant-associated proteins. Such surfactant was utilized for therapy in a limited number of patients and demonstrated its potential clinical utility in treatment of RDS in neonates (49). Strayer et al. (48) described potential antibodies against human surfactant proteins in serum from premature infants. These investigators detected antibodies in approximately one third of the patients in their study, irrespective of their treatment with exogenous human surfactant. The investigators utilized an ELISA assay in which the plates were coated with crude surfactant as the plating antigen.

Unfortunately, the interpretation of these studies is complicated by the high level of SP-A in the surfactant used as the primary antigen and the presence of the strong blood group A determinants now known to be present on the carbohydrate moieties of the human SP-A. Since the ELISA described by Strayer et al. (48) would likely detect both protein and blood group A antigenic epitopes, it is not surprising that "surfactant" antibodies were detected in a large number of infants.

The presence of anti–SP-B and SP-C antibodies were assessed in sera from patients enrolled in the clinical trials for both Survanta and for Calf Lung Surfactant Extract (CLSE). Both preparations contain bovine SP-B and SP-C (50), as well as phospholipids, but contain no detectable SP-A. Chida (51) reported the presence of antisurfactant protein antibodies in a number of premature infants but found no difference in the titer of the antibodies in the infants who received exogenous surfactant replacement as compared with placebo. In this study, antibodies were assessed in ELISA using bovine lung extracts as the plating antigen. Although interaction between the infant serum and the surfactant preparation were noted, the studies were likely complicated by the potential nonspecific association between immunoglobulins and the uniquely hydrophobic surfactant proteins utilized in the plating assay. In similar assays in our own laboratory, we demonstrated nonspecific binding of immunoglobulins to the hydrophobic surfactant proteins contained within the bovine lung or surfactant extracts and found reactivity in such assays with serum from normal individuals and newborn infants. Because of these analytical difficulties, we utilized a Western blot analysis to detect antibodies specific to SP-B or SP-C (52). Since the proteins (SP-B and SP-C) are separated from the lung lipids on the nitrocelluose support, nonspecific absorption of immunoglobulins were minimized. The specificity of the antibody against SP-B and SP-C could be readily determined by electrophoretic separation of the antigens, under reduced and unreduced conditions, wherein bovine SP-B migrates at 8700 reduced and 18,000–36,000 unreduced, and SP-C migrates at 3500 and 7000, respectively. Under these assay conditions, reactivity of rabbit polyclonal antisera against SP-B and SP-C was readily visualized (29). We were unable to identify antibodies in sera from more than 2000 premature infants treated with Survanta (52). In a more limited number of patients, we were unable to detect antibodies against SP-B or SP-C in the serum of premature infants who were treated with CLSE (J. A. Whitsett et al., unpublished observations). The lack of detectable antibody against the hydrophobic surfactant proteins SP-B and SP-C after surfactant replacement therapy for RDS is likely related to the relative conservation of amino acid sequence of the low molecular weight hydrophobic surfactant proteins, the low levels of protein in the extracts, the short duration of treatment, or intratracheal route of exposure. As seen in Fig. 1, the active peptides comprising SP-B and SP-C are predicted to be relatively weak antigens. The relatively weak antigenicity of these sites and the high amount of lipid associated with the proteins may also reduce the antigenic determinants exposed to the immune system. At present, there is no evidence that significant antigenic risks are associated with surfactant replacement therapy in neonates. The relative paucity of antigenic sites, the small amounts of surfactant proteins given in the preparation, the short duration of therapy, the relative immaturity of the immune system of premature infants, and limitations in the sensitivity of the assays may also have contributed to the failure to detect circulating antibodies against the SP-B and SP-C present in Survanta or CLSE.

SP-A and SP-A antibodies were also described in a series of adult patients with alveolar proteinosis and idiopathic pulmonary fibrosis using an ELISA assay. Kuroki et al. (53) demonstrated the activity of antisera against proteins in the serum of these patients; however, the size of the proteins reacting with the SP-A antibodies was distinct from SP-A, suggesting that the antibodies may react with antigenic sites shared between SP-A and the serum proteins (9). Thus, although an intriguing concept, there is no clear evidence of antibodies or circulating SP-A in these patients, and the concept that antibodies or circulating immune complexes may contribute to disease remains to be more fully elucidated.

IV. Conclusions

Antibodies have been generated against SP-A, SP-B, and SP-C in laboratory animals that react with both polypeptide or carbohydrate domains of these molecules or their precursors. In vivo, antibodies generated against the active SP-B polypeptide cause severe lung injury, pulmonary edema, and respiratory failure, which raises the possibility that antibodies against surfactant proteins may play a role in the pathogenesis of lung disease or injury. Although preliminary studies suggest the possible presence of either SP-A or other surfactant protein antibodies in patients with RDS irrespective of their treatment with exogenous surfactant, analytical problems related to the specificity of the antigenic determinants of surfactant components, and particularly the cross reactivity of SP-A with blood group A–dependent epitopes, raises questions regarding the presence of specific antisurfactant protein antibodies in patients with RDS. Likewise, the insolubility of SP-B and SP-C and their nonspecific interactions with immunoglobulins may have contributed to the detection of immune complexes or circulating antibodies in clinical studies. At present, there is no clear evidence that antisurfactant protein antibodies are generated after therapy or contribute to lung disease in neonatal RDS or adults with lung disease. The hypothesis that antisurfactant protein antibodies may contribute to the pathogenesis of either acute or chronic lung disease remains an intriguing question that merits further investigation as the analytic tools and reagents required for careful assessment of antisurfactant antibodies and immune complexes are refined.

References

1. Hawgood S, Shiffer K. Structures and properties of the surfactant-associated proteins. Annu Rev Physiol 1991; 53:375–394.
2. Weaver TE, Whitsett JA. Function and regulation of expression of pulmonary surfactant-associated proteins. Biochem J 1991; 273:249–264.
3. White RT, Damm D, Miller J, et al. Isolation and characterization of the human pulmonary surfactant apoprotein gene. Nature 1985; 317:361–363.
4. Katyal SL, Singh G, Locker J. Characterization of a second human pulmonary surfactant-associated protein SP-A gene. Am J Respir Cell Mol Biol 1992; 6:446–452.
5. Voss T, Eistetter H, Schäfer KP. Macromolecular organization of natural and recombinant lung surfactant protein SP 28-36: Structural homology with the complement factor C1q. J Mol Biol 1988; 201:219–227.
6. Kuroki Y, Mason RJ, Voelker DR. Pulmonary surfactant apoprotein A structure and modulation of surfactant secretion by rat alveolar type II cells. J Biol Chem 1988; 263:3388–3394.
7. Drickamer K, Dordal MS, Reynolds L. Mannose-binding proteins isolated from rat liver contain carbohydrate-recognition domains linked to collagenous tails. J Biol Chem 1986; 261:6878–6887.
8. Haurum JS, Thiel S, Haagsman HP, et al. Studies on the carbohydrate-binding characteristics of human pulmonary surfactant-associated protein-A and comparison with two other collectins—mannan-binding protein and conglutinin. Biochem J 1993; 293:873–878.
9. Stahlman MT, Gray ME, Ross GF, et al. Human surfactant protein-A contains blood group-A antigenic determinants. Pediatr Res 1992; 31:364–371.
10. Coulombe PA, Bendayan M. Lung surfactant-associated proteins and type IV collagen share common epitopes. Am Rev Respir Dis 1989; 140:1040–1044.
11. Jameson BA, Wolf H. The antigenic index: a novel algorithm for predicting antigenic determinants. Comput Appl Biosci 1988; 4:181–186.
12. Rice WR, Ross GF, Singleton FM, et al. Surfactant-associated protein inhibits phospholipid secretion from type II cells. J Appl Physiol 1987; 63:692–698.
13. Dobbs LG, Wright JR, Hawgood S, et al. Pulmonary surfactant and its components inhibit secretion of phosphatidylcholine from cultured rat alveolar type II cells. Proc Natl Acad Sci USA 1987; 84:1010–1014.
14. Haagsman HP, Elfring RH, Vanbuel BLM, Voorhout WF. The lung lectin surfactant protein-A aggregates phospholipid vesicles via a novel mechanism. Biochem J 1991; 275:273–276.
15. Khoor A, Gray ME, Hull WM, et al. Developmental expression of SP-A and SP-A mRNA in the proximal and distal respiratory epithelium in the human fetus and newborn. J Histochem Cytochem 1993; 9:1311–1319.

16. Weaver TE, Ross G, Daugherty C, Whitsett JA. Synthesis of surfactant-associated protein, 35,000, in fetal lung. J Appl Physiol 1986; 61:694–700.
17. Whitsett JA, Hull W, Ross G, Weaver T. Characteristics of human surfactant-associated glycoproteins A. Pediatr Res 1985; 19:501–508.
18. Phelps DS, Floros J, Taeusch HWJ. Post-translational modification of the major human surfactant-associated proteins. Biochem J 1986; 237:373–377.
19. Voorhout WF, Veenendaal T, Haagsman HP, et al. Intracellular processing of pulmonary surfactant protein-B in an endosomal/lysosomal compartment. Am J Physiol 1992; 263:L479–L486.
20. Williams MC, Hawgood S, Schenk DB, et al. Monoclonal antibodies to surfactant proteins SP28–36 label canine type II and nonciliated bronchiolar cells by immunofluorescence. Am Rev Respir Dis 1988; 137:399–405.
21. Walker SR, Williams MC, Benson B. Immunocytochemical localization of the major surfactant apoproteins in type II cells, Clara cells, and alveolar macrophages of rat lung. J Histochem Cytochem 1986; 34:1137–1148.
22. Voorhout WF, Veenendaal T, Haagsman HP, et al. Surfactant protein A is localized at the corners of the pulmonary tubular myelin lattice. J Histochem Cytochem 1991; 39:1331–1336.
23. Ryan RM, Morris RE, Rice WR, et al. Binding and uptake of pulmonary surfactant protein (SP-A) by pulmonary type II epithelial cells. J Histochem Cytochem 1989; 37:429–440.
24. Weaver TE, Lin S, Bogucki B, Dey C. Processing of surfactant protein-B proprotein by a cathepsin-D–like protease. Am J Physiol 1992; 263:L95–L103.
25. Weaver TE, Whitsett JA. Processing of hydrophobic pulmonary surfactant protein B in rat type II cells. Am J Physiol 1989; 257:L100–L108.
26. O'Reilly MA, Weaver TE, Pilot-Matias TJ, et al. In vitro translation, post-translational processing and secretion of pulmonary surfactant protein B precursors. Biochim Biophys Acta 1989; 1011:140–148.
27. Hawgood S, Latham D, Borchelt J, et al. Cell-specific posttranslational processing of the surfactant-associated protein SP-B. Am J Physiol 1993; 264:L290–L299.
28. Fan BR, Bruni R, Taeusch HW, et al. Antibodies against synthetic amphipathic helical sequences of surfactant protein–SP-B detect a conformational change in the native protein. FEBS Lett 1991; 282:220–224.
29. Whitsett JA, Hull WM, Ohning B, et al. Immunologic identification of a pulmonary surfactant-associated protein of molecular weight = 6000 daltons. Pediatr Res 1986; 20:744–749.
30. Suzuki Y, Kogishi K, Fujita Y, et al. A monoclonal antibody to the 15,000 dalton protein associated with porcine pulmonary surfactant. Exp Lung Res 1986; 11:61–73.
31. Strayer DS, Merritt TA, Makunike C, Hallman M. Antigenicity of low molecular weight surfactant species. Am J Pathol 1989; 134:723–732.
32. Voorhout WF, Weaver TE, Haagsman HP, et al. Biosynthetic routing of pulmonary surfactant proteins in alveolar type II cells. Microsc Res Tech 1993; 26:366–373.
33. Vorbroker DK, Dey C, Weaver TE, Whitsett JA. Surfactant protein-C precursor is palmitoylated and associates with subcellular membranes. Biochim Biophys Acta 1992; 1105:161–169.

34. Keller A, Eistetter HR, Voss T, Schäfer KP. The pulmonary surfactant protein-C (SP-C) precursor is a type-II transmembrane protein. Biochem J 1991; 277:493–499.
35. Farrell PM, Bourbon JR, Notter RH, et al. Relationships among surfactant fraction lipids, proteins and biophysical properties in the developing rat lung. Biochim Biophys Acta 1990; 1044:84–90.
36. Nogee LM, DeMello DE, Dehner LP, Colten HR. Deficiency of pulmonary surfactant protein B in congenital alveolar proteinosis. N Engl J Med 1993; 328:406–410.
37. Vorbroker DK, Nogee LM, Whitsett JA. Aberrant processing of surfactant protein C in hereditary surfactant protein B deficiency. Am J Physiol. In press.
38. Beers MF, Wali A, Eckenhoff MF, et al. An antibody with specificity for surfactant protein C precursors: Identification of pro-SP-C in rat lung. Am J Respir Cell Mol Biol 1992; 7:368–378.
39. Oetomo SB, deLey L, Curstedt T, et al. Distribution of endotracheally instilled surfactant protein SP-C in lung-lavaged rabbits. Pediatr Res 1991; 29:178–181.
40. Grossman G, Nilsson R, Robertson B. Scanning electron microscopy of epithelial lesions induced by artificial ventilation of the immature neonatal lung; the prophylactic effect of surfactant replacement. Eur J Pediatr 1986; 145:361–367.
41. Jobe A, Ikegami M, Jacobs H, et al. Permeability of premature lamb lungs to protein and the effect of surfactant on that permeability. J Appl Physiol 1983; 55:169–176.
42. Jeffries AL, Coates G, O'Brodovich H. Pulmonary epithelial permeability in hyaline membrane disease. N Engl J Med 1984; 311:1075–1080.
43. Kobayashi T, Nitta K, Takahashi R, et al. Activity of pulmonary surfactant after blocking the associated proteins SP-A and SP-B. J Appl Physiol 1991; 71:530–536.
44. Strayer DS, Hallman M, Merritt TA. Immunogenicity of surfactant. 2. Porcine and bovine surfactants. Clin Exp Immunol 1991; 83:41–46.
45. Robertson B, Kobayashi T, Ganzuka M, et al. Experimental neonatal respiratory failure induced by a monoclonal antibody to the hydrophobic surfactant-associated protein SP-B. Pediatr Res 1991; 30:239–243.
46. Suzuki Y, Robertson B, Fujita Y, Grossmann G. Respiratory failure in mice caused by a hybridoma making antibodies to the 15 kDa surfactant apoprotein. Acta Anaesthesiol Scand 1988; 32:283–289.
47. Fujita Y, Kogishi K, Suzuki Y. Pulmonary damage induced in mice by a monoclonal antibody to proteins associated with pig pulmonary surfactant. Exp Lung Res 1988; 14:247–260.
48. Strayer DS, Merritt TA, Lwebuga-Mukasa J, Hallman M. Surfactant-anti-surfactant immune complexes in infants with respiratory distress syndrome. Am J Pathol 1986; 122:353–362.
49. Hallman M, Merritt A, Schneider H, et al. Isolation of human surfactant from amniotic fluid and a pilot study of its efficacy in respiratory distress syndrome. Pediatrics 1983; 71:473–482.
50. Whitsett JA, Ohning BL, Ross G, et al. Hydrophobic surfactant-associated protein in whole lung surfactant and its importance for biophysical activity in lung surfactant extracts used for replacement therapy. Pediatr Res 1986; 20:460–467.
51. Chida S, Phelps DS, Soll RF, Taeusch HW. Surfactant proteins and antisurfactant

antibodies in sera from infants with respiratory distress syndrome with and without surfactant treatment. Pediatrics 1991; 88:84–89.

52. Whitsett JA, Hull WM, Luse S. Failure to detect surfactant protein-specific antibodies in sera of premature infants treated with Survanta, a modified bovine surfactant. Pediatrics 1991; 87:505–510.
53. Kuroki Y, Tsutahara S, Shijubo N, et al. Elevated levels of lung surfactant protein-A in sera from patients with idiopathic pulmonary fibrosis and pulmonary alveolar proteinosis. Am Rev Respir Dis 1993; 147:723–729.

Part Four

CLINICAL USE OF SURFACTANT FOR PREVENTION AND TREATMENT OF LUNG DISEASE

15

Techniques for Administering Surfactant

ALAN H. JOBE
Harbor–UCLA Medical Center
University of California, Los Angeles, School of Medicine
Los Angeles, California

I. Introduction

The instillation techniques presently used effectively to treat respiratory distress syndrome (RDS) were selected empirically based on the techniques used to treat preterm animal models of RDS (1). Two treatment strategies have been tested and approved for infants at risk for or with RDS (2). Surfactant can be given in the delivery room as soon as possible following delivery and intubation as a single bolus into the endotracheal tube followed by mechanical ventilation to infants at risk of developing RDS (3). For infants with RDS, surfactant is given by a variety of bolus injection schemes that include positioning the chest of the infant in an effort to optimize distribution. These treatment procedures were ritualized for the purposes of clinical trials of each of the surfactants such that each surfactant in currant use is given by a somewhat different technique (4–6). However, the essence of the treatment technique for infants with RDS is the instillation of boluses of surfactant into the proximal or distal trachea with positioning of the chest. The only clinical trial comparing treatment techniques found that there are no differences in the short-term efficacy if the surfactant dose was divided into two or four aliquots for administration or if two or four chest-positioning maneuvers were used (6). Although treatment techniques were not developed systematically, the different techniques are probably very similar in net result in terms of efficacy of treatment to decrease the incidence of air leak and death from RDS (2). Nevertheless, many clinicians are not satisfied with the present treatment techniques, and they modify treatment methods. Part of the dissatisfaction results from the need to take the infant off the ventilator for the instillation procedure (Survanta and Curosurf) or the need to administer manually the surfactant with inspiration (Exosurf) (4–6). These procedures when combined with handling of the infant can result in cyanosis, bradycardia, and reflux of surfactant up the endotracheal tube (7,8). These transient physiological disturbances in most cases result from acute airway obstruction with the surfactant suspension fluid, with foam generated by the mixing of surfactant with gas in the airways, and from vagal reflex effects of the instillation and handling. Although the cyanosis and bradycardia can be disturbing, more concerning are the reports of changes in cerebral blood flow velocities and electrocortical depression following surfactant treatments (9–11). Although long-term adverse effects of the treatment procedures have not been documented, attempts to simplify and improve treatment techniques are justified.

II. The Goals of Treatment Techniques

The goals of surfactant therapy are to achieve short-term decreases in lung-related injury such as pulmonary interstitial emphysema and pneumothorax and to decrease long-term lung-related morbidity (bronchopulmonary dysplasia) and death (2). At the clinical level, the goals of treatment techniques are to get the surfactant into an infant's lungs with as little physiological disturbance as possible in a manner that will promote the achievement of the overall goals of surfactant treatment. This clinical treatment goal may conflict with the ultimate goal of an optimum pulmonary outcome without bronchopulmonary dysplasia. Although not based on experimental evidence, intuitively it would seem that at the level of the alveolus the primary goal of a treatment technique is to achieve as uniform a distribution of surfactant as possible. If distribution was perfectly uniform, then expansion of the lung should be uniform and result in normal alveolar expansion. The physiological result should be decreased oxygen and pressure needs (12). In contrast, if the distribution of surfactant was primarily to one lobe or one lung, then that lung volume would expand. If pressures were not decreased, that inflated lung would overexpand and potentially be injured (13). If the pressures were decreased, the untreated lung would lose whatever gas volume it was receiving and become more atelectatic. At the alveolar level, alveoli are interdependent in that if a group of alveoli collapse, the adjacent alveoli may overinflate and distort (14) (Fig. 1). The frequent occurrence of bronchopulmonary dysplasia following surfactant treatment may result in part from the

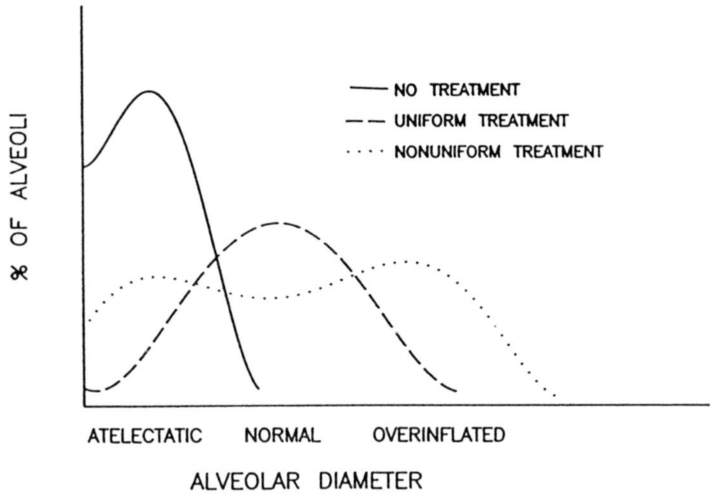

Figure 1 Idealized representation of alveolar size distributions. Alveoli in the surfactant-deficient lung would be atelectatic or very small unless very high ventilatory pressures are used. Following a uniformly distributed surfactant treatment, alveoli would expand uniformly to a larger mean diameter. If a surfactant treatment was not uniform, some alveoli would not expand, whereas others could overexpand with mechanical ventilation.

nonhomogeneous distribution of surfactant, resulting in focal injury as a result of nonuniform inflation of the lung.

III. Measurements of Surfactant Distribution

Measurements of the adequacy of surfactant distribution depend on the resolution of the evaluation. At the extremes, distribution can be evaluated at the lobar or the alveolar level. Unilateral surfactant instillations and unilateral chest film changes have been reported, almost certainly as a result of endotracheal tube placement in a mainstem bronchus (15). Surfactant does reach the alveolar level. The increase in lung volumes following surfactant treatment to approach those of a mature lung require alveolar expansion (14). If alveolar expansion did not occur, lung volumes could not become as large as they do after surfactant treatment. By similar logic, the rapid improvement in oxygenation in experimental models of RDS and in some infants to levels approaching that of a normal lung indicate alveolar deposition of surfactant (16). Robertson and Enhorning (17) mixed iron-dextran with surfactant and found the iron-dextran in the alveoli of preterm rabbits after pharyngeal deposition of the surfactant at birth. Subsequently, Obladen et al. (18) demonstrated by autoradiography that dipalmitoyl phosphatidylcholine instilled into the airways of adult rabbits was found in alveoli, and Geiger et al. (19) also found aerosolized surfactant lipid in alveoli and type II cells. Following airway instillation at birth in preterm rabbits, Winter et al. (20) found only 34% of the radiolabeled surfactant associated with alveoli and adjacent tissue. No other measurements of the efficiency of delivery of surfactant to the alveoli are available.

Most experimental studies of surfactant distribution have used radiolabeled surfactant components (primarily dipalmitoyl phosphatidylcholine) or other easily measured substances mixed with surfactant. The distribution of the material then has been measured by external scanning of radioactivity (21), autoradiograms of lung slices (22), or the content of the marked material in lung pieces of various sizes (23). Each technique has different strengths and weaknesses, giving only partial information about surfactant distribution. External scanning has low resolution because of the superposition of the entire thickness of the lungs. In the only attempt to measure distribution in infants, Charon et al. (21) mixed ^{99}Tc-sulfur colloid with surfactant and treated eight infants using a four-bolus, four-position treatment technique. They found relatively homogeneous distributions in all infants that did not correlate with clinical response. Subsequently, van der Bleck et al. (24) reported that microaggregated ^{99}Tc-albumin mixed with surfactant appeared to be uniformly distributed by external scanning of the lungs of saline-lavaged rabbits. However, when the lungs were divided into 200 pieces and distribution per price was measured, the distribution was not homogeneous. The technique of dividing the lungs into pieces and measuring the amount of surfactant or a marker that distributes with surfactant in each piece of lung has the advantage of being quantitative (23). However, the lung pieces do not provide information about alveolar distribution. For example, if the preterm human lung at 32 weeks' gestational age was cut into 200 pieces for a distribution measurement, each piece would contain about 200,000 alveoli (25). Therefore, even if distribution to lung pieces is homogeneous, significant inhomogeneities are almost inevitable at the alveolar level.

IV. Variables that Affect Surfactant Distribution

A. Surfactant Itself

Surfactant has the biophysical properties of adsorption to an air-fluid interface and rapid spreading over a surface. Therefore, it is logical to anticipate that surfactant will facilitate its own distribution by this spreading behavior. Davis et al. (26) used external scanning to measure the kinetics of surfactant or saline distribution to the lungs of saline-lavaged piglets following instillation of a single 3.3 ml/kg dose. They found that surfactant began to distribute within 5 sec of dosing, with substantial distribution to the five lung fields that were imaged within 20 sec. The distribution remained relatively uniform for the duration of the experiment. In contrast, saline did not distribute as rapidly and multiple filling defects were noted on the scans. These results demonstrate rapid spreading of surfactant with a more uniform ultimate distribution than for saline alone. However, the external scanning technique cannot resolve the homogeneity of distribution to small lung volumes (24). Kharasch et al. (22) compared surfactant and saline as carriers to spread pentamidine in the lungs of hamsters following airway instillation of 0.25 ml/kg volumes. After 4 hr of spontaneous ventilation, the lungs were removed, sliced, and autoradiograms were used to demonstrate distribution patterns. Surfactant resulted in 40% of the lung areas being labeled versus 21% for the saline-treated animals. These two studies demonstrate that surfactant facilitates its own distribution within the lungs. However, Oetomo et al. (27) treated single lobes of rabbit lungs with surfactant and found virtually no migration to other lobes after 10 hr of spontaneous ventilation. This result demonstrates that although surfactant can spread within a bronchial distribution, it does not spread between bronchi. Therefore, theoretically the most uniform distribution would be achieved if each bronchus at each branching level received surfactant in proportion to the surface area that the bronchus served. There have been no studies evaluating if distribution is dependent on the type of surfactant. However, surfactants containing the surfactant proteins SP-B and SP-C adsorb and spread more rapidly and thus might be anticipated to self-distribute better (28).

B. Age at Treatment

In preterm rabbits, lung injury occurs within minutes of the initiation of mechanical ventilation, and this injury can be prevented by surfactant treatments that cause a more uniform expansion of the lungs (29). Clinically, infants treated shortly after delivery seem to have better pulmonary outcomes than infants treated after a period of mechanical ventilation for RDS (30,31). In preterm lambs, mixing of surfactant with fetal lung fluid resulted in a more homogeneous distribution of surfactant than did a treatment after 23 min of mechanical ventilation (23) (Fig. 2). In the lambs treated after a period of ventilation, lung inflation correlated with quantity of surfactant recovered from the lung pieces. Based on visual inspection, lung pieces that were fully aerated contained 5.4 times more surfactant than did atelectatic pieces. Pulmonary blood flow was decreased to the pieces receiving the highest amounts of surfactant, suggesting overinflation in the situation where surfactant distribution was less uniform. In contrast, Heldt et al. (32) reported that surfactant distribution and compliance responses were not as good after treatment of preterm rabbits at birth than after 15 min of ventilation. This result may be dependent on the treatment technique or the differences resulting from treating the very small preterm rabbits.

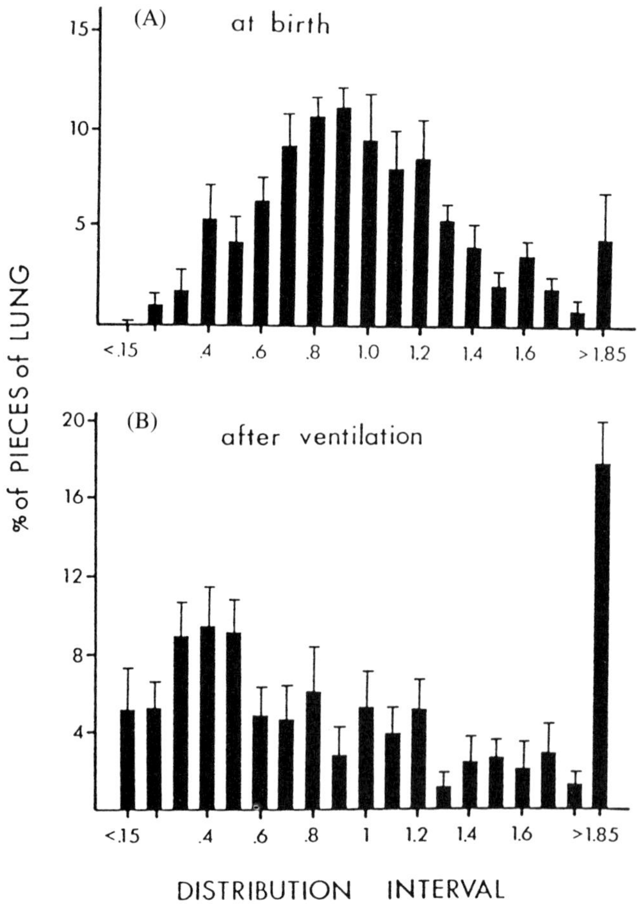

Figure 2 Distribution of surfactant to the lungs of preterm lambs at delivery and before ventilation (A) and after 23 min of mechanical ventilation (B). Preterm lambs were treated with 100 mg/kg radiolabeled natural sheep surfactant at birth or after mechanical ventilation. The lungs were then removed and cut into about 100 pieces each and the amount of surfactant per gram was measured for each piece. The mean amount of surfactant per gram was normalized to 1 and the distribution of the pieces about the mean were grouped in 10% intervals. Treatment at birth resulted in a more uniform distribution. (Redrawn from ref. 23; used with permission.)

C. Volume and Concentration of Surfactant

The surfactants used clinically are given as suspensions in volumes that range from 2.5 to 5.0 ml/kg. Intuitively, the larger the volume administered, the more likely multiple bronchi will be filled, and the better the distribution is likely to be. The problem is that large volumes are much more likely to cause airway obstruction, respiratory distress, cyanosis, and other undesirable side effects. The effects of volume and concentration of surfactant have been studied more thoroughly than other aspects of the treatment techniques. Gillard et al. (33) found that instillation of surfactant in 1.5 ml/kg saline into normal ventilated rabbits resulted in a very nonuniform distribution. Increasing surfactant concentration did not improve the distribution. The same amount of surfactant suspended in 15 ml/kg saline resulted in a quite homogeneous distribution. In contrast, with oleic acid–induced lung injury, the distribution was volume independent and reasonably uniform. This result was interpreted to mean that with severe lung injury, the alveoli are flooded and provide a fluid volume to facilitate surfactant distribution. Oetomo et al. (27) also found that the distribution of surfactant to the healthy lung was volume dependent. Using a single lung treatment technique in adult rabbits, about 4.5 ml/kg surfactant suspension gave a much less uniform lung distribution than did about 9 ml/kg. Similar observations were also made in the saline-lavaged rabbit model of RDS/lung injury by van der Bleek et al. (24). They found very poor distributions in unlavaged and lavaged rabbits when surfactant was instilled in volumes of 2.4 ml/kg. The distribution was only marginally improved when a suspension volume of 8 ml/kg was used. Distribution improved significantly when a suspension volume 16 ml/kg was instilled, and the distribution did not depend on surfactant concentration. These results are discouraging in relation to clinical practice, since volumes in excess of 10 ml may be required to improve distribution. The alveolar pulmonary edema associated with RDS (34) may decrease the volume by the same mechanism reported for oleic acid injury (33). However, large volumes are not realistic for clinical practice, and some nonhomogeneity of surfactant no doubt is an inevitable consequence of the present treatment techniques.

D. Time Interval for Surfactant Administration

If surfactant distribution is improved by increasing the treatment volume and the administration of large volumes over short treatment intervals results in respiratory complications, a logical approach on first impression would be to deliver surfactant to the lungs more slowly. Although this has not been tried with large volumes, a number of clinicians are administering the presently used volumes of 2.5 to 5.0 ml/kg over longer periods to avoid respiratory complications. This approach has been evaluated in two animal models of RDS. Segerer et al. (35) recently reported that 4 ml/kg of a surfactant suspension given as a bolus via the endotracheal tube in 10 sec to saline-lavaged rabbits resulted in a reasonably uniform distribution to the 50–70 lung pieces that were analyzed. In contrast, infusion of the same volume of surfactant over 45 min via a pressure-monitoring channel in an endotracheal tube resulted in an extremely nonhomogeneous distribution. The bolus-treated rabbits had a brisk and sustained response to surfactant, whereas the infused rabbits had no response. Ueda et al. (36) studied two techniques of bolus treatment and a slow infusion of surfactant in preterm lambs with RDS. One treatment technique delivered 25% of the 4 ml/kg dose of surfactant sequentially to the upper lobes and lower lobes together with the chest-positioning technique that is used clinically for Survanta (6). The second technique was to give half of the dose in the left lateral position and the other half in the right lateral position. The infusion-treated group received 2 ml/kg surfactant in the right lateral position over 15 min followed by 2 ml/kg in the left lateral position over 15 min. All three groups of lambs demonstrated improvements in Po_2 and lung mechanics, although the responses were not as large with surfactant infusion. The bolus treatments delivered surfactant quite uniformly to the different lobes of the sheep lung, whereas infusion resulted primarily in upper lobe localization (Fig. 3). The animals received a second treatment 2 hr after the initial treatment, and the second treatment localized to the same lung pieces that received the majority of the surfactant with the initial treatments. This result indicates that the first treatment will determine primarily which lung volumes will open, and the second treatment will tend to treat the same lung volumes that were initially treated. Pulmonary blood flow and distribution of ventilation also were measured. Blood flow was relatively uniform across the lung pieces of the bolus-treated animals. In contrast, blood flow decreased to the lung pieces that received the most surfactant by infusion. This result is consistent with overinflation of those lung regions receiving the most surfactant in circumstances where the overall distribution is nonuniform. The advantage of decreased acute respiratory symptoms using an infusion technique is counterbalanced by the very poor distribution of surfactant.

E. Style of Ventilation

Surfactant distributes to the lungs by bulk movement of the suspension down the airways and by spreading. The style of ventilation immediately following treatment could impact the distribution. In clinical practice conventional tidal volume ventilation is routinely used following surfactant treatments. Walther et al. (37) reported that surfactant instilled into the airways of preterm lambs distributed similarly with conventional or high-frequency ventilation. In contrast, Heldt et al. (32) found that high-frequency ventilation seemed to delay surfactant delivery to distal air spaces in preterm rabbits. Given this conflicting information,

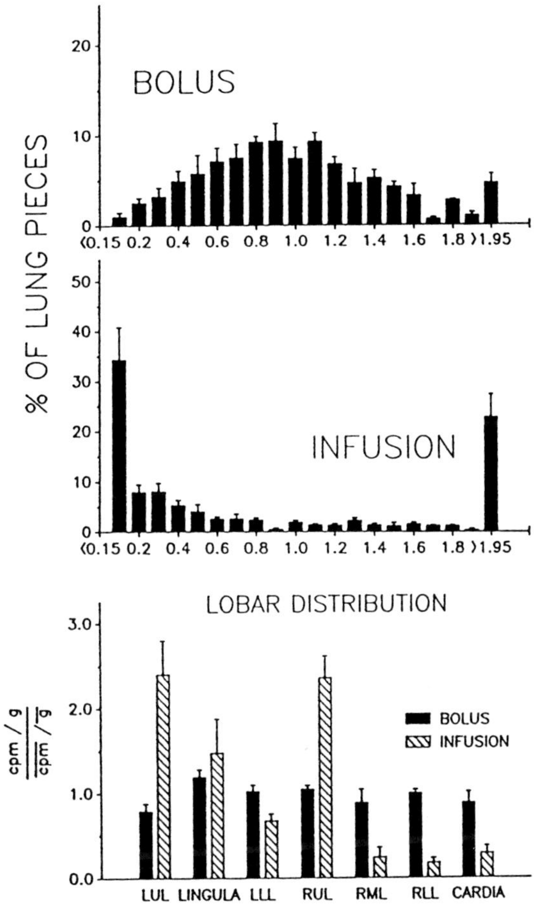

Figure 3 Mean distribution of surfactant by a bolus technique in comparison with a 30-min infusion to preterm ventilated lamb lungs. The 100 mg/kg bovine lung extract surfactant (Survanta®) was radiolabeled and the amount of surfactant recovered in lung pieces or by lobe was measured. Bolus treatment resulted in about 40% of the lung pieces containing within ±25% of the mean amount of surfactant. In contrast, infusion resulted in 7% of the pieces of lung receiving within ±25% of the mean. The majority of the infused surfactant was found in the upper lobes. (Redrawn from ref. 36; used with permission.)

new ventilation strategies must be assumed to potentially impact surfactant treatment techniques and distribution.

V. Aerosolized Surfactant

The initial clinical trials in the 1960s of the treatment of RDS with dipalmitoyl phosphatidylcholine as surfactant used aerosols and were inconclusive as to beneficial effects (38,39). The subsequent experimental demonstrations of surfactant treatment effects used pharyngeal or tracheal instillation techniques (1). Despite the effectiveness of surfactant instillation, aerosolized surfactant remains attractive because the variables of instillation technique, patient manipulation, and the deposition of a large volume of fluid in the lungs over a short period of time would be avoided. Shannon et al. (40) demonstrated that pressure-volume curves improved when dipalmitoyl phosphatidylcholine was aerosolized into excised dog lungs, although Ikegami et al. (41) reported that dipalmitoyl phosphatidylcholine or natural surfactant delivered via an ultrasonic space nebulizer had little effect on saline-lavaged rat lungs. Although Marks et al. (42) demonstrated in 1983 that surfactant could be aerosolized with preservation of surface activity, the efficacy of aerosolized surfactant has been tested only recently. Zelter et al. (43) found that aerosolized Exosurf had very little effect on acute oleic acid injury in sheep. In contrast, preterm lambs given aerosolized natural sheep surfactant or Survanta had improved compliances and pressure volume curves (44). In adult rabbits with lung injury induced with N-nitroso-N-methylurethane, aerosolized surfactant modestly improved lung function and was superior to instilled surfactant (45). Lewis et al. (46) also reported that aerosolized Survanta improved the respiratory function of saline-lavaged sheep relative to an untreated comparison group. The provocative result consistently reported by Lewis et al. (44–46) was that the responses noted in the different models occurred despite a lung parenchymal deposition of between 0.5 and 2.0 mg/kg surfactant. This dose is very small compared with the routine clinical dose of 100 mg/kg. The most likely explanation for the physiological responses despite the small dose delivered was that the aerosolized surfactant had a better distribution to the lung parenchyma than did the instilled surfactant (Fig. 4). In an adult respiratory distress syndrome (ARDS) model of oxygen toxicity in ventilated baboons, aerosolized Exosurf delayed the onset of respiratory deterioration and decreased shunt (47). These physiological effects were associated with a preservation of the alveolar epithelium (48). There have been a number of studies that demonstrated aerosolized surfactant can be effective.

A number of questions and problems remain to be evaluated. The small lung parenchymal doses achieved by Lewis et al. (44–46) result inevitably from the inefficiencies of aerosol delivery systems. Large particles will impact on the

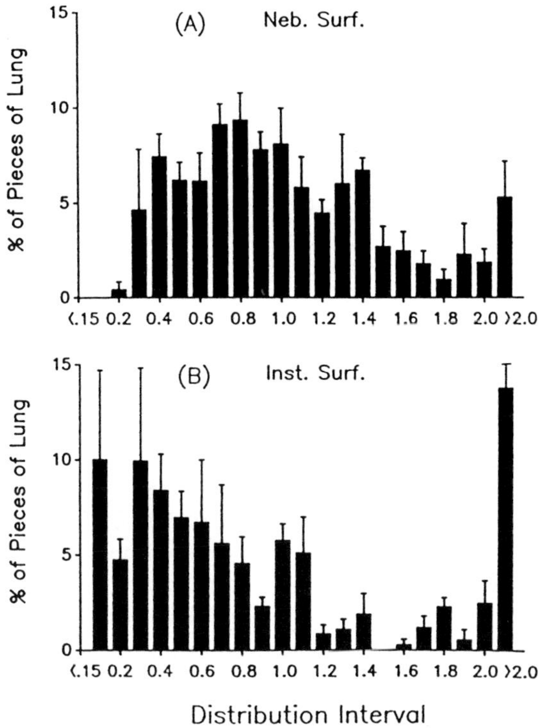

Figure 4 Distribution of radioactive nebulized surfactant and instilled surfactant to saline-lavaged adult sheep lungs. The aerosolized surfactant resulted in a more uniform distribution around the normalized mean value of 1 than did the instilled surfactant. (From ref. 46; used with permission.)

circuit and not clear the endotracheal tube, and very small particles will not settle in the lungs and be exhaled. Respirable particles of about 2 μm are thought to be ideal (49). Although particles of this size can be generated by a number of aerosolizers, jet nebulizers generally require flow rates of 6–10 L/min for optimal performance. A 1-kg infant with RDS being ventilated with a tidal volume of 10 ml at 40 breaths/min has a minute volume of 400 ml. Assuming no dilution of the aerosol by ventilator circuit gas and an 8 L/min aerosol generator, the maximum efficiency of delivery would be 0.4 L/8 L, or 5%. Efficiency can be improved by the location of the aerosolizer in the circuit (50), by timing aerosolization to the respiratory cycle (45), by changes in circuit design (51), and by increasing tidal volumes and dwell time of the aerosol in the lungs (52). However, a critical factor for treatment of preterm infants is a better matching of aerosol generation rate to minute ventilation. Devices that can perform at very low flow rates are not currently available. Other technical aspects of aerosolization of surfactant also need to be carefully evaluated for each surfactant, device, and ventilator. Surfactant tends to foam on aerosolization, and surfactant aerosols interfere with any valves or measuring devices on the expiratory circuit, requiring the use of filters. The encouraging aspect of the available information about aerosolized surfactant is that it can be effective at low doses; however, presently available devices make even those doses difficult to achieve.

Aerosolized surfactant is not a solution to the problem of nonuniform distribution. In the uniformly injured or immature lung, aerosolized surfactant seems to distribute more uniformly than does instilled surfactant (44,46). However, aerosolized surfactant will only go to ventilated lung volumes. Lewis et al. (13) found that with total lung lavage of adult sheep, the lobar distribution of aerosolized surfactant was quite uniform across lobes. Twenty percent was deposited in the right upper lobe. If the right upper lobe was not lavaged to yield a nonuniform lung injury model, 50% of both ventilation and surfactant went to the right upper lobe. Trajan et al. (52) found that in normal lungs, the areas of high ventilation received less aerosol than did regions of low ventilation, perhaps because increased residence time was required for aerosol deposition. Lewis and McCary (51) have extended the saline lavage model of ARDS by generating lobes with different amounts of lung injury. Following saline lavage to yield uniform surfactant deficiency, they instilled HCl into selected lobes to further injure those lobes. Although instilled surfactant was recovered from the most injured lobes, aerosolized surfactant was preferentially excluded from the most injured lobes. The physiological effect was that by treating the less injured lung, gas exchange and pressure requirements decreased more with aerosolization than with instillation.

VI. Conclusions

Aerosolized surfactant will become a clinical option only after devices and delivery techniques have been improved. Furthermore, aerosolized surfactant must be at least as effective as the presently used instillation techniques to be justifiable clinically. Surfactant could be delivered to the lungs by other devices. Niven et al. (53) found that nozzle extensions on metered-dose inhalers could increase the efficiency of delivery of those devices. Surfactant could be delivered as a dry powder to avoid the problems associated with the volume of vehicle in the presently available surfactant suspensions. Surfactant also could be used to deliver other agents to the lungs, such as antibiotics and antoxidants (22). However, enthusiasm for new treatment techniques must be tempered by the recognition that surfactant as presently used is a very effective therapy (2). Effective in this context means not only an initial physiological response to treatment (increase in oxygenation and decrease in ventilatory support), but also a comparable effect on pneumothorax, bronchopulmonary dysplasia, and death.

Acknowledgment

This review was supported in part by Grants HD 11932 and HD 12714.

References

1. Jobe AH, Ikegami M. Surfactant for the treatment of respiratory distress syndrome. Am Rev Respir Dis 1987; 136:1256–1275.
2. Soll RF, McQueen MC. Respiratory distress syndrome. In: Sinclair JC, Bracken MB, eds. Effective Care of the Newborn Infant. Oxford University Press, 1992:325–358.
3. Enhorning G, Shennan A, Possmayer F, et al. Prevention of neonatal respiratory distress syndrome by tracheal instillation of surfactant: A randomized clinical trial. Pediatrics 1985; 76:145–153.
4. Collaborative European Multicenter Study Group. Surfactant replacement therapy for severe neonatal respiratory distress syndrome: An international randomized clinical trial. Pediatrics 1988; 82:683–691.
5. Phibbs RH, Ballard RA, Clements JA, et al. Initial clinical trial of Exosurf, a protein-free synthetic surfactant, for the prophylaxis and early treatment of hyaline membrane disease. Pediatrics 1991; 88:1–8.
6. Zola EM, Gunkel JH, Chan RK, et al. Comparison of three dosing procedures for administration of bovine surfactant to neonates with respiratory distress syndrome. J Pediatr 1993; 122:453–459.
7. Zola EM, Overbach AM, Gunkel JH, et al. Treatment investigational new drug experience with Survanta (Beractant). Pediatrics 1993; 91:546–551.
8. Horbar JD, Wright LL, Soll RF, et al. A multicenter randomized trial comparing two surfactants for the treatment of neonatal respiratory distress syndrome. J Pediatr 1993; 123:757–765.
9. Jorch G, Rabe H, Garbe M, et al. Acute and protracted effects of intratracheal surfactant application on internal carotid blood flow velocity, blood pressure and carbondioxide tension in very low birth weight infants. Eur J Pediatr 1989; 148:770–773.
10. van de Bor M, Ma EJ, Walther FJ. Cerebral blood flow velocity after surfactant instillation in preterm infants. J Pediatr 1991; 118:285–287.
11. Hellstrom-Westas L, Bell AH, Skov L, et al. Cerebroelectrical depression following surfactant treatment in preterm neonates. Pediatrics 1992; 89:643–647.
12. Jobe AH. Pulmonary surfactant therapy. N Engl J Med 1993; 328:861–868.
13. Lewis JF, Ikegami M, Jobe AH, Absolom D. Physiologic responses and distribution of aerosolized surfactant (Survanta®) in a nonuniform pattern of lung injury. Am Rev Respir Dis 1993; 147:1364–1370.
14. Fujiwara T. Surfactant replacement in neonatal RDS. In: Robertson B, van Golde

LMG, Battenburg JJ, eds. Pulmonary Surfactant. Amsterdam: Elsevier Science, 1982; 479–503.
15. Edwards DK, Hilton SW, Merritt TA, et al. Respiratory distress syndrome treated with human surfactant: radiographic findings. Radiology 1985; 157:329–334.
16. Jobe AH, Ikegami M, Glatz T, et al. Duration and characteristics of treatment of premature lambs with natural surfactant. J Clin Invest 1981; 67:370–375.
17. Robertson B, Enhorning G. The alveolar lining of the premature newborn rabbit after pharyngeal deposition of surfactant. Lab Invest 1974; 31:54–59.
18. Obladen M, Brendlein F, Krempien B. Surfactant substitution. Eur J Pediatr 1979; 131:219–228.
19. Geiger K, Gallagher ML, Hedley-Whyte J. Cellular distribution and clearance of aerosolized dipalmitoyl lecithin. J Appl Physiol 1975; 39:759–766.
20. Winter I, Scott JE, Oulton MR, et al. Autoradiographic localization and effects of exogenous radioactively labelled surfactant in the lung of the prematurely delivered fetal rabbit. Biol Neonate 1991; 60:292–302.
21. Charon A, Taeusch HW, Fitzgibbon C, et al. Factors associated with surfactant treatment response in infants with severe respiratory distress syndrome. Pediatrics 1989; 83:348–354.
22. Kharasch VS, Sweeney TD, Fredberg J, et al. Pulmonary surfactant as a vehicle for intratracheal delivery of technetium sulfur colloid and pentamidine in hamster lungs. Am Rev Respir Dis 1991; 144:909–913.
23. Jobe AH, Ikegami M, Jacobs H, Jones S. Surfactant and pulmonary blood flow distributions following treatment of premature lambs with natural surfactant. J Clin Invest 1984; 73:848–856.
24. van der Bleek J. Plotz FB, van Overbeek M, et al. Distribution of exogenous surfactant in rabbits with severe respiratory failure: The effect of volume. Pediatr Res 1993; 34:154–158.
25. Hislop AA, Wigglesworth JS, Desai R. Alveolar development in the human fetus and infant. E Hum Dev 1986; 13:1–11.
26. Davis JM, Russ GA, Metlay L, et al. Short-term distribution kinetics of intratracheally administered exogenous lung surfactant. Pediatr Res 1992; 31:445–450.
27. Oetomo SB, Lewis J, Ikegami M, Jobe AH. Surfactant treatments alter endogenous surfactant metabolism in rabbit lungs. J Appl Physiol 1990; 68:1590–1596.
28. Hall SB, Venkitaraman AR, Whitsett JA, et al. Importance of hydrophobic apoproteins as constituents of clinical exogenous surfactants. Am Rev Respir Dis 1992; 145:24–30.
29. Robertson B. Pathology and pathophysiology of neonatal surfactant deficiency. In: Robertson B, van Golde LMG, Batenburg JJ, eds. Pulmonary Surfactant. Amsterdam: Elsevier Science, 1984:383–418.
30. Kendig JW, Notter RH, Cox C, et al. A comparison of surfactant as immediate prophylaxis and as rescue therapy in newborns of less than 30 weeks gestation. N Engl J Med 1991; 324:865–871.
31. Kattwinkel J, Bloom BT, Delmore P, et al. Prophylactic administration of calf lung surfactant extract is more effective than early treatment of respiratory distress syndrome in neonates 29 through 32 weeks gestation. Pediatrics 1993; 92:90–98.
32. Heldt GP, Merritt A, Golembeski E, et al. Distribution of surfactant, lung

compliance, and aeration of preterm rabbit lungs after surfactant therapy and conventional and high-frequency oscillatory ventilation. Pediatr Res 1992; 31:270–275.

33. Gilliard N, Richman PM, Merritt TA, Spragg RG. Effect of volume and dose on the pulmonary distribution of exogenous surfactant administered to normal rabbits or to rabbits with oleic acid lung injury. Am Rev Respir Dis 1990; 141:743–747.
34. Jackson JC, MacKenzie AP, Chi EY, et al. Mechanisms for reduced total lung capacity at birth and during hyaline membrane disease in premature newborn monkeys. Am Rev Respir Dis 1990; 142:413–419.
35. Sergerer H, van Gelder W, Angenent FWM, et al. Pulmonary distribution and efficacy of exogenous surfactant in lung-lavaged rabbits are influenced by the instillation technique. Pediatr Res 1993; 34:490–494.
36. Ueda T, Ikegami M, Rider ED, Jobe AH. Distribution of surfactant and ventilation in surfactant treated preterm lambs. J Appl Physiol 1994; 76:45–55.
37. Walther FJ, Kuipers IM, Gidding CEM, et al. A comparison of high-frequency oscillation superimposed onto backup mechanical ventilation and conventional mechanical ventilation on the distribution of exogenous surfactant in premature lambs. Pediatr Res 1987; 22:725–729.
38. Robillard E, Alarie Y, Dagenais-Perusse P, et al. Microaerosol administration of synthetic dipalmitoyl lecithin in the respiratory distress syndrome: A preliminary report. Can Med Assoc J 1964; 90:55–57.
39. Chu J, Clements JA, Cotton EK, et al. Neonatal pulmonary ischemia: clinical and physiological studies. Pediatrics 1967; 40:709–782.
40. Shannon DC, Kazemi H, Merril EW, et al. Restoration of volume-pressure curves with lecithin fog. J Appl Physiol 1970; 28:470–473.
41. Ikegami M, Hesterberg T, Nozaki M, Adams FH. Restoration of lung pressure-volume characteristics with surfactant: comparison of nebulization versus instillation and natural versus synthetic surfactant. Pediatr Res 1977; 11:178–182.
42. Marks LB, Notter RH, Oberdorster G, McBride JT. Ultrasonic and jet aerosolization of phospholipids and the effects on surface activity. Pediatr Res 1983; 17:742–747.
43. Zelter M, Escudier BJ, Hoeffel JM, Murray JF. Effects of aerosolized artificial surfactant on repeated oleic acid injury in sheep. Am Rev Respir Dis 1990; 141:1014–1019.
44. Lewis JF, Ikegami M, Jobe AH, Tabor B. Aerosolized surfactant treatment of preterm lambs. J Appl Physiol 1991; 70:869–876.
45. Lewis J, Ikegami M, Higuchi R, et al. Nebulized vs. instilled exogenous surfactant in an adult lung injury model. J Appl Physiol 1991; 71:1270–1276.
46. Lewis JF, Tabor B, Ikegami M, et al. Lung function and surfactant distribution in saline-lavaged sheep given instilled vs. nebulized surfactant. J Appl Physiol 1993; 74:1256–1264.
47. Simonson SG, Huang YC, Pracica PJ, et al. Exogenous surfactant improves oxygenation in hyperoxic lung injury. Am Rev Respir Dis 1992, 145:A609.
48. Fracica PJ, Piantadosi CA, Young SL, Crapo JD. Artificial surfactant diminishes pathologic injury in hyperoxia in primates. Am Rev Respir Dis 1992, 145:A610.
49. Raabe OG. Deposition and clearance of inhaled particles. In: Occupational Lung

Diseases, eds. Gee JBL, Morgan WKC, Brooks SM. New York: Raven Press, 1984:1–38.
50. O'Doherty MJ, Thomas SHL, Page CJ, et al. Delivery of a nebulized aerosol to a lung model during mechanical ventilation. Am Rev Respir Dis 1992; 146:383–388.
51. Lewis JF, McCaig L. Aerosolized versus instilled exogenous surfactant in a nonuniform pattern of lung injury. Am Rev Respir Dis 1993; 148:1187–1193.
52. Tajan M, Logus JW, Enns EG, Man SFP. Relationship between regional ventilation and aerosol deposition in tidal breathing. Am Rev Respir Dis 1984; 130:64–70.
53. Niven RW, Kacmarek RM, Brain JD, Peterfreund RA. Small bore nozzle extensions to improve the delivery efficiency of drugs from metered dose inhalers: Laboratory evaluation. Am Rev Respir Dis 1993; 147:1590–1594.

16

Biochemical Prediction of Response to Surfactant Therapy in the Newborn Infant

MIKKO HALLMAN, JACK SILLS, and KRISTINA BRY
University of California, Irvine
School of Medicine
Irvine, California

T. ALLEN MERRITT
University of California, Davis,
Medical Center
Davis, California

I. Introduction

Surfactant deficiency is a primary cause of respiratory distress syndrome (RDS) in newborn infants. Analysis of the airway specimens is an investigative approach to clarify the development of the surfactant system and to study the effect of therapies during the course of RDS. Biochemical analysis of surfactant components in lung effluent may help to predict the response to exogenous surfactant therapy. The present review on exogenous surfactant treatment response focuses on newborn infants with RDS. Current data indicates that RDS is a spectrum of diseases, with variable degrees of surfactant system immaturity, with secondary surfactant dysfunction, and with variable involvement of the surfactant system in respiratory failure.

II. Studies on Fetal Surfactant Maturity

The degree of surfactant maturity before birth predicts the response to exogenous surfactant therapy. There are similarities in surfactant regulation between human and several animal species (1,2). However, in the human fetus, saturated phosphatidylcholine (SPC) is found in large amounts in lung tissue much earlier in gestation than in other species (3). Human fetuses establish biochemical surfactant maturity at a mean gestational age of 85% of term (range 60–100%) (4), whereas, in animal species, the variability is small, with surfactant maturity being attained at 90–98% of term gestational age (2). Unlike other species, the prematurity rate in human species is quite high (4–20% depending on the population). Diseases leading to preterm birth influence maturation, further complicating the assessment of fetal lung maturity and the responsiveness to exogenous surfactant therapy (5).

Maturity of surfactant is most often estimated to ensure elective delivery without iatrogenic RDS. There is a need to evaluate fetal lung maturity in order to individualize treatment and to avoid unnecessary surfactant therapy at birth. For a test to predict lung immaturity, a predictive value is critical (number of correct predictions of immature result/number of all immature test results). The second desirable feature of the test is a high sensitivity (the number of correct immature test results/number of all immature fetuses).

Screening tests such as the foam stability test, optical density at 650 nm and semiquantitative measurement of phosphatidylglycerol (PG) tend to have a low positive predictive value and high sensitivity. On the other hand, quantitative tests such as the L/S ratio and saturated phosphatidylcholine (SPC) concentration have a high positive predictive value, especially when the cutoff value has been set low. The high predictive value of the test, however, tends to be associated with low sensitivity (6).

The accuracy of the test results for fetal lung maturity is inversely related to gestational age. (7,8). The accuracy figures may be distorted, however, since there is a significant reporting bias that additionally is dependent on gestational age. In elective close to term deliveries, the fetuses with immature or transitional lung profiles are not delivered as a rule, whereas high-risk fetuses are often delivered early regardless of the test result because of serious fetomaternal disease or spontaneous preterm birth. The documented trend toward increased incidence of false immature test results at low gestational age may be caused by the reporting bias. The incidence of a false mature test result increases at low gestational ages (Fig. 1).

In very early gestations (e.g., 28 weeks or less), infants regardless of a "mature" surfactant profile tend to have a spectrum of lung diseases diagnosed as transient respiratory distress, retained lung fluid syndrome, pulmonary maladaptation syndrome, or RDS. At gestations of less than 28 weeks, the incidence of RDS is generally at least 50%. Although the predictive value of lung maturity tests are higher than the prediction based on gestational age alone, the practical benefits of fetal lung maturity measurements may be outweighed by the costs and risks of amniocentesis in very early gestations. In cases of rupture of the fetal membranes, biochemical screening of vaginal pool fluid for surfactant is indicated. (9).

According to three studies, routine treatment with surfactant at birth of

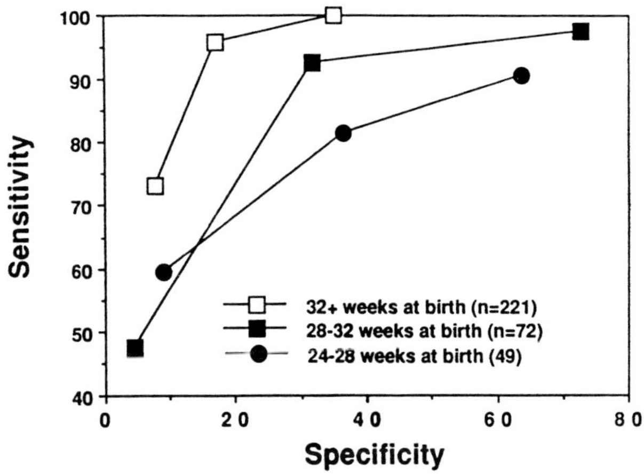

Figure 1 Influence of the gestational age on the receiver operating characteristic curves of the L/S ratio and phosphatidylglycerol (PG) in predicting presence or absence of RDS. The symbols connected by line indicate the characteristic of the test as a function of the following cutoff values for negative test result: L/S ratio >1.4, undetectable PG (left), L/S ratio ≥2, undetectable PG, and L/S ratio ≥2 and positive PG (right). All infants were born within 48 hr after the recovery of the amniotic fluid specimen.

infants at less than 30 weeks of gestation results in unnecessary treatment in 37–54% of cases (10–12). Prophylactic treatment of infants with false lung immaturity was decreased to 18% when lung maturity was diagnosed prior to treatment. (13). Knowledge on fetal surfactant maturity even in early gestation would therefore be helpful in deciding on the treatment practices during early life.

III. Surfactant Dysfunction in RDS

The systems maintaining pulmonary gas exchange and ventilation are interrelated; that is, a severe disturbance in any of these systems affects pulmonary surfactant function adversely. Likewise, lack of surfactant function severely impairs lung homeostasis. Besides surfactant deficiency, prematurity is associated with a spectrum of functional and structural features that cause cardiopulmonary insufficiency. These include increased alveolar-capillary permeability, immaturity of transport across alveolar epithelial cells, structural immaturity of the lung, and deficient ventilation (unstable chest wall, diaphragmatic fatigue, and immature defense systems). (14–19).

The immediate causes of surfactant dysfunction are complex. These include

(1) lack of adequate surfactant secretion due to immaturity; (2) abnormalities in surfactant secretion, recycling, or compartmentation or excessive uptake of surfactant into lung parenchyma (type II cell damage/immaturity); (3) dilution of extracellular surfactant by alveolar edema fluid; (4) increased minimum surface tension caused by inhibitors of surface activity (20); (5) excessive degradation of essential surfactant components by proteases and phospholipases (21); and (6) inactivation of the surfactant complex by oxygen free radicals. The potential importance of these various mechanisms in causing surfactant dysfunction during the course of RDS remains to be studied.

IV. Diagnosis of Surfactant Deficiency After Birth

The following sources may be used for biochemical assessment of surfactant responsiveness: (1) amniotic fluid at birth (5,6); (2) gastric or retropharyngeal aspirate shortly after birth (22); (3) airway specimens (AS) recovered during airway suctioning of intubated patients (23); or (4) bronchoalveolar lavage (BAL) obtained during bronchoscopy (24). Postmortem BAL and other pathological specimens have been used to characterize the surfactant system (25–30).

Table 1 lists methods used in diagnostic studies. A number of other supplementary biochemical tests define the host defense systems (e.g., protease-antiprotease system, antioxidant defense system) that are likely to influence surfactant responsiveness. With the exception of the mature surfactant protein SP-C, other surfactant components can be quantitatively measured. However, most studies deal only with a few major surfactant components.

Table 1 Biochemical Analysis of the Airway Specimens

Approach	Reference
Concentration of surfactant component in AS	Gerdes et al. (80)
Surfactant component/reference component	Gluck et al. (22) Hallman et al. (120) Obladen and Gluck (121) Shelley et al. (122)
Concentration of surfactant component in ELF	Hallman et al. (41)
Fractionation of AS before analysis (studies of surfactant aggregates, inhibitors of surfactant function)	Ikegami et al. (53) Hallman et al. (41)
Probes attached to exogenous surfactant (distribution of exogenous surfactant, pool size, and half-life studies)	Hallman et al. (35) Charon et al. (37) Hallman et al. (41)

A. Definition of Surfactant Responsiveness

The degree of responsiveness to exogenous surfactant can be evaluated on the basis of acute effect and on the basis of intermediate or long-term outcomes. Acute responsiveness is defined as an improvement in gas exchange, a decrease in the distending pressures or an improvement in lung mechanics within a few hours to a few days after the therapy. Intermediate responsiveness to exogenous surfactant deals with the duration and requirement of mechanical ventilation and supplementary oxygen <28 days after surfactant treatment and with the incidence of complications (lung ruptures, patent ductus arteriosus). The long-term outcome measures include the incidence of chronic lung disease and/or the incidence of death 4 weeks after birth or at 36–38 weeks' postmenstrual age. Biochemical surfactant diagnostics are principally associated with acute responsiveness, as the surfactant system is in a dynamic state with a fairly short turnover time and a variety of confounding variables, such as gestational age and extrapulmonary diseases, influence the outcome.

B. Comment on Methods

Unlike in animal studies, in newborn infants, only small-volume AS recovered during routine suctioning of the airways is available for surfactant studies. Arguably a small-volume BAL represents the surfactant lining of a selective population of airways and air spaces. According to experimental studies, there is a close similarity in the phospholipid composition of a small-volume and quantitative BAL (31). Retention of exogenous surfactant within the central airways is a potential cause for misjudgment of lung effluent results. This problem is decreased when the first specimens recovered during suctioning of the airways after surfactant supplementation are excluded from analysis (32). Another problem is the lack of consistency in the amount of surfactant recovered in AS.

Surfactant is measured by quantitating a surfactant component on the basis of a reference compound. The most frequently used index is the SPC/sphingomyelin ratio or the L/S ratio (22). Phosphatidylcholine is also expressed on the basis of serum-derived protein or the total protein in AS (33). A conventional approach is to analyze the concentration of surfactant in BAL. This method is complicated by the fact that in BAL return, the fraction representing epithelial lining fluid (ELF) is not constant. In general, the amount of ELF in BAL or in AS increases in high-permeability lung edema, causing an overestimate of the surfactant concentration. In order to decrease this source of variability, the concentration of the surfactant component in ELF is estimated by measuring the concentrations of a freely permeable molecule such as urea in both serum and airway specimens. The concentration of surfactant in ELF is then calculated as follows: $(\text{surfactant component})_{\text{ELF}} = (\text{surfactant component})_{\text{BAL}} \times (\text{urea})_{\text{serum}}/$

(urea)$_{BAL}$; where (surfactant component)$_{ELF}$ and (surfactant component)$_{BAL}$ are concentrations of surfactant in ELF and in BAL, respectively.

A delay between lavage fluid instillation and the recovery of BAL allows significant diffusion of urea into the lavage fluid, causing underestimation of surfactant concentration (24,34). This problem is decreased when the time period between the application of the lavage fluid and the recovery of the specimen is shortened (i.e., <15 sec). In severe lung diseases, the concentration of surfactant in ELF may be nonuniform, and thus the concentration reflects the mean value of the respiratory units sampled.

The sum of extra- and intracellular surfactant pools has been estimated by the dilution method according to the Fick principle. A label is attached to exogenous surfactant: PG or deuterium-labeled dipalmitoyl phosphatidylcholine (DPPC) have been used (35,36). The method is also useful for clearance rate analysis, as well as for analysis of surfactant distribution (37). The sources for error of pool size measurements include lack of complete mixing and dissimilarity of the clearance pathways of endogenous and exogenous surfactant pools. In experimental studies, the gold standard for extracellular surfactant quantitation is postmortem lavage (38,39).

V. Predictive Accuracy of the Airway Specimens

A. Diagnosis of RDS

Surfactant indices measured in airway specimens shortly after birth are as accurate as amniotic fluid specimens in the diagnosis of RDS. However, the receiver operating characteristic curve for surfactant indices changes as a function of neonatal age, reflecting accumulation of surfactant complex within the airways after birth in RDS. Thus, the cutoff value of the L/S ratio increases during the first day of life (23). Both the concentration and the distribution of PG among the other surfactant phospholipids are low in RDS. Unlike other surfactant components, PG does not increase until recovery is evident or until 30–32 weeks of postmenstrual age. However, the positive predictive value of PG is lower than that of the L/S ratio. Increasing the sensitivity of the PG assay does not appear to improve the predictive value, since the number of false-negative test results increases as a result of trace quantities of PG present in a number of biological materials. Both SP-A and SP-B, deficient at birth in RDS, may be useful in diagnosis of RDS (40,41).

Besides RDS, a variety of lung diseases in newborn infants are associated with abnormalities in surfactant phospholipids and with surfactant dysfunction. These include wet lung syndrome and RDS type II (pulmonary maladaptation syndrome). In lung hypoplasia (Potter's syndrome, diaphragmatic hernia) and often in congenital pneumonia in premature infants, a low L/S ratio and a low or undetectable PG level are found at birth (42). In evolving postasphyxia syndrome with respiratory failure, severe meconium aspiration syndrome, and pneumonia, the L/S ratio, PG, SP-A, and SP-B levels decrease (43), as in adult RDS (44,45).

B. Association with the Severity of Respiratory Failure

Table 2 shows the association between various surfactant indices and the severity of respiratory failure in RDS. The relationship is studied in 290 airway specimens obtained from 61 infants during the first 4 weeks of life. The conceptional age at birth ranged between 24 and 30 weeks. Infants treated with human surfactant (both rescue and prophylactic) and placebo were studied (41). As seen, there is lack of a close linear association between surfactant indices and respiratory failure. The test results based on quantitation of the concentration of surfactant component in AS are not associated with the degrce of respiratory failure in the present series. The L/S ratio and the concentration of surfactant component in ELF had a low but significant association with the degree of respiratory failure. The low association between the concentration of a surfactant component in ELF and the degree of respiratory failure is in part explained by the fact that infants with a high concentration of surfactant in ELF generally have a mild respiratory

Table 2 Relationship Between Surfactant Indices and the Degree of Respiratory Failure Expressed as Arterial-Alveolar PO_2 Difference

	0–28 days			12–24 hr		
Index	no. of AS	*r*	*P*	no. of infants	*r*	*P*
$(PC)_{AS}$	290	−0.109	>0.1	61	−0.206	>0.1
$(PC)_{ELF}$	288	−0.265	<0.001	60	−0.250	0.05
$(SPC)_{ELF}$	283	−0.298	<0.001	59	−0.410	<0.01
Ln $(PC)_{ELF}$	288	−0.528	<0.001	60	−0.645	<0.001
Ln $(SPC)_{ELF}$	283	−0.568	<0.001	59	−0.652	<0.001
SP-A/SPC	283	−0.071	>0.1	59	−0.098	>0.1
SPC/PC	283	−0.337	<0.001	59	−0.177	>0.1
PC/Protein	290	−0.185	<0.01	61	−0.292	<0.05
Ln SP-A/SPC	280	−0.120	<0.05	59	−0.164	>0.1
Ln (PC/Protein)	290	−0.496	<0.001	61	−0.433	<0.001
Ln (SPC/Protein)	283	−0.597	<0.001	59	−0.428	<0.001

The two correlation coefficients (r_{0-28} days vs r_{12-24} hr) did not significantly differ from each other (Z transformation, normal distribution).
Source: Data from ref. 41; with permission.

failure, and among these infants there is no detectable association between surfactant indices and respiratory failure.

Surfactant inhibitors decrease surface activity. They include fibrin(ogen), fibrin monomer, iron-saturated transferrin, albumin, so-called 110-kDa surfactant inhibitor, hemoglobin, meconium, lyso-PC, lactocyl ceramide, bilirubin, and cationic amino acids (46–49,41,50–52). As shown by Ikegami et al., surfactant inhibitor decreases the surface activity in RDS, and may be responsible for the delay in weaning from the respirator (53). The quantitation of the concentration of total nonsedimentable protein, albumin or transferrin in ELF, is a suitable screening method for surfactant inhibitors that decrease the minimum surface tension. Surfactant inhibition is particularly evident when the concentration of surfactant is low and when there is a deficiency in surfactant proteins (41,54,55). The nonsedimentable protein concentration in ELF bears a weak but significant positive association with the degree of the respiratory failure (41).

The ratio between a surfactant component and a nonsedimentable protein takes into consideration both the concentration of surfactant and its inhibitor, making it an attractive biochemical screening method for surfactant function in respiratory failure (33). As shown in Table 2, the correlation between the degree of respiratory failure and surfactant indices recovered during the neonatal period, increases in the following order: $(PC)_{AS}$, SP-A/PC ratio, $(PC)_{ELF}$, L/S ratio, PC/protein ratio, In $(PC)_{ELF}$, In PC/protein ratio, In $(SPC)_{ELF}$, and in SPC/protein ratio.

The association with the degree of respiratory failure in RDS is strengthened when several surfactant indices are combined. In multiple regression analysis, each of the following variables bears a significant association with the degree of respiratory failure: In $(PC)_{ELF}$, SP-A/SPC ratio, PC/SPC ratio, and (nonsedimentable protein)$_{ELF}$. According to multiple regression model, these four indices explained nearly 50% of the variability in the degree of respiratory failure. Each of the four indices represent an individual surfactant characteristic, or a property of the nonsedimentable fraction of ELF, affecting the surface activity. During the first day of life, ln $(SPC)_{ELF}$ correlates with the ventilatory index ($r = -0.65$), because in conventionally treated infants with severe respiratory failure, the concentration of surfactant in ELF was low, and in surfactant-treated infants the opposite was true. The (nonsedimentable protein)$_{ELF}$ correlated with the degree of respiratory failure during days 1–7 of life ($r = 0.31$) when serum-derived proteins accumulate in ELF, inhibiting the surfactant function.

The individual variability in the association between the surfactant indices and the degree of respiratory failure is considerable. Postmenstrual age or postnatal age do not explain the variability (41). Airway specimens during the neonatal period from a single infant, analyzed for saturated phosphatidylcholine/sphingomyelin ratio, correlated closely with the degree of respiratory failure, whereas in few other infants no such association was found (35).

Extracellular surfactant can be fractionated by differential centrifugation or on density gradients (56–58). Ultraheavy, heavy and light subtypes are obtained by isopycnic sucrose gradient centrifugation. The ultraheavy and heavy subtypes have good surface activities and contain SP-A and SP-B. (59). Light subtype is not surface active and contains very small quantities of surfactant proteins, whereas the phospholipid composition is similar in the different surfactant forms (59–62, 56,57,63). Conversion from heavy to light subtypes requires cyclic surface area cycling and the action of a protease enzyme, tentatively identified as a serine protease (57,64). SP-B is degraded during the heavy to light subtype conversion (61); addition of SP-A may inhibit that conversion (65).

At term birth, the extracellular surfactant consists of heavy subtypes. They are precursors for the light subtypes that appear during air breathing of a term rabbit within a few hours after term birth (66). Thus, the increase in surfactant in ELF at the onset of air breathing (67) is associated with activation of the metabolic conversion into light surfactant subtype that has poor surface activity.

Surfactant inactivation and clearance of inactivated surfactant complex is likely to occur in RDS. It may depend on ventilatory treatment practices (68), on the variable presence of proteolytic enzymes (69), or on the presence of oxygen free radicals ($OH\cdot$, $ONOO^-$, OCl^-) that can change the aggregate structure in vitro (70,71). The biochemical composition of surfactant is likely to influence the rate of inactivation too. Besides surfactant inhibition, the inactivation of surfactant as it is converted from heavy to light subtypes is likely to affect the surfactant function in RDS.

A study of 95 airway specimens from 24 infants with RDS for the distribution of the aggregate fractions, recovered by differential centrifugation, revealed no association with the degree of respiratory failure, surfactant supplementation, or postnatal age. However, the cell-free specimens were frozen before separation of the subtypes; freezing is likely to affect the aggregate size. Whatsoever, in severe respiratory failure, the sedimentable surfactant complex was frequently not surface active in vitro (M. Hallman, unpublished). In addition, inactivated surfactant frequently contained very small quantities of SP-A and SP-B. It is unclear at present whether in these cases there is an accelerated rate of subtype conversion or whether as a result of inadequate endogenous secretion, intracellular uptake, or inadequate recycling, the surface activity is not maintained. The experimental data available (58) raise the possibility that in lung damage major changes take place in macroaggregate structure of surfactant in ELF and that these changes may be responsible for deterioration of surfactant function.

C. Association with the Outcome

We studied 50 infants with RDS, who were born with a mean gestation of 26 weeks. Altogether 74% of the infants received exogenous natural surfactant, the rest received placebo. Poor outcome was defined as neonatal death due to respiratory failure or diagnosis of chronic lung disease at 4 weeks of age. Low $(SPC)_{ELF}$ during days 0–2 of life and high $(\text{nonsedimentable protein})_{ELF}$ during days 4–7 were significantly associated with poor outcome. Low $(SPC)_{ELF}$ was associated with lack of surfactant substitution ($p < 0.001$), whereas both low gestational age at birth and lack of surfactant substitution were associated with high concentration of nonsedimentable protein.

Among the surfactant indices studied, SP-A/SPC ratio was the best predictor of poor outcome during 0–7 first days of life. Low SP-A/SPC ratio (25 < ng/nmol) significantly predicted the odds of dying, when both the gestational age at birth and surfactant substitution were considered as confounding variables. It is unlikely that the remarkable association between SP-A and the outcome is due to surface tension–lowering properties of SP-A, since SP-A was a poor predictor of the actual degree of respiratory failure (see Table 2). As described, SP-A has immunomodulatory properties, particularly effects on pulmonary macrophage defense system (72). Regulation of SP-A by hormones, growth factors and cytokines, is different from other surfactant components (73,74). Very low SP-A during early life may reflect compromised host-defense system in infants with a high risk of dying or developing chronic lung disease.

VI. Factors Affecting Response to Surfactant Therapy

Preterm infants with severe RDS have alveolar surfactant pool sizes estimated to contain 2–10 μmol SPC, whereas at term the pool size approaches 100 μmol/kg (27,35,75). Synthetic rates and secretory kinetics of surfactant PC seem to be similar in preterm and term animals (38). Recycling pathways are also active at all ages studied to date, and the surfactant used for treatment is involved in recycling (76). Surfactant treatments do not adversely affect synthetic and secretory pathways by feedback inhibition (35,38). The treatment doses of exogenous surfactant are rapidly cleared from the air spaces by an apparently unsaturable mechanism, so that regardless of the dose (maximum studied 400 mg/kg) only a fraction of exogenous surfactant administered (10–50 mg/kg) can be lavaged from the airways of immature animals a few hours after surfactant administration (76,77).

A. Factors Associated with Exogenous Surfactant

The metabolic effects caused by exogenous surfactant depend on the quality and quantity of the exogenous surfactant applied to the airways, and may in part be responsible for the differences in the acute and intermediate outcome between a synthetic and a natural surfactant currently used in clinical practice (78).

In small preterm infants with RDS, exogenous human surfactant increases the concentration of SPC in ELF in a dose-dependent manner (Fig. 2). Assuming

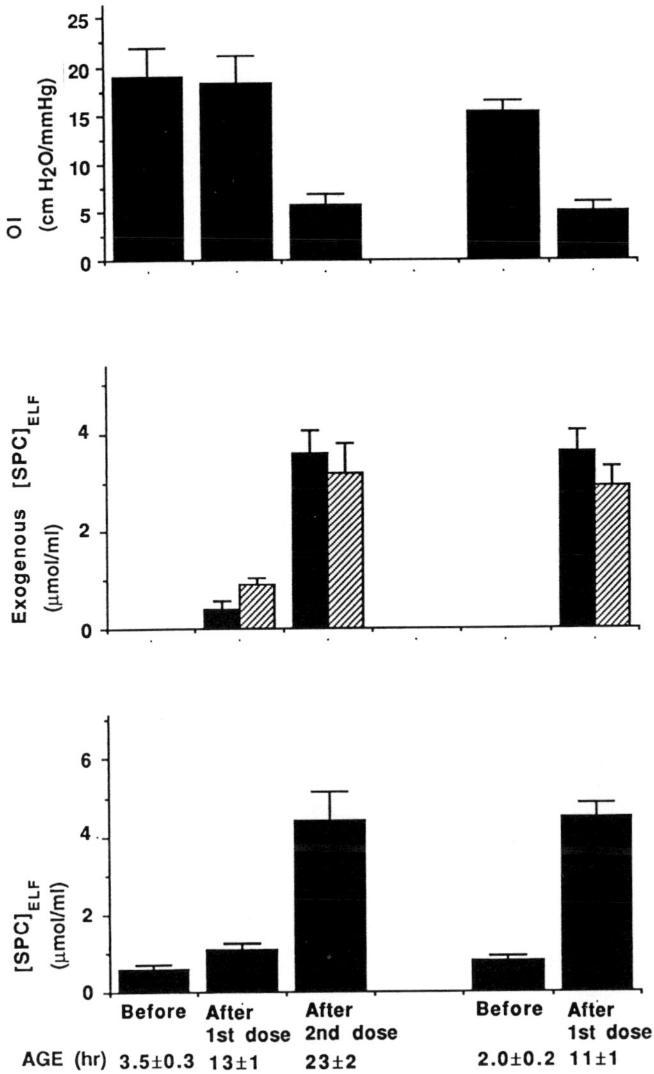

Figure 2 Effect of exogenous human surfactant on the concentration of saturated phosphatidylcholine in epithelial lining fluid, $[SPC]_{ELF}$ (mean + SE). The results are shown separately in infants who required one dose of surfactant (70 mg/kg, n = 6), and in infants who required two doses (n = 5), because one dose did not abolish severe respiratory failure. Exogenous $[SPC]_{ELF}$ was calculated either as a difference between post- and presurfactant $[SPC]_{ELF}$, assuming that endogenous $[SPC]_{ELF}$ increases at a rate of 15 nmol/ml/hr (black bars), or using phosphatidylglycerol as a marker of exogenous surfactant (35), and taking into consideration the differences in the half-lives of SPC (46 hr) and phosphatidylglycerol (31 hr) (36) (stippled bars).

that endogenous SPC accumulates into ELF at a similar slow rate as in infants who do not require surfactant, the calculated increase in SPC is almost exclusively due to exogenous surfactant. Contribution of exogenous surfactant to the increase in ELF levels is somewhat less, when the estimate is based on the exogenous surfactant marker. In infants requiring one dose of human surfactant (70 mg/kg), the concentration of surfactant in ELF increases more and the severity of RDS decreases more than in infants requiring two doses of surfactant. In infants requiring two doses of surfactant, the dose-concentration relationship is biphasic: possibly the first dose is rapidly cleared from the airways or trapped within atelectatic air spaces.

Administration of PG-containing natural surfactant to small preterm infants with RDS increases phosphatidylinositol secretion into ELF (35). This takes place concomitant with the elimination of exogenous surfactant PG that proceeds with a half-life of 30 hr. Surfactant PG interacts with SP-B and SPC to improve surface adsorption (79). It is likely that phosphatidylinositol or other acidic lipids are important constituents of PG-devoid surfactant in RDS.

According to Chida et al. (40), treatment of RDS with cow lung surfactant that contains no SP-A (Survanta) leads to initially high SP-B levels in these infants' airway aspirates relative to untreated infants. By day 3, however, the levels in untreated infants had increased to be similar to those of surfactant-treated infants. No difference was found in concentrations of SP-A. Others (41) report that within 1 day following treatment of infants with RDS with an SP-A–containing surfactant, the ratio between SP-A and SP-C fell from 145 ng/nmol to a mean of 70 ng/nmol and remained unchanged for 7 days. During the first 7 days of life in surfactant recipients, $(\text{SP-A})_{\text{ELF}}$ was significantly higher than in placebo-treated infants. Gerdes et al. (80) measured the concentrations of SP-A and SP-B in airway aspirates in preterm neonates with RDS treated with a synthetic surfactant (Exosurf) or with placebo. Surfactant substitution had no effect on SP-B levels. However, significantly higher concentrations of SP-A were observed by 2 days after surfactant treatment, and the higher SP-A levels were maintained through the sixth day of life.

In immature lambs, endogenously synthesized SP-A incorporated to the large aggregate fraction within 4 hr after surfactant administration. This surfactant fraction was superior to treatment surfactants in improving the compliance of immature rabbits' lungs (60). It appears that the immature lung is effectively remodeling exogenous surfactant, although the mechanisms remain unknown.

The acute treatment response following exogenous natural surfactants tends to be faster and more extensive than the response of various protein-free surfactants. A comparison between bovine surfactant (Survanta) and synthetic surfactants (Exosurf and surfactant aggregates containing DPPC, PG, and palmitic acid) reinforces that finding (60). The large aggregate fraction isolated from the airways following administration of bovine surfactant was more effective in improving the compliance of immature rabbits than the parent surfactant, or than the large aggregate fractions following administration of synthetic surfactants. Thus, the remodeling capacity of the endogenous surfactant system in the immature lung may be limited depending on the exogenous surfactant.

B. Surfactant Responsiveness Among Infants with Biochemical Surfactant Maturity

A subgroup of small preterm infants who have high L/S ratio, detectable PG (>2% of total phospholipid), and prominent phosphatidylinositol develop RDS despite biochemical surfactant maturity (81). It has been proposed that the respiratory failure in these cases is due to lung edema, delayed clearance of lung fluid, and the presence of surfactant inhibitors in ELF. Segerer et al. (82) studied 16 preterm infants who had accelerated surfactant maturity but nonetheless had clinical respiratory distress. Ten of these 16 infants responded rapidly to bovine surfactant substitution. Thus, exogenous surfactant substitution was an effective treatment in these particular cases of RDS, perhaps by restoring the surface activity and contributing toward the clearance of lung fluid. Other therapies (fluid restriction, closure of patent ductus arteriosus, continuous distending pressure, mechanical ventilation) are also effective in relieving the respiratory failure and increasing the concentration of $(SPC)_{ELF}$.

The surfactant system is "mature" at birth in term or postterm infants developing meconium aspiration syndrome or pneumonia. Many of the infants with meconium aspiration or pneumonia have responded favorably to exogenous surfactant therapy (83,84), although the response has been less than in RDS. The basis of this response may be due to relief of meconium-induced or serum protein–induced surfactant inhibition (20), of airway obstruction, relieved by exogenous surfactant (85), or of surfactant system damage, characteristic of ARDS (44). The surfactant status of patients supplemented with surfactant was not documented. Therefore, it is unclear whether biochemical changes indicative of surfactant system damage were present.

C. Factors Decreasing Responsiveness to Exogenous Surfactant

Several factors have been associated with poor responsiveness to exogenous surfactant (86,87). In severe high-permeability lung edema, poor responsiveness is likely to be associated with rapid clearance of surfactant from the airways (88), a high distribution volume of surfactant, high protein concentration in ELF, and poor distribution of surfactant (36). In addition, inflammation and damage of alveolar cells are likely to perturb surfactant metabolism and to decrease the responsiveness. Exogenous surfactant given for pulmonary hypoperfusion syndromes (severe PPHN, severe cases lung hypoplasia, shock, congenital cardiac diseases) may not be efficacious either.

Exogenous surfactant treatment in congenital alveolar proteinosis associated with a genetic defect in SP-B had no beneficial effect (89,90). In the infants with a defective "surfactant gene," gene therapy using transfection of viral plasmids or lung transplantation are future treatments. Genetic polymorphism of surfactant genes potentially affect the risk of RDS and the responsiveness of surfactant therapy (30).

D. Conditions Promoting Efficacy of Exogenous Surfactant

Prenatal Factors

The antenatal and intrapartum management of high-risk pregnancies influences surfactant responsiveness. Attempts to decrease prematurity rate have been unsuccessful. The second most effective way to prevent RDS and potentially improve surfactant responsiveness is to decrease the lung immaturity. Glucocorticoid given in threatened premature birth decreases the incidence of RDS and of other diseases caused by immaturity. Treatment of animals with glucocorticoid and thyrotropin-releasing hormone (TRH), epidermal growth factor (EGF), fibroblast-pneumonocyte factor, or other drugs accelerates fetal lung maturity (2,91,92). Glucocorticoid and TRH, administered together, appear to be more efficacious in decreasing chronic lung disease than glucocorticoid alone (93).

According to animal studies, administration of glucocorticoid or combination of glucocorticoid and TRH to the mother before preterm birth has multiple beneficial effects on lung immaturity. These include a decrease in alveolar-capillary permeability following birth (94), acceleration of the development of air spaces and pulmonary connective tissue (95), acceleration of the maturity of the surfactant system (2), activation of Cl^- transport across alveolar epithelium (96) and increase in the activity of the antioxidant enzymes (97). Prenatal glucocorticoid treatment improves dose-responsiveness to surfactant (94).

A randomized double-blind trial of dexamethasone treatment (0.5 mg/kg $\times$ 4 every 8 hr) in threatened preterm birth on 25th to 31st week of gestation was performed to determine whether prenatal dexamethasone (DEX) treatment improves the outcome of the preterm infant when exogenous surfactant is available for treatment of RDS. Of the infants born 1–14 days after the initial DEX/placebo treatment, the DEX-treated infants had lower incidence of RDS and fewer infants required natural surfactant for treatment of RDS (98). DEX treatment increased $(SP\text{-}A)_{ELF}$ and SP-A/SPC ratio during the first day of life, decreased the concentration of nonsedimentable protein in ELF during first 2 days of life, and had no detectable effect on the concentration surfactant phospholipids in ELF. There was no difference in dose requirements between DEX and placebo groups. Following DEX, the recipients of exogenous surfactant had a more striking acute response to surfactant. In addition, DEX-treated infants who were ventilated during the first day of life had a closer association between ln $(SPC)_{ELF}$ and the degree of respiratory failure (Fig. 3).

On the basis of current evidence, DEX-induced improvement in surfactant responsiveness is associated with decrease in high-permeability lung edema, and decrease in lung water content (lowered alveolar capillary permeability, decreased flux of serum proteins to ELF) rather than with an increase in surfactant phospholipids in ELF (94). Some placebo-treated infants had high surfactant phospholipid concentration in ELF despite respiratory failure (see Fig. 3), and the lipid-protein complex recovered from the airways was not surface active, suggesting excessive inactivation or inadequate metabolism of surfactant.

Management of RDS

Acute responsiveness to exogenous surfactant is maximal before the first breath or very soon after birth (12,99,101). The decrease in surfactant responsiveness is associated with an increase in the contamination of ELF with proteinaceous surfactant inhibitors and with deterioration of exogenous surfactant distribution. Current evidence supports the superiority of early rescue (mean age 2 hr) over late (mean age ≥3 hr) rescue therapy in decreasing the incidence of pneumothoraces and improving survival without BPD. However, the evidence that prophylactic therapy is superior to early rescue therapy is lacking (101).

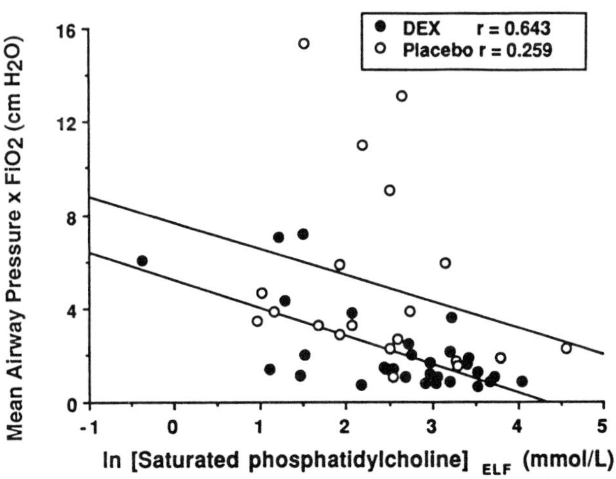

Figure 3 The relationship between $[SPC]_{ELF}$ and the degree of respiratory failure during 12 and 24 hr of life. The infants participated in a randomized trial involving dexamethasone (DEX) administration in threatened preterm birth. All infants were born within 1–14 days after the onset of DEX/Placebo.

A low rate of fluid intake increases surfactant responsiveness in RDS (102). In BAL-induced surfactant deficiency in rabbits, low fluid intake (1–4 ml/kg/hr) compared with high fluid intake (10–20 ml/kg/hr) increases the concentration of SPC in ELF and decreases the amount of nonsedimentable proteins which increase the minimum surface tension (103).

The methods of ventilation in RDS have been extensively studied (104). According to prospective clinical trial results, initial weaning of Fio_2, followed by weaning of the distending pressures as soon as lung compliance increases, was associated with improved acute responsiveness, low incidence of barotrauma, and an improved 28-day survival without BPD (102). Similar results were obtained from paralyzed, mechanically ventilated rabbits with surfactant deficiency and high-permeability lung edema induced by BAL. Weaning of animals following natural surfactant substitution using efficient ventilation with high tidal volume (TV 11 ml/kg) and normocarbia was compared with early weaning of peak inspiratory pressures (TV 9 ml/kg) and allowance of moderate hypercarbia (Pco_2 45–55 mmHg). Efficient ventilation ("high" TV and "low" Pco_2) increased the efficacy of surfactant. In addition, it paradoxically lowered mean airway pressure requirements compared with low TV and high Pco_2. In addition, efficient ventilation decreased $[\text{nonsedimentable protein}]_{ELF}$ ($p = 0.04$), increased the distribution of heavy and ultraheavy surfactant subtypes (82 vs 59% of total surfactant in BAL) and tended to increase $(SPC)_{ELF}$. (105).

High continuous distending pressures improved responsiveness to surfactant (106,107). Weaning of high distending pressures is important too, since excessively high pressures may produce barotrauma, increase pulmonary vascular resistance, and cause abnormal ventilation-perfusion ratios (108).

Combination of Other Therapies with Surfactant Supplementation

ExtraCorporeal membrane oxygenator (ECMO) is used for treatment of mainly near-term or term infants with severe respiratory failure resistant to conventional therapy. Supplementation of exogenous surfactant to infants in ECMO is associated with an increase in the concentrations of SP-A in airway specimens and shortened treatment requirement for ECMO (43, 109). A minority of the infants had RDS, and most of the patients fulfilled the criteria of adult RDS (ARDS). The infants did not receive surfactant prior to ECMO. It is unknown at present whether "the lung rest" by ECMO was actually priming the effect of exogenous surfactant or whether early surfactant supplementation ameliorates respiratory failure, decreasing the requirement of ECMO.

PPHN is often associated with surfactant deficiency (110). Although exogenous synthetic surfactant has apparently reduced pulmonary vascular resistance in RDS (111), the attempts of surfactant therapy in PPHN have not been successful (112). Vasodilators, particularly inhaled nitric oxide (NO), have improved the gas exchange in PPHN and decreased pulmonary vascular resistance with little effect on systemic perfusion (113). Surfactant supplementation has acutely increased the gas exchange in some infants treated with NO (B. Turbow et al., unpublished results). However, NO may induce left-to-right shunt through patent ductus arteriosus, and its metabolites, $ONOO^-$, NO_2, and nitric acid, are toxic. $ONOO^-$ has been reported to catalyze oxidative inactivation of surfactant in vitro (114).

Surfactant supplementation improves gas exchange and increases lung compliance (108,115). This acute decrease in disease severity has not consistently been translated into lowering of the incidence or severity of chronic lung disease (101). Besides pulmonary surfactant, other defense systems in the immature lung are deficient and may become further compromised during intensive care. Protease/antiprotease imbalance (69), deficient antioxidative capacity (19), deficient SP-A (41), and abnormal cytokine responses (116) are among the phenomena correlating with high odds of BPD. The surfactant complex is a carrier of several antioxidant enzymes and other minor components. However, surfactants commercially available for treatment are devoid of antioxidant enzymes and hydrophilic surfactant proteins. In experimental studies, surfactant has proven to be an efficacious carrier for targeting of antibiotics and antioxidants (117–119). It remains to be studied whether this property of surfactant can be utilized for improving the therapeutic efficacy.

Acknowledgments

This work was supported by HL/HD 35036 and FDA 000112 from the U.S. Public Health Service and by the Orange County Infant Care Specialists.

References

1. Mendelson CR, Johnston JM, McDonald P, Snyder. Multihormonal regulation of surfactant synthesis by human fetal lung in vitro. J Clin Endocrinol Metab 1981; 53:307–317.
2. Post M, Smith BT. Hormonal control of surfactant metabolism. In: Robertson B, Van Golde LMG, Batenburg JJ, eds. Pulmonary Surfactant. From Molecular Biology to Clinical Practice. Amsterdam: Elsevier, 1992:379–424.
3. Clements JA, Tooley WH. Kinetics of surface-active material in the fetal lung. In: Hodson WA, ed. Development of the Lung. New York: Marcel Dekker, 1977:349–366.
4. Gluck L, Kulovich MV, Borer RC Jr, et al. The diagnosis of the respiratory distress syndrome (RDS) by amniocentesis. Am J Obstet Gynecol 1971; 109:440–445.
5. Gluck L, Kulovich MV. Lecithin/sphingomyelin ratios in amniotic fluid in normal and abnormal pregnancy. Am J Obstet Gynecol 1973; 115:539–546.

6. Hallman M. Antenatal diagnosis of lung maturity. In: Robertson B, Van Golde LMG, Batenburg JJ, eds. Pulmonary Surfactant. From Molecular Biology to Clinical Practice. Amsterdam: Elsevier, 1992:425–458.
7. Schluetter MA, Phibbs RH, Creasy RK, et al. Antenatal prediction of graduated risk of hyaline membrane disease by amniotic fluid foam test for surfactant. Am J Obstet Gynecol 1979; 134:761–767.
8. Hunink, MGM, Richardson DK, Doubilet PM, Begg CB. Testing for fetal pulmonary maturity. ROC analysis involving covariates, verification bias, and combination testing. Med Decis Making 1990; 10:201–211.
9. Lewis DF, Towers CV, Major CA, et al. Use of amniostat-FML in detecting the presence of phosphatidylglycerol in vaginal pool samples in preterm premature rupture of membranes. Am J Obstet Gynecol 1993; 169:573–576.
10. Dunn MS, Shennan AT, Zayack, Possmayer F. Bovine surfactant replacement therapy in neonates of less than 30 week's gestation: a randomized controlled trial of prophylaxis versus treatment. Pediatrics 1991; 87:377–386.
11. Kendig JW, Notter RH, Cox C, et al. A multicenter randomized trial comparing preventilatory and post-ventilatory surfactant therapy for the respiratory distress syndrome. N Engl J Med 1991; 324:865–871.
12. Kattwinkel J, Bloom BT, Delmore P, et al. Prophylactic administration of calf lung surfactant extract (CLSE) is more effective than early treatment of respiratory distress syndrome in neonates of 29 through 32 weeks' gestation. Pediatrics 1993; 92:90–98.
13. Merritt TA, Hallman M, Berry C, et al. Randomized, placebo-controlled trial of human surfactant given at birth versus rescue administration in very low birth weight infants with lung immaturity. J Pediatr 1991; 118:581–94.
14. Jobe A, Ikegami M. Surfactant for the treatment of respiratory distress syndrome. Am Rev Respir Dis 1987; 136:1256–1275.
15. Chapman DL, Widdicombe JH, Bland D. Developmental differences in the rabbit lung epithelial cell NA^+, K^{+-}ATPase. Am J Physiol 1990; 259:L481–L487.
16. Walters DV, Ramsden CA, Olver RE. Dibutyryl cAMP induces a gestation-dependent absorption of fetal lung liquid. J Appl Physiol 1990; 68:2054–2059.
17. Schellenberg J-C, Liggins GC, Kitterman JA, Lee CH. Elastin and collagen in the fetal sheep lung. II. Relationship to mechanical properties of the lung. Pediatr Res 1987; 22:339–343.
18. Bryan AC, Bryan MH. Control of respiration in the newborn. In: Thibeault DW, Gregory GA, eds. Neonatal Pulmonary Care. Norwalk, CT: Appleton-Century-Crofts. 1989:33–48.
19. Frank L. Antioxidants, nutrition, and bronchopulmonary dysplasia. Clin Perinatol 1992; 19:541–562.
20. Moses D, Holm BA, Spitale P, et al. Inhibition of pulmonary surfactant by meconium. Am J Obstet Gynecol 1991; 164:477–481.
21. Pison U, Tam EK, Caughey GH, Hawgood S. Proteolytic inactivation of dog lung surfactant-associated proteins by neutrophil elastase. Biochim Biophys Acta 1989; 992:251–257.
22. Gluck L, Kulovich MV, Eidelman AL, et al. Biochemical development of surface activity in mammalian lung. IV. Pulmonary Lecithin synthesis in the human fetus

and the newborn and etiology of respiratory distress syndrome. Pediatr Res 1972; 6:81–99.
23. Hallman M. Lung surfactant in respiratory distress syndrome. Acta Anesth Scand 1991; 35(S95):15–21.
24. Hallman M, Maasilta P, Kivisaari L, Mattson K. Changes in surfactant in bronchoalveolar lavage fluid after hemithorax irradiation in patients with mesothelioma. Am Rev Respir Dis 1990; 141:998–1005.
25. Fujiwara T, Adams FH, Schadder A. Fetal lamb amniotic fluid: Relationship of lipid composition to surface tension. J Pediatr 1964; 65:824–830.
26. Gluck L, Motoyama EK, Smits HL, Kulovich MV. The biochemical development of surface activity in mammalian lung. I. The surface-active phospholipids; the separation and distribution of surface-active lecithin in the lung of the developing rabbit fetus. Pediatr Res 1967; 1:237–246.
27. Adams FH, Fujiwara T, Emmanouilides GC. Lung phospholipids of human fetuses and infants with and without hyaline membrane disease. J Pediatr 1970; 77:833–841.
28. King, RJ, Clements JA. Surface active materials from dog lung. II. Composition and physiological correlations. Am J Physiol 1972; 223:715–726.
29. Rider ED, Ikegami M, Jobe AH. Localization of alveolar surfactant clearance in rabbits lung cells. Am J Physiol 1992; 263:L201–L209.
30. Floros J, Karinch AM. Genetics of neonatal lung disease in relation to the surfactant protein genes. In: Robertson B, Taeusch HW, eds. Surfactant Therapy for Lung Disease. New York: Marcel Dekker, 1994:95–106.
31. Hallman M, Arjomaa P, Tahvanainen J, Lachmann B, Spragg R. Endobronchial surface active phospholipids in various pulmonary diseases. Eur J Respir Dis 1985; 142:37–47.
32. Ashton MR, Postle AD, Hall MA, et al. Turnover of exogenous artificial surfactant. Arch Dis Child 1992; 67:383–387.
33. Hallman M. Treatment of established respiratory distress syndrome with surfactant. In Ekelund et al., eds. Surfactant and the respiratory tract. Amsterdam: Elsevier, 1988:187–195.
34. Effros RM, Murphy C, Ozker MK, Hacker A. Kinetics of urea exchange in air-filled and fluid-filled rat lungs. Am J Physiol 1992; 263:L619–L626.
35. Hallman M, Merritt TA, Pohjavuori M, Gluck L. Effect of surfactant substitution on lung effluent phospholipids in respiratory distress syndrome: Evaluation of surfactant phospholipid turnover, pool size, and the relationship to severity of respiratory failure. Pediatr Res 1986; 20:1228–1235.
36. Hallman, Merritt TA, Bry K. The fate of exogenous surfactant in neonates with respiratory distress syndrome. Clin Pharmacokinet 1994; 26:215–232.
37. Charon A, Taeusch W, Fitzgibbon C, et al. Factors associated with surfactant treatment response in infants with severe respiratory distress syndrome. Pediatrics 1989; 83:348–354.
38. Jobe A. Metabolism of endogenous surfactant and exogenous surfactants for replacement therapy. Semin Perinatol 1988; 12:231–244.
39. Robertson B, Kobayashi T, Ganzuka M, et al. Experimental neonatal respiratory failure induced by monoclonal antibody to the hydrophobic surfactant-associated protein SP-B. Pediatr Res 1991; 30:239–243.

40. Chida S, Phelps DS, Cordle C, et al. Surfactant-associated proteins in tracheal aspirates of infants with respiratory distress syndrome after surfactant therapy. Am Rev Respir Dis 1988; 137:943–947.
41. Hallman M, Merritt TA, Akino T, Bry K. Surfactant protein A, phosphatidylcholine and surfactant inhibitors in epithelial lining fluid: Correlation with surface activity, severity of respiratory distress syndrome and outcome of small premature infants. Am Rev Respir Dis 1991; 144:1376–1384.
42. Hallman M, Arjomaa P, Romu M, Tahvanainen J. The lung profile in diagnosis of fetal and neonatal surfactant defects. In: Vignali M, Cosmi EV, Luerti M, eds. Diagnosis and Treatment of Fetal Lung Immaturity: Proceedings of the International Workshop. Milan: Masson Italia Editori, 1986:41–49.
43. Lotze A, Whitsett JA, Kammerman LA, et al. Surfactant protein A concentrations in tracheal aspirate fluid from infants requiring extracorporeal membrane oxygenation. J Pediatr 1990; 116:435–440.
44. Hallman M, Spragg R, Harrell JH, et al. Evidence of surfactant abnormality in respiratory failure. Study of bronchoalveolar lavage phospholipids, surface activity, phospholipase activity, and plasma myoinositol. J Clin Invest 1982; 70:673–683.
45. Gregory TJ, Longmore WL, Moxley MA, et al. Surfactant chemical composition and biophysical activity in acute respiratory distress syndrome. J Clin Invest 1991; 88:1976–1981.
46. Taylor FB, Abrams ME. Effect of surface active lipoprotein on clotting and fibrinolysis, and of fibrinogen on surface tension of surface active lipoprotein. Am J Med 1965; 40:346–350.
47. Ikegami M, Jobe A, Jacobs H, Lam R. A protein from airways of premature lambs that inhibits surfactant function. J Appl Physiol 1984; 57:1134–1142.
48. Seeger W, Elssner A, Günther A, et al. Lung surfactant phospholipids associate with polymerizing fibrin: loss of surface activity. Am J Respir Cell Mol Biol 1993; 9:213–220.
49. Holm BA, Notter RH. Effects of hemoglobin and red blood cell membrane lipids on the biophysical and physiological activity of pulmonary surfactant. J Appl Physiol 1987; 63:1434–1442.
50. Rauvala H, Hallman M. Glycolipid accumulation in bronchoalveolar space in adult respiratory distress syndrome. L Lipid Res 1984; 25:1257–1262.
51. Sun B, Curstedt T, Robertson B. Surfactant inhibition in experimental meconium aspiration. Acta Pediatr 1993; 82:182–189.
52. Holm BA. Surfactant inactivation in adult respiratory distress syndrome. In: Robertson B, Van Golde LMG, Batenburg JJ, eds. Pulmonary Surfactant. From Molecular Biology to Clinical Practice. Amsterdam: Elsevier, 1992:665–684.
53. Ikegami M, Jacobs H, Jobe AH. Surfactant function in respiratory distress syndrome. J Pediatr 1983; 102:443–447.
54. Venkitaraman AR, Hall SB, Whitsett JA, et al. Enhancement of biophysical activity of synthetic phospholipid—Lung surfactant apoprotein admixtures by plasma proteins. Chem Phys Lipids 1990; 57:49–57.
55. Cockshutt AM, Weitz J, Possmayer, et al. Pulmonary surfactant-associated protein A enhances the surface activity of lipid extract surfactant and reverses inhibition by blood proteins in vitro. Biochemistry 1990; 29:8424–8429.

56. Magoon MW, Wright JR, Baritussio A, et al. Subfractionation of lung surfactant. Implications for metabolism and surface activity. Biochim Biophys Acta 1983; 750:18–31.
57. Gross NJ, Narine KR. Surfactant subtypes in mice: metabolic relationship and conversion in vitro. J Appl Physiol 1989; 67:414–421.
58. Lewis JR, Ikegami M, Jobe AH. Altered surfactant function and metabolism in rabbits with acute lung injury. J Appl Physiol 1990; 69:2303–2310.
59. Wright JR, Benson BJ, Williams MC, et al. Protein composition of rabbit alveolar surfactant subfractions. Biochim Biophys Acta 1984; 791:320–332.
60. Ikegami M, Ueda T, Absolom D, et al. Changes in exogenous surfactant in ventilated preterm lamb lungs. Am Rev Respir Dis 1993; 148:837–844.
61. Veldhuizen RAW, Inchley K, Hearn SA, et al. Degradation of surfactant-associated protein B (SP-B) during *in vitro* conversion of large to small surfactant aggregates. Biochem J 1993; 295:141–147.
62. Keough KMW. Physical chemistry of pulmonary surfactant in the terminal air spaces. In: Robertson B, Van Golde LMG, Batenburg JJ, eds. Pulmonary Surfactant. From Molecular Biology to Clinical Practice. Amsterdam: Elsevier, 1992:109–164.
63. Yamada T, Ikegami M, Tabor BL, Jobe AH. Effects of surfactant protein-A on surfactant function in preterm ventilated rabbits. Am Rev Respir Dis 1990; 142:754–757.
64. Gross NJ, Schultz RM. Requirements for extracellular metabolism of pulmonary surfactant: Tentative identification of serine protease. Am J Physiol 1992; 262: L446–L453.
65. Higuchi R, Lewis JF, Ikegami M. In vitro conversion of surfactant subtypes is altered in alveolar surfactant isolated from injured lungs. Am Rev Respir Dis 1992; 145:1416–1420.
66. Bruni R, Baritussio A, Quaglini D, et al. Postnatal transformations of alveolar surfactant in the rabbit: changes in pool size, pool morphology and isoforms of the 32-38 kDa apolipoproteins. Biochim Biophys Acta 1988; 958:255–267.
67. Jacobs H, Jobe A, Ikegami M, Jones S. Accumulation of surfactant following delivery and ventilation of premature lambs. Exp Lung Res 1985; 8:125–140.
68. Massaro D, Clerch L, Temple D, et al. Surfactant deficiency in rats without a decreased amount of extracellular surfactant. J Clin Invest 1983; 71:1536–1543.
69. Merritt TA, Cochrane CG, Holcomb K, et al. Elastase and proteinase inhibitor activity in tracheal aspirates during RDS: The role of inflammation in the pathogenesis of bronchopulmonary dysplasia. J Clin Invest 1983; 72:656–666.
70. Ryan SF, Ghassibi Y, Liau DF. Effects of activated polymorphonuclear leukocytes upon pulmonary surfactant in vitro. Am J Respir Cell Biol 1991; 4:33–41.
71. Merritt TA, Amirkhanian JD, Helbock H, et al. Reduction of the surface-tension-lowering ability of surfactant after exposure to hypochlorous acid. Biochem J 1993; 295:19–22.
72. Van Iwaarden JF, Van Golde LMG. Pulmonary surfactant and lung defense: interactions of surfactant proteins with phagocytic cells and pathogens. In: Robertson B, Taeusch HW, eds. Surfactant Therapy for Lung Disease. New York: Marcel Dekker. 1994:75–91.

73. Weaver TE, Whitsett JA. Function and regulation of expression of pulmonary surfactant-associated proteins. Biochem J 1991; 273:249–264.
74. Ballard PL, Liley HG, Gonzales LW. Interferon-gamma and synthesis of surfactant components by cultured human fetal lung. Am J Respir Cell Mol Biol 1990; 2:137–143.
75. Jacobs H, Jobe A, Ikegami M, Conaway D. The significance of reutilization of surfactant phosphatidylcholine. J Biol Chem 1983; 258:4159–4165.
76. Pettenazzo A, Jobe A, Ikegami M, Seidner S. Clearance of treatment doses of surfactant. Effect of lipid extraction and aggregate sizes. Biol Neonate 1988; 53:23–31.
77. Oguchi K, Ikegami M, Jacobs H, Jobe A. Clearance of large amounts of natural surfactants and liposomes of dipalmitoylphosphatidylcholine from the lungs of rabbits. Exp Lung Res 1985; 9:221–35.
78. Horbar JD, Wright LL, Soll RF, et al. A multicenter randomized trial comparing two surfactants for the treatment of neonatal respiratory distress syndrome. J Pediatr 1993; 123:757–766.
79. Hawgood S, Benson BJ, Schilling J, et al. Nucleotide and amino acid sequences of pulmonary surfactant protein SP18 and evidence for cooperation between SP18 and SP28-36 in surfactant lipid adsorption. Proc Natl Acad Sci USA 1987; 84:66–70.
80. Gerdes J, Whitsett J, Long W. Elastase activity and surfactant protein concentration in tracheal aspirates from neonates receiving synthetic surfactant. J Pediatr 1992; 120:S34–S39.
81. Kankaanpaa K, Hallman M. Respiratory distress syndrome in very low birth weight infants with occasionally normal surfactant phospholipids. Eur J Pediatr 1982; 139:31–34.
82. Segerer H, Stevens P, Schadow B, et al. Surfactant substitution in ventilated very low birth weight infants: Factors related to response types. Pediatr Res 1991; 30:591–96.
83. Auten R, Notter RH, Kendig JW, et al. Surfactant treatment of full-term newborns with respiratory failure. Pediatrics 1991; 87:101–107.
84. Khammash H, Perlman M, Wojtulewicz J, Dunn M. Surfactant therapy in full-term neonates with severe respiratory failure. Pediatrics 1993; 92:135–139.
85. Enhorning G, Holm BA. Disruption of pulmonary surfactant's ability to maintain openness of a narrow tube. J Appl Physiol 1993; 74:2922–2927.
86. Hallman M, Merritt TA, Kari A, Bry K. Factors affecting surfactant responsiveness. Ann Med 1991; 23:693–698.
87. Jobe AH. Pulmonary surfactant therapy. N Engl J Med 1993; 328(12):861–868.
88. Wilkinson A, Jenkins PA, Jeffrey JA. Two controlled trials of dry artificial surfactant: Early effects and later outcome in babies with surfactant deficiency. Lancet 1985; 2:287–291.
89. Nogee LM, DeMello DE, Dehner LP, Colten HR. Brief report: Deficiency of pulmonary surfactant protein B in congenital alveolar proteinosis. N Engl J Med 1993; 328:406–410.
90. Hamvas A, Cole FS, deMello D, et al. Inherited surfactant protein-B (SP-B) deficiency: Effects of surfactant replacement. Pediatr Res 1993; 33:328A.

91. Schellenberg J-C, Liggins GC, Kitterman JA, Lee CCH. Sympathectomy and β-adrenergic blockade during lung maturation stimulated by TRH and cortisol in fetal sheep. J Appl Physiol 1993; 75:141–147.
92. Moya FR, Gross I. Combined hormonal therapy for the prevention of respiratory distress syndrome and its consequences. Semin Perinatol 1993; 17:267–274.
93. Ballard RA, Ballard RL, Creasy RK, et al. Respiratory disease in very-low-birthweight infants after prenatal thyrotropin-releasing hormone and glucocorticoid. Lancet 1992; 339:510–515.
94. Ikegami M, Berry D, ElKady T, et al. Corticosteroids and surfactant change lung function and protein leaks in the lungs of ventilated premature rabbits. J Clin Invest 1987; 79:1371–1378.
95. Schellenberg J-C, Liggins GC, Stewart AW. Growth, elastin concentration, and collagen concentration of perinatal rat lung: effects of dexamethasone. Pediatr Res 1987; 21:603–607.
96. Ballard PL. Hormonal regulation of pulmonary surfactant. Endocrinol Rev 1989; 10:165–181.
97. Frank L, Lewis P, Sosenko IRS. Dexamethasone stimulates fetal rat lung antioxidant enzyme activity in parallel with surfactant stimulation. Pediatrics 1985; 75:569–574.
98. Kari A, Hallman M, Eronen M, et al. Prenatal dexamethasone treatment in conjunction with rescue therapy of human surfactant—A randomized placebo-controlled multicenter study. Pediatrics 1994; 93:730–736.
99. Enhorning G, Grossman G, Robertson B. Tracheal deposition of surfactant before the first breath. Am Rev Respir Dis 1973; 107:921–927.
100. Jobe A, Ikegami M, Glatz T, et al. Duration and characteristics of treatment of premature lambs with natural surfactant. J Clin Invest 1981; 67:370–375.
101. Merritt TA, Soll RF, Hallman M. Overview of exogenous surfactant replacement therapy. J Intens Care Med 1993; 8:205–228A
102. Hallman M, Merritt TA, Bry K, Berry C. Association between neonatal care practices and efficacy of exogenous human surfactant: Results of a bicenter randomized trial. Pediatrics 1993; 91:552–560.
103. Hallman M, Barsotti M, Chundu V, et al. Relationship between fluid intake and the responsiveness to surfactant. Pediatr Res 1990; 27:305A.
104. DeLemos RA. Ventilator strategies in relation to surfactant replacement. In: Robertson B, Taeusch HW, eds. Surfactant Therapy for Lung Disease. New York: Marcel Dekker, 1994.
105. Goldstein M, Hallman M, Slivka S, Stevens J. Surfactant responsiveness: comparison of two ventilation strategies. Am Rev Respir Dis 1993; 147:A719.
106. Rider ED, Jobe AH, Ikegami M, Sun B. Different ventilation strategies alter surfactant responses in preterm rabbits. J Appl Physiol 1992; 73:2089–2096.
107. Lachmann B. Open up the lung and keep the lung open. Intens Care Med 1992; 18:319–321.
108. Goldsmith LS, Greenspan JS, Rubenstein SD, et al. Immediate improvement in lung volume after exogenous surfactant: Alveolar recruitment versus increased distension. J Pediatr 1991; 119:424–428.
109. Lotze A, Knight GR, Martin GR, et al. Improved pulmonary outcome after

exogenous surfactant therapy for respiratory failure in term infants requiring extracorporeal membrane oxygenation. J Pediatr 1993; 122:161–268.
110. Hallman M, Kankaanpää K. Evidence of surfactant deficiency in persistence of pulmonary hypertension. Eur J Pediatr 1980; 134:129–134.
111. Kaapa P, Seppanen M, Kero P, Saraste M. Pulmonary hemodynamics after synthetic surfactant replacement in neonatal respiratory distress syndrome. J Pediatr 1993; 123:115–119.
112. Fujiwara T, Robertson B. Pharmacology of exogenous surfactant. In: Robertson B, Van Golde LMG, Batenburg JJ, eds. Pulmonary Surfactant. From Molecular Biology to Clinical Practice. Amsterdam: Elsevier 1992:561–592.
113. Kinsella JP, Neish SR, Shaffer E, Abman SH. Low dose inhalational nitric oxide therapy in persistent pulmonary hypertension of the newborn. Lancet 1992; 340:819–820.
114. Matalon S, Myles C, Ischiropoulos H, et al. Peroxynitrite inhibition of surface activity of surfactant mixtures. Am Rev Respir Dis 1993; 147:A490.
115. Svenningsen NW. Pulmonary functional residual capacity and lung mechanics in surfactant-treated infants. Semin Perinatol 1992; 16:181–185.
116. Groneck P, Reuss D, Gotze-Speer B, Speer CP. Effects of dexamethasone on chemotactic activity and inflammatory mediators in tracheobronchial aspirates of preterm infants at risk for chronic lung disease. J Pediatr 1993; 122:938–944.
117. Kharasch VS, Sweeney TD, Fredberg J, et al. Pulmonary surfactant as a vehicle to intratracheal delivery of technetium sulfur colloid and pentamidine in hamster lungs. Am Rev Respir Dis 1991; 144:909–913.
118. Davis JM, Rosenfeld WN, Koo H-C, Gonenne A. Pharmacologic Interactions of exogenous lung surfactant and recombinant human Cu/Zn superoxide dismutase. Pediatr Res 1994; 35:37–44.
119. Walther FJ, David-Cu R, Supnet MC, et al. Uptake of antioxidants in surfactant liposomes by cultured alveolar type II cells is enhanced by SP-A. Am J Physiol 1993; 265:L330–L339.
120. Hallman M, Feldman BH, Kirkpatrick E, et al. Absence of phosphatidylglycerol (PG) in respiratory distress syndrome in the newborn. Study of the minor surfactant phospholipids in newborns. Pediatr Res 1977; 11:714–720.
121. Obladen M, Gluck L. RDS and tracheal phospholipid composition in twins: Independent of gestational age. J Pediatr 1977; 90:799–802.
122. Shelley SA, Kovacevic M, Paciga JE, Balis JU. Sequential changes of surfactant phosphatidylcholine in hyaline-membrane disease of the newborn. N Engl J Med 1979; 300:112–116.

17

Prediction of Mechanical Responses to Surfactant Therapy

JON GOERKE
University of California, San Francisco
San Francisco, California

I. Introduction

A. Overview

The purpose of this chapter is to relate the surface activity of pulmonary surfactant, lung tissue forces, and any applied ventilatory pattern to resultant lung mechanics. Because this is more than a back of the envelope calculation, we have created a special computer program to calculate a model for our discussion. As we proceed we hope to make the point that surfactant properties, tissue forces, and ventilator settings interact in important ways, and that no one of them can be considered in isolation. This effort is made all the more necessary by the continued introduction of new and potentially effective surfactant substitutes for use in treating the respiratory distress syndrome of the newborn and other clinical problems (1–3). A means of connecting in vitro surfactant and tissue behavior to overall lung mechanics would therefore be very useful. We hope to convince the reader that this model can provide a bridge between this book's Chapter 1 by Schürch and Bachofen (9) dealing with surfactant properties and Chapter 7 by Cotton and Olsson (21), dealing with lung mechanics in the respiratory distress syndrome.

B. Background

We have known about the role of surface forces in the lung since von Neergaard's seminal publication of 1929 (4), in which he demonstrated the important contribution of alveolar surface tension to lung retractile force. He did this by showing that inflation pressures were remarkably decreased when the alveolar air-water interface was abolished by fluid filling. In his paper, von Neergaard explicitly invoked the law of Laplace: $P = 2\ \gamma/r$, where P is the pressure gradient across a spherical interface, γ is surface tension, and r is the radius of curvature. This law, sometimes in a more general form, continues to underlie any discussion of alveolar mechanics (5), and it is still the basis for what is described below.

II. Description of the Model

A. Surfactant Properties Included in the Model

Since the time of von Neergaard we have come to realize that a number of surfactant properties influence lung mechanics, and we must consider some of these. In particular, new in vitro techniques to measure surfactant behavior have allowed us to assess kinetic properties that had not been quantitatively considered before (6–8). Of course, the ability to generate a low, quasi-static surface tension upon compression is the first and most important consideration for any surfactant. A quantitative statement of this ability is the surfactant's surface tension–area isotherm that describes just how such low tensions are achieved. Monolayer compressibility at a surface tension of 15 mN/m can be calculated directly from such isotherms, and is given by $C = (dA/d\gamma)\ /\ A$, where $(dA/d\gamma)$ is the inverse slope of the surface tension (Y axis) versus area (X axis) isotherm at area A corresponding to surface tension 15 mN/m. The best lung surfactants will have a very low compressibility in this region; that is, only a very small decrease in alveolar area on expiration will be necessary in order to drive surface tension down to the very low level where it promotes alveolar stability. This is reflected in the surface tension versus area isotherm being steep in the usual operating region between surface tensions of 0 and 30 mN/m. On the other hand, an abnormally high compressibility will require that expiration be continued to lower alveolar areas (and of course, volumes, too) to reach comparably low surface tensions. For the model below, we have assumed a compression (and expansion) isotherm nearly identical to that described by Schürch and Bachofen in Figure 8A of Chapter 1 (9). We believe that data obtained with the captive bubble surfactometer apparatus are the most reliable (6,8). We also take into account the rapidity with which surfactant in the bulk forms a monolayer. Here we use an adsorption rate constant, k_{ads}, described in the relation $dn = k_{ads}\ A\ (\gamma - \gamma_{eq})\ dt$, where dn is the increment of material entering the monolayer, A is the area of the monolayer, γ is the instantaneous surface tension, γ_{eq} is the equilibrium surface tension for the surfactant in question, and dt is the time increment. The relation states that surfactant entry into the film occurs only when film surface tension is above the equilibrium value, a finding that is confirmed in surface balance experiments. This process is well demonstrated in Fig. 5 of Chapter 1 (9). The desorption rate constant, k_{des}, is described by a similar relation, dn = k_{des} A $(\gamma - \gamma_{eq})$ dt. The desorption equation states in an analogous fashion that desorption occurs only when $\gamma < \gamma_{eq}$. When $\gamma < \gamma_{eq}$, only the adsorption equation is used, and dn is positive, and conversely for desorption. Since there are no published values using these particular equations, we chose values for the normal state so as to achieve reasonably normal lung mechanics, and then varied these values for pathological states. The key role for γ_{eq} should be emphasized: It forms the dividing line between adsorption and desorption of surfactant.

B. Major Characteristics of the Surfactant/Ventilation Model

The model to be described is a minimalist one: It considers only the bare necessities and even simplifies those. It was written for the Macintosh II family of computers (Apple, Cupertino, CA) using the "G" language of LabVIEW (National Instruments, Austin, TX), which was designed initially for data collection and manipulation but serves admirably as a modeling medium. Its easy display of graphical output is particularly convenient for this task.

C. Specific Features Included in the Model

Input to and Relationships in the Model

As intimated above, the model considers input and functions related to surface and tissue phenomena and to ventilatory interventions.

First, we consider the following surface-related features. In addition to the assumed surfactant isotherm and surface compliance mentioned above, we chose to fix the radius of the alveolar ring opening at 51.3 μm. We also decided not to consider monolayer collapse during overcompression, inasmuch as alveolar area seems not to decrease much below functional residual capacity (FRC) in vivo (10), and collapse would be limited to the end of expiration following relatively rare breaths to total lung capacity (TLC). We postulate an equilibrium surface tension for lung surfactant of 25 mN/m, close to that measured in in vitro systems (11) and demonstrated in Fig. 5 of Chapter 1 (9). We keep track of the amount of surfactant in the interface as an intermediate and output variable, and we use values of 5.0 m/(cm^2 mN sec) for normal k_{ads} and 1 $\times$ 10^{-6} m/(cm^2 mN sec) for normal k_{des}.

As to lung tissue forces, we consider these to be represented by an assumed pressure-volume fluid–filling curve (12–15). We are aware that in so doing, we are ignoring the fact that different shapes during air and fluid filling mean that tissue forces are not identical in the two states (10,16). This same relationship also presupposes a limiting maximum volume for the alveolus (2.03×10^{-6} cm^3). Practically speaking, this limits the alveolar radius to values less than 80 μm.

Alveolar volume and area are calculated as for a sector of a sphere. Airway and tissue resistances to flow are taken to be a single constant, 1×10^8 cmH_2O sec/cm^3, which (unrealistically) does not vary with volume.

The model is driven by an impressed pressure wave, with the program choosing suitable values of alveolar radius for calculating pressures that match the target wave with a specifiable error (normally 0.01 cmH_2O). The pressure wave is described by a frequency (normal = 1/sec), inspiratory/expiratory time ratio (0.3/0.7), peak inspiratory pressure (32 cmH_2O on a TLC breath, 10 cmH_2O on subsequent tidal breaths), and end-expiratory pressure (4 cmH_2O). The overall character of the wave was chosen to match the profile of pressure-driven infant respirators.

Output of the Model

For output we calculated the time course of inflation pressure, alveolar volume, alveolar area, alveolar radius, amount of surfactant in the monolayer, and the surface tension of monolayer. Suitable plots of these variables were provided at the end of each run for immediate inspection, and a table of values was stored on disk as an Excel spreadsheet file (Microsoft, Redmond, WA) for further analysis and paper plots.

D. Features Not Included in the Model

A more complete model would not be necessary to illustrate the essential contributions of lung surfactant to lung mechanics. It is important to realize, however, what we have left out, since some of these features will modify surfactant's overall effect. Here are the caveats.

We have first of all considered only pressure-driven respirations, inasmuch as these represent the normal breathing mode and much of ventilatory therapy. A volume-driven pattern, for example, might prove more efficient in treating slow surfactant adsorption.

Any contribution of alveolar duct or conducting airway to volume and pressure behavior have been ignored, even though these would be substantial, particularly at high surface tensions. The closely associated expandability of alveolar opening rings, an important determinant of both alveolar and alveolar duct behavior, is also not included.

Only one size of alveolar has been tested, whereas smaller or larger ones would have behaved quantitatively differently. In this same context, interdependence between adjacent alveolar units has not been considered, although this phenomenon might well ameliorate the effect of surfactant deficiencies arising in a fraction of alveoli within an interdependent group (17).

As mentioned above, the treatment of resistance is physiologically naive, and there has been no attempt to include viscoelastic behavior.

More to the point, some aspects of surfactant itself have not been considered: (1) variability of the surfactant isotherm with inspiration and expiration (expansion and compression), and as might occur with occupancy of the monolayer by a changing mixture of surfactant components; (2) possible selective adsorption rates of different surfactant components; (3) surfactant inhibition, except as is reflected in the parameters used; and (4) concentration of surfactant in the aqueous subphase and its influence on adsorption rate.

III. Results from Running the Model

Caveats aside, how does the model perform under "normal" and pathological settings of the parameters?

A. Normal Baseline Behavior for Comparison

Figure 1 shows the typical pressure pattern driving the model. The alveolus is first inflated from the "airless" (flat bubble) state to TLC. This is followed by deflation to the predetermined end-expiratory pressure (at FRC) and then by one to four tidal

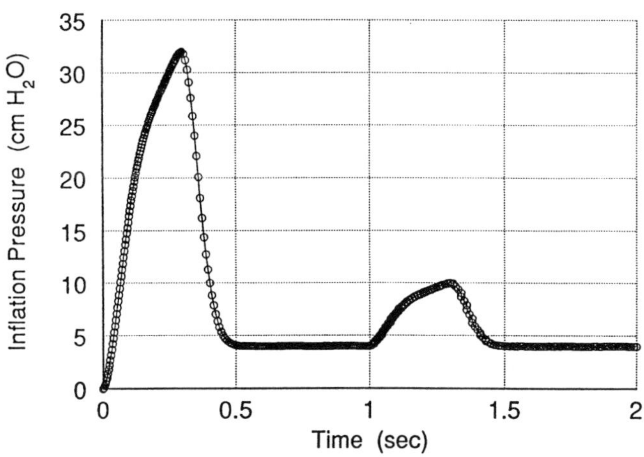

Figure 1 Inflation pressure waveform driving the model. The first breath is usually an inspiration to a pressure of 32 cmH_2O followed by deflation to an end-expiratory pressure of 4 cmH_2O (so-called TLC breath). Thereafter a variable number of tidal breaths cycle between this end-expiratory pressure and a peak inspiratory pressure of either 10 or 32 cmH_2O. The basic rate is 60 breaths/min. Individual points in this figure and most others are 0.03 sec apart during inspiration and 0.07 sec apart during expiration.

breaths. The discrete steps taken during inspiration (0.03 sec) and expiration (0.07 sec) give a qualitative impression of the rate of change of variables in this and other plots. The resultant pressure-volume (PV) curve is shown in Figure 2, where the tidal volume loop shows only a minimal hysteresis at most. Note the rapidity of volume change in the initial inflation, centered on a pressure of approximately 17 cmH_2O. The obviously large pressure-volume hysteresis of the TLC loop is primarily due to surface tension differences during inspiration versus expiration as is shown below. Though not explicitly shown, the workings of the model assures us that the lung is kept from overinflation by restraining tissue forces: above the hemispherical shape; the lung would otherwise expand without limit.

Figure 3 shows how volume and alveolar radius change with time. The volume tracing is not surprising (except for our choice of a tidal volume nearly two times normal), but the early radial dance may seem so. Starting with an infinite radius in the flat alveolus at time zero, the radius *falls* with inflation until the hemisphere is reached and then behaves in a more dignified manner by rising and falling with volume during tidal breathing. Note that minimum alveolar radius occurs at the time of the greatest slope in the volume-time curve. This region of the plot is the model equivalent of alveolar "opening," not exactly a step change, but a very fast one nevertheless. We show the forces behind these volume and radius effects in Figure 4. This shows a maximal working amount of surfactant being *rapidly* recruited into the monolayer during inspiration to TLC, and the *very slow* decrease in that amount during tidal breathing. No further surfactant recruitment will occur until another large breath supervenes, implying

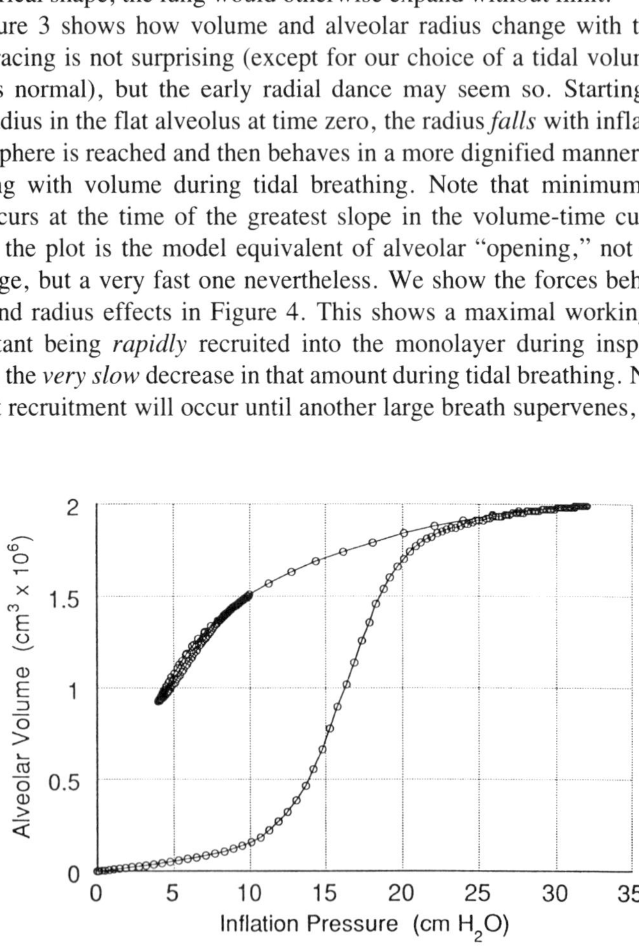

Figure 2 Normal surfactant: Pressure-volume diagram describing a TLC breath followed by a tidal breath for a normal alveolus driven by the pressure wave of Fig. 1.

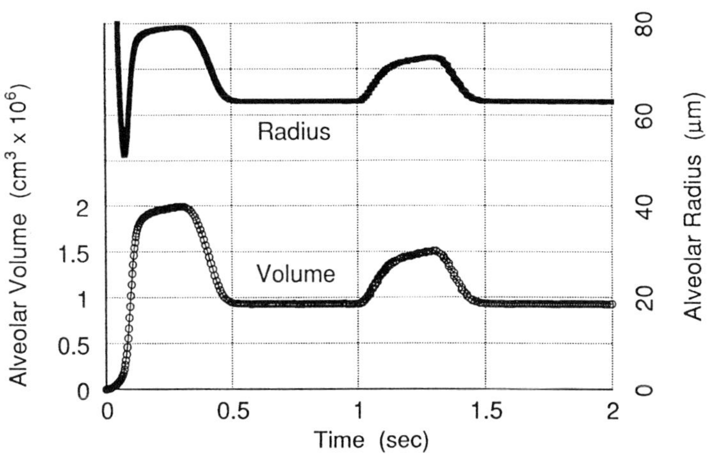

Figure 3 Normal surfactant: Radius and volume of the normal alveolus depicted in Figs. 1, 2, and 4 versus time.

that surface surfactant turnover is normally a slow process. All during the first inspiration, surface tension sits at the equilibrium value, because surfactant is adsorbing as fast as the alveolar area is changing, keeping its surface concentration constant. Once area begins decreasing with expiration; however, the very much slower exit of material from the monolayer allows surfactant concentration

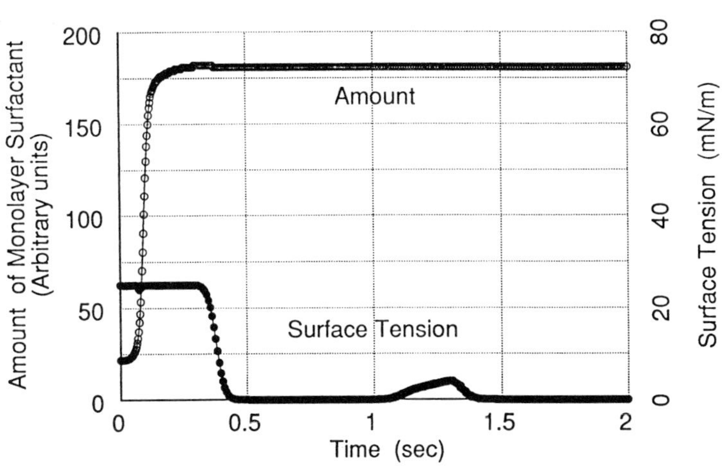

Figure 4 Normal surfactant: Amount of surfactant and surface tension in the monolayer of the normal alveolus depicted in Figs. 1, 2, and 3 versus time.

to increase and hence surface tension to decrease. In the normal lung, this probably produces near-zero surface tensions. During the tidal breath, area increases slightly, but no new surfactant can adsorb, because surface tension is still below the equilibrium value of 25 mN/m. Thus, during tidal breathing in this model, surface tension cycles between 0 and about 10 mN/m.

B. Selected Surfactant Abnormalities

Nonideal Surfactant Isotherms

Now we will discuss some pathological states. Using surface tension–area isotherms with surface compressibilities ranging from 0.005 to 0.02 m/mN at a surface tension of 15 mN/m, we were able to show a moderate decrease in FRC at the higher compressibilities (results not shown). When surface compressibility was higher than 0.02 m/mN, FRC fell much lower, indicating the importance of this factor in mechanical performance. The publication of isotherms with high compressibilities on the first compression, even with improvement on subsequent compressions (see Figs. 4 and 5 of ref. 2) makes one retrospectively question the experimental methods used to obtain these data (18). The surfactants themselves may have been perfectly functional in such studies, but either the effective concentration employed or the surface balances used may have been inadequate. As can be seen in Figures 3 and 6 of Chapter 1 (9), values of surface compliance

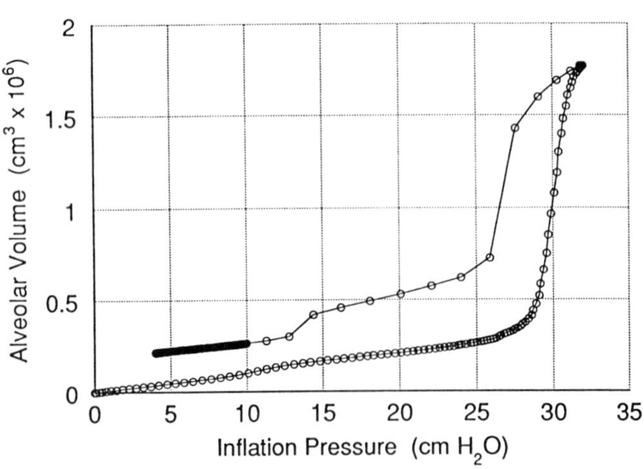

Figure 5 Slowly adsorbing surfactant: Pressure-volume diagram describing a TLC breath followed by four tidal breaths for an alveolus with slowly adsorbing surfactant. It is driven by a pressure waveform similar to that of Fig. 1, but with four tidal breaths. The adsorption rate constant, k_{ads}, is 5×10^{-5}.

in the neighborhood of 0.007 m/mN are obtainable on the first monolayer compression in the captive bubble surfactometer with satisfactory surfactants.

Slow Adsorption

Abnormally slow surfactant adsorption to the air-water interface can be devastating to lung function, particularly with our above "normal" ventilatory pattern. The next two figures tell the story for a low adsorption rate constant ($k_{ads} = 5 \times 10^{-5}$, our "normal" $k_{ads} = 5.0$) in an alveolus taken first to 32 cmH_2O and then cycled between 4 and 10 cmH_2O for "tidal" breathing. Figure 5 is the PV loop (cf. Fig. 2), and it shows alveolar opening to be delayed until a pressure of 30 cmH_2O has been applied. This opening is transient, however, and the alveolus closes again at about 27 cmH_2O and stays closed during tidal breathing. In Figure 6 (cf. Fig. 4), we see the cause of this malfunction: Only a small fraction of a working monolayer has been recruited during the first breath, and even with area compression during expiration, surface tension remains above 9 mN/m at "FRC." At this juncture, k_{ads} looks to be an extremely important property by which to judge a lung surfactant, but see below.

Rapid Desorption

Equally deleterious to lung function is an unstable monolayer, characterized by a higher than normal surface desorption rate (e.g., $k_{des} = 2 \times 10^{-4}$ versus normal $k_{des} = 1 \times 10^{-6}$). Figure 7 shows the PV diagram (cf. Fig. 2) for the same

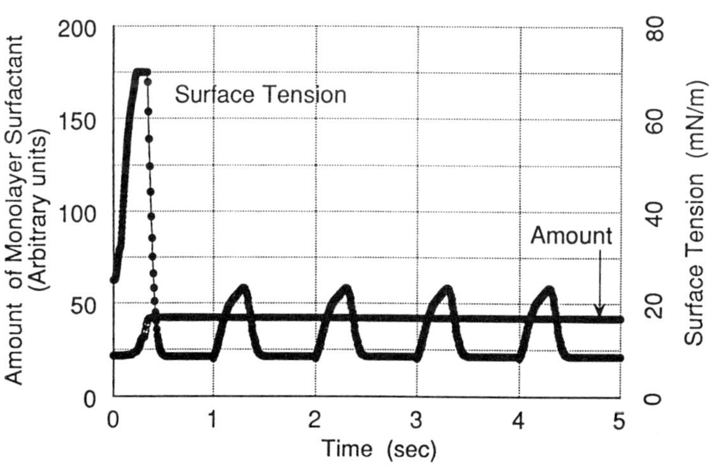

Figure 6 Slowly adsorbing surfactant: Amount of surfactant and surface tension in the monolayer of the alveolus with slowly adsorbing surfactant depicted in Fig. 5 versus time.

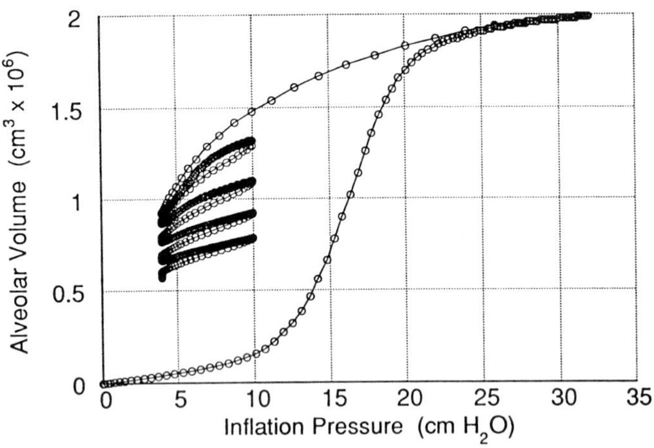

Figure 7 Rapidly desorbing surfactant: Pressure-volume diagram describing a TLC breath followed by four tidal breaths for an alveolus with rapidly desorbing surfactant. The model is driven by a pressure waveform similar to that of Fig. 1, but with four tidal breaths. The desorption rate constant, k_{des}, is 2×10^{-4}.

ventilatory pattern as above: One high-pressure breath followed by four tidal breaths. TLC is achieved with ease, but once FRC is reached, the monolayer literally slips away during tidal breathing, with FRC eventually decreasing to ineffective values even lower than shown after the first four tidal breaths. Again, the reasons behind this performance can be seen in the surface amount and surface tension time plots (Fig. 8; cf. Fig. 4) in which monolayer surfactant decreases as surface tension rises. It is also instructive to see the relative effects of surface desorption rate, k_{des}, on the amount of surfactant lost from the monolayer in four tidal breaths. Figure 9 is such a plot, showing that much above $k_{des} = 2 \times 10^{-5}$, replacement of such losses by frequent breaths to TLC would result in an unsatisfactorily high surfactant turnover. Clearly, surfactant monolayer stability must be a critical parameter for lung function if desorbed material cannot easily reenter the monolayer.

Soluble Detergent–like Behavior

This behavior can be either good or bad. By combining rapid adsorption with rapid desorption, one creates a fascinating kind of surfactant, one example of which is a common, water-soluble laundry detergent. This product gets into clothing fabric easily, and leaves with equal facility (hopefully taking the dirt with it). Figure 10 shows what might happen if such agents were to replace our natural surfactant in the lung. Experiments doing just this have been performed

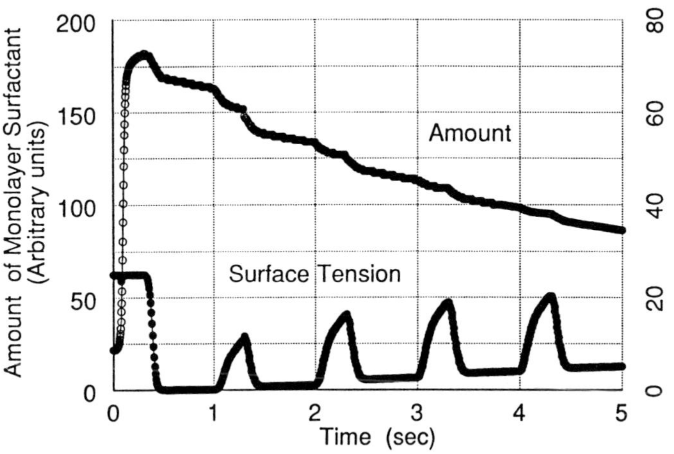

Figure 8 Rapidly desorbing surfactant: Amount of surfactant and surface tension in the monolayer of the alveolus with rapidly desorbing surfactant depicted in Figs. 7 and 9 versus time.

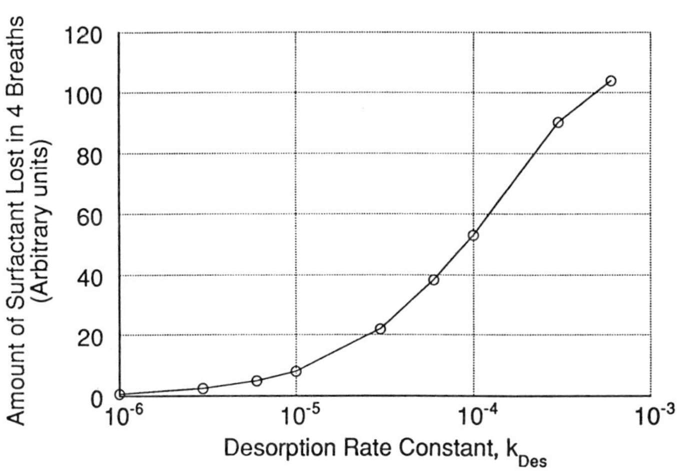

Figure 9 Rapidly desorbing surfactant: Amount of surfactant lost in the first 4 tidal breaths from the monolayers of alveoli with variously desorbing surfactants versus desorption rate, k_{des}.

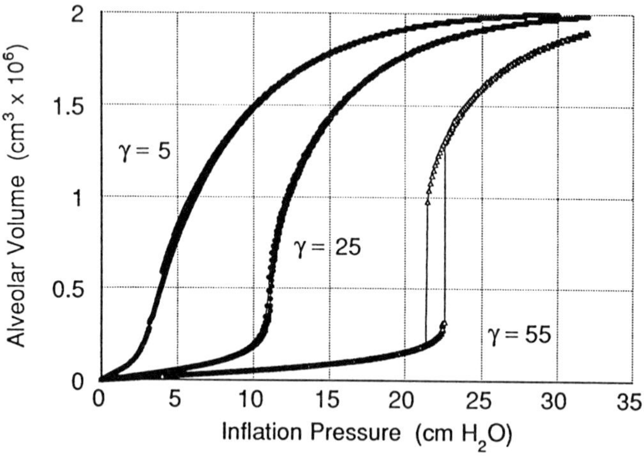

Figure 10 Detergent-like behavior: Pressure-volume diagrams describing ventilation between pressures of 32 and 4 cmH_2O for alveoli with surfactants that both adsorb and desorb rapidly. The pressure waveform is similar to that of Fig. 1, but with no tidal breaths. Equilibrium surface tension (indicated on the graph as γ in mN/m) differs for the three breaths. The breath at $\gamma = 55$ mN/m shows appreciable hysteresis, whereas it was minimal for the other two curves. Point interval for all curves was 0.00015 sec on inspiration and 0.00035 sec on deflation to achieve greater resolution for these plots than for all others.

since the 1950s (12,15,19) and have taught us much about surfactant function in the lung. Examples of detergent curves from Hoppin et al. (20) are reproduced in Chapter 7 (21). In our Figure 10, the rapid adsorption and desorption result in constant, equilibrium surface tensions (γ_{eq}) of 5, 25 and 55 mN/m. In our examples, the single TLC PV loops shown for the lower two surface tensions show minimal hysteresis.

In the case of $\gamma = 55$ mN/m, a return to an inflating pressure of 0.5 cmH_2O is also recorded, because there was evident hysteresis. In these particular examples, airway/tissue resistance was set to zero so as to eliminate flow as a cause of hysteresis. We begin to see a real, abrupt "opening" of the alveolus at the highest surface tension because of inaccessible reverse curvatures in the PV diagram. Such jumping behavior could have been eliminated, and the reverse curvature shown, by stepwise volume inflation of this alveolus, and this can be demonstrated by inflating isolated lungs. This latter phenomenon is well demonstrated in Figures 1 and 3 of Chapter 7 (21), where data from Hoppin et al. (20) and Clements et al. (22), respectively, have been plotted. Soluble detergent–like behavior at this high end of this scale ($\gamma = 55$ mN/m) is a reasonable mimic of the situation obtaining in lungs that are very surfactant deficient. Presumably in these lungs such proteins and unsaturated lipids as are present in the alveolar subphase enter and leave the interface with relative ease, never allowing the surface tension to be driven below 55 or so mN/m. The result would be a collapsed lung that could be opened only with extremely high inflating pressures.

The $\gamma = 25$ mN/m curve of Figure 10, on the other hand, might represent a lung surfactant that adsorbed well but was unstable when compressed below its equilibrium value (γ_{eq}), or equivalently, it could represent a lung surfactant that could not be compressed below its equilibrium surface tension. The $\gamma = 25$ mN/m curve also suggests that an end-expiratory pressure in the neighborhood of 12 cmH_2O combined with an EIP about 3 cmH_2O higher might produce reasonably normal values for FRC and tidal volume, and a model run (not shown) bears this out. Somewhere between a γ_{eq} of 5 and 25 mN/m is an interesting region, perhaps populated by the perfluorinated substances used in fluorocarbon-breathing therapy (23,24). These substances have a low surface tension against air (25). If no other substantial force–contributing interfaces were present in inflated alveoli, ventilation with γ near 25 mN/m is a possibility, as indicated above.

C. Selected Ventilatory Patterns for Treating Surfactant Malfunctions

Increasing Peak Inspiratory Pressure to the Pressure at Normal TLC to Treat Slow Surfactant Adsorption

By referring to Figure 2, it is easy to visualize the PV loops that would result from ventilating the model from 0 to 32 cmH_2O and then between 4 and 32 cmH_2O using normal surfactant parameters. This mode of therapy is a natural for situations where surfactant is slowly, but eventually completely, adsorbing to the air-water interface. The PV diagram for the untreated situation, with $k_{ads} = 5 \times 10^{-5}$, is shown above in Figure 5, and the same alveolus ventilated to 32 cmH_2O is shown in Figure 11. As can be seen, FRC is rising with each breath, and very few seconds of ventilation will be required to reach a normal-appearing curve. This is important, because one could then switch to tidal breathing and maintain normal mechanics for several minutes until it was necessary to "recharge" the system again with a few more breaths to high peak-inspiratory pressure. Continual application of such high peak inspiratory pressures in patients would lead to bronchopulmonary dysplasia (1). Again, the action behind this favorable result is shown in the time courses of surfactant amount and surface tension displayed in Figure 12. Compare this with the untreated situation shown in Figure 6. In only five breaths, we have recruited more than half the surfactant to the monolayer necessary to ensure normal function. Figure 13 illustrates the effect of such therapy at different values of k_{ads}. The open circles plot FRC after the first breath at each adsorption rate, and the closed circles plot the rise in FRC

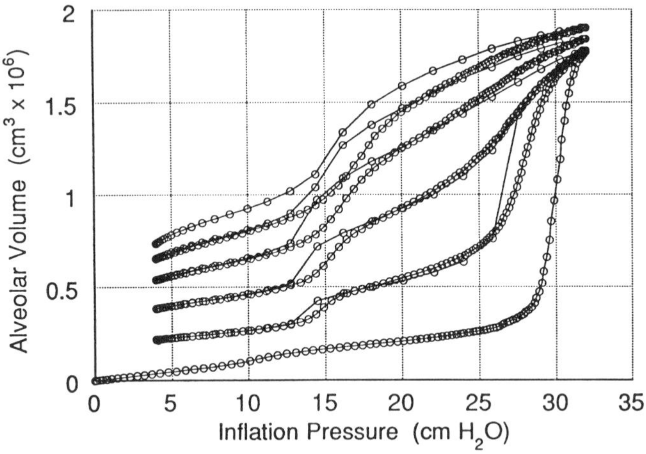

Figure 11 Treated slow adsorption: Pressure-volume diagram describing five sequential breaths to TLC for an alveolus with slowly adsorbing surfactant. It is driven by a pressure waveform similar to the first breath of Fig. 1. The adsorption rate constant, k_{ads}, is 5×10^{-5}.

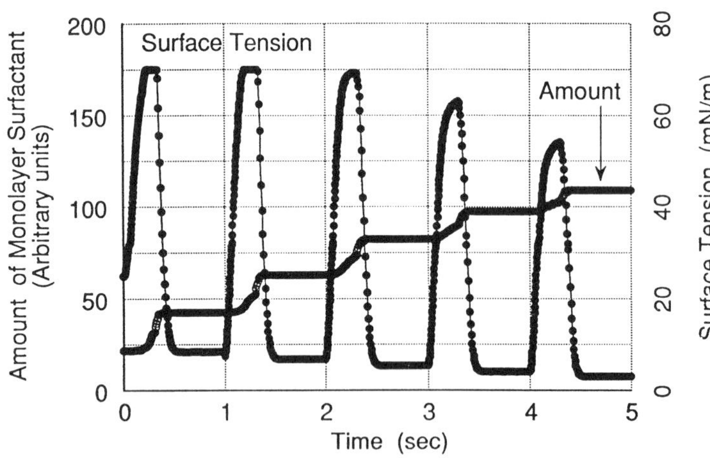

Figure 12 Treated slow adsorption: Amount of surfactant and surface tension in the monolayer of the alveolus with slowly adsorbing surfactant depicted in Fig. 11 versus time.

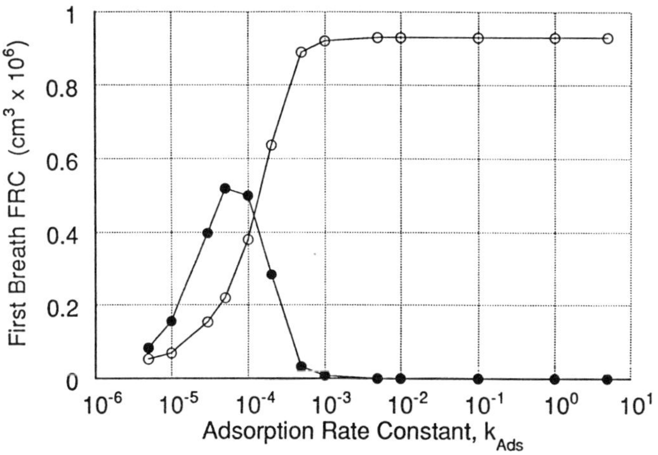

Figure 13 Treated slow adsorption: The open circles plot FRC after the first breath to 32 cmH_2O over a range of adsorption rates, k_{ads}. The closed circles plot the rise in FRC over the subsequent four breaths to the same high inflation pressure for the same set of k_{ads}.

over the subsequent four cycles. It appears that a normal FRC could be easily achieved with a few breaths, even with adsorption rates slower than that of Figures 11 and 12. It is interesting that a plot of first breath FRC versus surfactant amount is nearly linear up to a normal FRC value (data not shown), reflecting how tightly coupled FRC is to surfactant amount.

Varying End-Expiratory Pressure with Normal Surfactant

This pattern of model ventilation provides one breath from 0 to 32 cmH_2O, followed by four breaths between sets of end-expiratory pressures (EEP) ranging from 2 to 20 cmH_2O and peak-inspiratory pressures (PIP) 6 cmH_2O higher, all using normal surfactant parameters. This scheme effectively aborts deflation at a higher "FRC" (end-expired volume) for each run. A more clinically effective pattern would have tried to maintain ventilation reasonably constant at each setting by increasing both frequency and PIP to counteract the progressively lower tidal volumes inherent in this scheme. The effect of the entire set can be seen by following the upper, deflation PV curve of Figure 2 but substituting FRC for volume and EEP for pressure.

Figure 14 shows an interesting byproduct of varying EEP: Higher EEPs are generally associated with decreasing losses from the interface over the first four tidal breaths. Note that even the highest rate of loss represents only 0.5% of a full

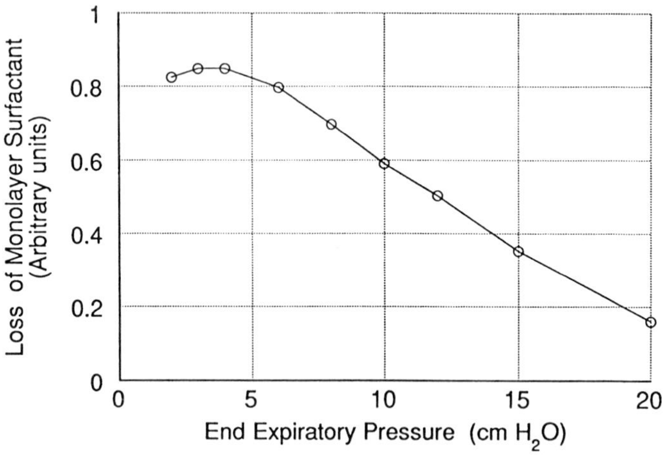

Figure 14 Normal surfactant, varying end-expiratory pressure: Loss of monolayer surfactant during the first four tidal breaths following an initial breath to 32 cmH_2O versus end-expiratory pressure. The model is driven by a pressure waveform similar to that of Fig. 1 but with four tidal breaths.

alveolar monolayer in four breaths. In retrospect, our choice of 10^{-6} for a normal k_{des} may have still been slightly high, since this would have produced more rapidly decreasing FRCs and lung compliances (26,27) and more rapidly desorbing alveolar monolayers (28) than have been measured. One also finds that these decreased losses at higher EEP are associated with elevations in the maximum and minimum surface tensions during tidal breathing; in fact it is these higher surface tensions that cause the lower losses, since the rate of surface loss is taken to be proportional to the difference between γ and γ_{eq}. Note that if γ were to become greater than γ_{eq}, the loss would be succeeded by a gain, as we shall see below.

Increasing End-Expiratory Pressure to Treat Increased Desorption Rate

One can indeed replace a potential loss by a gain by using increased end-expiratory pressure. Consider our case of a high desorption rate ($k_{des} = 2 \times 10^{-4}$) using the same single large breath followed by four tidal breaths as before, but employing an EEP of 8 cmH_2O. The PV diagram of Figure 15 tells the story. Compare it with Figure 7, where k_{des} is the same, but EEP = 4 cmH_2O, and FRC continues to decrease with each breath. With increased EEP, FRC rapidly comes to a steady-state at a normal level, which is associated here with a normal tidal volume because of our choice of a somewhat elevated PIP as well. Further increases in EEP would be counterproductive, providing unnecessarily higher values of FRC.

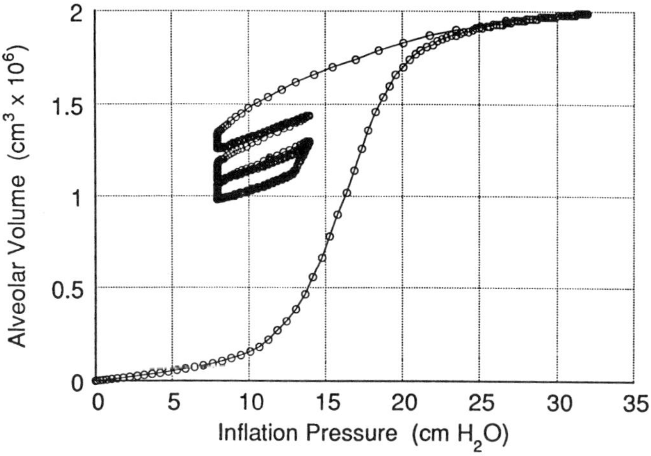

Figure 15 Treated rapid desorption: Pressure-volume diagram describing one breath to TLC followed by four tidal breaths down to an end-expiratory pressure of 8 cmH_2O, for an alveolus with rapidly desorbing surfactant. The desorption rate constant, k_{des}, is 2×10^4.

By inspecting plots of surfactant amount over the first few tidal cycles at this same k_{des} and EEP (Fig. 16), one can see that there is no net loss of surfactant in the steady state. It is evident, however, that a substantial surfactant turnover may have arisen as new surfactant material adsorbs during inspiration and is lost during expiration. We say "may have arisen" because some claim that material lost from the interface must be repackaged by type II cells before it can reenter the monolayer (29), and others have evidence that it can respread (30). Note that in this case the increments of monolayer surfactant occur when surface tension has apparently risen to γ_{eq}, but has actually been kept from rising further by ensuing rapid adsorption.

The favorable behavior here with the application of EEP in situations with rapidly desorbing surfactant mirrors the favorable response of patients with the respiratory distress syndrome to the same maneuver (31). Even the decrease in dynamic compliance would be predicted as one climbs to higher and higher points on the PV curve (21).

Varying Respiratory Frequency

Keeping other ventilatory parameters constant and varying the frequency of respirations would be expected to interact most strongly with those properties of the system that determine its time constant: resistance and compliance. Because we rather naively kept resistance constant throughout the whole range of inflation,

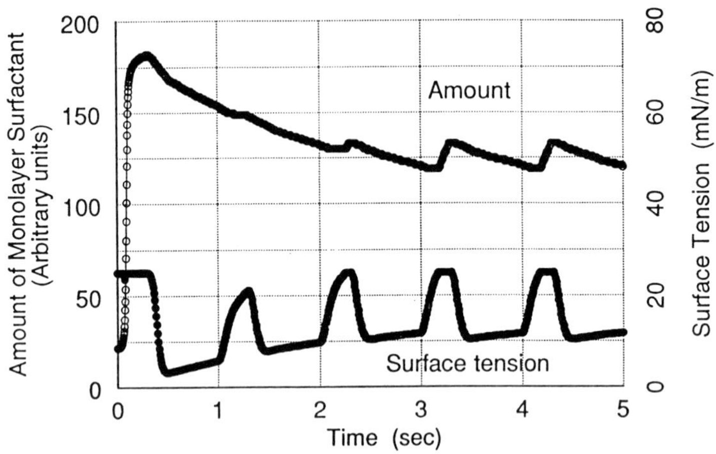

Figure 16 Treated rapid desorption: Amount of surfactant and surface tension in the monolayer of the alveolus with rapidly desorbing surfactant depicted in Fig. 15 versus time.

it would be pointless to report detailed results from varying either frequency or resistance. We did find, as one might have expected, that increased resistance per se was associated with an increased hysteresis of PV curves. This finding is mentioned merely to remind the reader that airway/tissue resistance to volume change is an important contributor to hysteresis, although normally paling in comparison with surface tension–area hysteresis as a cause. Because lung compliance varies so severely with lung inflation, becoming very low at high lung volumes, and because our resistances were not appropriately strong functions of volume, we did not pursue further the interaction of frequency and volume or compliance.

Varying the Inspiratory/Expiratory Time Ratio

Increasing the inspiratory/expiratory time ratio in the model yielded the expected results in cases of slow adsorption (low k_{ads}): consistently higher monolayer surfactant amounts and higher values of FRC (data not shown). One would expect similar results from changing the shape of the inflation pressure curve to prolong the time spent at PIP. Where adsorption was not impaired, monolayer surfactant amounts were maximal and mechanics were not affected.

IV. Conclusions

Getting enough surfactant into the interface and keeping it there should be the overall goals of therapy designed to ameliorate surfactant deficiencies.

The ill effects of low adsorption rate, seen as increased alveolar opening pressures in the most severe cases, should be treatable by intermittent periods of higher than normal peak inspiratory pressures.

The companion surfactant kinetic anomaly, a high desorption rate, should be treatable by maintaining higher than normal end-expiratory pressures. Of these two kinetic difficulties, rapid desorption and its concomitant, mechanical instability would seem to be the more serious. One should keep in mind that adequate means of testing retrieved or exogenous surfactants for this difficulty in vitro have only recently been described, and that all available therapeutic products probably have not yet been tested in this way.

As a general principle, a ventilatory pattern appropriate to a given surfactant should be used both in testing exogenous surfactants and in treating patients with them, since common ventilatory maneuvers can compensate for a wide range of surfactant deficiencies.

Acknowledgments

This work was supported by NIHLBI Grant No. 24075. The author is grateful to Dr. John A. Clements for discussions during developing the model and for his helpful comments regarding this manuscript.

References

1. Walther FJ, Taeusch HW. Pathophysiology of neonatal surfactant insufficiency: Clinical aspects. In: Robertson B, van Golde LMG, Batenburg JJ, eds. Pulmonary Surfactant: From Molecular Biology to Clinical Practice. Amsterdam: Elsevier, 1992:485–524.
2. Fujiwara T, Robertson B. Pharmacology of exogenous surfactant. In: Robertson B, van Golde LMG, Batenburg JJ, eds. Pulmonary Surfactant: From Molecular Biology to Clinical Practice. Amsterdam: Elsevier, 1992:561–592.
3. Smith BT. Clinical experience with modified natural surfactant. In: Robertson B, van Golde LMG, Batenburg JJ, eds. Pulmonary Surfactant: From Molecular Biology to Clinical Practice. Amsterdam: Elsevier, 1992:593–604.
4. von Neergaard K. Neue Auffassungen über einen Grundbegriff der Atemmechanik. Die Retraktionskraft der Lunge, abhängig von der Oberflächenspannung in den Alveolen. Z Gesampte Exp Med 1929; 66:373–394.
5. Goerke J. Surfactant and lung mechanics. In: Robertson B, van Golde LMG, Batenburg JJ, eds. Pulmonary Surfactant: From Molecular Biology to Clinical Practice. Amsterdam: Elsevier, 1992:165–192.
6. Schürch S, Bachofen H, Goerke J, Possmayer F. A captive bubble method

reproduces the in situ behavior of lung surfactant monolayers. J Appl Physiol 1989; 67:2389–2396.

7. Schürch S, Bachofen H, Goerke J, Green F. Surface properties of rat pulmonary surfactant studied with the captive bubble method: Adsorption, hysteresis, stability. Biochim Biophys Acta 1992; 1103:127–136.
8. Putz G, Goerke J, Schürch S, Clements JA. Evaluation of a pressure-driven captive bubble surfactometer. J Appl Physiol 1994; 76:1417–1424.
9. Schürch S, Bachofen H. Biophysical aspects in the design of a therapeutic surfactant. In: Robertson B, Taeusch HW, eds. Surfactant Therapy for Lung Disease. New York: Dekker, 1995:3–32.
10. Wilson TA, Bachofen H. A model for mechanical structure of the alveolar duct. J Appl Physiol 1982; 52:1064–1070.
11. Putz G, Goerke J, Clements JA. Surface activity of rabbit pulmonary surfactant subfractions at different concentrations in a captive bubble. J Appl Physiol 1994; 77:597–605.
12. Radford EP Jr. Recent studies of mechanical properties of mammalian lungs. In: Remington JW, ed. Tissue Elasticity. Washington, DC: American Physiological Society, 1957:177–190.
13. Mead J, Whittenberger JL, Radford EP Jr. Surface tension as a factor in pulmonary volume-pressure hysteresis. J Appl Physiol 1957; 10:191–196.
14. Bachofen H, Hildebrandt J, Bachofen M. Pressure-volume curves of air- and liquid-filled excised lungs—Surface tension in situ. J Appl Physiol 1970; 29:422–431.
15. Valberg PA, Brain JD. Lung surface tension and air space dimensions from multiple pressure-volume curves. J Appl Physiol 1977; 43:730–738.
16. Hoppin FG Jr, Hildebrandt J. Mechanical properties of the lung. In: West JB, ed. Lung Biology in Health and Disease. Bioengineering Aspects of the Lung. Vol. 3. New York: Dekker, 1977:83–162.
17. Mead J, Takishima T, Leith D. Stress distribution in lungs: A model of pulmonary elasticity. J Appl Physiol 1970; 28:596–608.
18. Putz G, Goerke J, Taeusch HW, Clements JA. Comparison of captive- and pulsating-bubble surfactometers using lung surfactants. J Appl Physiol 1994; 76:1425–1431.
19. Bachofen H, Gehr P, Weibel ER. Alterations of mechanical properties and morphology in excised rabbit lungs rinsed with a detergent. J Appl Physiol 1979; 47:1002–1010.
20. Hoppin FG Jr, Stothert JC Jr, Greaves IA, et al. Lung recoil: Elastic and rheological properties. In: Macklem PT, Mead J, Fishman P, Geiger SR, eds. Handbook of Physiology, Sect. 3: The Respiratory System, Vol. III. Bethesda, MD: American Physiological Society, 1986:195–215.
21. Cotton RB, Olsson T. Lung mechanics in respiratory distress syndrome: In: Robertson B, Taeusch HW, eds. Surfactant Therapy for Lung Disease. New York: Dekker, 1995:121–149.
22. Clements JA, Hustead RF, Johnson RP, Gribetz I. Pulmonary surface tension and alveolar stability. J Appl Physiol 1961; 16:444–450.
23. Kylstra JA, Paganelli CV, Lanphier EH. Pulmonary gas exchange in dogs ventilated with hyperbarically oxygenated liquid. J Appl Physiol 1966; 21:177–184.

24. Curtis SE, Peek JT, Kelly DR. Partial liquid breathing with perflubron improves arterial oxygenation in acute canine lung injury. J Appl Physiol 1993; 75:2696–2702.
25. Schürch S, Goerke J, Clements JA. Direct determination of surface tension in the lung. Proc Natl Acad Sci USA 1976; 73:4698–4702.
26. Mead J, Collier C. Relation of volume history of lungs to respiratory mechanics in anesthetized dogs. J Appl Physiol 1959; 14:669–678.
27. Young SL, Tierney DF, Clements JA. Mechanism of compliance change in excised rat lungs at low transpulmonary pressure. J Appl Physiol 1970; 29:780–785.
28. Schürch S, Goerke J, Clements JA. Direct determination of volume- and time-dependence of alveolar surface tension in excised lungs. Proc Natl Acad Sci USA 1978; 75:3417–3421.
29. Goerke J, Clements JA. Alveolar surface tension and lung surfactant. In: Macklem PT, Mead J, eds. Handbook of Physiology. The Respiratory System. Vol. III. Washington, DC: American Physiological Society, 1986:247–261.
30. Fleming BD, Keough KM. Surface respreading after collapse of monolayers containing major lipids of pulmonary surfactant. Chem Phys Lipids 1988; 49:81–86.
31. de Lemos RA, Gerstmann DR, Coalson JJ. Ventilation of the surfactant-deficient lung. In: Robertson B, van Golde LMG, Batenburg JJ, eds. Pulmonary Surfactant: From Molecular Biology to Clinical Practice. Amsterdam: Elsevier, 1992:525–538.

18

Augmentation of Exogenous Surfactant Treatments with Lung Maturational Agents

STEVEN R. SEIDNER
University of Texas Health Science Center at San Antonio
San Antonio, Texas

I. Introduction

If neonatal respiratory distress syndrome (RDS) is viewed as primarily surfactant deficiency, then it would seem redundant to use glucocorticoids or other lung maturational agents to augment the effects of a large dose of instilled surfactant. Some physicians may take this view and be tempted to abandon the use of prenatal lung maturational agents (e.g., maternal glucocorticoids) now that postnatal surfactant therapy is readily available. However, lung maturational agents may modify several components of neonatal RDS that are independent of the surfactant system, as well as some essential components of surfactant that are currently not optimized following exogenous surfactant therapy. In addition, "lung" maturational agents may accelerate development of nonpulmonary organs that are associated with both RDS and the subsequent outcomes of preterm newborns.

Exogenous surfactant therapy is usually administered to premature neonates during either the canalicular or saccular stage of lung development. Mature alveoli are not yet present and the existing terminal air spaces have relatively thick walls which have limited distensibility even after surface tension is lowered with exogenous surfactant. Capillaries are less numerous and more distant from potential air spaces than later in gestation resulting in increased anatomical and physiological dead spaces.

II. Components of Immaturity that Persist Following Instilled Surfactant

A. Protein Permeability in Underdeveloped Lungs Before and After Birth

In addition to having decreased surface areas of the potential air spaces and capillary beds, premature lungs subjected to the extrauterine environment and ventilation are unable to maintain optimal barriers to serum proteins. The pulmonary microvasculature normally has a limited permeability to proteins and other macromolecules with an apparent pore size in utero of 90–150 Å in immature and mature fetal lambs, a permeability that does not change significantly following birth in full-term, spontaneously breathing newborns (1,2). In contrast to the endothelium of the microvasculature, the alveolar epithelium of the developing fetus, prior to delivery and ventilation, is nearly impermeable to macromolecules with an apparent pore size of only 5–12 Å (3–5). In spontaneously breathing full-term lambs, this epithelium becomes transiently more permeable during the early postnatal course with an increase in the apparent pore size to 35–56 Å (4). Subsequently, after several hours of rapid lung water and sodium absorption, the pore size decreases toward the nearly impermeable state of the unventilated fetus and normal adult. In premature animals requiring positive-pressure ventilation, permeabilities of the pulmonary epithelium to proteins and other macromolecules are higher and more persistent (6–8). In addition, the pulmonary endothelium becomes markedly more permeable to proteins after preterm delivery in surfactant-deficient fetuses of various species (9,10). These abnormal endothelial and epithelial leaks of proteins into the lungs also increase with decreasing gestational age and with increasing peak pressure requirements on the ventilator (9–11). However, this correlation does not necessarily mean that positive-pressure ventilation per se causes the abnormal leakage of serum proteins into preterm lungs. In fact, chest wall restriction that limited overexpansion of the lungs in young full-term rabbits and lambs prevented the usual protein permeability increases seen with increasing levels of positive-pressure ventilation (12,13).

In premature newborns with RDS, regional overexpansion of terminal air spaces is potentiated by overly compliant chest walls and regions of atelectasis in the supporting adjacent airspaces. End-expiratory collapse and the lack of hysteresis in surfactant-deficient lungs further complicate the maldistribution of terminal airspace expansion. Even if structural and biochemical immaturity were not present, it would be necessary for an exogenous surfactant treatment to reach all terminal airspaces to totally prevent the abnormalities usually seen. This is probably not practically possible and animal studies show that exogenous surfactant can improve but not totally correct abnormal leakage of serum proteins from the pulmonary microvasculature into the lung interstitium and air spaces (6). Reductions in both the endothelial and epithelial protein leaks following exogenous surfactant therapy are significantly correlated with reductions in the required peak pressures which probably reflect the degree of regional collapse and overexpansion (Fig. 1). In addition, surfactant-treated newborn lambs at 122 days gestational age had significantly higher protein leaks in their lungs than untreated newborn lambs with much lower endogenous surfactant at 135 days' gestational age despite nearly identical pressure requirements for ventilation (9). Mature lambs at 146 days gestational age had still lower recoveries of radiolabeled albumin that leaked from the intravascular compartment into the air

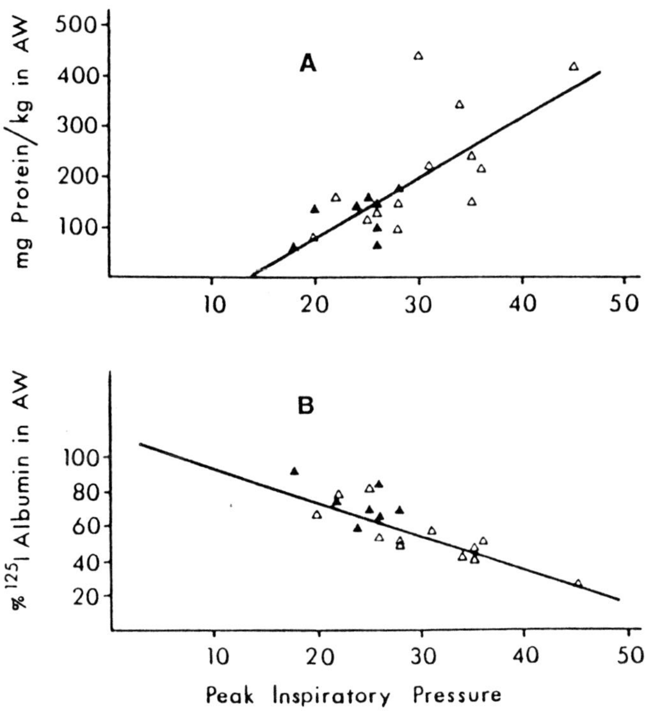

Figure 1 Linear regressions for the correlations of peak inspiratory pressures used for mechanical ventilation of 136-day gestational age preterm lambs (in cmH_2O) versus milligrams protein per kilograms of body weight recovered from alveolar wash (A) and versus percentage of instilled ^{125}I-albumin recovered from alveolar wash (B). Lambs not treated with surfactant are indicated by open triangles; lambs treated with surfactant are indicated by solid triangles. (From ref. 6; used with permission.)

spaces despite being overventilated with similar peak pressures. In fact, the net flux of intravascular radiolabeled albumin to the air spaces progressively increased by 5.8-fold with decreasing gestational age (Fig. 2).

The importance of this abnormality in humans was demonstrated by Jefferies et al. (14), who by measuring lung clearance rates and deposition of aerosolized ^{99m}technetium diethylenetriaminepentaacetate (DTPA) showed increased pulmonary epithelial permeability to solutes in human infants with RDS and a longer duration of the increased permeability in those that later developed bronchopulmonary dysplasia (BPD). Seidner et al. (15) showed that even exogenous surfactant

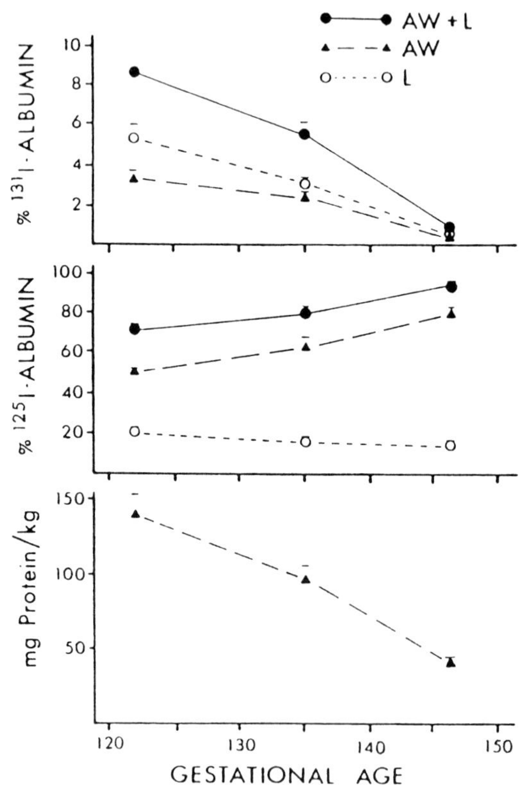

Figure 2 Measurements of protein permeability versus gestational age in mechanically ventilated newborn lambs. Means ± standard errors for percent recoveries of intravascularly injected ^{131}I-albumin and intratracheally instilled ^{125}I-albumin from alveolar washes (AW), postwash lung tissue (L), and the total lung (AW + L) are shown versus gestational age. Values for all measurements for each group are different from values for all measurements for other groups ($p<0.05$), except for the recovery of ^{125}I-albumin in L which was not different. (From ref. 9; used with permission.)

treatments did not prevent this phenomenon in chronically ventilated preterm baboons. One might hope that the increased influx of serum proteins into the lungs and air spaces during RDS would be partially balanced by a concurrently increased ability of these proteins to leave the air spaces and interstitial tissues and reenter the vascular space (6,9–11,16). However, coagulation of proteins within the air spaces may prevent their egress and contribute to the formation of the classic "hyaline membranes." Immunofluorescent studies of the lungs of babies who died of RDS have shown fibrin to be the main component of these hyaline membranes that also contain other serum proteins and cellular debris (17,18). Surfactant has thromboplastic activity and may also inhibit fibrinolysis, so it may actually aggravate the problem (19,20). Following coagulation of proteins in the air spaces, surfactant may either be sequestered in the fibrin clots or inhibited by soluble serum proteins (20–28). It is, therefore, not surprising that both endogenous surfactant and exogenous surfactant therapy show progressive declines in their ability to lower surface tension in premature humans and animals with RDS during the first hours of life (22,29). Fibrin monomer (22,23) and a 110-kDa surfactant inhibitor protein found in the lungs of preterm lambs and human infants with RDS (24,29) are potent inhibitors of surfactant function.

B. Fetal Lung Fluid Flux in Immature Lungs

The epithelium of the fetal lung, which is predominantly secretory, must dramatically change during the perinatal period and become predominantly absorptive with the onset of ventilation. Although secretion of fetal lung fluid by the respiratory tract during fetal life is driven by active chloride secretion into the air spaces, the predominant ion movement during perinatal lung water resorption is active sodium transport from air spaces toward the interstitium. In the last few days prior to labor in a full-term gestation, the lung fluid secretion rate decreases by about 50% and air space fluid volume decreases from 25 to 18 ml/kg (30). The process of labor further decreases lung water content in both rabbit pups and newborn lambs (31,32). Hormonally, these effects are paralleled by increases in serum catecholamines during perinatal adaptation and can be mimicked in utero with physiological doses of β-adrenergic agonists or instilled cyclic adenosine monophosphate (cAMP) analogues (33–39) and with pharmacological systemic doses of arginine vasopressin or atrial natriuretic factor (38–42). However, β-receptor blockade does not affect the ability of labor and birth to decrease lung water (43,44) so several mechanisms must be acting concurrently and interchangeably to stimulate cAMP.

With preterm delivery, postnatal clearance of fetal lung fluid is slower than at full term (8, 45–47). Many factors interact to slow reabsorption of fetal lung fluid in preterm newborns and exogenous surfactant therapy will not affect most of these (Table 1). As already discussed, there is more fetal lung fluid present during the late second and early third trimester than at full term. In preterm

Table 1 Factors Prolonging Lung Water Clearance in Preterms

Increased amounts of fetal lung fluid
Absence or decreased duration of labor
Decreased numbers of β-adrenergic receptors
Decreased numbers of sodium channels
Decreased activity of Na-K ATPase
Decreased surface area of absorptive epithelium
Increased epithelial and endothelial protein permeabilities
Decreased serum protein concentrations
Increased surface tension in surfactant-deficient airspaces
Increased pulmonary vascular resistance

rabbits, lung water content was about 25% greater after preterm delivery at 28 days' gestation than after delivery at 31 days' full-term gestation (46).

Preterm deliveries in humans also may not allow adequate periods for the benefits of the labor-associated reductions in fetal lung fluid. Cesarean sections prior to or shortly after the onset of labor may preclude the normal reductions seen prior to birth (labor decreased extravascular lung water by 45% in near-term lambs when compared with similar animals that did not experience labor [32]). In addition, the responsiveness to epinephrine during labor is progressively decreased with decreasing gestational age (48), and the concentration of β-adrenergic receptors is reduced until late in gestation (49–51). Even the post β-adrenergic receptor effects of cAMP analogues are reduced with decreasing gestational age (37).

Several mechanisms of ion transport may account for the changes seen with maturation. Fetal rats showed a marked increase in mRNA for the apical sodium channels of distal lung epithelium during the saccular stage of development (52) and further key developmental studies on these apical channels should become available in the near future, since the molecular probes are currently being developed. On the basolateral membrane of the epithelium, sodium transport is regulated by Na^+-K^+-ATPase activity and developmental differences could be regulated by changes in either pump number or pump activity. In fetal rabbits, sodium pump number (determined by the number of ouabain-binding sites) was the same in fetal and newborn cells, whereas the turnover number (determined by ouabain-sensitive $^{86}Rb^+$ uptake) was four times greater in newborn cells (53) indicating that an increase in Na^+-K^+-ATPase activity is chiefly responsible for the increases in sodium transport across the basolateral membrane. Interestingly, further increases in activity that occur postnatally appear to be chiefly due to increases in pump number (53).

Another major factor in the decreased capacity of preterm newborns to rapidly absorb fetal lung fluid is the decreased surface area of the distal lung epithelium and the progressively increased distances of the capillaries from the air spaces with decreasing gestational age. O'Brodovich speculates that the bronchioles, which occupy a much higher percentage of the surface area during the canalicular and saccular stages of lung development, may be primarily responsible for chloride and fetal lung liquid secretion, and that the distal lung epithelium is primarily responsible for active sodium transport (54).

Other factors that may increase lung water in the postnatal preterm infant are increased vascular leaks of protein into the lung interstitium and air spaces (discussed in the previous section), decreased serum protein contents, increased surface tensions in the alveoli, decreased lymphatic drainage, and/or increased pulmonary vascular resistance. Bland showed that total serum protein content decreased with decreasing gestational age and correlated with the occurrence of RDS (55). Raj et al. used micropuncture in isolated lungs of immature fetal rabbits to show that increased surface tensions in the alveoli, which may result from surfactant deficiency and/or surfactant inhibition, led to increased extravascular lung water content (56). These increased surface tensions may still occur in many alveoli after exogenous surfactant therapy, because distribution at the alveolar level is probably not uniform. Bland et al. showed that lung lymph flow, lymph protein flow, and pleural liquid drainage all increased in response to respiratory distress and pulmonary edema in preterm lambs with RDS (8) suggesting that lymphatic drainage is able to partially compensate for increased lung liquid and protein contents in preterm animals. (See also Chapter 10).

Studies in very premature lambs (57) have shown that maldistribution of instilled surfactant increases with delayed administration. In addition, synergistic contributions of maldistribution and surfactant inhibition would probably be increasingly apparent with decreasing gestational age due to the very high leaks of proteins (10). Lung maturational agents could potentially ameliorate the negative effects of exogenous surfactant maldistribution by several mechanisms. First, a maturational agent could stimulate the synthesis of endogenous surfactant components and partially reduce the regional deficiency of the underinstilled areas. Second, a maturational agent might reduce protein permeability of the endothelium and epithelium and, therefore, reduce the inhibition of surface activity by serum proteins in the undertreated airspaces. Finally, acceleration of structural maturation of the lungs might help prevent the problem by improving the initial distribution of the instilled surfactant treatment.

C. Functional and Structural Immaturity of Nonpulmonary Organs

RDS is caused primarily by the immature milieu of underdeveloped lungs, but many extrapulmonary organs play fundamental roles in its pathophysiology, eventual severity, and resolution; for example, patent ductus arteriosus (PDA).

Exogenous surfactant therapy may affect shunting across the PDA following rapid decreases in pulmonary vascular resistance (58,59). In the pre–surfactant era, surgical ligation or closure with indomethacin decreased ventilatory requirements and/or the incidence of BPD (60–62). In the current era of widespread surfactant use, surfactant treatment has sometimes been associated with a higher incidence of clinically significant PDA but not delayed subsequent closure (63). This topic is covered in more extensive detail in Chapter 25.

Lower systemic blood pressures in preterm newborns and large degrees of left-to-right shunting across the PDA may result in decreased perfusion of immature kidneys and profoundly impact on the diuresis that is associated with resolution of the pulmonary edema associated with RDS. Similarly, other common complications of prematurity and large PDA shunts such as intraventricular hemorrhage and necrotizing enterocolitis may cause significant hypotension, acidosis, and renal ischemia leading to worsening or delayed resolution of RDS.

III. Potential Lung Maturational Agents

A. Glucocorticoids

Glucocorticoid Effects on Lung Function and Structure

Endogenous glucocorticoids are a major factor in the fetal transition from a developing lung wherein growth gives way to differentiation and structural maturation. Since their reduction by fetal hypophysectomy or adrenalectomy retarded normal fetal lung morphogenesis (64–66), it was logical to hypothesize that supplementation with exogenous glucocorticoids could accelerate fetal lung development. In fetal rabbits injected at various times in gestation with 1 mg of cortisol, airway branching, flattening of lining epithelial cells, and volume increases of potential air spaces were all accelerated by approximately 1.5 days when compared with saline-injected littermates (67). In nonhuman primates, potential air spaces had increased distensibility and reduced interstitial volumes when antenatal glucocorticoids were administered (68,69). Rhesus monkeys (*Macaca mulatta*) at 67–85% fullterm gestation had an 11% increase in their collagen to elastin ratios following 3 days of antenatal betamethasone exposure when compared with controls (84). However, the number of alveoli per unit volume was reduced, as was the mean surface area of the lungs in the betamethasone-treated monkeys with the larger air spaces. Similarly, antenatal administration of glucocorticoids to pregnant rats diminished the normal postnatal increases in alveolarization and gas exchange surface areas of the lungs (70).

As reviewed by Ballard (71), several studies have also shown that treatment with antenatal glucocorticoids accelerated the appearance of lamellar bodies in future type II pneumocytes. Kauffman et al. showed that in mice exposed transplacentally to dexamethasone, glucocorticoid-induced changes in lung structure occurred more rapidly and with lower doses than required for accelerated appearance of lamellar bodies in type II cells (72). In preterm rhesus monkeys, Mitzner et al. (73) showed that antenatal betamethasone increased maximal lung capacities to a similar degree following either air or saline pressure-volume curves suggesting that surface tension effects did not play a major role. Several studies have found minimal surfactant-related effects on fetal lung after maternal treatment with glucocorticoids (68,73–75). In addition, other studies showed that following the onset of ventilation, antenatal betamethasone did not increase surfactant phosphatidylcholine pool sizes, and that static compliance was affected more by surfactant than glucocorticoids, whereas total lung conductance was increased more following glucocorticoids than after surfactant (10,76).

Most importantly, studies in both preterm rabbits and sheep show that antenatal glucocorticoids potentiate the beneficial effects of surfactant on lung function (75,77). In mechanically ventilated preterm rabbits whose mothers received antenatal glucocorticoids, maximal lung volumes and dynamic compliances were improved after low doses of exogenous surfactant to levels that could not be obtained even after high doses of exogenous surfactant in the absence of antenatal glucocorticoids (75). Complementary beneficial effects on maximal lung volumes, dynamic compliances, and ventilatory requirements were also seen in mechanically ventilated preterm lambs treated with antenatal glucocorticoids and postnatal exogenous surfactant despite equivalent saturated phosphatidylcholine air space pool sizes in the two groups (77).

Glucocorticoid Effects on Lung Protein Permeability

In both preterm rabbits and lambs, antenatal glucocorticoids have been shown to reduce the net fluxes of radiolabeled albumin from the intravascular space into the lung tissue and potential airspaces (10,11,77–79). These postglucocorticoid reductions in transvascular protein fluxes were accompanied by improvements in lung function and decreasing peak pressure requirements during mechanical ventilation. In preterm rabbits, but not lambs, antenatal maternal glucocorticoids also increased the leak of radiolabeled albumin out of the air spaces, which could have been related to increased air space volumes or decreased coagulation and sequestering of proteins in airspace hyaline membranes. Unfortunately, alveolar fibrin deposition was not studied in these animals. In preterm rabbits, exogenous surfactant caused a relatively larger improvement in lung protein permeability than antenatal glucocorticoids suggesting that the reductions in intravascular protein leaks and subsequent pulmonary edema following therapy are mostly due to decreases in regional overdistension of the immature air spaces and their associated capillaries. However, the studies in preterm lambs delivered at 128 days' gestation suggest that additional modulation of endothelial or neutrophil mediators of capillary permeability play a very significant role. In this species, the transvascular flux of radiolabeled albumin was significantly higher in surfactant-treated control lambs on lower peak inspiratory pressures than it was in glucocorticoid-treated lambs that did not receive surfactant and required significantly higher peak pressures for adequate ventilation (77). In addition, exogenous surfactant did not further reduce the protein leak in the lungs of glucocorticoid-treated lambs despite reducing their peak inspiratory pressure requirements by 45%. These differences between species emphasize the variability of glucocorticoid effects, which may also act differently at different gestations.

Glucocorticoid Effects on Ion Transport and Absorption of Fetal Lung Fluid

Antenatal glucocorticoids alone probably cannot accelerate the maturational transition from a fluid-secreting fetal lung to a fluid-absorbing postnatal lung in preterm animals. However, in combination with triiodothyronine (T_3), antenatal hydrocortisone caused a striking transition to lung liquid reabsorption in response to fetal epinephrine infusion in very preterm fetal lambs (80). Glucocorticoids appear to be critical, since neither epinephrine alone nor in combination with T_3 caused the response. The mechanism appears to be related to increased synthesis of either critical components of the apical sodium channels and/or of the intracellular signaling pathway, since the response was blunted by blocking the sodium channels with amiloride (81) or by inhibiting protein synthesis with instilled cycloheximide (82). A recent in vitro study suggested that glucocorticoids alone could promote the maturation of transepithelial sodium transport in distal pulmonary epithelium (83). However, these results may have been affected by oxygen concentrations that regulate liquid secretion of fetal lung in vitro (84).

Glucocorticoid Effects on SP-A

Glucocorticoid effects on surfactant protein (SP-A) gene expression vary with development, species, and dose. Their influence is potentially important since SP-A appears relatively late in normal development and is not contained in clinically approved surfactant preparations. As reviewed extensively by Mendelson et al. (85), Ballard (86), and Gross (87), glucocorticoids have a dose-dependent biphasic response in cultured midgestation human fetal lung explants with stimulatory effects on SP-A gene expression at dexamethasone concentrations below 10 nM and inhibitory effects at higher concentrations. While increasing the rate of gene transcription, SP-A may decrease mRNA and protein levels of SP-A by decreasing mRNA stability in a dose-dependent manner (88). In cultured lung explants of nonhuman primates, explants removed at midgestation had SP-A mRNA inhibited to a much greater degree by high concentrations of dexamethasone than did explants removed in the latter half of the third trimester (89).

Results of in vivo studies have also varied with the dose used, the stage of development, and the species studied. Both newly synthesized intracellular and secreted SP-A levels were increased 2.5 and 4.5 times, respectively, by dexamethasone in the postnatal rat, with mRNA levels elevated an average of 1.4 times control. Dose response for mRNA was continuous and for apoprotein was maximal at 2 mg/kg (90). SP-A protein and mRNA in the fetal lung increased when 1 mg/kg was given to the pregnant rats prior to day 18 but not later in gestation (91). However, SP-A protein was not increased in the lung lavage of preterm lambs infused antenatally with cortisol (77).

Direct effects of antenatal glucocorticoids on the distribution of postnatally instilled surfactant have not been reported, but the potentiation of surfactant dose-response with regard to dynamic compliances and maximal lung volumes on PV curves in steroid-treated lungs suggests that distribution might be significantly improved with glucocorticoid therapy (75).

Maturational Effects of Glucocorticoids on Nonpulmonary Organs

Perhaps the most compelling argument for the use of antenatal glucocorticoids or other "lung" maturational agents in conjunction with exogenous surfactant is that they also may accelerate maturation of other organ systems aside from the lungs. Antenatal glucocorticoids have been shown in various studies to affect the incidence of several major problems associated with prematurity to a much greater extent than seen after exogenous surfactant alone.

Intraventricular Hemorrhage

In a large meta-analysis, antenatal administration of glucocorticoids in clinical trials prior to surfactant use reduced the odds ratio of intraventricular hemorrhage (IVH) to 0.5 (0.28–0.85 95% confidence intervals) (92). In infants delivered before 28 weeks' gestation who did not receive exogenous surfactant, antenatal glucocorticoids were associated with a 3% incidence of severe IVH (grade 3 or 4), whereas placebo treatment was associated with a 25% incidence (93). In a retrospective analysis of two large multicenter trials of multidose exogenous surfactant treatments, antenatal glucocorticoids reduced the incidence of grade 3 or 4 IVH from 25 to 7% in the surfactant-treated infants and from 23 to 11% in those not receiving surfactant (94). All four groups were born at mean gestational ages of 27 weeks. In another retrospective analysis of an exogenous surfactant trial, antenatal glucocorticoids reduced the overall incidence of IVH from 19 to 6% in those newborns who received surfactant (95). In a placebo-controlled, randomized, double-blind study of antenatal glucocorticoids using rescue treatment with exogenous surfactant if needed, antenatal glucocorticoids were associated with a significant reduction in the overall incidence of all IVH from 28 to 10% (96). If only those babies who delivered from 24 hr to 2 weeks after the glucocorticoid or placebo treatments were analyzed, the difference was even more striking with a reduction from 46 to 10%. Interestingly, a different preparation of exogenous surfactant was used in each of the above three studies, but each yielded similar results with regard to the glucocorticoid-associated reductions in IVH.

Necrotizing Enterocolitis

In the large meta-analysis previously mentioned, antenatal administration of glucocorticoids in trials prior to surfactant use also reduced the odds ratio of necrotizing enterocolitis (NEC) to 0.35 (0.18–0.68, 95% confidence intervals) (92). A reanalysis of the Collaborative Study on Antenatal Steroid Therapy revealed that the incidence of NEC was reduced from 7% with placebo treatment to 2% with antenatal glucocorticoids (93). There are few data on how the combination of antenatal glucocorticoids and postnatal surfactant treatment may affect the incidence of NEC.

Patent Ductus Arteriosus

The data on the effects of antenatal glucocorticoids with regard to the incidence of patent ductus arteriosus (PDA) have been variable. Isolated ductal rings from fetal lambs had greater oxygen-induced contraction and less dilatation by prostaglandin E_2 (PGE_2) when exposed to antenatal glucocorticoids (11). However, although several studies found reductions in the incidence of PDA with antenatal glucocorticoids in the pre–surfactant era (97–99), the meta-analysis of Crowley et al. (92) and a study of infants delivered before 28 weeks' gestation who did not receive exogenous surfactant (93) showed no reductions with antenatal glucocorticoids. Similarly, the retrospective analyses of two surfactant databases showed conflicting results, with a 50% reduction in the incidence of PDA with antenatal glucocorticoids in one (94) and no significant change in the other (100).

Circulatory Stability

Several studies have shown increases in systemic blood pressures and a decreased requirement for inotropic support in preterm newborns following exposure to antenatal glucocorticoids (97,101,102). Similarly, fetal sheep treated with hydrocortisone and delivered prematurely had higher aortic blood pressures than controls (103). In addition, a single dose of 0.25 mg/kg dexamethasone given postnatally to very preterm human newborns was associated with increases in blood pressure 8–12 hr later (104).

Glucocorticoid Effects on Antioxidants

Antioxidant enzyme activities increase rapidly and in parallel with saturated phospholipid content in the lungs during the latter part of fetal life in rodents, lambs, and humans (105–108). Antenatal glucocorticoids have been shown to accelerate the increases of superoxide dismutase, catalase, and glutathione peroxidase in fetal rats and lambs (109,110). Clerch et al. showed that glucocorticoid effects on catalase were regulated at the level of gene transcription. Increases seen in response to postnatal hyperoxia were mediated posttranscriptionally by increased catalase mRNA stability (111). In addition, antenatal glucocorticoids have increased survival of both preterm and term rats in hyperoxia with a stimulatory effect on subsequent antioxidant enzyme levels in one study (112) and no effect on subsequent levels in another (113).

Glucocorticoid Effects on RDS in Human Preterm Newborns

In 1972, the first randomized, placebo-controlled trial of betamethasone in 282 pregnant women threatening premature delivery was reported by Liggins and Howie (114). Women in the glucocorticoid group received two 12-mg doses of betamethasone 24 hr apart. Reductions in neonatal mortality and the incidence of RDS with antenatal glucocorticoids led to continuation of their trial and numerous other trials by other investigators. By the time of Crowley's meta-analysis in 1990, 12 major trials were analyzed, and Liggins and Howie had randomized a total of 1135 women with 1070 cases reported (92). Of the 12 trials analyzed by Crowley, only two failed to show significant reductions in RDS, and the overall odds ratio for RDS was 0.5 following antenatal glucocorticoids, with 95% confidence intervals of 0.4–0.6 (Fig. 3) (114–125). In the two trials not showing significant effects of antenatal glucocorticoids on RDS, one was complicated by small numbers and only a 7% incidence of RDS in controls (119), whereas the other was complicated by small numbers as well as three different glucocorticoid regimens (subgroups received either hydrocortisone, methylprednisolone, betamethasone, or placebo) (125). A subsequent trial to the meta-analysis in infants delivered before 28 weeks' gestation who did not receive exogenous surfactant showed no decreased incidence of RDS with antenatal glucocorticoids, but the study was complicated by relatively low numbers and a greater proportion of female newborns in the placebo group (26/40 versus 15/33 in the glucocorticoid group) (93). In addition, although the numbers were insufficient for statistical significance the preterm infants with RDS after antenatal glucocorticoids tended toward less severe disease having 25% lower ventilatory pressure requirements despite the increased proportion of males in that group. In a retrospective analysis of two large multicenter trials of multidose exogenous surfactant treatments, antenatal glucocorticoids reduced the incidence of RDS-related mortality from 20% (111/566) to 6% (3/46) in those not receiving surfactant and from 7% (40/555) to 0% (0/57) in those that were treated with exogenous surfactant (94). In another retrospective analysis of an exogenous surfactant trial, antenatal glucocorticoids significantly reduced the overall incidence of RDS from 40% (33/83) to 12% (2/16) and the incidence of moderate-severe RDS from 25% to 0% in singleton pregnancies (95). In a placebo-con-

Study	Treated n	Treated (%)	Control n	Control (%)	Odds ratios and 95% CI: Numerical
Liggins & Howie (1972)	49/532	(9·21)	84/538	(15·61)	0·56 (0·39–0·80)
Block *et al.* (1977)	5/69	(7·25)	12/61	(19·67)	0·34 (0·12–0·94)
Schutte *et al.* (1979)	11/64	(17·19)	17/58	(29·31)	0·51 (0·22–1·18)
Taeusch *et al.* (1979)	7/56	(12·50)	14/71	(19·72)	0·60 (0·23–1·52)
Doran *et al.* (1980)	4/81	(4·94)	10/63	(15·87)	0·29 (0·10–0·88)
Teramo *et al.* (1980)	3/38	(7·89)	3/42	(7·14)	1·11 (0·21–5·83)
Gamsu *et al.* (1989)	7/131	(5·34)	16/137	(11·68)	0·45 (0·19–1·05)
Collaborative Group (1981)	42/371	(11·32)	59/372	(15·86)	0·68 (0·45–1·03)
Morales *et al.* (1986)	30/121	(24·79)	63/124	(50·81)	0·33 (0·20–0·56)
Papageorgiou *et al.* (1979)	7/71	(9·86)	23/75	(30·67)	0·28 (0·13–0·63)
Morrison *et al.* (1978)	6/67	(8·96)	14/59	(23·73)	0·33 (0·13–0·87)
Schmidt *et al.* (1984)	9/34	(26·47)	10/31	(32·26)	0·76 (0·26–2·20)
Typical odds ratio					0·49 (0·41–0·60)

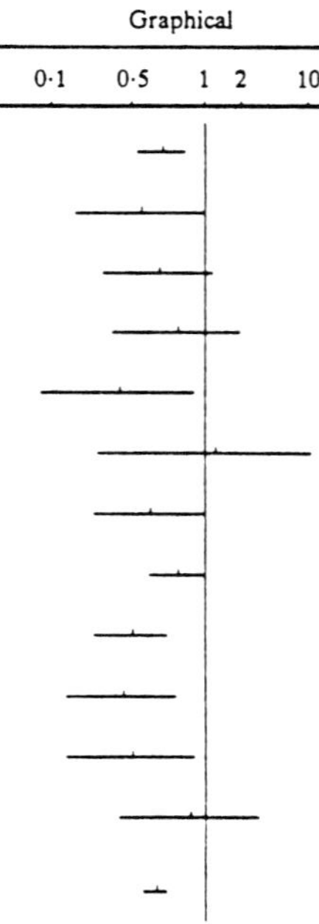

Figure 3 Meta-analysis of effect of antenatal glucocorticoids on the overall incidence of respiratory distress syndrome in 12 clinical trials (refs 129–140). (From ref. 92; used with permission.)

trolled, randomized, double-blind study of antenatal glucocorticoids and exogenous surfactant if needed, antenatal glucocorticoids were associated with a significant reduction in the incidence of RDS from 79% (30/38) to 44% (18/41) in those preterm infants born 1–14 days following treatment with prenatal dexamethasone or placebo (96). Therefore, it appears that both exogenous surfactant and antenatal glucocorticoids are required for maximal reductions in mortality and severity of RDS.

Although selected benefits of antenatal glucocorticoid therapy have been generally accepted, there has been much controversy over which subgroups might benefit most from its use. A summary of the subgroup findings from Crowley's meta-analysis is shown in Figure 4. There is good evidence that the optimal benefit from antenatal glucocorticoids is obtained when delivery occurs >24 hr and <7 days after the first maternal dose, but limited numbers also suggest that there may also be benefits when delivery occurs within 24 hr of treatment initiation or more than 7 days afterwards.

Controversy also persists over which gestational age infants benefit from antenatal glucocorticoids. Although the use of antenatal glucocorticoids in large trials had the greatest impact on the incidence of RDS from 30 to 34 weeks' gestational age, effects on the severity of RDS in the very immature babies delivered at <30 weeks were often not reported and may be difficult to evaluate in different clinical settings. In the meta-analysis of Crowley (see Fig. 4), there appears to be a very marked effect in this highest risk group (92). In the

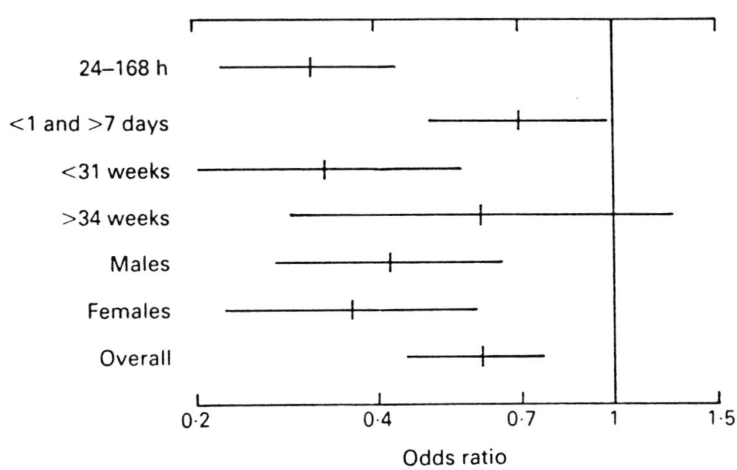

Figure 4 Odds ratios and 95% confidence intervals for the incidence of respiratory distress syndrome in subgroups of meta-analysis. Analyses of the interval between glucocorticoid administration and delivery, the gestational age at delivery, and the infant gender are shown. (From ref. 92; used with permission.)

retrospective analysis of two large multicenter trials of multidose exogenous surfactant treatments, the mean gestational age was only 27 weeks in all groups, and there was no mortality from RDS when both surfactant and antenatal glucocorticoids were utilized (94).

Gender effects on antenatal glucocorticoid responsiveness have also been strongly debated. Antenatal glucocorticoids improved female outcome but were not associated with any significant effect on the incidence of RDS in male infants in the Collaborative Trial (121). In contrast, the data of Liggins and Howie showed a much greater improvement in male infants (114). The meta-analysis of Crowley yields similar improvements for males and females (see Fig. 4). The retrospective analysis of Farrell et al. in preterm surfactant-treated infants showed that male infants of 29 weeks' mean gestational age had a higher incidence of RDS than females of similar age, but that the male incidence of severe RDS was reduced significantly from 35 to 9% when antenatal glucocorticoids were utilized in combination with postnatal surfactant treatment (95).

Potential adverse effects of antenatal glucocorticoids have been hypothesized and often used by obstetricians as contraindications for therapy but little supportive evidence has been found. Increased risks for adrenal suppression and/or infection in treated infants have not been seen in the vast majority of trials. Pulmonary function tests at 6–9 years of age in treated infants were not different from controls (126). Similarly, long-term neurodevelopmental outcome was not adversely affected in treated infants (101,127). From the maternal standpoint, pulmonary edema can occur when antenatal glucocorticoids are used in combination with tocolytic agents, but it does not occur when antenatal glucocorticoids are used alone (it does occur with tocolytics such as ritodrine alone) (128,129). There is some evidence that the risk of maternal infection may be increased when antenatal glucocorticoids are used with premature rupture of the membranes (117), but other studies showed no increased risk (120–22,124). In addition, there is no evidence that antenatal glucocorticoids hinder the ability to diagnose maternal infection. Glucocorticoid therapy may complicate diabetic control and diagnosis (130). Detailed consideration of the evidence has led a broadly based National Institutes of Health–Child Health and Human Development Institute Consensus panel to recommend in 1994 that antenatal glucocorticoids be used for essentially all women at risk of delivering an infant at risk of RDS (W. Taeusch, personal communication).

B. Thyrotropin-Releasing Hormone and Thyroid Axis Hormones Alone or in Combination with Glucocorticoids

Human fetal serum concentrations of thyroid-stimulating hormone (TSH) peak between 20 and 24 weeks of gestation and total thyroxine (T_4) markedly increases from a mean of 2 μg/dl at 20 weeks' gestational age to 9 μg/dl at

30 weeks (71,131). In addition, triiodothyronine (T_3) is not detected in fetal serum until about 30 weeks' gestation, and premature infants who develop RDS also have lower levels of circulating thyroid hormones than unaffected infants (132–135). Therefore, numerous investigators have studied the potential of prenatal treatment with thyroid hormone to accelerate lung maturation in preterm animals and humans. Several different pharmacological strategies have been used, since thyroid hormones do not readily cross the placenta. These include maternal administration of transplacental thyroid stimulants such as analogues or thyrotropin-releasing hormone (TRH) and ultrasound-guided administration of T_4 or T_3 into either the amniotic cavity or the fetus during the antenatal period (136).

Thyroid Hormone Effects on Lung Function and Structure

In postnatal developing rat lungs, supplemental thyroid hormones accelerated the increase of the surface to volume ratios and surface areas in the gas exchange saccules, whereas thyroid inhibition with propylthiouracil slowed the normal postnatal development (137). In preterm rabbits, fetal administration of thyroid hormones induced structural maturation of the lungs as determined by pressure-volume curves and histological evaluations (138,139). The combined use of thyroid hormones and glucocorticoids also accelerated the cellular differentiation of type II cells in cultured human fetal lungs (140), increased the lung volumes and deflation stabilities in preterm fetal lambs (51), and improved the dynamic compliances in mechanically ventilated preterm rabbits (141). In preterm rabbits, when exogenous surfactant was administered postnatally, the combination of antenatal TRH and glucocorticoids improved dynamic compliances and ventilatory efficiency index more than surfactant alone or than antenatal glucocorticoids plus postnatal surfactant (141). However, in preterm lambs, the combination of antenatal TRH and glucocorticoids did not show a significant improvement over antenatal glucocorticoids alone regardless of postnatal surfactant use (77). It is important to note that postnatal surfactant administration in combination with antenatal hormonal regimens improved lung function over that seen with hormonal treatments not accompanied by surfactant in all the groups in both studies.

Interestingly, there may be an important role to factors other than T_3 and T_4 in some of the effects seen in the above studies using TRH. TRH has neurotransmitter as well as neuroendocrine effects and also stimulates release of prolactin. An analogue of TRH neurotransmitter function (DN1417) that has much weaker neuroendocrine functions gave similar results to TRH when administered antenatally to preterm rabbits (142). In addition, prolactin supplementation was required to see the beneficial effects of glucocorticoids plus thyroid hormones on lung volumes in preterm fetal lambs (143).

TRH Effects on Lung Protein Permeability

Antenatal maternal TRH alone decreased the transvascular albumin flux to the air spaces in preterm rabbits by 2.4-fold, whereas the combination of antenatal TRH plus postnatally instilled surfactant resulted in a sevenfold decrease from that seen in control rabbits treated with neither TRH nor surfactant (141). However, although albumin leaks decreased relatively more than the ventilatory requirements of these rabbits after antenatal glucocorticoids, albumin leaks decreased more proportionately to decreases in the ventilatory requirements after antenatal TRH. In a study of TRH dose-response in glucocorticoid-treated preterm rabbits, TRH (independent of dose) appeared to augment the reductions in transvascular albumin leaks seen following antenatal glucocorticoids when compared with untreated controls (144). However, in preterm lambs, antenatal TRH did not affect the significant reductions seen with antenatal glucocorticoids (77). Therefore, it appears that the effects of antenatal TRH on lung protein permeability occur as a secondary phenomenon to reduced requirements for positive-pressure ventilation.

Thyroid Hormone Effects on Ion Transport and Absorption of Fetal Lung Fluid

Thyroidectomy in fetal lambs prevented the normal reabsorptive response of the distal lung epithelium to epinephrine infusions (36,80), and intravenous administration of T_3 plus hydrocortisone for 3 days restored the response to epinephrine, which did not occur when either hormone was administered in the absence of the other (80). In addition, cessation of the combination therapy reversed the response in 24–48 hr and instillation of the protein synthesis inhibitor cycloheximide into the fetal lung liquid blunted the effect suggesting a hormonal mechanism mediated by synthesis of proteins critical to sodium channel structure, sodium channel density, or the phophorylation/activation of those channels (82). Subsequent studies with proximal and distal fetal rat lung explants concluded that only distal lung epithelium contributes to this process and that amiloride-sensitive sodium transport is critical to the accelerated hormonal maturation (81).

Thyroid Hormone Effects on SP-A and Other Surfactant Components

As reviewed by Ballard (86) and Gross (87), thyroid hormones do not appear to have major effects on SP-A expression in midgestation human fetal lung explants. However, in preterm lambs, antenatal therapy with TRH plus glucocorticoids resulted in a fivefold increase in SP-A protein recovered from postnatal lung lavage when compared with lambs treated with single or no hormonal therapy (77). There are no reports concerning the effects of thyroid hormone stimulation with regard to postnatal distribution of instilled surfactant.

Other Pulmonary Effects of Thyroid Hormones

Fetal rabbits treated antenatally with T_3 and fetal lambs infused with TRH both showed enhancement of β-adrenergic–binding capacities in their lungs (51,145), whereas hypothyroidism decreased β-adrenergic receptor binding in fetal rats (146). In contrast, T_3 and TRH antagonized the stimulatory effect of antenatal glucocorticoids on fetal rat lung antioxidant enzyme activity and suppressed the normal prenatal surge in antioxidant enzyme induction (147,148). However, this seemingly negative effect may be species specific, since antenatal TRH did not inhibit glucocorticoid stimulation of antioxidant enzymes in preterm lambs (110).

Thyroid Hormone Effects on RDS and Lung Disease in Human Preterm Newborns

Clinical trials evaluating lung maturational effects of antenatal thyroid stimulation have employed one of two strategies. The first group of trials have evaluated the effects of intra-amniotic infusions of T_3 or T_4 in high-risk preterm pregnancies. These are reviewed in detail by Romaguera et al. (136), but the clinically relevant efficacy of these trials are generally difficult to interpret because of relatively low numbers of very low birth weight infants, the unpredictable fetal absorption of thyroid hormones from amniotic fluid, the frequent use of indirect measures of amniotic fluid phospholipid indices, and the lack of postnatal surfactant use. One recent study in 82 women showed that intra-amniotic T_4 appeared to enhance fetal lung maturity as effectively as intramuscular maternal dexamethasone (149). Increases in human newborn blood levels of T_4 and rT_3 have also been shown when delivery occurs within 5 days of intra-amniotic therapy with T_4 (150).

The second group of larger trials have compared the effects of administering TRH in combination with glucocorticoids to mothers threatening preterm delivery. These studies are reviewed comprehensively by Moya et al. (151). Maternal doses of TRH used in these studies (400 μg intravenously) cross the placenta and significantly elevate fetal T_3, T_4, and prolactin levels (152). In the first two published trials, therapy with TRH plus betamethasone significantly reduced the incidence of chronic lung injury when compared with therapy with betamethasone alone (18% vs 44% in the study of Ballard et al. [153] and 8% vs 24% in the study of Morales et al. [154]). However, addition of TRH to the antenatal glucocorticoid therapy did not decrease the incidence of RDS to a degree that reached statistical significance. Further meta-analysis of combined trials did reveal significant reductions in RDS as well (151). No differences have been reported in the incidence of intraventricular hemorrhage or necrotizing enterocolitis, but patent ductus arteriosus was actually more common among TRH-exposed infants in the trial of Ballard et al. despite the decreased incidence of chronic lung disease (153). Unfortunately, neither of these studies evaluated infants receiving postnatal surfactant therapy.

C. Cyclic AMP Agonists, Phosphodiesterase Inhibitors, and β-Adrenergic Agonists

Both β-adrenergic agonists and cAMP stimulation have been shown to stimulate (1) surfactant phosphatidylcholine secretion, (2) surfactant-associated protein gene expression, (3) the transition from lung fluid secretion to lung fluid absorption, and (4) control of breathing (71,85–87). Unfortunately, the evaluation of this family of mediators as potential antenatal lung maturational agents in vivo has been extremely difficult for several reasons. First, cAMP is a very ubiquitous mediator with multiple effects on many organs (some desirable and some not). Second, β-adrenergic agonists have been used as tocolytics, and it is difficult to determine whether benefits seen after antenatal maternal therapy are due to direct effects on fetal lungs or due to increased exposure of the lungs to endogenous glucocorticoids and/or other factors following increased fetal time in utero. Finally, tachyphylaxis and increased secretion of surfactant components may cause early beneficial effects to eventually lead to deleterious consequences (i.e., decreased fetal lung fluid and increased loss of surfactant into amniotic fluid would not be desirable goals if delivery was not imminent). Therefore, it is unlikely that this group of agents, will ever be considered for widespread use as antenatal maturational agents. However, since β-adrenergic agonists are still widely used as tocolytic agents, we will review some of the pertinent studies. In addition, for the reasons described above, these agents might still be useful during the early postnatal course in preterm babies at high risk for RDS and could be delivered via either the systemic route or co-instilled with exogenous surfactant therapy.

Studies in fetal rats, rabbits, and lambs have shown a progressive increase in β-adrenergic receptor density and maximal binding during the latter part of gestation (50,155,156), and in fetal lambs the doubling of maximal binding capacity in the third trimester corresponded to the onset of surfactant flux into the tracheal fluid (156). As reviewed by Ballard (71), numerous in vivo and in vitro studies have shown that β-adrenergic agonists, cAMP analogues, and phosphodiesterase inhibitors can stimulate surfactant phosphatidylcholine secretion and de novo synthesis. However, when fetal rabbits were injected antenatally with the β-adrenergic agonist isoxsuprine, the increased L/S ratio in the fetal lung fluid and the lowered surface tension on the bubble surfactometer were accompanied by a significant decrease in the number of lamellar inclusions in the type II pneumocytes (157). Interestingly, β-adrenergic receptor blockade reduced perinatal surfactant secretion into fetal lung fluid, but postnatal release following air expansion was not affected (44). The other major effect of β-adrenergic agonists and stimulants of cAMP is to stimulate reabsorption of fetal lung fluid and the fetal rabbits injected antenatally with isoxsuprine also had significantly less fetal lung fluid at the time of birth (157). When fetal lambs had terbutaline instilled into their fetal lung fluid, the net secretion of fetal lung fluid decreased over time and lung liquid absorption became predominant (33). When aminophylline was added to the instilled terbutaline, it potentiated the effect; but aminophylline instilled in the absence of terbutaline had no significant effect suggesting low baseline levels of endogenous cAMP (33).

As reviewed by Mendelson et al. (85), Ballard (86), and Gross (87), stimulants of cAMP strongly induce SP-A gene expression in fetal lung explants of various species, including midgestation human tissues. In lung explants cultured from nonhuman primates at varying stages of development, cAMP stimulation of SP-A mRNA levels progressively decreased from midgestation until the latter half of the third trimester (89). This decreased sensitivity to cAMP at advancing gestational ages coincided with preculture increases in baseline SP-A gene expression to relatively high levels during the latter stages of gestation.

In human studies, both aminophylline and ritodrine have been given to mothers antenatally in an attempt to improve the mortality and morbidity from RDS (158). However, in the aminophylline study, there were no data on ventilatory variables in the preterm infants and other discrepancies in the data were also noted (71). In a meta-analysis of data from 890 women who participated in 16 methodologically acceptable trials of β-adrenergic therapy, ritodrine delayed delivery for up to 48 hr but did not improve perinatal mortality or morbidity from RDS (159). In a multicenter, randomized, controlled trial from Canada, similar results were found (160).

D. Growth Factors

One of the most actively growing areas of lung research in the past few years has been the study of polypeptide growth factors or cytokines. The majority of these have primarily paracrine (cell-cell) effects, although endocrine and autocrine effects may also play critical roles. Many of the epithelial-mesenchymal interactions that play essential roles in growth and differentiation are mediated by a delicate balance of these substances. It is highly likely that the lung maturational agents of the next generation will be found within this class of mediators. As examples we will review some of the preclinical benefits which have been described in vitro and occasionally in vivo for epidermal growth factor, transforming growth factor α, bombesin-like peptides, hepatocyte growth factor, and keratinocyte growth factor. Many other growth factors such as fibroblast pneumocyte factor, interferon γ, insulin-like growth factors, and platelet-derived growth factors have promising roles as well.

Epidermal Growth Factor (EGF) and Transforming Growth Factor α (TGF-α)

EGF and TGF-α belong to a large family of distinct EGF-related proteins, including urokinase, tissue plasminogen activator, clotting factors, vaccinia virus growth factor, and the receptor for low-density lipoprotein. The identifying feature of this protein family is a stretch of six cysteine residues spaced at defined intervals within a sequence of approximately 40 amino acids. As reviewed by Ryan et al. (161), TGF-α binds with a much higher affinity than EGF to the EGF receptor (110-fold in the chicken) and not surprisingly is sometimes more potent than EGF. There is also evidence that EGF and TGF-α may interact with different sites on the EGF receptor and/or cause different conformational changes in the receptor leading to variable subsequent regulation of tyrosine kinase activity. The potential importance of EGF in lung development is suggested by a 10-fold rise in amniotic fluid EGF levels between 30 and 40 weeks' gestational age in humans (162).

In developing human airway epithelium, immunostaining for EGF which was present in the late first and early second trimester in tracheal epithelium was absent in that location by 24 weeks of gestation (163). However, from 18 weeks until term, tracheal submucosal glands had scattered immunostaining. Bronchiolar epithelium did not have EGF immunostaining unless chronic lung disease was present, suggesting a role for EGF in the process of both normal and abnormal regeneration (163). Injection of fetal rabbits with EGF accelerated morphological maturation of alveolar type II cells and improved deflation stability on pressure-volume curves (164). Administration of EGF to fetal lambs decreased lung liquid secretion (165), induced epithelial hyperplasia in both trachea and bronchi, accelerated alveolarization and lamellar body formation in the distal lung epithelium, and improved postnatal lung function in one study (166), but in a later study did not have any significant effect in the absence of other hormonal therapy (143). EGF also stimulated phospholipid synthesis in a dose-dependent manner and antioxidant enzymes in an oxygen-dependent manner in fetal rat lung explants (167,168) and stimulated SP-A synthesis in human fetal lung tissue explants (169). In rhesus monkeys, four treatments of antenatal EGF over a 7-day period given via the intraperitoneal route alone or via both the intraperitoneal and intra-amniotic routes simultaneously stimulated type II cell and tracheal mucous secretory cell differentiation, increased concentrations of SP-A and phosphatidylglycerol in amniotic fluid, and increased immunostaining for SP-A in distal lung epithelium (170,171). However, three doses of EGF in a subsequent study did not stimulate epithelial proliferation or seem to improve postnatal lung function in the same primate model (172). Therefore, it is still unknown whether EGF has a physiological role as a lung maturational agent.

In contrast to EGF, TGF-α immunostaining was present in airway epithelial cells at all levels, including the bronchioles from 10 to 22 weeks of gestation in lung tissues from human abortuses, suggesting that it may play an even more important role than EGF in distal air space growth and development (173). However, in vivo studies have not yet been reported in preterm animals and will be necessary to evaluate its potential use as a lung maturational agent.

Bombesin-like Peptides

Mammalian homologues of the 14 amino acid frog skin peptide bombesin have been termed bombesin-like peptides (BLPs). The main BLP in humans is the 27 amino acid "gastrin-releasing peptide" (GRP), which shares the highly conserved C-terminus that is required for immunogenicity and high-affinity binding to physiological receptors (174). BLPs appear in pulmonary neuroendocrine cells as soon as the cells are detectable at 8–9 weeks' gestation in human fetal lungs, and transient expression of GRP mRNA is found during mid-gestation in a proximal to distal fashion that parallels the growth of fetal airways (175). Lungs of preterm infants with RDS have low levels of BLPs and low numbers of BLP-positive pulmonary neuroendocrine cells (176–178). Administration of bombesin to fetal mice in utero led to increased lung growth and maturation by both biochemical and ultrastructural analyses (179). In addition, anti-BLP monoclonal antibody blocked endogenous fetal lung maturation in utero (180) and in serum-free human lung organ cultures (179). Studies of postnatal lung function in preterm animals treated antenatally have not yet been reported.

Hepatocyte Growth Factor and Keratinocyte Growth Factor

In the past, several investigators showed that fibroblast-conditioned media could stimulate DNA synthesis in alveolar epithelial cells, but until recently no specific growth factors had been identified (181–183). Subsequently, medium conditioned by human adult lung fibroblasts stimulated DNA synthesis in and proliferation of fetal rat type II pneumocytes, with the stimulatory activity being localized to two soluble heparin-binding growth factors, hepatocyte growth factor (HGF) and keratinocyte growth factor (KGF) (184).

HGF, which is also called scatter factor, is a mitogen that is found in a variety of tissues, including embryonic lung fibroblasts (185). Its cDNA reveals no homology with known growth factors but is about 38% identical to plaminogen (186). HGF binds specifically to plasma membranes isolated from lung tissue (187) and immunostaining for HGF is positive in tracheal, bronchial, and bronchiolar epithelium as well as in intra-alveolar macrophages and endothelial cells (188).

KGF is a member of the fibroblast growth factor family, also known as FGF-7, and is an epithelial cell-specific heparin-binding growth factor (189). Unlike EGF and TGF-α, which significantly retarded terminal differentiation when stimulating proliferation in human keratinocytes, KGF was able to stimulate proliferation and not disrupt markers for terminal differentiation (190). Most impressively, a single intratracheal injection of recombinant human KGF caused a prominent dose-dependent proliferation of type II pneumocytes in adult rats with a lesser effect on the bronchiolar epithelium and no effect on large airways (191). Administration of KGF has not been studied yet in vivo in preterm animals, but KGF mRNA expression was spontaneously induced in cultured midgestation fetal human lung explants with relatively stable levels of KGF receptor mRNA throughout (192). Furthermore, dexamethasone, which has been shown to inhibit SP-A expression, significantly decreased KGF mRNA expression at 10^{-7} and 10^{-8} M concentrations (192).

IV. Conclusions and Future Directions

There is clear evidence that surfactant is necessary but not sufficient for maximizing lung function in immature lungs. Structural immaturity and the resulting dysfunction of gas exchange in terminal air spaces of underdeveloped lungs, increased leaks of protein inhibitors and procoagulants into the air spaces, and delayed reabsorption of fetal lung fluid create major barriers to normalizing lung function with instilled surfactant. Absence of SP-A from clinically available preparations of exogenous surfactant and maldistribution of instilled treatments may also maintain surfactant-deficient characteristics in many terminal air spaces. Strategies to accelerate lung maturation both structurally and physiologically will be necessary to further impact on RDS and BPD. Maternally administered antenatal glucocorticoids have been the most extensively studied and proven of these agents in both animals and humans. Antenatal stimulants of thyroid hormones, enhancers of cyclic AMP, and various growth factors have also significantly accelerated varying aspects of lung maturation.

However, the clinical experience with antenatal glucocorticoids has revealed some major obstacles to its usefulness and possibly to all antenatal therapies. Maternal presentation at too advanced a stage of labor to permit the necessary time interval for antenatal glucocorticoid therapy and fear by many obstetricians of increased maternal risks have severely limited its use despite the belief of most that it is efficacious. In fact, only 8% of the preterm pregnancies enrolled in the multidose Survanta trials received antenatal glucocorticoid therapy (94), and the Neonatal Network found only a 16% utilization before premature deliveries of babies from 500 to 1500 g (193). Therefore, it may be critical to either develop antenatal therapies which can be administered shortly before delivery or to develop early postnatal strategies to accelerate the extrauterine maturation of the lungs and other organs.

Meta-analysis of the maternal glucocorticoid trials showed evidence for some efficacy at intervals <24 hr prior to delivery (Crowley et al. [92]) and recent studies have evaluated the administration of ultrasound-guided fetal injections with glucocorticoids and/or thyroid hormones only 15 hr prior to delivery (Dr. A. H. Jobe, personal communication). Early postnatal therapy would significantly increase the number of premature babies eligible for treatment and would allow an initial screening for the subgroup most likely to benefit. We have recently shown that suboptimal pulmonary responses to exogenous surfactant can be augmented with early postnatal dexamethasone in preterm baboons of borderline viability (194), but we are hesitant to extend this therapy too hastily to humans, since there was also evidence of disrupted alveolarization in the treated animals. Postnatal therapies may often require exposure to higher pharmacological doses when compared with the physiological doses often received by the fetus after transplacental therapies. Postnatal agents to accelerate lung maturation could also be co-instilled with surfactant when systemic effects are not desired. In the future, transient postnatal stimulation of desired mediators or their receptors may be modulated via gene therapy with lung specific promoters or antisense oligonucleotides may be used to downregulate gene expression of specific inhibitors. The natural ability of liposomes to associate with surfactant aggregates may prove useful for many of these future therapies.

References

1. Boyd RDH, Hill JR, Humphreys PW, et al. Permeability of lung capillaries to macromolecules in fetal and newborn lambs and sheep. J Physiol (Lond) 1969; 201:567–588.
2. Normand ICS, Olver RE, Reynolds EOR, Strang LB. Permeability of lung capillaries and alveoli to non-electrolytes in the foetal lamb. J Physiol (Lond) 1971; 219:303–330.
3. Anderson TM, Boyd RDH, Platt HS, Strang LBS. Composition of alveolar liquid in the foetal lamb. J Physiol (Lond) 1969; 204:159–168.
4. Egan EA, Olver RE, Strang LB. Changes in non-electrolyte permeability of alveoli and the absorption of lung liquid at the start of breathing in the lamb. J Physiol (Lond) 1975; 244:161–179.
5. Olver RE, Schneeberger EE, Walters DV. Epithelial solute permeability, ion transport and tight junction morphology in the developing lung of the fetal lamb. J Physiol (Lond) 1981; 315:395–412.
6. Jobe A, Ikegami M, Jacobs H, et al. Permeability of premature lamb lungs to protein and the effect of surfactant on that permeability. J Appl Physiol 1983; 55:169–176.
7. Sundell HW, Harris TR, Cannon JR, et al. Lung water and vascular permeability-surface area in premature newborn lambs with hyaline membrane disease. Circ Res 1987; 60:923–932.
8. Bland RD, Carlton DP, Scheerer RG, et al. Lung fluid balance in lambs before and after premature birth. J Clin Invest 1989; 84:568–576.
9. Jobe A, Jacobs H, Ikegami M, Berry D. Lung protein leaks in ventilated lambs: Effect of gestational age. J Appl Physiol 1985; 58:1246–1251.
10. Ikegami M, Jobe AH, Seidner S, Yamada T. Gestational effects of corticosteroids and surfactant in ventilated rabbits. Pediatr Res 1989; 25:32–37.
11. Ikegami M, Berry D, Elkady T, et al. Corticosteroids and surfactant change lung function and protein leaks in the lungs of ventilated premature rabbits. J Clin Invest 1987; 79:1371–1378.

12. Hernandez LA, Peevy KJ, Moise AA, Parker JC. Chest wall restriction limits high airway pressure-induced lung injury in young rabbits. J Appl Physiol 1989; 66:2364–2368.
13. Carlton DP, Cummings JJ, Scheerer RG, et al. Lung overexpansion increases pulmonary microvascular protein permeability in young lambs. J Appl Physiol 1991; 69:577–583.
14. Jefferies AL, Coates G, O'Brodovich H. Pulmonary epithelial permeability in hyaline-membrane disease. N Engl J Med 1984; 311:1075–80.
15. Seidner S, Cox W. Pulmonary clearance of ^{99m}technetium diethylene-triamine pentacetate during acute and chronic lung injury in preterm baboons. Am Rev Respir Dis 1993; 147(Suppl):A421.
16. Robertson B, Berry D, Curstedt T, et al. Leakage of protein in the immature rabbit lung; effect of surfactant replacement. Respir Physiol 1985; 61:265–276.
17. Gitlin D, Craig JM. The nature of the hyaline membrane in asphyxia of the newborn. Pediatrics 1956; 17:64–71.
18. Gajl-Peczalska K. Plasma protein composition of hyaline membrane in the newborn as studied by immunofluorescence. Arch Dis Child 1964; 39:226–231.
19. Higuchi M, Hirano H, Maki M. The thromboplastic activity of lung surfactant in amniotic fluid and its application to prenatal assessment of fetal lung maturity. Tohoku J Exp Med 1981; 133:267–273.
20. Tierney DF, Johnson RP. Altered surface tension of lung extracts and lung mechanics. J Appl Physiol 1965; 20:1253–60.
21. Ikegami M, Jobe A, Glatz T. Surface activity following natural surfactant treatment in premature lambs. J Appl Physiol 1981; 51:306–312.
22. Seeger W, Stohr G, Wolf HRD, et al. Alteration of surfactant function due to protein leakage: Special interaction with fibrin monomer. J Appl Physiol 1985; 58:326–338.
23. Seeger W, Stohr G, Wolf HRD, et al. Interaction of alveolar surfactant with plasma-derived proteins, especially fibrin monomer, as causative principle of surfactant dysfunction. Prog Respir Res 1984; 18:208–213.
24. Ikegami M, Jobe A, Jacobs H, Lam R. A protein from airways of premature lambs that inhibits surfactant function. J Appl Physiol 1984; 57:1134–1142.
25. Ikegami M, Jobe A, Berry D. A protein that inhibits surfactant in respiratory distress syndrome. Biol Neonate 1986; 50:121–129.
26. Seeger W, Gunther A, Thede C. Differential sensitivity of SP-B- and SP-C-based synthetic surfactants to the inhibitory effect of fibrinogen—Implications for surfactant replacement therapy. Am Rev Respir Dis 1990; 141(Suppl):A538.
27. Fuchimukai T, Fujiwara T, Takahashi A, Enhorning G. Artificial pulmonary surfactant inhibited by proteins. J Appl Physiol 1987; 62:429–437.
28. Seidner S, Ikegami M, Yamada T, et al. Decreased surfactant dose-response following the onset of mechanical ventilation in preterm rabbits. Pediatr Res 1989; 25(Suppl):326A.
29. Jacobs H, Jobe A, Ikegami M, et al. Premature lambs rescued from respiratory failure with natural surfactant: Clinical and biophysical correlates. Pediatr Res 1982; 16:424–429.
30. Dickson KA, Maloney JE, Berger PJ. Decline in lung liquid volume before labor in fetal lambs. J Appl Physiol 1986; 61:2266–2272.

31. Bland RD, Bresack MA, McMillan DD. Labor decreases the lung water content of newborn rabbits. Am J Obstet Gynecol 1979; 135:364–367.
32. Bland RD, Hansen TN, Haberkern CM, et al. Lung fluid balance in lambs before and after birth. J Appl Physiol 1982; 53:992–1004.
33. Chapman DL, Carlton DP, Cummings JJ, et al. Intrapulmonary terbutaline and aminophylline decrease lung liquid in fetal lambs. Pediatr Res 1991; 29:357–361.
34. Lawson EE, Brown ER, Torday JS, et al. The effect of epinephrine on tracheal fluid flow and surfactant efflux in fetal sheep. Am Rev Respir Dis 1978; 118:1023–1026.
35. Walters DV, Olver RE. The role of catecholamines in lung liquid absorption at birth. Pediatr Res 1978; 12:239–242.
36. Barker PM, Brown MJ, Ramsden CA, et al. The effect of thyroidectomy in the fetal sheep on lung liquid reabsorption induced by adrenaline or cyclic AMP. J Physiol (Lond) 1988; 407:373–383.
37. Walters DV, Ramsden CA, Olver RE. Dibutyrl cAMP induces a gestation-dependent absorption of fetal lung liquid. J Appl Physiol 1990; 68:2054–2059.
38. Perks AM, Cassin S. The effects of arginine vasopressin and other factors on the production of lung liquid in fetal goats. Chest 1982; 81:63S–65S.
39. Perks AM, Cassin S. The effects of arginine vasopressin and epinephrine on lung liquid production in fetal goats. Can J Physiol Pharmacol 1989; 67:491–498.
40. Ross MG, Ervin G, Leake RD, et al. Fetal lung liquid regulation by neuropeptides. Am J Obstet Gynecol 1984; 150:421–425.
41. Wallace J, Hooper S, Harding R. Regulation of lung liquid secretion by arginine vasopressin in fetal sheep. Am J Physiol 1990; 258 (Reg Integ Comp Physiol 27):R104–R111.
42. Castro R, Ervin MG, Ross MG, et al. Ovine fetal lung response to atrial natriuretic factor. Am J Obstet Gynecol 1989; 161:1337–1343.
43. Chapman DL, Carlton DP, Cummings JJ, et al. Propranolol does not prevent absorption of lung liquid in fetal lambs during labor. FASEB J 1990; 14:A4111.
44. McDonald JV, Gonzales LW, Ballard PL, et al. Lung β-adrenoreceptor blockade affects perinatal surfactant release but not lung water. J Appl Physiol 1986; 60:1727–1733.
45. Egan EA, Dillon WP, Zorn S. Fetal lung liquid absorption and alveolar epithelial solute permeability in surfactant deficient, breathing fetal lambs. Pediatr Res 1984; 18:566–570.
46. Bland RD. Dynamics of pulmonary water before and after birth. Acta Pediatr Scand 1983; 305(Suppl):12–20.
47. Aherne W, Dawkins MJR. The removal of fluid from the pulmonary airways after birth in the rabbit, and the effect on this of prematurity and pre-natal hypoxia. Biol Neonate 1964; 7:214–229.
48. Brown MJ, Olver RA, Ramsden CA, et al. Effects of adrenaline and of spontaneous labour on the secretion and absorption of lung liquid in the fetal lamb. J Physiol (Lond) 1983: 344:137–152.
49. Cheng JB, Goldfein A, Ballard PL, Roberts JM. Glucocorticoids increase pulmonary β-adrenergic receptors in fetal rabbit. Endocrinology 1980; 107:1646–1648.
50. Whitsett JA, Manton MA, Darovec-Beckerman C, et al. β-Adrenergic receptors in

the developing rabbit lung. Am J Physiol 1981; 240 (Endocrinol Metab 3:E351–E357.
51. Warburton D, Parton L, Buckley S, et al. Combined effects of corticosteroid, thyroid hormones, and β-agonist on surfactant, pulmonary mechanics, and β-receptor binding in fetal lamb lung. Pediatr Res 1988; 24:166–170.
52. O'Brodovich H, Canessa C, Ueda J, et al. Expression of the epithelial Na^+ channel in the developing rat lung. Am J Physiol 1993; 265 (Cell Physiol):C491–C496.
53. Chapman DL, Widdicombe JH, Bland RD. Developmental differences in rabbit lung epithelial cell Na^+-K^+-ATPase. Am J Physiol 1990; 259 (Lung Cell Mol Physiol 3):L481–L487.
54. O'Brodovich H. Epithelial ion transport in the fetal and perinatal lung. Am J Physiol 1991; 261 (Cell Physiol 30):C555–C564.
55. Bland RD. Cord-blood total protein level as a screening aid for the idiopathic respiratory-distress syndrome. N Engl J Med 1972; 287:9–13.
56. Raj JU. Alveolar liquid pressure measured by micropuncture in isolated lungs of mature and immature fetal rabbits. J Clin Invest 1987; 79:1579–1588.
57. Jobe A, Ikegami M, Jacobs H, Jones S. Surfactant and pulmonary blood flow distributions following treatment of premature lambs with natural surfactant. J Clin Invest 1984; 73:848–856.
58. Fujiwara T, Maeta H, Chida S, et al. Artificial surfactant therapy in hyaline membrane disease. Lancet 1980; 1:55–59.
59. Clyman RI, Jobe A, Heymann M, et al. Increased shunt through the patent ductus arteriosus after surfactant replacement therapy. J Pediatr 1982; 100:101–107.
60. Kitterman JA, Edmunds LH Jr, Gregory GA, et al. Patent ductus arteriosus in premature infants:incidence, relation to pulmonary disease, and management. N Engl J Med 1972; 287:473–477.
61. Mahony L, Carnero V, Brett C, et al. Prophylactic indomethacin therapy for patent ductus arteriosus in very-low-birthweight infants. N Engl J Med 1982; 306:506–510.
62. Merritt TA, Harris JP, Roghmann K, et al. Early closure of the patent ductus arteriosus in very-low-birthweight infants: a controlled trial. J Pediatr 1981; 99:281–286.
63. Heldt GP, Pesonen E, Merritt TA, et al. Closure of the ductus arteriosus and mechanics of breathing in preterm infants after surfactant replacement therapy. Pediatr Res 1989; 25:305–310.
64. Liggins GC, Schellenberg J-C, Finberg K, et al. The effects of $ACTH_{1\text{-}24}$ or cortisol on pulmonary maturation in the adrenalectomized ovine fetus. J Dev Physiol 1985; 7:105–111.
65. Crone RK, Davis P, Liggins GC, Reid L. The effects of hypophysectomy, thyroidectomy, and postoperative infusion of cortisol or adrenocorticotrophin on the structure of the ovine fetal lung. J Dev Physiol 1983; 5:281–288.
66. Pinkerton KE, Kendall JZ, Randall GC, et al. Hypophysectomy and porcine fetal lung development. Am J Respir Cell Mol Biol 1989; 1:319–328.
67. Kikkawa Y, Kaibara M, Motoyama EK, et al. Morphologic development of fetal rabbit lung and its acceleration with cortisol. Am J Pathol 1971; 64:423–433.
68. Kessler DL, Truog WE, Murphy JH, et al. Experimental hyaline membrane disease in the premature monkey. Effects of antenatal dexamethasone. Am Rev Respir Dis 1982; 126:62–69.

69. Beck JC, Mitzner W, Johnson JWC, et al. Betamethasone and the rhesus fetus:effect on lung morphometry and connective tissue. Pediatr Res 1981; 15:235–240.
70. Massaro GD, Massaro D. Formation of alveoli in rats: postnatal effect of prenatal dexamethasone. Am J Physiol 1992; 263 (Lung Cell Mol Physiol 7):L37–L41.
71. Ballard PL. Monographs in Endocrinology. Vol 28: Hormones and Lung Maturation. Berlin: Springer-Verlag, 1986.
72. Kauffman SL. Acceleration of canalicular development in lungs of fetal mice exposed transplacentally to dexamethasone. Lab Invest 1977; 36(4):395–401.
73. Mitzner W, Johnson WC, Scott R, et al. Effect of betamethasone on pressure-volume relationship of fetal rhesus monkey lung. J Appl Physiol 1979; 47:377–382.
74. Fiascone JM, Jacobs HC, Moya FR, et al. Betamethasone increases pulmonary compliance in part by surfactant-independent mechanisms in preterm rabbits. Pediatr Res 1987; 22:730–735.
75. Seidner S, Pettenazzo A, Ikegami M, Jobe A. Corticosteroid potentiation of surfactant dose response in preterm rabbits. J Appl Physiol 1988; 64:2366–2371.
76. Gladstone IM, Mercurio MR, Devenny SG, Jacobs HC. Antenatal steroids, postnatal surfactant, and pulmonary function in premature rabbits. J Appl Physiol 1989; 67:1377–1382.
77. Ikegami M, Polk D, Tabor B, et al. Corticosteroid and thyrotropin-releasing hormone effects on preterm sheep lung function. J Appl Physiol 1991; 70:2268–2278.
78. Rider ED, Jobe AH, Ikegami M, et al. Antenatal betamethasone dose effects in preterm rabbits studied at 27 days gestation. J Appl Physiol 1990; 68:1134–1141.
79. Tabor BL, Rider ED, Ikegami M, et al. Dose effects of antenatal corticosteroids for induction of lung maturation in preterm rabbits. Am J Obstet Gynecol 1991; 164:675–681.
80. Barker PM, Markiewicz M, Parker KA, et al. Synergistic action of triiodothyronine and hydrocortisone on epinephrine-induced reabsorption of fetal lung liquid. Pediatr Res 1990; 27:588–591.
81. Krochmal-Mokrzan EM, Barker PM, Gatzy JT. Effects of hormones on potential difference and liquid balance across explants from proximal and distal fetal rat lung. J Physiol (Lond) 1993; 463:647–665.
82. Barker PM, Walters DV, Markiewicz M, Strang LB. Development of the lung liquid reabsorptive mechanism in fetal sheep: synergism of triiodothyronine and hydrocortisone. J Physiol (Lond) 1991; 433:435–449.
83. Cott GR, Rao AK. Hydrocortisone promotes the maturation of Na+-dependent ion transport across the fetal pulmonary epithelium. Am J Respir Cell Mol Biol 1993; 9:166–171.
84. Barker PM, Gatzy JT. Effect of gas composition on liquid secretion by explants of distal lung of fetal rat in submersion culture. Am J Physiol 1993; 265 (Lung Cell Mol Physiol 9):L512–L517.
85. Mendelson CR, Alcorn JL, Gao E. The pulmonary surfactant protein genes and their regulation in fetal lung. Semin Perinatol 1993; 17:223–232.
86. Ballard PL. Hormonal regulation of pulmonary surfactant. Endocrine Rev 1989; 10:165–181.
87. Gross I. Regulation of fetal lung maturation. Am J Physiol 1990; 259 (Lung Cell Mol Physiol 3):L337–L344.

88. Boggaram V, Smith ME, Mendelson CR. Posttranscriptional regulation of surfactant protein-A messenger RNA in human fetal lung in vitro by glucocorticoids. Mol Endocrinol 1991; 5:414–423.
89. Seidner SR, Smith ME, Mendelson CR. Developmental changes in hormonal regulation of surfactant protein-A (SP-A) gene expression in lung tissues of fetal baboons. Pediatr Res 1993; 33(Suppl):57A.
90. Floros J, Phelps DS, Harding HP, et al. Postnatal stimulation of rat surfactant protein A synthesis by dexamethasone. Am J Physiol 1989; 257 (Lung Cell Mol Physiol 1):L137–L143.
91. Schellhase DE, Shannon JM. Effects of maternal dexamethasone on expression of SP-A, SP-B, and SP-C in the fetal rat lung. Am J Respir Cell Mol Biol 1991; 4:304–312.
92. Crowley P, Chalmers I, Keirse MJNC. The effects of corticosteroid administration before preterm delivery: An overview of the evidence from controlled trials. Br J Obstet Gynaecol 1990; 97:11–25.
93. Garite TJ, Rumney PJ, Briggs GG, et al. A randomized, placebo-controlled trial of betamethasone for the prevention of respiratory distress syndrome at 24 to 28 weeks' gestation. Am J Obstet Gynecol 1992; 166:646–651.
94. Jobe AH, Mitchell BR, Gunkel JH. Beneficial effects of the combined use of prenatal corticosteroids and postnatal surfactant on preterm infants. Am J Obstet Gynecol 1993; 168:508–513.
95. Farrell EE, Silver RK, Kimberlin LV, et al. Impact of antenatal dexamethasone administration on respiratory distress syndrome in surfactant-treated infants. Am J Obstet Gynecol 1989; 161:628–633.
96. Kari MA, Hallman M, Eronen M, et al. Prenatal dexamethasone treatment in conjunction with rescue therapy of human surfactant: A randomized placebo-controlled multicenter study. Pediatrics 1994; 93:730–736.
97. Bauer CR, Morrison JC, Poole WK, et al. A decreased incidence of necrotizing enterocolitis after prenatal glucocorticoid therapy. Pediatrics 1984; 73:682–688.
98. Clyman RI, Mauray F, Roman C, et al. Glucocorticoids alter the sensitivity of the lamb ductus arteriosus to prostaglandin E_2. J Pediatr 1981; 98:126–128.
99. Papageorgiou AN, Doray J, Ardila R, Kunos I. Reduction of mortality, morbidity, and respiratory distress syndrome in infants weighing less than 1000 grams by treatment with betamethasone and ritodrine. Pediatrics 1989; 83:493–497.
100. Andrews EB, White AD, Weinberg JM, et al. Antenatal steroids and neonatal outcomes in infants receiving surfactants in the Exosurf treatment IND. Pediatr Res 1992; 31(Suppl):241A.
101. Leviton A, Kuban KC, Pagano M, et al. Antenatal corticosteroids appear to reduce the risk of postnatal germinal matrix hemorrhage in intubated low birth weight newborns. Pediatrics 1993; 91:1083–1088.
102. Moise AA, Wearden ME, Welty SE, et al. Antenatal steroids reduce the need for blood pressure support in extremely premature infants. Section on Perinatal Pediatrics Program for Scientific Sessions 1993:12–13.
103. Stein HM, Oyama K, Martinez A, et al. Effects of corticosteroids in preterm sheep on adaptation and sympathoadrenal mechanisms at birth. Am J Physiol 1993; 264:E763–E769.

104. Fauser A, Pohlandt F, Bartmann P, Gortner L. Rapid increase of blood pressure in extremely low birth weight infants after a single dose of dexamethasone. Eur J Pediatr 1993; 152:354–356.
105. Frank L, Sosenko IRS. Prenatal development of lung antioxidant enzymes in four species. J Pediatr 1987; 110:106–110.
106. Tanswell AK, Freeman BA. Pulmonary antioxidant enzyme maturation in the fetal and neonatal rat. I. Developmental profiles. Pediatr Res 1984; 18:584–587.
107. Walther FJ, Wade AB, Warburton D, Forman HJ. Ontogeny of antioxidant enzymes in the fetal lamb lung. Exp Lung Res 1991; 17:39–45.
108. Autor AP, Frank L, Roberts RJ. Developmental characteristics of pulmonary superoxide dismutase: Relationship to idiopathic respiratory distress syndrome. Pediatr Res 1976; 10:154–158.
109. Frank L, Lewis PL, Sosenko IRS. Dexamethasone stimulation of fetal rat lung antioxidant enzyme activity in parallel with surfactant stimulation. Pediatrics 1985; 75:569–574.
110. Walther FJ, Ikegami M, Warburton D, Polk DH. Corticosteroids, thyrotropin releasing hormone, and antioxidant enzymes in preterm lamb lungs. Pediatr Res 1991; 30:518–521.
111. Clerch LB, Iqbal J, Massaro D. Perinatal rat lung catalase gene expression: influence of corticosteroid and hyperoxia. Am J Physiol 1991; 260 (Lung Cell Mol Physiol 4):L428–L433.
112. Frank L. Prenatal dexamethasone treatment improves survival of newborn rats during prolonged high O_2 exposure. Pediatr Res 1992; 32:215–221.
113. Keeney SE, Mathews MJ, Rassin DK. Antioxidant enzyme responses to hyperoxia in preterm and term rats after prenatal dexamethasone administration. Pediatr Res 1993; 33:177–180.
114. Liggins GC, Howie RN. A controlled trial of antepartum glucocorticoid treatment for prevention of the respiratory distress syndrome in premature infants. Pediatrics 1972; 50:515–525.
115. Block MF, Kling OR, Crosby WM. Antenatal glucocorticoid therapy for the prevention of respiratory distress syndrome in the premature infant. Obstet Gynecol 1977; 50:186–190.
116. Schutte MF, Treffers PE, Koppe JG, et al. The clinical use of corticosteroids for acceleration of foetal lung maturity. Ned Tijschr Geneeskd 1979; 123:420–427.
117. Taeusch HW, Frigoletto F, Kitzmiller J, et al. Risk of respiratory distress syndrome after prenatal dexamethasone treatment. Pediatrics 1979; 63:64–72.
118. Doran TA, Swyer P, MacMurray B, et al. Results of a double-blind controlled study on the use of betamethasone in the prevention of respiratory distress syndrome. Am J Obstet Gynecol 1980; 136:313–320.
119. Teramo K, Hallman M, Raivio KO. Maternal glucocorticoid in unplanned premature labor. Pediatr Res 1980; 14:326–329.
120. Gamsu HR, Mullinger BM, Donnai P, Dash CH. Antenatal administration of betamethasone to prevent respiratory distress syndrome in preterm infants: Report of a UK multicentre trial. Br J Obstet Gynaecol 1989; 96:401–410.
121. Collaborative Group on Antenatal Steroid Therapy. Effect of antenatal dexameth-

asone administration on the prevention of respiratory distress syndrome. Am J Obstet Gynecol 1981; 141:276–287.
122. Morales WJ, Diebel D, Lazar AJ, Zadrozny D. The effect of antenatal dexamethasone administration on the prevention of respiratory distress syndrome in preterm gestations with premature rupture of membranes. Am J Obstet Gynecol 1986; 154:591–595.
123. Papageorgiou AN, Desgranges MF, Masson M, et al. The antenatal use of betamethasone in the prevention of respiratory distress syndrome: A controlled double-blind study. Pediatrics 1979; 63:73–79.
124. Morrison JC, Whybrew WD, Bucovaz ET, Schneider JM. Injection of corticosteroids into mother to prevent neonatal respiratory distress syndrome. Am J Obstet Gynecol 1978; 131:358–366.
125. Schmidt PL, Sims ME, Strassner HT, et al. Effect of antepartum glucocorticoid administration upon neonatal respiratory distress syndrome and perinatal infection. Am J Obstet Gynecol 1984; 148:178–186.
126. Wiebicke W, Poynter A, Chernick V. Normal lung growth following antenatal dexamethasone treatment for respiratory distress syndrome. Pediatr Pulmonol 1988; 5:27–30.
127. MacArthur BA, Howie RN, Dezoete IA, Elkins J. Cognitive and psychosocial development of 4-year-old children whose mothers were treated antenatally with betamethasone. Pediatrics 1981; 68:638–643.
128. Elliot HR, Abdulla U. Pulmonary edema associated with ritodrine infusion and betamethasone administered in premature labor. Br Med J 1978; 2:799–800.
129. Philipsen T, Eriksen PS, Lynggard F. Pulmonary edema following ritodrine-saline infusion in premature labor: A case report. Am J Obstet Gynecol 1978; 3:341–342.
130. Miodovnik M, Peros N, Holroyde JC, Siddiqi TA. Treatment of premature labor in insulin-dependent diabetic women. Obstet Gynecol 1985; 65:621–627.
131. Fisher DA, Klein AH. Thyroid development and disorders of thyroid function in the newborn. N Engl J Med 1981; 304:702–712.
132. Klein AH, Foley B, Foley TP, et al. Thyroid function studies in cord blood from premature infants with and without RDS. J Pediatr 1981; 98:818–820.
133. Hadeed AJ, Asay LD, Klein AH, Fisher DA. Significance of transient postnatal hypothyroxinemia in premature infants with and without respiratory distress syndrome. Pediatrics 1981; 68:494–498.
134. Cuestas RA, Lindall A, Engel RR. Low thyroid hormones and respiratory distress syndrome of the newborn: Studies on cord blood. N Engl J Med 1976; 295:297–302.
135. Dhanireddy R, Smith YF, Hamosh M, et al. Respiratory distress syndrome in the newborn: Relationship to serum prolactin, thyroxine, and sex. Biol Neonate 1983; 43:9–15.
136. Romaguera J, Ramirez M, Adamsons K. Intra-amniotic thyroxine to accelerate fetal maturation. Semin Perinatol 1993; 17:260–266.
137. Massaro D, Teich N, Massaro GD. Postnatal development of pulmonary alveoli: modulation in rats by thyroid hormones. Am J Physiol 1986;250 (Reg Integ Comp Physiol 19):R51–R55.
138. Wu B, Kikkawa Y, Orzalesi MM, et al. The effect of thyroxine on the maturation of fetal rabbit lungs. Biol Neonate 1973; 22:161–168.

139. Church J, Khafayan E, Chechani V, et al. Transplacental stimulation of fetal lung maturation: Effect of triiodothyronine in the female and male rabbit fetus. Biol Neonate 1987; 52:157–165.
140. Gonzales LW, Ballard PL, Ertsey R, Williams MC. Glucocorticoids and thyroid hormones stimulate biochemical and morphological differentiation of human fetal lung in organ culture. J Clin Endocrinol Metab 1986; 62:678–691.
141. Ikegami M, Jobe AH, Pettenazzo A, et al. Effects of maternal treatment with corticosteroids, T3, TRH, and their combinations on lung function of ventilated preterm rabbits with and without surfactant treatments. Am Rev Respir Dis 1987; 136:892–898.
142. Devaskar UP, deMello DE, Ackerman J. Effect of maternal administration of thyrotropin-releasing hormone or DN1417 on functional and morphologic fetal rabbit lung maturation and duration of survival after premature delivery. Biol Neonate 1991; 59:346–351.
143. Schellenberg JC, Liggins GC, Manzai M, et al. Synergistic hormonal effects on lung maturation in fetal sheep. J Appl Physiol 1988; 65:94–100.
144. Tabor BL, Ikegami M, Jobe AH, et al. Dose response of thyrotropin-releasing hormone on pulmonary maturation in corticosteroid-treated preterm rabbits. Am J Obstet Gynecol 1990; 163:669–676.
145. Das DK, Ayromlooi J, Bandyopadhyay D, et al. Potentiation of surfactant release in fetal lung by thyroid hormone action. J Appl Physiol 1984; 56(6):1621–1626.
146. Whitsett JA, Darovec-Beckerman C, Pollinger J, Moore JJ Jr. Ontogeny of beta-adrenergic receptors in the rat lung: effects of hypothyroidism. Pediatr Res 1982; 16:381–387.
147. Sosenko IRS, Frank L. Thyroid hormone depresses antioxidant enzyme maturation in fetal rat lung. Am J Physiol 1987; 253 (Reg Integ Comp Physiol 22):R592–R598.
148. Chen Y, Whitney PL, Frank L. Negative regulation of antioxidant enzyme gene expression in the developing fetal rat lung by prenatal hormone treatments. Pediatr Res 1993; 33:171–176.
149. Barkai G, Reichman B, Lusky A, et al. The effect of thyroxine and corticosteroids upon amniotic fluid fluorescence polarization: A randomized controlled study. J Perinat Med 1992; 20:459–464.
150. Dudenhausen JW. Alternatives to antenatal glucocorticoid treatment for the prevention of respiratory distress syndrome. J Perinat Med 1987; 15:453–459.
151. Moya FR, Gross I. Combined hormonal therapy for the prevention of respiratory distress syndrome and its consequences. Semin Perinatol 1993; 17:267–274.
152. Moya F, Mena P, Heusser F, et al. Response of the maternal, fetal, and neonatal pituitary-thyroid axis to thyrotropin-releasing hormone. Pediatr Res 1986; 20:982–986.
153. Ballard RA, Ballard PL, Creasy RK, et al. Respiratory disease in very-low-birthweight infants after prenatal thyrotropin-releasing hormone and glucocorticoid. Lancet 1992; 339:510–515.
154. Morales WJ, O'Brien WF, Angel JL, et al. Fetal lung maturation: The combined use of corticosteroids and thyrotropin-releasing hormone. Obstet Gynecol 1989; 73:111–116.
155. Whitsett JA, Manton MA, Darovec-Beckerman C, Adams K. Current concepts. II.

β-adrenergic receptors and catecholamine sensitive adenylate cyclase in the developing rat lung. Life Sci 1981; 28:339–345.
156. Warburton D, Parton L, Buckley S, et al. β-receptors and surface active material flux in fetal lamb lung: Female advantage. J Appl Physiol 1987; 63:828–833.
157. Enhorning G, Chamberlain D, Contreras C, et al. Isoxsuprine-induced release of pulmonary surfactant in the rabbit fetus. Am J Obstet Gynecol 1977; 129:197–202.
158. Hadjigeorgiou E, Kitsiou S, Psaroudakis A, et al. Antipartum aminophylline treatment for prevention of the respiratory distress syndrome in premature infants. Am J Obstet Gynecol 1979; 135:257–260.
159. King JF, Grant AM, Keirse MJNC, Chalmers I. Beta-mimetics in preterm labour: An overview of the randomized controlled trials. Br J Obstet Gynaecol 1988; 95:211–222.
160. The Canadian Preterm Labor Investigators Group. Treatment of preterm labor with the beta-adrenergic agonist ritodrine. N Engl J Med 1992; 327:308–312.
161. Ryan RM, Finkelstein JN. Growth factors and pulmonary epithelia. In: Brody JS, Center DM, Tkachuk VA. Signal Transduction in Lung Cells. New York: Marcel Dekker, 1993:263–291.
162. Haigh RS, D'Souza W, Micklewright L, et al. Human amniotic fluid urogastrone (epidermal growth factor) and fetal lung phospholipids. Br J Obstet Gynaecol 1989; 96:171–178.
163. Stahlman MT, Orth DN, Gray ME. Immunocytochemical localization of epidermal growth factor in the developing human respiratory system and in acute and chronic lung disease in the neonate. Lab Invest 1989; 60:539–547.
164. Catterton WZ, Escobedo MB, Sexson WR, et al. Effect of epidermal growth factor on lung maturation in fetal rabbits. Pediatr Res 1979; 13:104–108.
165. Kennedy KA, Wilton P, Mellander M, et al. Effect of epidermal growth factor on lung liquid secretion in fetal sheep. J Dev Physiol 1986; 8:421–423.
166. Sundell HW, Gray ME, Serenius FS, et al. Effects of epidermal growth factor on lung maturation in fetal lambs. Am J Pathol 1980; 100:707–726.
167. Gross I, Dynia DW, Rooney SA, et al. Influence of epidermal growth factor on fetal rat lung development in vitro. Pediatr Res 1986; 20:473–477.
168. Price L, Chen Y, Frank L. Epidermal growth factor increases antioxidant enzyme and surfactant system development during hyperoxia and protects fetal rat lungs in vitro from hyperoxic toxicity. Pediatr Res 1993; 34:577–585.
169. Whitsett JA, Weaver TE, Lieberman MA, et al. Differential effects of epidermal growth factor and transforming growth factor-β on synthesis of $M_R = 35{,}000$ surfactant-associated protein in fetal lung. J Biol Chem 1987; 262:7908–7913.
170. Plopper CG, St. George JA, Read LC, et al. Acceleration of alveolar type II cell differentiation in fetal rhesus monkey lung by administration of EGF. Am J Physiol 1992; 262 (Lung Cell Mol Physiol 6):L313–L321.
171. St George JA, Read LC, Cranz DL, et al. Effect of epidermal growth factor on the fetal development of the tracheobronchial secretory apparatus in rhesus monkey. Am J Respir Cell Mol Biol 1991; 4:95–101.
172. Goetzman BW, Read L, Plopper CG, Styne DM. Postnatal administration of epidermal growth factor (EGF) and lung function in prematurely delivered rhesus monkeys. Pediatr Res 1991; 29(Suppl):333A.

173. Strandjord TP, Clark JH, Hodson WA, et al. Expression of transforming growth factor-α in mid-gestation human fetal lung. Am J Respir Cell Mol Biol 1993; 8:266–272.
174. Sunday ME, Kaplan LM, Motoyama E, et al. Biology of disease: Gastrin-releasing peptide (mammalian bombesin) gene expression in health and disease. Lab Invest 1988; 59:5–24.
175. Spindel ER, Sunday ME, Hofler H, et al. Transient elevation of messenger RNA encoding gastrin-releasing peptide, a putative pulmonary growth factor in human fetal lung. J Clin Invest 1987; 80:1172–1179.
176. Stahlman MT, Kasselberg AG, Orth DN, Gray ME. Ontogeny of neuroendocrine cells in human fetal lung: II. An immunohistochemical study. Lab Invest 1985; 52:52–60.
177. Johnson DE, Lock JE, Elde RP, Thompson TR. Pulmonary neuroendocrine cells in hyaline membrane disease and bronchopulmonary dysplasia. Pediatr Res 1982; 16:446–454.
178. Ghatei MA, Sheppard MN, Henzen-Logman S, et al. Bombesin and vasoactive intestinal polypeptide in the developing lung: Marked changes in acute respiratory distress syndrome. J Clin Endocrin Metab 1983; 57:1226–1232.
179. Sunday ME, Hua J, Dai HB, et al. Bombesin increases fetal lung growth and maturation in utero and in organ culture. Am J Respir Cell Mol Biol 1990; 3:199–205.
180. Sunday ME, Hua J, Reyes B, et al. Anti-bombesin monoclonal antibodies modulate fetal mouse lung growth and maturation in utero and in organ cultures. Anat Rec 1993; 236:25–32.
181. Everett MM, King RJ, Jones MB, Martin HM. Lung fibroblasts from animals breathing 100% oxygen produce growth factors for alveolar type II cells. Am J Physiol 1990; 259 (Lung Cell Mol Physiol 3):L247–L254.
182. Stiles AD, Smith BT, Post M. Reciprocal autocrine and paracrine regulation of growth of mesenchymal and alveolar epithelial cells from fetal lung. Exp Lung Res 1986; 11:165–177.
183. Tanswell AK. Cellular interactions in pulmonary oxygen toxicity in vitro: I. Hyperoxic induction of fibroblast factors which alter growth and lipid metabolism of pulmonary epithelial cells. Exp Lung Res 1983; 5:23–36.
184. Panos RJ, Rubin JS, Aaronson SA, Mason RJ. Keratinocyte growth factor and hepatocyte growth factor/scatter factor are heparin-binding growth factors for alveolar type II cells in fibroblast-conditioned medium. J Clin Invest 1993; 92:969–977.
185. Rubin JS, Chan AM-L, Bottaro DP, et al. A broad-spectrum human lung fibroblast-derived mitogen is a variant of hepatocyte growth factor. Proc Natl Acad Sci USA 1991; 88:415–419.
186. Tashiro K, Hagiya M, Nishizawa T, et al. Deduced primary structure of rat hepatocyte growth factor and expression of the mRNA in rat tissues. Proc Natl Acad Sci USA 1990; 87:3200–3204.
187. Tajimo J, Higuchi O, Mizuno K, Nakumura T. Tissue distribution of hepatocyte growth factor receptor and its exclusive down-regulation in a regenerating organ after injury. J Biochem 1992; 111:401–406.

188. Wolf HK, Zarnegar R, Michalopoulos GK. Localization of hepatocyte growth factor in human and rat tissues: An immunohistochemical study. Hepatology 1991; 14:488–494.
189. Rubin JS, Osada H, Finch PW, Taylor WG, Rudikoff S, Aaronson SA. Purification and identification of a newly identified growth factor specific for epithelial cells. Proc Natl Acad Sci USA 1989; 86:802–806.
190. Marchese C, Rubin J, Ron D, et al. Human keratinocyte growth factor activity on proliferation and differentiation of human keratinocytes: Differentiation response distinguishes KGF from EGF family. J Cel Physiol 1990; 144:326–332.
191. Ulich TR, Yi ES, Longmuir K, et al. Keratinocyte growth factor is a growth factor for type II pneumocytes in vivo. J Clin Invest 1994; 93:1298–1306.
192. Dekowski SA, Foust RJ, Panos RJ. Dexamethasone inhibits keratinocyte growth factor (KGF) mRNA expression in human fetal lung explants. Pediatr Res 1994; 35(Suppl):65A.
193. Hack M, Horbar JD, Malloy MH, et al. Very low birthweight outcomes of the NIH-CHD Neonatal Network. Pediatrics 1991; 87:587–597.
194. Seidner SR, Coalson JJ, McCurnin DC, Correll D. Clinical responses to early postnatal dexamethasone in surfactant-treated male baboons of borderline viability. Pediatr Res 1994; 35(Suppl):254A.

19

Clinical Trials of Surfactant Therapy in the Newborn

ROGER F. SOLL
University of Vermont College of Medicine
Burlington, Vermont

I. Clinical Trials of Surfactant Therapy

In the first clinical trials of surfactant substitution, aerosols of dipalmitoyl phosphatidylcholine (DPPC) were administered to preterm infants with respiratory distress syndrome (RDS). Although Robillard (1) reported that aerosolized DPPC alleviated the severity of RDS, Chu and coworkers (2) noted improvement only in compliance but little clinical improvement in treated infants. The lack of significant clinical effect with surfactant treatment led Chu and coworkers to hypothesize that pulmonary ischemia rather than surfactant deficiency was the major problem in RDS.

The studies of Enhorning and coworkers (3–5) and Adams et al. (6) documented the beneficial effects of natural surfactant given as a liquid instilled into the tracheae of premature animals. These studies served as the impetus toward attempting the first successful clinical trials.

Fujiwara et al. (7) were the first to successfully treat preterm infants with a modified surfactant extract. The initial study of Surfactant-TA involved 10 preterm infants studied consecutively without a control group. The treated infants represented a diverse group of neonates; gestational age ranged from 28 to 33 weeks of gestation and birth weight ranged between 1150 and 2143

g. All infants had severe RDS requiring assisted ventilation. Infants received a single intratracheal dose of Surfactant-TA between 4 and 33 hr of age. The infants responded to surfactant treatment within 3 hr demonstrating increased arterial oxygenation, improved alveolar-arterial oxygen difference, and decreased ventilatory support, oxygen requirement, and carbon dioxide retention. Improvement in the radiographic features of RDS was also reported. Fujiwara and coworkers found that infants exhibited a sustained response to surfactant treatment despite being treated after respiratory failure had occurred. Two infants involved in the study died during the neonatal period. Fujiwara cautioned that a high incidence of PDA was noted in treated infants (9 of 10 infants).

Since this initial experience, 33 randomized controlled clinical trials of surfactant replacement involving over 6000 infants have been reported. Trials have been conducted using either synthetic or natural surfactant products. In general, these trials have utilized two approaches to treatment: prophylactic administration of surfactant to high-risk premature infants (prevention trials) or administration of surfactant to premature infants with moderate to severe RDS (rescue or treatment trials). The hypothetical advantages of both approaches have been described, and both approaches have their advocates. Prevention trials offer the theoretical advantage of replacing surfactant before the onset of respiratory disease, decreasing the need for ventilatory support and avoiding the secondary barotrauma that results from even short periods of assisted ventilation (8). Another advantage of prophylactic administration may be improved distribution. Surfactant may distribute more homogeneously when given immediately at birth into lungs still filled with fluid (9) leading to improved response and decreasing the risk of lung injury. The possible advantage of rescue therapy is clear; rescue trials offer the advantage of treating only those infants who have the clinical signs of RDS, eliminating the potential risks and costs of treating surfactant sufficient infants who do not have RDS.

The following discussion of randomized controlled trials performed with surfactant therapy include overview analyses performed by the Cochrane Centre (10a,18,18a,121–123) and are updated from the discussion of Respiratory Distress Syndrome (10) in *Effective Care of the Newborn*. All available data from randomized controlled trials of surfactant have been included. The studies of modified or unmodified natural surfactant extracts are discussed separately from the studies of synthetic preparations. For the overview analyses, only trials with similar treatment strategies (prophylactic administration of surfactant or surfactant treatment of established RDS) are grouped together. Results from the overview analyses are given for pneumothorax, patent ductus arteriosus, intraventricular hemorrhage, bronchopulmonary dysplasia, survival without bronchopulmonary dysplasia (or the converse, bronchopulmonary dysplasia (BPD) or death) and mortality.

Results of the analyses are expressed as an "odds ratio" for individual studies and a "typical odds ratio" to express the results of the overview analysis. The odds ratio is the odds of an event occurring in the treated group compared with the same odds in the control group. For example, if mortality is reported in 20 out of a total of 100 infants treated with surfactant, the odds of dying after surfactant treatment is derived by comparing the number of infants who die (20) against the number of surviving infants (100–20). The odds of dying is, therefore, 20/(100–20), or 0.25. If 40 out of 100 infants in the control group die, the odds of dying without treatment would be 40/(100–40), or 0.67. The ratio of these odds would be 0.25/0.67, or 0.38. In the discussion, the odds ratio is presented with the 95% confidence interval. Odds ratio's of less than 1 suggest a decreased risk or odds of experiencing an adverse outcome. The typical odds ratio is derived by pooling data from similar trials using the methods of Collins and coworkers (11). A summary of the results of the overview analyses of randomized controlled trials is given in Table 1.

A. Natural Surfactant Extract

Prophylactic Administration of Natural Surfactant Extract

Eight trials have evaluated the prophylactic use of natural surfactant extract in infants at high risk of developing RDS (Table 2) (18). The first trial of prophylactic administration of a natural surfactant extract was conducted by Enhorning et al. (12). Seventy-two infants less than 30 weeks' gestation were

Table 1 Meta-analysis of Randomized Controlled Trials of Surfactant Replacement Therapy

		Natural surfactant extract		Synthetic surfactant
Prophylactic treatment	N	ODDS RATIO (95% CI)	N	ODDS RATIO (95% CI)
pneumothorax	8	0.31 (0.22–0.44)	5	0.64 (0.45–0.89)
patent ductus arteriosus	8	1.16 (0.89–1.50)	6	1.27 (1.03–1.57)
intraventricular hemorrhage	8	0.95 (0.73–1.24)	4	0.99 (0.73–1.21)
bronchopulmonary dysplasia	7	0.88 (0.67–1.15)	5	1.09 (0.80–1.47)
mortality	8	0.60 (0.42–0.85)	7	0.67 (0.52–0.88)
Selective treatment	N	ODDS RATIO (95% CI)	N	ODDS RATIO (95% CI)
pneumothorax	12	0.34 (0.27–0.44)	4	0.52 (0.42–0.65)
patent ductus arteriosus	12	0.96 (0.79–1.18)	3	0.73 (0.60–0.88)
intraventricular hemorrhage	10	0.94 (0.76–1.15)	2	0.77 (0.62–0.97)
bronchopulmonary dysplasia	10	1.01 (0.81–1.27)	3	0.68 (0.46–0.99)
mortality	11	0.59 (0.47–0.74)	5	0.65 (0.50–0.82)

Cl, confidence interval. Soll RF, Cochrane Centre Neonatal Module.

Table 2 Randomized Controlled Trials of Prophylactic Administration of Natural Surfactant Extract

Author	N	Surfactant preparation (dosage)	Frequency of administration	Entry criteria	Outcome
Enhorning et al. (1985)	72	Calf lung lavage (75–100 mg)	Single	GA < 30 wks	↓ IVH ↓ Death ↓ BPD/Death
Kwong et al. (1985)	27	Calf lung surfactant extract (Infasurf) (90 mg)	Single	GA 24–28 wks Antenatal steroids <24 hrs	None
Merritt et al. (1986)	60	Human amniotic fluid extract (60 mg)	Multiple	GA 24–29 wks Immature phospholipid	↓ Pneumothorax ↓ Death ↓ BPD/Death
Kendig et al. (1988)	65	Calf lung surfactant extract (90 mg)	Single	GA 25–29 wks Required intubation in delivery room	↓ Pneumothorax
Shennan and Dunn (1989)	56	Calf lung surfactant extract (75–100 mg)	Single	GA < 29 wks	↓ Pneumothorax
Soll et al. (1990)	156	Survanta (100 mg/kg)	Single	GA 24–30 wks BW 750–1250 g Stabilized <15 min	↓ Pneumothorax ↑ NEC
Dunn et al. (1990)	122	Calf lung surfactant extract (75–100 mg)	Multiple	GA < 30 wks	↓ Pneumothorax ↑ Severe BPD
Hoekstra et al. (1991)	430	Survanta (100 mg/kg)	Multiple	GA 23–29 wks BW 600–1250 g Stabilized ≤15 min	↓ Pneumothorax ↑ Death

BW, birth weight; GA, gestational age.

enrolled and randomly assigned to either a single intratracheal dose of calf lung lavage (75 mg/kg) or control treatment. Treatment was administered prior to the onset of spontaneous breathing. Significant improvement in respiratory status was noted in the 72 hr after treatment. Fewer treated infants had intraventricular hemorrhage and more infants who received treatment survived.

Other prevention trials using a single dose of natural surfactant extract similar to the calf lung lavage tested by Enhorning have been reported. Kwong et al. (13) enrolled infants between 24 and 28 weeks' gestation who had not received a complete course of antenatal steroids. Twenty-seven infants were randomized immediately before birth to receive either calf lung surfactant extract (CLSE) or saline as a single intratracheal instillation prior to the onset of breathing. Although respiratory status improved in the 48 hr after treatment, no other improvement in clinical outcome was demonstrated. In a similar study, Kendig et al. (14) enrolled 65 infants between 25 and 29 weeks' gestation. Infants received either a single intratracheal dose of CLSE or saline control. Infants given prophylactic CLSE demonstrated improved respiratory status, but these improvements were not sustained. A decreased incidence of pneumothorax was associated with prophylactic treatment. Shennan et al. (15) conducted a study of prophylactic surfactant administration similar in design to their original trial (12). Results of this trial were less impressive than the original study; a decrease in pneumothorax was noted, but no improvement was noted in intraventricular hemorrhage or mortality.

One study has evaluated the use of multiple doses of CLSE. Dunn et al., (16) enrolled 122 infants of less than 30 weeks' gestational age. Infants randomized to surfactant could receive multiple doses of CLSE if they demonstrated continued respiratory distress (defined as an increase in oxygen requirement of 10%). Using this treatment approach, surfactant-treated infants demonstrated fewer pneumothoraces and fewer surfactant-treated infants developed severe BPD (defined as oxygen therapy at 36 weeks' adjusted gestational age).

Surfactant derived from human amniotic fluid extract has been tested in the prevention of RDS. Merritt et al. (17) studied 60 infants between 24 and 29 weeks' gestation. Infants were included in the final analysis only if they had an immature lung profile. Infants could receive multiple doses of surfactant if the infant required increasing supplemental oxygen or ventilatory support. Surfactant treatment not only improved the initial respiratory course, it also improved overall survival and survival without bronchopulmonary dysplasia.

Two trials have utilized prophylactic administration of a modified natural surfactant extract (19,20). Soll et al. (20) enrolled infants between 24 and 30 weeks' gestational age. Infants were treated with either a single dose of Survanta or air placebo if they weighed between 750 and 1250 g at birth and could be successfully intubated and stabilized. Unlike previous prophylactic trials, infants were routinely ventilated for up to 10 min prior to treatment. A decrease in the requirement for supplemental oxygen was noted in the treated group. Improvement in clinical outcome was limited to a decrease in pneumothoraces. An increase in the incidence of necrotizing enterocolitis was noted. A multicenter trial of prophylactic Survanta treatment has been reported by Soll et al. (19). This trial was similar in design to the trial of Soll et al. (20) except that infants of lower birth weight were eligible (600–1250 g) and multiple doses of Survanta were administered. The trial noted a significant decrease in the incidence of pneumothorax and mortality. An increase in the incidence of patent ductus arteriosus was noted in this trial.

Overview Analysis of Prophylactic Administration of Natural Surfactant Extract

The trials of prophylactic administration of natural surfactant extracts all report decreased the need for supplemental oxygen or ventilatory support early in the course of RDS (48–72 h). However, response is not always sustained and many of the trials resorted to a treatment approach which allowed for the administration of multiple doses of surfactant (17,19,21). Although many individual trials reported significant improvement in outcome, the results are not always consistent. Overview analysis allows for an estimate of the effect of prophylactic natural surfactant on clinical outcome. The results of the overview analysis from the Cochrane Centre Neonatal Module are given in Table 1 (18).

The majority of trials (six of nine) of prophylactic surfactant reported a decrease in the incidence of pneumothorax (14,20). The overview analysis demonstrates that prophylactic administration of natural surfactant extract is associated with a highly significant decrease in the odds of pneumothorax (typical odds ratio 0.31, 95% confidence level 0.22–0.44).

Evidence from animal experiments and early experience with surfactant replacement raised the concern that surfactant replacement might be associated with increased shunt through the patent ductus arteriosus (PDA). Only one of the nine studies of prophylactic administration of natural surfactant extract reported an increase in hemodynamically significant patent ductus arteriosus (19). The typical estimate suggests no effect of prophylactic administration of natural surfactant extract on the risk of PDA (typical odds ratio 1.16, 95% confidence level 0.89–1.50). Definitive conclusions regarding the role of prophylactic natural surfactant extracts on PDA cannot be made based on this evidence, since in most of the clinical trials, the diagnosis of PDA was loosely defined (diagnosis of PDA based on clinical diagnosis without specific echocardiographic or Doppler criteria or timing of studies).

Prophylactic administration of natural surfactant extract has no apparent impact on the incidence of intraventricular hemorrhage (IVH). Only the study of Enhorning et al. (12) noted a decrease in the overall incidence of IVH. No study noted any impact on the more severe grades of hemorrhage. In the eight trials which reported on IVH, the overview analysis does not demonstrate any beneficial effect of prophylactic natural surfactant on the odds of any IVH (typical odds ratio 0.95, 95% confidence level 0.73–1.24).

Prophylactic administration of natural surfactant extract does not decrease the risk of BPD in treated infants. For the purpose of most studies, BPD was diagnosed in all infants requiring supplemental oxygen at 28–30 days of age. For the purpose of this discussion, the incidence of BPD is given for all randomized infants, not only for survivors. No individual study could demonstrate a decrease in the absolute incidence of BPD in treated infants, and the typical estimate does not suggest a significant effect of prophylactic natural surfactant extracts in decreasing the odds of BPD (typical odds ratio 0.88, 95% confidence level 0.67–1.15). However, more infants survive without the complication of BPD. When the combined outcome of BPD or death during the first 28 days of life is evaluated, a significant improvement in outcome is noted with prophylactic surfactant treatment (typical odds ratio 0.64, 95% confidence level 0.49–0.84).

Mortality data are available from all nine randomized controlled trials of prophylactic administration of natural surfactant extracts. Several of these trials, using a variety of natural surfactant extracts, were able to demonstrate a significant reduction in mortality (12,17,19). The typical estimate suggests that a significant decrease in the odds of mortality occurs with prophylactic administration of natural surfactant (typical odds ratio 0.60, 95% confidence level 0.42–0.85).

Treatment of Established RDS with Natural Surfactant Extract

The first successful clinical experience with natural surfactant extract treatment of established RDS was the original trial of Fujiwara et al. (7). Twelve randomized controlled trials of natural surfactant extract in the treatment of RDS followed Fujiwara's initial experience (Table 3). Five studies evaluated the modified natural surfactant extract Surfactant-TA. Gitlin et al. (22) studied 41 infants weighing between 1000 and 1500 g with RDS requiring assisted ventilation and supplemental oxygen. Infants were randomly assigned to a single dose of Surfactant-TA or saline control and treated between 5 and 8 hr of age. Significant differences in the arterial/alveolar oxygen ratio (a/A O_2 ratio) and requirement for assisted ventilation (decrease in mean airway pressure) were noted during the 48 hr after treatment. The treated infants experienced fewer pneumothoraces and fewer days in supplemental oxygen. In this small population, no difference in long-term clinical outcome was noted.

Raju et al. (23) conducted a similar study of single-dose Surfactant-TA in infants with established RDS. A broader weight range of infants was included

Table 3 Randomized Controlled Trials of Natural Surfactant Extract in the Treatment of RDS

Author	N	Surfactant preparation (dosage)	Frequency of administration	Entry criteria	Outcome
Hallman et al. (1985) (27)	45	Human amniotic fluid extract (60 mg/kg)	Multiple	BW <1500 g RDS requiring assisted ventilation, FiO_2 ≥0.6 immature lung profile, age <10 hr	↓ Pneumothorax ↓ BPD ↓ BPD/death
Gitlin et al. (1987) (22)	41	Surfactant-TA (100 mg/kg)	Single	BW 1000–1500 g RDS requiring assisted ventilation, FiO_2 ≥0.4, age <8 hr	↓ Pneumothorax
Raju et al. (1987) (23)	30	Surfactant-TA (100 mg/kg)	Single	BW 751–1750 g RDS requiring assisted ventilation, FiO_2 ≥0.5, MAP ≥8 cmH_2O a/A ratio ≤0.24, age <6 hr	↓ Pneumothorax ↓ Death ↑ PDA
Collaborative Group (1988) (29)	146	Curosurf (porcine lung extract) (200 mg/kg)	Single	BW 700–2000 g RDS requiring assisted ventilation, FiO_2 ≥0.6, age 2–15 hr	↓ Pneumothorax ↓ Death ↓ BPD/death
Soll et al. (1988) (24)	31	Surfactant-TA (100 mg/kg)	Single	BW 750–1750 g RDS requiring assisted ventilation, FiO_2 ≥0.4, age 3–6 hr	None

Horbar et al. (1989) (31)	159	Survanta (100 mg/kg)	Single	BW 750–1750 g RDS requiring assisted ventilation, $FiO_2 \geq 0.4$, age 3–6 hr	↓ Pneumothorax
Gortner (1990) (30)	69	SF-RI 1 (bovine lung extract) (50 mg/kg)	Multiple	GA 25–30 wks Assisted ventilation, age ≤1 hr	↓ BPD/death
Horbar et al. (1990) (32)	104	Survanta (100 mg/kg)	Single	BW 750–1750 g RDS requiring assisted ventilation, $FiO_2 \geq 0.4$, age 3–6 hr	↑ IVH
Lang (1990) (28)	59	Human amniotic fluid extract (70–105 mg)	Multiple	GA 24–32 wks BW ≤1500 g RDS requiring assisted ventilation, $FiO_2 > 0.8$, age ≤12 hr	↓ Pneumothorax
Fujiwara et al. (1990) (26)	100	Surfactant-TA (120 mg/kg)	Single	BW 750–1750 g RDS requiring assisted ventilation, $FiO_2 \geq 0.4$, MAP ≥7 cmH_2O No IVH ≥ grade 2	↓ Pneumothorax ↓ IVH ↓ BPD/death
Chen et al. (1990) (25)	18	Surfactant-TA (120 mg/kg)	Single	RDS requiring assisted ventilation, evidence of surfactant deficiency	None
Liechty et al. (1991) (33)	798	Survanta (100 mg/kg)	Multiple	BW 600–1750 g RDS requiring assisted ventilation, $FiO_2 \geq 0.4$, age <8 hr	↓ Pneuomothorax ↓ Death

BW, birth weight; GA, gestational age.

in this study, but the entry criteria for severity of RDS were more stringent (assisted ventilation with $FiO_2 > 0.5$, MAP > 8 cmH_2O and a/A O_2 ratio <0.24). Infants less than 6 hr of age were enrolled and randomized to a single dose of Surfactant-TA or saline placebo. Treated infants demonstrated significant improvement in oxygenation and decreased requirement for ventilatory support during the 72 hr after treatment. Fewer pneumothoraces and deaths were noted in the surfactant-treated infants. An increased incidence of patent ductus arteriosus was associated with treatment.

A small pilot study of Surfactant-TA was conducted at five European centers. Soll et al. (24) studied 31 infants weighing 750–1750 g with RDS requiring assisted ventilation and supplemental oxygen of greater than 40%. Although acute improvement was noted, no significant clinical effect was reported. Chen et al. (25) demonstrated improved ventilatory status in a small study of Surfactant-TA in infants with established RDS.

After their initial experience with Surfactant-TA, Fujiwara et al. (26) conducted a larger randomized controlled trial of Surfactant-TA at 21 centers in Japan. Infants weighing 750–1750 g were enrolled if they had RDS requiring assisted ventilation and supplemental oxygen. Infants (n = 100) received either a single dose of Surfactant-TA (120 mg/kg) or placebo treatment with air. Significant improvement in both early and late outcome measures was noted. Treatment with Surfactant-TA significantly decreased the incidence of pneumothorax, intraventricular hemorrhage, and BPD or death at 28 days.

Other natural surfactant products have been tested in the treatment of established RDS. Hallman et al. (27) tested a surfactant preparation obtained from an extract of human amniotic fluid. Fifty-three infants weighing less than 1500 g with severe RDS defined by radiographic and clinical criteria (assisted ventilation, $FiO_2 > 0.6$) were enrolled at two centers. The initial treatment was given at approximately 5 hr of age, and retreatment was given if the requirement for supplemental oxygen or assisted ventilation increased. Of the 53 infants originally enrolled, 45 are included in the final analysis (exclusions included sepsis or cardiac disease mimicking RDS). Treated infants demonstrated significant improvement in oxygenation and decreased need for respiratory support. Significantly fewer pneumothoraces were noted in treated infants. The overall incidence of bronchopulmonary dysplasia as well as the combined incidence of BPD or death at 28 days was significantly decreased in surfactant-treated infants.

Lang et al. (28) studied human amniotic fluid extract in a population similar to the infants studied by Hallman et al. (27). The clinical impact of surfactant treatment is less substantial in Lang and coworkers' study. Fewer surfactant treated infants had pneumothoraces, but no other clinical benefit was noted.

Two natural surfactant extracts have been studied exclusively in Europe. Robertson and coworkers conducted a collaborative trial of Curosurf, a porcine lung extract, at eight European centers (29). A broad range of infants (birth weight 700–2000 g) were studied if they had RDS requiring assisted ventilation and supplemental oxygen of 60% or greater. Infants were randomized to either Curosurf (200 mg/kg) or sham treatment. Infants who received Curosurf demonstrated a significant reduction in pneumothoraces or death. Fewer infants were noted to have BPD or death at 28 days of age. Gortner et al. (30) studied multiple doses of a bovine lung extract SF-RI1 (Alveofact). Infants between 25 and 30 weeks' gestation were enrolled. Although described as a prevention trial by the authors, infants were eligible only if intubated and on assisted ventilation at 1 hr of life. Gortner and coworkers noted a decrease in BPD or death at 28 days in association with surfactant treatment.

The most extensively tested natural surfactant preparation in the treatment of established RDS is Survanta (Ross Laboratories). Survanta is a modified bovine surfactant extract similar in composition to Surfactant-TA. Survanta has been tested in multicenter collaborative trials both in Europe and the United States (31–33). Two identical single dose trials of Survanta in treating established RDS have been reported (31,32). Infants weighing between 750 and 1750 g with RDS requiring respiratory support were enrolled at centers in the United States and Europe. In the US Trial, Horbar et al. (31) demonstrated improved oxygenation and decreased requirement for respiratory support. Fewer pneumothoraces occurred in Survanta-treated infants. The European trial of Horbar et al. (32) also demonstrated early improvement in various respiratory parameters. No other clinical benefit of surfactant treatment could be demonstrated. Unlike other studies of Survanta, the European trial noted a significant increase in intraventricular hemorrhage in surfactant treated infants.

A large multicenter trial using multiple doses of Survanta in treating established RDS has been reported by Liechty et al. (33). Infants with birth weights between 600 and 1750 g were enrolled if they had RDS requiring assisted ventilation and supplemental oxygen of 40% or greater. Infants were randomized to multiple doses of Survanta or sham air treatment prior to 8 hr of age. The study demonstrated a decrease in pneumothoraces in surfactant treated infants. Multiple doses of Survanta also led to a decrease in mortality in treated infants.

Overview Analysis of Natural Surfactant Extract in the Treatment of Established RDS

As was noted in the prophylactic trials of natural surfactant extract, the treatment of RDS with natural surfactant extract universally led to improvement in the need for supplemental oxygen and ventilatory support early in the course of RDS. Treatment with both single and multiple doses has been shown to be effective in reducing major complications related to prematurity and respiratory distress. Although many trials have reported significant clinical improvement, results are not always consistent. Overview analysis of the 12 trials of natural surfactant extract in the treatment of RDS allows for an estimate of the effect of surfactant on clinical outcome of infants with RDS (see Table 1) (18a).

All 12 of the trials of natural surfactant extract reported data on the incidence of pneumothorax. Eight reported a decrease in pneumothorax in surfactant treated infants (22,23,26–29,31,33). The typical estimate of effect supports a substantial and highly significant reduction in the odds of pneumothorax in surfactant treated infants (typical odds ratio 0.34, 95% confidence level 0.27–0.44).

The original experience reported by Fujiwara et al. (7) raised concern regarding an increase in shunting through the patent ductus arteriosus. Of the randomized controlled trials, only the study of Raju et al. (23) demonstrated an increased risk of PDA (odds ratio 6.28, 95% confidence level 1.52–25.97). The overview analysis does not suggest any effect of surfactant treatment on PDA (typical odds ratio 0.96, 95% confidence level 0.79–1.18).

The single-dose study of Survanta conducted in Europe (32) raised concern regarding an increased risk of intraventricular hemorrhage regarding both the risk of any IVH and the risk of severe IVH (grade 3–4). An overview analysis of the effect of natural surfactant extract on all intraventricular hemorrhage and severe IVH does not support the concerns raised by the European study. Data on IVH are available on 10 trials (22–24,26,27,29–33). Only the European single dose study of Survanta of Horbar et al. (32) noted an increased risk of IVH (odds ratio 3.74, 95% confidence level 1.73, 8.09). The multicenter trial of Surfactant-TA conducted by Fujiwara et al. (26) noted a decreased risk of IVH associated with surfactant treatment (odds ratio 0.23, 95% confidence level 0.10, 0.52). Overall, treatment of established RDS with natural surfactant extract appears to have little impact on either all IVH (typical odds ratio 0.94, 95% confidence level 0.76–1.15) or severe IVH (typical odds ratio 0.91, 95% confidence level 0.72–1.14).

The overall risk of BPD is not decreased with natural surfactant extract treatment. Hallman et al. (27) reported the only trial which demonstrated a decreased risk of BPD (odds ratio 0.23, 95% confidence level 0.06, 0.94). The overview analysis of the 10 trials which reported on BPD (22–28,32,33) does not suggest an effect of natural surfactant treatment on the risk of BPD (typical odds ratio 1.01, 95% confidence level 0.81, 1.27).

Mortality is reduced in infants with RDS who were treated with natural surfactant extract. Three trials demonstrated a significant reduction in mortality (23,29,33). The overview analysis from 11 trials demonstrates a significant decrease in the risk of mortality in surfactant treated infants (typical odds ratio 0.59, 95% confidence level 0.47–0.74).

An analysis of the incidence of either BPD or death at 28 days of age suggests a significant effect of natural surfactant extract treatment. Of the 10 studies with available data (22–24,26–28,30,31,33), four trials demonstrated a significant reduction in BPD or death at 28 days in surfactant treated infants (26,27,30,33). The typical estimate suggests a significant reduction in the risk of BPD or death at 28 days (typical odds ratio 0.66, 95% confidence level 0.53, 0.82).

B. Synthetic Surfactant

Prophylactic Administration of Synthetic Surfactant

The first attempts at surfactant replacement used synthetic preparations of dipalmitdyl phosphatidylcholine (DPPC). The original trials of DPPC alone were unsuccessful, since neither the surfactant (DPPC alone) nor the route of administration were effective. For the purposes of this discussion, only the recent trials of complex synthetic surfactants are included.

A wide variety of synthetic products have been tested during the past decade (Table 4). Halliday et al. (34) tested a saline suspension of DPPC and high-density lipoprotein (HDL). In vitro studies demonstrated the ability of this surfactant to adsorb and spread rapidly (35). The investigators studied 100 infants between 25 and 33 weeks' gestation. Infants were randomized to receive either intratracheal DPPC/HDL or manual ventilation with air. Treated infants fared no better than control infants regarding both immediate and long-term clinical outcome.

A synthetic surfactant composed of DPPC and phosphatidylglycerol (PG) has been tested in the United Kingdom. Morley et al. (35a) first studied a dry synthetic mixture of DPPC/PG in infants less than 34 weeks gestation. In this nonrandomized study, no sustained improvement improvement in respiratory status was reported. Fewer infants who received DPPC/PG died.

The results of this clinical experience with dry powder DPPC/PG have not been corroborated in other studies. Wilkinson et al. (36) conducted a randomized controlled trial of dry DPPC/PG in both the prevention and treatment of RDS in premature infants (≤31 weeks' gestation). In this small trial, infants given prophylactic dry DPPC/PG had similar outcomes as did untreated controls.

The Ten Centre Study Group (37) used a saline suspension of DPPC and PG called Artificial Lung Expanding Compound (ALEC). The Ten Centre Study randomized 328 infants between 25 and 29 weeks' gestation to either ALEC or 1 ml of saline. Treatment was administered in the delivery room by injecting the surfactant suspension into the hypopharynx of the infant. In those infants who failed to breathe spontaneously, intubation and resuscitation was followed by a repeat treatment via the endotracheal tube. Infants who remained intubated could be given up to two more doses during the first 24 hr of life. No immediate benefit

Table 4 Randomized Controlled Trials of Prophylactic Administration of Synthetic Surfactant

Author	N	Surfactant preparation (dosage)	Frequency of administration	Entry criteria	Outcome
Halliday et al. (1984) (34)	100	DPPC/HDL (30 mg/3 mg)	Single	GA 25–33 wks Neonatologist present	None
Wilkinson et al. (1985) (36)	32	DPPC/PG Powder (25 mg)	Single	GA ≤31 wks	None
Ten Centre Study (1987) (37)	308	ALEC (DPPC/PG in saline) (100 mg)	Multiple	GA 25–29 wks Neonatologist present	↓ Death
Bose et al. (1990) (40)	385	Exosurf Neonatal (5 ml/kg, 67.5 mg DPPC/kg)	Single	BW 700–1350 g	↓ BPD/death
Corbet et al. (1990) (41)	446	Exosurf Neonatal (5 ml/kg, 67.5 mg DPPC/kg)	Single	BW 700–1100 g	↓ Pneumothorax ↓ Death
Phibbs et al. (1991) (42)	74	Exosurf Neonatal (5 ml/kg, 67.5 mg DPPC/kg)	Single	GA ≤ 34 wks BW 700–1350 g	None
Stevenson et al. (1992) (43)	215	Exosurf Neonatal (5 ml/kg, 67.5 mg DPPC/kg)	Single	BW 500–700 g	↓ Pneuomothorax

BW, birth weight; GA, gestational age.

of surfactant treatment was reported. Treated infants did demonstrate a significant decrease in severe intracranial hemorrhage and neonatal mortality. No adverse effects were reported.

The most widely tested of synthetic surfactant products is Exosurf Neonatal (Burroughs-Wellcome). Exosurf Neonatal is composed primarily of DPPC, but it also contains hexadecanol (an alcohol) and tyloxapol (a nonionic surfactant). Hexadecanol and tyloxapol are not found in naturally occurring surfactant, and they have been added to aid in spreading and dispersion of the surfactant. Exosurf Neonatal has been successfully tested in animal models (38,39). Tooley et al. (39) demonstrated improved pressure-volume characteristics in the lungs of premature rabbits treated with Exosurf. Lung compliance is improved in premature lambs given intratracheal Exosurf (38). The effects of Exosurf Neonatal in animal models is significantly better than saline control, but not equivalent to treatment with a crude natural surfactant extract (39).

Four randomized controlled trials have evaluated the use of a single intratracheal prophylactic dose of Exosurf Neonatal in infants at risk of developing RDS (40–43). The results from these studies are favorable but not consistent. Phibbs et al. (42) studied Exosurf Neonatal in both the prevention and treatment of RDS. In the prevention trial, 74 infants of birth weights of 700–1350 g were randomized to Exosurf Neonatal or control treatment. Significant reduction in the requirement for ventilatory support was noted in the 72 hr after treatment. No other substantial clinical effect was noted. Two large multicenter trials evaluated prophylactic Exosurf in a similar population of premature infants. Corbet et al. (41) and Bose et al. (40) studied Exosurf Neonatal in infants with birth weights of 700–1100 g and 700–1350 g, respectively. Both trials reported early decreased need for supplemental oxygen and ventilatory support. In the study of Corbet et al. (41), fewer pneumothoraces were noted in treated infants and mortality was significantly decreased. Bose et al. (40) did not demonstrate an improvement in overall mortality, but the number of surviving infants without bronchopulmonary dysplasia was increased.

Stevenson et al. (43) studied a single dose of prophylactic Exosurf in infants with birth weights of 500–700 g. Only a reduction in pneumothorax was noted. Studies are currently evaluating whether prophylactic treatment and possible retreatment with Exosurf Neonatal is superior to single-dose prophylactic treatment.

Overview Analysis of Prophylactic Administration of Synthetic Surfactant

The immediate effect of synthetic surfactant administration may not be as pronounced as the immediate effect of natural surfactant extracts. Only the trials using Exosurf Neonatal have reported acute improvement in the requirement for supplemental oxygen or ventilatory support. Although the requirement for supplemental oxygenor ventilatory support is increased with Exosurf treatment, the magnitude of this response may not be as great as the initial response seen in infants treated with natural surfactant extract. As was noted in the overviews of other surfactant trials, results may not be consistent across studies. Overview analysis allows for an estimate of the clinical impact of prophylactic synthetic surfactant on pneumothorax, PDA, intraventricular hemorrhage, BPD, and death (see Table 1) (122).

Data are available from five trials regarding the incidence of pneumothoraces. Two studies demonstrated a significant decrease in pneumothoraces associated with treatment (41,43). The overview analysis suggests a significant decrease in the risk of pneumothorax with prophylactic administration of synthetic surfactant (typical odds ratio 0.64, 95% confidence level 0.45–0.89).

No individual trial of prophylactic administration of synthetic surfactant reported any effect of treatment on the incidence of patent ductus arteriosus. As noted in the discussion of natural surfactant extracts, PDA was never a primary outcome variable in these studies and the diagnosis of PDA was made based on clinical judgment, not rigorous evaluation through sequential echocardiographic or Doppler studies. Although no individual study noted an increased incidence of PDA, the typical estimate suggests that prophylactic synthetic surfactant leads to a slight increase in the risk of clinically significant ductal shunting (typical odds ratio 1.27, 95% confidence level 1.03, 1.57).

The Ten Centre Study Group (37) reported a decrease in intracranial hemorrhage in treated infants. However, this study did not use the classification system commonly used in the other trials and, therefore, data from the Ten Centre Study Group is not included in the overview analysis. Four trials (34,40,41,43) reported their overall incidence of intraventricular hemorrhage using the criteria of Papile et al. (43a). None of these studies demonstrated a decrease in intraventricular hemorrhage. The typical estimate derived from the data from these four trials does not suggest any effect of prophylactic synthetic surfactant on intraventricular hemorrhage (typical odds ratio 0.94, 95% confidence level 0.73, 1.21).

The incidence of bronchopulmonary dysplasia is not decreased by prophylactic administration of synthetic surfactant. In this discussion, bronchopulmonary dysplasia (BPD) is defined as the need for supplemental oxygen at 28 days of life with or without radiographic support. Estimates are calculated based on all enrolled infants, not only for infants who survived until 28 days. Five trials reported data on the incidence of bronchopulmonary dysplasia (34,36,40,41,43). No individual trial noted a decreased incidence of BPD in treated infants. The overview analysis does not suggest any impact of prophylactic synthetic surfactant on BPD (typical odds ratio 1.09, 95% confidence level 0.80, 1.47). Only three studies report data on the combined outcome of BPD or death at 28 days (40,41,43). Overview analysis of these three studies does not conclusively support a reduction in BPD or death (typical odds ratio 0.82, 95% confidence level 0.63–1.08).

Prophylactic administration of synthetic surfactant leads to a significant decrease in mortality. Data on mortality are available from all seven studies. Two trials demonstrated a decrease in overall mortality. In the Ten Centre Study (37), mortality was decreased from 30% in control infants to 19% in ALEC-treated infants (odds ratio 0.56, 95% confidence level 0.33, 0.94). In the study of Corbet et al. (41), mortality was decreased from 22% in control infants to 13% in Exosurf-treated infants (odds ratio 0.54, 95% confidence level 0.32–0.90). Overview analysis suggests that prophylactic administration of synthetic surfactant will significantly decrease the odds of mortality (typical odds ratio 0.67, 95% confidence level 0.52, 0.88).

Treatment of Established RDS with Synthetic Surfactant

Synthetic surfactant preparations have been used in the treatment of established RDS. The six randomized controlled trials using this approach are summarized in Table 5. Wilkinson et al. (36) evaluated the use of dry DPPC/PG in infants with established RDS. Infants of 31 weeks' gestation or less who did not require intubation in the delivery room (and therefore were not enrolled in the prevention study) were enrolled if they subsequently had an immature lecithin/sphingomyelin ratio and developed RDS requiring assisted ventilation. Neither immediate nor long-term benefit could be demonstrated with surfactant treatment.

With the exception of the trial done by Wilkinson et al. (36), all other trials of synthetic surfactant treatment of RDS utilized Exosurf Neonatal (42,44–47). Phibbs et al. (42) studied the effect of a single dose of Exosurf Neonatal in infants weighing 650 g or more who had RDS requiring assisted ventilation and supplemental oxygen. Requirements for ventilatory support decreased significantly during the 72 hr after treatment. No other clinical benefit was noted.

Four large multicenter trials studied the effect of multiple doses of Exosurf Neonatal in the treatment of RDS (44–47). These trials evaluated a wide range of infants with established RDS. Long et al. (45) and the Canadian Pediatric Study Group (44) evaluated very low birth weight infants with RDS (birth weight criteria: Long et al., 700–1350 g; Canadian Study 750–1249 g). Infants were enrolled if they had RDS requiring assisted ventilation, had an arterial/alveolar oxygen ratio less than 0.22, and were between 2 and 24 hr of age. Both trials reported significant improvement in respiratory status during the first week of life. Long et al. (45) reported a decrease in mortality in surfactant treated infants. In both studies, a significant decrease in the incidence of pneumothorax and BPD or death at 28 days of age was noted. Long et al. (45) reported an increased incidence of apnea in surfactant-treated infants.

Table 5 Randomized Controlled Trials of Synthetic Surfactant in the Treatment of RDS

Author	N	Surfactant preparation (dosage)	Frequency of administration	Entry criteria	Outcome
Wilkinson et al. (1985) (36)	24	DPPC/PG (powder) (25 mg)	Single	GA ≤31 wks RDS requiring assisted ventilation, L/S ratio <1.8	↓ BPD/death (personal communication)
Canadian Exosurf Study (1990) (44)	342	Exosurf Neonatal	Multiple	BW 750–1249 g RDS requiring assisted ventilation, a/A ratio <0.22, Age 2–24 hr	↓ Pneumothorax ↓ Death ↓ BPD/death
Long et al. (1991) (46)	1232	Exosurf Neonatal (75 mg/kg)	Multiple	BW ≥1250 g (Canada) BW >1350 g (US) RDS requiring assisted ventilation, a/A ratio <0.22, Age 2–24 hr	↓ Pneumothorax ↓ IVH ↓ BPD ↓ Death ↓ BPD/Death ↑ Apnea
Phibbs et al. (1991) (42)	105	Exosurf Neonatal (75 mg/kg)	Single	BW ≥650 g RDS requiring assisted ventilation, FiO_2 >0.4, Age 4–24 hr	None
Long et al. (1991) (45)	419	Exosurf Neonatal (75 mg/kg)	Multiple	BW 700–1350 g RDS requiring assisted ventilation, a/A ratio <0.22, Age 2–24 hr	↓ Pneumothorax ↓ Death ↓ BPPD/death ↑ Apnea
Smyth et al. (1991) (47)	221	Exosurf Neonatal (75 mg/kg)	Multiple	BW 500–749 g RDS requiring assisted ventilation, a/A ratio <0.22, Age 2–24 hr	None

BW, birth weight; GA, gestational age.

Larger infants with RDS were studied by the combined US and Canadian Exosurf Pediatric Study Group (46). Entry criteria were similar to the other Exosurf treatment studies, except infants with birth weights of more than 1250 g were enrolled. Treated infants demonstrated significant improvement in respiratory status as well as improvement in long-term clinical outcome. A significant reduction in pneumothorax, intraventricular hemorrhage, BPD, and neonatal death was noted. As seen with the smaller infants, an increase in apnea was noted.

Smyth et al. (47) have reported on extremely low birth weight infants weighing 500–749 g who met entry criteria similar to the other Exosurf treatment studies. No clinical improvement was associated with treatment. Complete data are not available from this study so it is not included in the overview analysis.

Overview Analysis of Synthetic Surfactant in the Treatment of Established RDS

Overview analyses of the trials of synthetic surfactant in the treatment of RDS support a small but significant benefit in virtually all clinical outcomes analyzed (see Table 1) (121).

The three trials which used multiple doses of Exosurf Neonatal all demonstrated a significant reduction in the incidence of pneumothorax (44–46). Overview analysis demonstrates a significant overall reduction in the risk of pneumothorax with synthetic surfactant treatment of infants with RDS (typical odds ratio 0.52, 95% confidence level 0.42, 0.65).

Three studies reported data on the incidence of PDA (42,45,46). In the North American study of Exosurf Neonatal which enrolled larger infants with RDS (46), a decrease in the risk of PDA was noted (odds ratio 0.72, 95% confidence level 0.57, 0.90). Unlike the studies of prophylactic synthetic surfactant treatment, overview analysis of the treatment trials suggests a reduction in the risk of PDA (typical odds ratio 0.73, 95% confidence level 0.60, 0.88).

Few data from these studies are available regarding the incidence of intraventricular hemorrhage. Only two of the Exosurf Neonatal studies have reported on this outcome (45,46). Neither study demonstrated an effect on the incidence of IVH. The overview analysis suggests that synthetic surfactant treatment reduces the risk of IVH in these infants (typical odds ratio 0.77, 95% confidence level 0.62, 0.97).

The overview analysis suggests that the incidence of bronchopulmonary dysplasia may be decreased in infants with RDS treated with synthetic surfactant. The typical estimate derived from three trials (36,45,46) suggests a small reduction in risk (typical odds ratio 0.68, 95% confidence level 0.46, 0.99). The risk of BPD or death at 28 days is also decreased with synthetic surfactant treatment. Two studies of Exosurf Neonatal were able to demonstrate decreased BPD or death (45,46). The overview analysis demonstrates a significant reduction in the risk of BPD or death at 28 days (typical odds ratio 0.56, 95% confidence level 0.45, 0.71).

Mortality is reduced by synthetic surfactant treatment of infants with RDS. The trial of Long et al. (45) demonstrated a significant reduction in the risk of mortality (odds ratio 0.47, 95% confidence level 0.30, 0.74). The trials of Phibbs et al. (42) and the North American study (46) demonstrated a marginal decrease in the risk of mortality. Overview analysis suggests a significant reduction in the risk of mortality (typical odds ratio 0.65, 95% confidence level 0.50, 0.82).

II. Timing of Treatment

A. Prophylactic Administration of Surfactant versus Surfactant Treatment of Established RDS

As the evidence grew that surfactant therapy was effective both in the prevention and treatment of RDS, investigators began to design trials that would compare these two approaches to treatment. The prophylactic approach may allow for more homogeneous distribution of surfactant and may minimize barotrauma but clearly involves treating more infants than does a selective approach in which only infants with established RDS receive treatment. To date, five trials comparing prophylactic administration of surfactant with surfactant treatment of RDS involving over 2200 infants have been reported (Table 6).

These studies are similar in that infants at high risk of developing RDS were randomized to prophylactic surfactant treatment administered shortly after birth (within 10 min of birth) or selective therapy if the infant developed signs of significant respiratory distress. The trials all utilized natural surfactant extracts. The major difference in these trials is in the specific selection criteria used for later selective treatment.

Dunn et al. (48) studied 182 infants 30 weeks' gestation or less. Infants were randomized to either prophylactic administration of a bovine surfactant extract (calf lung lavage) or surfactant administration only if the clinical course within the first 6 hr of life was compatible with RDS. A decrease in BPD was noted in the late treatment group.

Kendig et al. (49) compared the prophylactic administration of CLSE with expectant management of 479 infants between 24 and 29 weeks' gestation. Infants randomized to the late treatment group received CLSE if they had moderate or severe RDS requiring assisted ventilation with an $\mathrm{Fio_2} \geq 0.4$ and MAP ≥ 7 $\mathrm{cmH_2O}$. The group that received prophylactic CLSE had a significant decrease in the incidence of pneumothoraces and death.

Merritt et al. (50) have completed a trial which compared the prophylactic or treatment approach using human amniotic fluid extract. Infants 24–29 weeks' gestation were eligible for enrollment. If randomized to late treatment, an infant would receive surfactant if the infant required assisted ventilation ($\mathrm{Fio_2} \geq 0.5$

Table 6 Randomized Controlled Trials of Prophylactic Administration of Surfactant versus Surfactant Treatment of Established RDS

Author	N	Surfactant preparation	Entry criteria	Outcome
Dunn et al. (1991) (48)	182	Calf lung lavage (75–100 mg)	Ga <30 wks Treatment group given surfactant if clinical course compatible with RDS Age <6 hr	Treatment of RDS: ↓ BPPD
Kendig et al. (1991) (49)	479	Calf Lung surfactant extract (90 mg)	GA 24–29 wks Treatment group given surfactant if $FiO_2 \geq .4$ and MAP ≥7 cmH_2O	Prophylactic administration: ↓ Pneumothorax ↓ Mortality
Merritt et al. (1991) (50)	203	Human amniotic fluid surfactant extract	GA 24–29 wks Treatment group given surfactant if on assisted ventilation, $FiO_2 \geq .5$, and MAP ≥7 cmH_2O Age 2–12 hr	No difference
Egberts et al. (1993) (80)	147	Curosurf (Porcine lung surfactant extract)	GA 26–29 wks Treatment group given surfactant if on assisted ventilation, and $FiO_2 \geq 0.6$ Age 6–24 hr	No difference
Kattwinkel (1993) (80a)	1248	Calf lung surfactant extract	GA 29–33 wks Treatment group given surfactant if on assisted ventilation, and $FiO_2 > 0.3$	Prophylactic administration: ↓ BPD ↓ Mortality

and a MAP $\geq$ 7 cmH_2O) at 2–12 hr of age. In the intention-to-treat analysis, no differences emerged between the two approaches.

Egberts et al. (80) compared prophylactic administration of porcine lung surfactant to surfactant treatment in 147 infants between 26 and 29 weeks' gestation. Treatment was given to infants who required assisted ventilation and supplemental oxygen of 60% or greater. No important clinical differences between the two groups were demonstrated.

Kattwinkel et al. (80a) enrolled 1248 infants of slightly older gestation (gestational age 29–33 weeks). Infants were given prophylactic CLSE or selective treatment if the infant required greater than 30% supplemental oxygen. These investigators noted a small reduction in bronchopulmonary dysplasia and mortality associated with prophylactic treatment.

B. Overview Analysis of Trials Comparing Prophylactic Administration of Surfactant Versus Surfactant Treatment of Established RDS

The five trials which compared prophylactic administration of surfactant with selective surfactant treatment of symptomatic infants have divergent results (123). Four trials published data on the incidence of pneumothorax (48,49,80,80a). Kendig et al. (49) noted a marginal decrease in pneumothorax associated with prophylactic therapy (odds ratio 0.54, 95% confidence level 0.29–1.03), whereas the other trials noted no difference between treatment groups. Overview analysis suggests that prophylactic treatment may reduce the risk of pneumothorax (typical odds ratio 0.66, 95% confidence level 0.36–0.91).

All five trials reported data on bronchopulmonary dysplasia. Dunn et al. (48) noted an increased incidence of BPD in the infants given prophylactic surfactant (odds ratio 2.66, 95% confidence level 1.29–5.49). Kattwinkel (80a) noted a small reduction in the risk of developing BPD in the group receiving prophylactic surfactant. The other studies noted no difference in BPD. The typical estimate from these trials suggests no significant difference in the incidence of BPD.

Data on the combined outcome of BPD or death at 28 days are also reported in four trials. Dunn et al. (48) noted an increase in BPD or death in the group that received prophylactic surfactant (odds ratio 3.38, 95% confidence level 1.61–7.10). Kattwinkel (80a) demonstrated a small decrease in the risk of BPD or death in the prophylactically treated group (odds ratio 0.59, 95% confidence level 0.36–0.89). Kendig et al. (49) and Merritt et al. (50) reported no significant difference between these two groups. The overview analysis suggests no increased risk of developing BPD or death at 28 days in infants receiving prophylactic surfactant (typical odds ratio 0.90, 95% confidence level 0.71–1.13).

Both Kendig et al. (49) and Kattwinkel (80a) demonstrated a decrease in mortality in infants receiving prophylactic treatment. Neither Dunn et al. (48) Merritt et al. (50) nor Egberts et al. (80) reported any difference in mortality.

Overview analysis suggests a decrease in the risk of mortality associated with prophylactic treatment (typical odds ratio 0.72, 95% confidence level 0.52–0.98).

The current studies demonstrate that prophylactic administration of surfactant to infants at high risk of developing RDS results in a small reduction in mortality and a small increase in survival without BPD compared with selective surfactant treatment of infants with moderate RDS. In interpreting the clinical relevance of this data, several issues need to be addressed. The first issue relates to the time that surfactant treatment was administered to the selective group. The average time of treatment in the selective group varied greatly between the studies (in four of the studies, the mean age ranged from 2.9 to 7.4 hr of life). Data from subsequent trials suggests that earlier selective treatment (age less than 2 hr) may be more beneficial than delaying selective treatment (51). The number of infants in the prophylactic group receiving surfactant is almost twice that in the selective treatment group. Perhaps in order to optimize efficacy without increasing drug utilization, future studies will focus on early selective surfactant administration.

C. Early Treatment Versus Delayed Selective Treatment

As noted in the previous section, treatment choices are not confined to the two extremes of prophylactic administration in the delivery room or late treatment of severe established disease. In the largest randomized trial in neonatal medicine, the OSIRIS Collaborative Group (51) studied early treatment (less than 2 hr of age) compared with delayed selective treatment in 2690 premature infants at high risk of RDS. Earlier treatment led to a small but significant reduction in the risk of death or oxygen dependence at term-adjusted age (relative risk 0.84, 95% confidence level 6.76, 0.93).

III. Factors Affecting Response to Therapy

The immediate effects of therapy with surfactant are well documented and, in general, are positive. Acute improvement in pulmonary disease is demonstrated by many randomized, controlled trials, particularly those using natural surfactant extract. However, these immediate benefits do not directly translate into improvement in long-term outcome. Pneumothoraces are decreased with surfactant therapy, but other important outcome measures do not consistently improve with treatment. Although some of the failures in these studies can be ascribed to limitations of study design, many investigators have begun exploring other factors that may influence response to surfactant therapy and explain the variable effect of treatment.

Not all treated infants responded to surfactant therapy. Takeuchi et al. (52) analyzed the response to surfactant treatment in infants with established RDS.

In 17 of 191 infants (9%), no immediate effect of surfactant therapy was seen. Most of these infants who did not respond to surfactant treatment (12 of 17) had asphyxia (defined as an Apgar score of less than 3 at 1 min of life). In other reports, Fujiwara et al. (53) classified the response in 96 infants treated with Surfactant-TA (120 mg/kg). Immediate and sustained response was seen in 79% of infants, immediate response followed by relapse and recovery was seen in 16%, and poor or no response was seen in 6%. Among the subgroup of infants with birth weights of less than 1000 g, fewer infants (64%) exhibited immediate and sustained response to surfactant treatment.

Charon et al. (54) analyzed the response of infants enrolled in the Boston-Burlington study (22) and an additional 11 infants treated outside the randomized trial. They classified response in three categories: (1) lasting response (an a/A O_2 ratio ≥ 0.3 at 24 hr and no more than a 50% decrease from maximal response within 48 hr of treatment or extubation within 24 hr; (2) transient response (an a/A O_2 ratio ≥ 0.3 at 12 hr followed by a fall to $\geq$50% of the maximal response within 48 hr of treatment; and (3) absent response (an a/A O_2 ratio <0.3 at 24 hr after treatment). The responses of 29 infants treated with surfactant were categorized, and clinical factors that might influence response were analyzed. Sixteen infants (55%) had a lasting response to surfactant treatment, six (21%) exhibited a transient response, and seven (24%) had no response. No difference in birth weight, gestational age, sex, race, or time of treatment was noted in the infants in the three categories. Infants with absent response tended to have lower initial a/A O_2 ratio. A greater number of infants with a transient response had a hemodynamically significant PDA. Eight of the infants included in the analysis were studied with technitium-labeled surfactant. Although differences in distribution were seen, the pattern of distribution did not correlate with clinical response. These studies suggest that infants with more severe disease or infants who have experienced asphyxia may not respond optimally to surfactant therapy.

The degree of surfactant responsiveness will also be effected by the quality of the surfactant preparation. In animal models, natural surfactants are generally more effective than artificial surfactants in improving gas exchange, restoring the pressure-volume relationship, and increasing survival (55,56). Eleven tertiary care units which participate in the National Institute of Child Health and Human Development Neonatal Research Network conducted a comparison trial of synthetic surfactant (Exosurf Neonatal) and modified bovine surfactant extract (Survanta) (57). Premature infants ($n = 617$) weighing between 501 and 1500 g with established RDS were enrolled. Significant improvement in the initial respiratory course was noted in the group that received modified bovine surfactant extract. A smaller, single center, randomized trial came to similar conclusions (58). No major clinical differences were noted. Two other small trials were also unable to demonstrate major clinical differences (59,60).

Another issue affecting the responsiveness to surfactant therapy is which initial surfactant dose is most appropriate. The surfactant dose used in the majority of single-dose studies of modified surfactant extract (100–120 mg/kg) approximates 30 times the amount of surfactant estimated to make up the alveolar surfactant pool (61). Randomized, controlled trials have been conducted in Japan that demonstrate greater improvement when doses this large are administered. Konishi et al. (62) compared the efficacy of low-dose (60 mg/kg) versus high-dose (120 mg/kg) Surfactant-TA. Infants with severe RDS requiring ventilatory support were randomized to receive either low-dose or high-dose Surfactant-TA. An infant could be retreated if the MAP did not decrease from the pretreatment value or if the MAP increased to 10 cmH_2O or greater. Forty-seven infants whose birth weight was between 1000 and 1500 g were enrolled. The low-dose group (n = 23) and the high-dose group (n = 23) were similar in birth weight, gestational age, sex, Apgar score, disease severity, and time of treatment. Greater improvement was noted in the high-dose group regarding both early and late outcome measures. Significant improvement in outcome was noted in the high-dose group regarding IVH and BPD. Mortality was low in both groups.

Larger doses of surfactant have been used by other investigators. Robertson and coworkers (29) used a dose of porcine lung surfactant extract almost twice as large as the dose used in previous studies. The promising results from the experience of these investigators led to a large multicenter trial comparing high dose (200 mg/kg) to low dose (100 mg/kg) surfactant therapy in infants with established RDS (63). Although infants receiving the higher dose had better initial response to treatment, no major clinical differences were noted.

Another question is whether multiple doses of surfactant are needed to optimize clinical outcome. Rapid metabolism and inactivation of exogenous surfactant may lead to transient unsustained improvement in surfactant treated animals. Twenty percent of the treated neonates may have a transient response to surfactant administration (54). Retreatment may be important in optimizing response. Two studies have compared single-dose and multiple-dose treatment in infants with established RDS. Dunn et al. (21) studied infants with RDS between 30 and 36 weeks' gestational age. Infants could receive no surfactant therapy, a single dose of CLSE (100 mg/kg), or multiple doses of CLSE. Both the single-dose and the multiple-dose groups demonstrated improved oxygenation and ventilation, but no differences in clinical outcome were noted.

Speer et al. (64) studied 343 infants with established RDS requiring assisted ventilation and supplemental oxygen. Infants were randomized to receive a single dose of Curosurf (200 mg/kg) or multiple doses of Curosurf (initial dose 200 mg/kg followed by 100 mg/kg 12 and 24 hr after initial treatment if on assisted ventilation). Infants who received multiple doses had a decreased incidence of pneumothorax and neonatal death. Overview analysis of these two trials supports a reduction in the risk of pneumothorax (typical odds ratio 0.48, 95% confidence level 0.27–0.85), and mortality (typical odds ratio 0.59, 95% confidence level 0.34–1.02) with multiple-dose treatment. Although multiple-dose strategies appear to be most effective, the specific issues of exact timing, dosage, and retreatment criteria remain uncertain.

In summary, not all infants will respond to surfactant therapy. Response to treatment may be extremely variable. Retrospective analysis of several trials suggests that infants with perinatal asphyxia or severe respiratory distress at the time of treatment may demonstrate the poorest response. Relapse after an initial response may be due to pulmonary edema secondary to a hemodynamically PDA. Response may be affected by other therapies including prenatal steroids, timing of initial dose, size of initial dose, retreatment, and ventilatory management.

IV. Complications of Therapy

The benefits from surfactant therapy must be weighed against the actual and theoretical risks of its use in preterm infants. The risk of complications or adverse responses may result from either the surfactant, the mode of surfactant administration, the immediate effects on physiological stability, or other effects on complications of prematurity.

Theoretical risks of the use of natural surfactant products have focused on the possible transmission of infectious agents, including bovine spongiform encephalitis (BSE) in bovine-derived surfactants, other viral infections in swine, or HIV and hepatitis B infection from amniotic fluid in human surfactant. Organic solvent processing of phospholipids, terminal sterilization techniques, and screening of animal and human donors have been used to minimize these risks. Because BSE has not been recognized in cattle from New Zealand, isolation of surfactant (Survanta) from beef raised in this country minimizes the risk of transmission of this infection.

Proteins in surfactant preparations may elicit an immune response in infants. Surfactant protein A has been shown to have blood Group A antigenic recognition sites (65). While work assessing the potential immunogenicity of surfactant proteins continues, there has not been recognition of clinical disease or evidence of immunological injury from early surfactant therapy among the thousands of infants treated with natural surfactant extracts. (See also Chapter 14.)

Surfactants are administered into the airways either by direct instillation in the endotracheal tube with a catheter or by injection into the endotracheal tube using a sideport. The former technique requires that the infant is transiently removed from positive-pressure ventilation, whereas with the latter technique, the infant remains on positive-pressure ventilation. During 1189 dosing procedures with Survanta, Liechty et al. (33) found 329 (28%) instances of transient bradycardia or decrease in oxygen saturation (by more than 20%). Other adverse responses reported during surfactant administration have been reflux of surfactant up the endotracheal tube, decrease in transcutaneous P_{CO_2} or oxygen saturation, blood pressure, and cerebral blood flow alterations, tachycardia, gagging, and mucous plugging of the endotracheal tube.

An increased incidence of pulmonary hemorrhage has been suggested by some of the trials of surfactant therapy. In an analysis of infants weighing 600–1250 g, 3.4% of those given Survanta at birth developed evidence for pulmonary hemorrhage (19). Among infants treated with Survanta for established RDS (birth weights 600–1750 g), pulmonary hemorrhage occurred in 7.1% compared with 5.4% among placebo-treated infants (33). A similar rate of pulmonary hemorrhage has been noted in a study comparing synthetic and natural surfactant (57); however, a meta-analysis indicates that pulmonary hemorrhage is a condition particularly of extremely low birth weight infants and may occur more frequently in those treated with synthetic surfactant (66). The mechanisms responsible for pulmonary hemorrhage after surfactant administration are uncertain.

The relationship between surfactant administration and IVH is also being investigated. During and shortly after Survanta administration, van der Bor et al. (67) described a fall in anterior cerebral artery blood flow velocities. Thc Collaborative European Multicenter Study Group (76) found that those infants having a high arterial oxygen tension peak (>30 kPa) within 30 min of surfactant replacement also had a higher incidence of grade 1–2 intracranial hemorrhage when compared with infants with lesser increases in arterial oxygen tension peak. However, an association was also found between the magnitude of improvement in a/A O_2 at 24 hr after treatment and a lower incidence of both pneumothorax and severe IVH. Surprisingly, more of these infants have clinical evidence of a significant patent ductus arteriosus.

Other neonatal complications such as pneumonia, apnea, sepsis, and necrotizing enterocolitis have been reported in individual trials, but these are not noted in the vast majority of studies. Future studies will need to address these complications.

References

1. Yamada T, Ikegami M, Tabor BL, Jobe AH. (1990). Effects of surfactant protein-A on surfactant function in preterm ventilated rabbits. Am Rev Respir Dis 142:754–7.

1a. Robillard E, Alaire Y, Dagenais-Perusse P, et al (1964). Microaerosol administration of dipalmitoyl-lecithin in the respiratory distress syndrome: a preliminary report. Canadian Medical Association 90:55–57.

2. Yu SH, Wallace D, Bhavnani B, et al. (1988). Effect of reconstituted pulmonary surfactant containing the 6000-dalton hydrophobic protein on lung compliance of prematurely delivered rabbit fetuses. Pediatr Res 23:23–30.
2a. Chu J, Clements JA, Cotton EK, et al. (1967). Neonatal pulmonary ischemia. Part 1—Clinical and physiological studies. Pediatrics 40:709–782.
3. Enhorning G, Robertson B. (1972). Lung expansion in the premature rabbit fetus after tracheal deposition of surfactant. Pediatrics 50:58–66.
4. Enhorning G, Grossmann G, Robertson B. (1973). Tracheal deposition of surfactant before the first breath. Am Rev Respir Dis 107:921–927.
5. Enhorning G. Hill D, Sherwood G, et al. (1978). Improved ventilation of prematurely delivered primates following tracheal deposition of surfactant. Am J Obstet Gynecol 132:529–536.
6. Adams FH, Towers B, Osher AB, et al. (1978). Effects of tracheal instillation of natural surfactant in premature lambs. I. Clinical and autopsy findigs. Pediatr Res. 12:841–848.
7. Fujiwara T, Maeta H, Chida S, et al. (1980). Artificial surfactant therapy in hyaline membrane disease. Lancet 1:55–59.
8. Nilsson R, Grossman G, Robertson B. (1978). Lung surfactant and the pathogenesis of neonatal bronchiolar lesions induced by artificial ventilation. Pediatr Res 12:249–255.
9. Jobe A, Ikegami M, Jacobs M, Jones S, (1984). Surfactant and pulmonary blood flow distributions following treatment of premature lambs with natural surfactant. J Clin Invest 73:848–856.
10. Soll RF, McQueen MC. Respiratory Distress Syndrome. In Sinclair J and Bracken M (eds): *Effective Care of the Newborn.* Oxford University Press, Oxford, United Kingdom 1992.
10a. Soll RF. Single vs multiple dose surfactant for severe RDS. In Chalmers I, ed. Oxford Database of Perinatal Trials. May 12, 1992.
11. Collins R, Yusuf S, Peto R. (1985). Overview of randomized trials of diuretics in pregnancy. Br Med J 290:17–23.
12. Enhorning G, Shennan A, Possmayer F, et al. (1985). Prevention of neonatal respiratory distress syndrome by tracheal instillation of surfactant: A randomized clinical trial. Pediatrics 76:145–153.
13. Kwong M, Egan EA, Notter RH, Shapiro DL. (1985). Double blind clinical trial of calf lung surfactant extract for the prevention of hyaline membrane disease in extremely premature infants. Pediatrics 76:585–592.
14. Kendig JW, Notter RH, Cox C, Shapiro DL. (1988). Surfactant replacement therapy at birth: Final analysis of a clinical trial and comparisons with similar trials. Pediatrics 82:756–762.
15. Shennan A, Dunn M (1989). Surfactant replacement trials—the need to maintain concurrent placebo controls. Pediatr Res 25:231A.
16. Dunn M, Shennan A, Possmayer F (1990a). Bovine surfactant prophylaxis in infants less than 30 weeks gestation—A randomized controlled trial employing a multiple dose protocol. Pediatr Res 27:204A.
17. Merritt TA, Hallman M, Bloom BT, et al. (1986). Prophylactic treatment of very premature infants with human surfactant. New England J Med 315:785–790.

18. Soll, RF. Prophylactic Administration of Natural Surfactant Extract. In: Chalmers I, ed. Oxford Database of Perinatal trials. January 27, 1990. Updated August 29, 1990, January 29, 1991, July 24, 1991, November 21, 1991.

18a. Soll RF. Natural Surfactant Extract Treatment of RDS. In: Chalmers I, ed. Oxford Database of Perinatal Trials, January 27, 1990. Updated August 29, 1990, January 29, 1991, July 24, 1991, November 21, 1991.

19. Hoekstra RE, Jackson JC, Meyers TF, et al. (1991). Improved neonatal survival following multiple doses of bovine surfactant in very premature neonates at risk for respiratory distress syndrome. Pediatrics 88:10–18.

20. Soll RF, Hoekstra R, Fangman J, et al. (1990). Multicenter trial of single-dose modified surfactant extract (Survanta) for prevention of respiratory distress syndrome. Pediatrics 85:1092–1102.

21. Dunn MS, Shennan AT, Possmayer F (1990b). Single-versus multiple-dose surfactant replacement therapy in neonates at 30 to 36 weeks gestation with respiratory distress syndrome. Pediatrics 86:564–571.

22. Gitlin JD, Soll RF, Parad RB, et al. (1987). A randomized controlled trial of exogenous surfactant for the treatment of hyaline membrane disease. Pediatrics 79:31–37.

23. Raju TNK, Bhat R, McCulloch KM, et al. (1987). Double-blind controlled trial of single-dose treatment with bovine surfactant in severe hyaline membrane disease. Lancet 1:651–656.

24. Soll RF, Duc G, Minoli I, et al. (1988). European study of single dose Surfactant-TA (STA) for treatment of respiratory distress syndrome (RDS). Pediatr Res 23:525A.

25. Chen J-Y (1990). Exogenous surfactant for treatment of respiratory distress syndrome in premature infants. Formosan Med Assoc 89:110–114.

26. Fujiwara T, Konishi M, Chida S, et al. (1990). Surfactant replacement therapy with a single postventilatory dose of a reconstituted bovine surfactant in preterm neonates with respiratory distress syndrome: Final analysis of a multicenter, double blind, randomized trial and comparison with similar trials. Pediatrics. 86:753–764.

27. Hallman M, Merritt TA, Jarvenpaa AL, et al. (1985). Exogenous human surfactant for treatment of severe respiratory distress syndrome: A randomized prospective clinical trial. J Pediatr 106:963–969.

28. Lang MJ, Hall RT, Reddy NS, et al. (1990). A controlled trial of human surfactant replacement therapy for severe respiratory distress syndrome in very low birth weight infants. J Pediatr 116:295–300.

29. Collaborative European Multicentre Group (1991). Factors influencing the clinical response to surfactant replacement therapy in babies with severe respiratory distress syndrome. Eur J Pediatr 150:433–439.

30. Gortner L. (1990). A multicenter randomized controlled clinical trial of bovine surfactant for prevention of respiratory distress syndrome. Lung 168(Suppl):864–869.

31. Horbar JD, Soll RF, Sutherland JM, et al. (1989). A Multicenter randomized placebo-controlled trial of surfactant therapy for respiratory distress syndrome. N Engl J Med 320:959–965.

32. Horbar JD, Soll RF, Schachinger M, et al. (1990). A European multicenter randomized controlled trial of single dose surfactant therapy for idiopathic respiratory distress syndrome. Eur J Pediatr 149:416–423.

33. Liechty EA, Donovan E, Purohit D, et al. (1991). Reduction of neonatal mortality after multiple doses of bovine surfactant in low birthweight neonates with respiratory distress syndrome. Pediatrics 88:19–28.
34. Halliday HL, Reid MM, Meban C, et al. (1984). Controlled trial of artificial surfactant to prevent respiratory distress syndrome. Lancet 1:476–478.
35. Meban C (1981). Effect of lipids and other substances on the adsorption of dipalmitoylphosphatidylcholine. Pediatr Res 15:1029–1031.
35a. Morley CJ, Bangham AD, Miller N, et al (1981). Dry artificial lung surfactant and its effect on very premature babies. Lancet 1:64–68.
36. Wilkinson AR, Jenkins PA, Jeffrey JA. (1985). Two controlled trials of dry artificial surfactant: early effects and later outcome in babies with surfactant deficiency. Lancet 2:287–291.
37. Ten Centre Study Group (1987). Ten centre trial of artificial surfactant (artificial lung expanding compound) in very premature babies. Br Med J 294:991–996.
38. Durand DJ, Clyman RI, Heymann MA, et al. (1985). Effects of a protin-free, synthetic surfactant on the survival and pulmonary function of preterm lambs. J Pediatr 107:775–780.
39. Tooley WH, Clements JA, Muramatsu K, et al. (1987). Lung function in prematurely delivered rabbits treated with a synthetic surfactant. Am Rev Respir Dis 136:651–656.
40. Bose C, Corbet A, Bose G, et al., (1990). Improved outcome at 28 days of age for very low birth weight infants treated with a single dose of a synthetic surfactant. J Pediatr 117:947–953.
41. Corbet A, Bucciarelli R, Goldman S, et al. (1991). Decreased mortality rate among small premature infants treated at birth with a single dose of synthetic surfactant: A multicenter controlled trial. J Pediatr 118:277–284.
42. Phibbs RH, Ballard RA, Clements JA, et al. (1991). Initial clinical trial of Exosurf, a protein free synthetic surfactant, for the prevention and early treatment of hyaline membrane disease. Pediatrics 88:1–9.
43. Stevenson D, Walther F, Long W, et al. (1992). Controlled trial of a single dose of synthetic surfactant at birth in premature infants weighing 500–699 grams. J Pediatr 120:503–512.
43a. Papile LA, Burstein J, Burstein R, Koffler H (1978). Incidence and evolution of subependymal and intraventricular hemorrhage: A study of infants with birth weights less than 150 gm. J Pediatr 92:529–534.
44. Canadian Exosurf Pediatric Study Group (1990). Effects of two rescue doses of Exosurf, Pediatric in 342 750–1249 gram infants. Pediatr Res 27:200A.
45. Long W, Thompson T, Sundell H, et al. (1991a). Effects of two rescue doses of a synthetic surfactant on mortality rate and survival without bronchopulmonary dysplasia in 700–1350 gram infants with respiratory distress syndrome. J Pediatr 118:595–605.
46. Long W, Corbet A, Cotton R, et al. (1991b). A controlled trial of synthetic surfactant in infants weighing 1250 g or more with respiratory distress syndrome. N Engl J Med 325:1696–1703.
47. Smyth J, Allen A, Sankaran K, et al. (1991). Effects of two rescue doses of Exosurf. Neonatal in 221 500–749 gram infants. Pediatr Res 29:330A.

48. Dunn M, Shennan A, Zayack D, et al. (1991a). Bovine surfactant replacement therapy in neonates of less than 30 weeks gestation: A randomized controlled trial of prophylaxis versus treatment. Pediatrics 87:377–386.
49. Kendig JW, Notter RH, Cox C, et al. (1991). A comparison of surfactant as immediate prophylaxis and as rescue therapy in newborns of less than 30 weeks' gestation. N Engl J Med 324:865–871.
50. Merritt TA, Hallman M, Berry C, et al. (1991). Randomized, placebo-controlled trial of human surfactant given at birth versus rescue administration in very low birth weight infants with lung immaturity. J Pediat 118:581–594.
51. OSIRIS Collaborative Group (1992). Early versus delated neonatal administration of a synthetic surfactant—The judgment of OSIRIS. Lancet 340:1363–1369.
52. Takeuchi Y, Yasujimine K, Odo Y, et al. (PSF Collaborative Groups) (1986). Multifacility cooperative research on surfactant supplementation treatment of RDS. II. Investigation of control before and after PSF administration. Shusanki Igaki 16:1541–1548.
53. Fujiwara T, Konishi M, Chida S, et al. (1988). Factors affecting the response to a postnatal single dose of reconstituted bovine surfactant. In Lachmann B, ed. Surfactant Replacement Therapy in Neonatal and Adult Respiratory Distress Syndrome. Berlin: Springer-Verlag, pp 91–107.
54. Charon A, Taeusch HW, Fitzgibbon C, et al. (1989). Factors associated with surfactant treatment response in infants with severe respiratory distress syndrome. Pediatrics 83:348–354.
55. Cummings JJ, Holm BA, Hudak ML, et al. (1992). A controlled clinical comparison of four different surfactant preparations in surfactant-deficient preterm lambs. Am Rev Respir Dis 145:999–1004.
56. Ikegami M, Silverman J, Adams FH. (1979). Restoration of lung pressure-volume characteristics with various phospholipids. Pediatr Res 13:1377–1380.
57. Horbar JD, Wright LL, Soll RF, et al. (1993). A multicenter randomized trial comparing two surfactants for the treatment of neonatal Respiratory Distress Syndrome. J Pediatr 123:757–766.
58. Sebgal S, Ewing CK, Richards T, Taeusch HW (1994). Modified bovine surfactant (Survanta) vs. a protein-free surfactant (Exosurf) for treatment of RDS in preterm infants: a pilot study. J Natl Med Assoc 86:46–52.
59. Alvarado M, Hingre R, Hakanson D, Gross S (1993). Clinical trial of Survanta vs Exosurf therapy in infants <1500 g with respiratory distress syndrome (RDS). Pediatr Res 33:215A.
60. Pearlman SA, Leef KH, Stefano JL, et al. (1993). A randomized trial comparing Exosurf vs Survanta in the treatment of neonatal RDS. Pediatr Res 33:340A.
61. Jobe A, Ikegami M, Jacobs H, et al. (1983). Surfactant pool sizes and severity of RDS in prematurely delivered lambs. Am Rev Respir Dis 127:751–755.
62. Konishi M, Fujiwara T, Naito T, et al. (1988). Surfactant replacement therapy in neonatal respiratory distress syndrome. A multi-centre, randomized clinical trial: Comparison of high- versus low-dose surfactant TA. Eur J Pediatr 147:20–25.
63. Halliday HL, Tarnow-Mordi WO, Corcoran JD, et al. (1993). Multicentre randomized trial comparing high and low dose surfactant regimens for the treatment of respiratory distress syndrome (The Curosurf 4 Trial). Arch Dis Child 69:276–280.

64. Speer CP, Robertson B, Curstedt T, Halliday HL, et al. (1992). Randomized European multicenter trial of surfactant replacement therapy for severe neonatal respiratory distress syndrome: Single versus multiple doses of Curosurf. Pediatrics 89:13–20.
65. Stalhman MT, Gray ME, Ross GF, et al. (1992). Human surfactant protein-A contains blood group A antigenic determinants. Pediatr Res 31:364–71.
66. Raju TNK, Langenberg P (1993). Pulmonary hemorrhage and exogenous surfactant treatment: a meta-analysis. J Pediatr 123:603–610.
67. van de Bor M, Ma EJ, Walther FJ (1991). Cerebral blood flow velocity after surfactant instillation in preterm infants. J Pediatr 118:285–87.
68. Adams FH, Enhorning G (1966). Surface properties of lung extracts. I. A dynamic alveolar model. Acta Physiol Scand 68:23–27.
69. Avery ME, Mead J (1959). Surface properties in relation to atelectasis and hyaline membrane disease. Am J Dis Child 97:517.
70. Bartmann P, Jorch G, Phlandt F, et al. (1991). Antibody response to bovine surfactant in preterm infants. Pediatr Res 29:203A.
71. Bland RD. (1987). Pathogenesis of lung edema after premature birth. Adv Pediatr 34:175–222.
72. Chida S, Phelps D, Soll R, et al. (1991). Surfactant proteins and anti-surfactant antibodies in sera from infants with respiratory distress syndrome with and without surfactant treatment. Pediatrics 88:84–89.
73. Clark RH, Gestmann DR, Null DM, et al. (1992). Prospective randomized comparison of high-frequency oscillatory and conventional ventilation in respiratory distress syndrome. Pediatrics 89:5–12.
74. Coalson JJ, Kuehl TJ, Prihoda TJ, et al. (1988). Diffuse alveolar damage in the evolution of bronchopulmonary dysplasia. Pediatr Res 24:357–366.
75. Cockshutt AM, Weitz J, Possmayer F. Pulmonary surfactant-associated protein A enhances the surface activity of lipid extract surfactant and reverses inhibition by blood proteins in vitro. Biochemistry 29:8424–8429.
76. Collaborative European Multicenter Study Group (Robertson B) (1988). Surfactant replacement therapy for severe neonatal respiratory distress syndrome; an international randomized clinical trial. Pediatrics 82:683–691.
77. Davis JM, Russ G, Metlay L, Dickerson B, & Greenspan B. (1992). Short-term distribution of kinetics of intratracheally administered exogenous lung surfactant. Pediatr Res 31:445–450.
78. Dunn M, Zayack D, Edmonds J, et al. (1991b). Two year follow-up of infants enrolled in a randomized trial of surfactant replacement therapy-extension of original cohort due to concern about type II error. Pediatr Res 29:254A.
79. Egan EA, Notter RH, Kwong MS, et al. (1983). Natural and artificial lung surfactant replacement in premature lambs. *J Appl Physiol* 55:875–883.
80. Egberts J, deWinter JP, Sedin G, et al. (1993). Comparison of prophylaxis and rescue treatment with curosurf in babies less than 30 weeks gestation. A randomized trial. Pediatrics 92:768–774.
80a. Kattwinkel J, Bloom BT, Delmore P, et al (1993). Prophylactic administration of calf lung surfactant is more effective than early treatment of respiratory distress syndrome in neonates of 29 through 32 weeks' gestation. Pediatrics 92:90–98.

81. Enhorning G (1977). Pulsating bubble technique for evaluating pulmonary surfactant. J Appl Physiol 43:976–979.
82. Enhorning G. (1984). In search of an artificial pulmonary surfactant. Jpn Med Soc Biol Interface 15:73–81.
83. Fujiwara T, Konishi M, Chida S, et al. (1988). Factors affecting response to a postnatal single dose of exogenous surfactant. In: Jobe A, Taeusch W, eds. Surfactant Treatment of Lung Diseases. Report of the 96th Ross Conference on Pediatric Research, Columbus, OH, Ross Laboratories.
84. Gitlin JD, Parad R, Taeusch HW. (1984). Exogenous surfactant therapy in hyaline membrane disease. Semin Perinatol 8:272–282.
85. Golden J, Bejar R, Lohrer R, et al. (1992). Acute changes in cerebral blood flow velocities (CBFV) and intraventricular bleeds (IVH) after Exosurf Administration. Clin Res 40:65A.
86. Hall SB, Venkitaraman AR, Whitsett JA, et al. (1992). Importance of hydrophobic apoproteins as constituents of clinical exogenous surfactants. Am Rev Respir Dis 145:24–30.
87. Halliday HL, McClure G, McC Reid M. (1986). Growth and development two years after artificial surfactant replacement at birth. Early Hum Dev 113:323–327.
88. Hallman M (1989). The severity of RDS during the first two neonatal days in relationship to fluid intake. Acta Paediatr Scand 360(Suppl):93–100.
89. Hallman M, Kankaanpaa K (1980). Evidence of surfactant deficiency in persistence of fetal circulation. Eur J Pediatr 134:129–34.
90. Hallman M, Merritt TA, Schneider H, et al. (1981). Isolation of human surfactant from amniotic fluid and a pilot study of its efficacy in respiratory distress syndrome. Pediatrics 71:473–482.
91. Hallman M, Merritt TA, Pohjavuori M, et al. (1986). Effect of surfactant substitution on lung effluent phospholipids in respiratory distress syndrome: Evaluation of surfactant phospholipid turnover, pool size, and the relationship to severity of respiratory failure. Pediatr Res 20:1228–35.
92. Hallman M, Barsotti M, Chundu V, et al. (1990). Relationship between fluid intake and the responsiveness to surfactant. Pediatr Res 27:305A.
93. Hallman M, Merritt TA, Akino T, et al. (1991). Surfactant protein A, phosphatidylcholine and surfactant inhibitors in epithelial lining fluid: Correlation with surface activity, severity of RDS and outcome of small premature infants. Am Rev Respir Dis 144:1376–84.
94. Heldt GP, Merritt TA, Golenbeski D, et al. (1992). Distribution of surfactant, lung compliance and aeration of preterm rabbit lungs following surfactant therapy and conventional and high frequency oscillatory ventilation. Pediatr Res 31:270–275.
95. Holm BA, Venkitaram AR, Enhorning G, et al. (1990). Biophysical inhibition of synthetic lung surfactants. Chem Phys Lipids 52:243–250.
96. Ikegami M, Adams FH, Towers B, Osher AB. (1980). The quantity of natural surfactant necessary to prevent the respiratory distress syndrome in premature lambs. Pediatr Res 14:1082–1085.
97. Ikegami M, Jobe A, Glatz T, et al. (1981). Surface activity following natural surfactant treatment in premature lambs. J Appl Physiol 51:306–312.
98. Ikegami M, Jobe A, Jacobs H, Lam R. (1984). A protein from airways of premature

lambs that inhibits surfactant function. J Appl Physiol Respir Environ Exerc Physiol 57:1134–1142.

99. Ikegami M, Agata Y, Elkady T, et al. (1987). Comparison of four surfactants: In vitro surface properties and responses of preterm lambs to treatment at birth. Pediatrics 79:38–46.
100. Ikegami M, Jobe AH, Seidner S, Yamada T. (1989). Gestational effects of corticosteroids and surfactant in ventilated rabbits. Pediatr Res 25:32–37.
101. Jacobs H, Jobe A, Ikegami M, Glatz T, et al. (1982). Premature lambs rescued from respiratory failure with natural surfactant: clinical and biophysical correlates. Pediatr Res 16:424–429.
102. Jain L, Vidyasagar D, Raju TNK (1989). Developmental outcome of infants from surfactant trials. Pediatr Res 25:255A.
103. Jobe A, Ikegami M (1987). Surfactant for the treatment of respiratory distress syndrome. Am Rev Respir Dis 136:1256–75.
104. Jobe A, Ikegami M, Glatz T, et al. (1981). Duration and characteristics of treatment of premature lambs with natural surfactant. J Clin Invest 67:1373–1375.
105. Kawashima T, Chida S, Fujiwara T. (1987). Measurement of anti-PSF antibodies in RDS infants supplemented by the artificial pulmonary surfactant preparation (PSF) Shusanki Igaku 17:185–188.
106. Kobayashi T, Nitta K, Ganzuka M., et al. (1991). Inactivation of exogenous surfactant by pulmonary edema fluid. Pediatr Res 29:353–356.
107. Lachmann B. (1989). Animal studies of surfactant replacement therapy. Developmental Pharmacol Ther 13:164–172.
108. Lewis J, Ikegami M, Higuchi R, et al. (1991). Nebulized vs instilled exogenous surfactant in an adult lung injury model. J Appl Physiol 71:1270–1276.
109. Liu MY, Wang LM, Enhorning G. (1991). Pulmonary surfactant may secure free airflow through a narrow tube. J Appl Physiol 71:742–748.
110. Long W, Corbet A, Allen A, et al. (1992). Retrospective search for bleeding diathesis among premature newborn infants with pulmonary hemorrhage after synthetic surfactant treatment. J Pediatr 120:S45–S50.
111. Malcolm JD, Elliot CD. (1980). Interfacial tension from height and diameter of a single profile drop or captive bubble. Can J Chem Eng 58:151–153.
112. Meredeth KS, deLemos RA, Coalson JJ, et al. (1989). The role of lung injury in the pathogenesis of hyaline membrane disease in premature baboons. J Appl Physiol 66:2150–2158.
113. Merritt TA, Strayer DS, Hallman M, et al. (1989). Immunologic considerations Regarding Exogenous Surfactant in Surfactant Replacement Therapy. New York: Alan R. Liss, pp 145–162.
114. Morley CJ, Morley R. (1990), Follow-up of premature babies treated with artificial surfactant (ALEC). Arch Dis Child 65:667–69.
115. Morley C, Robertson B, Lachmann B, et al (1980). Artificial surfactant and natural surfactant. Comparison study of the effects on premature rabbit lungs. Arch Dis Child 55:758–765.
116. Moses D, Holm BA, Spitale P, Liu M, et al. (1991). Inhibition of pulmonary surfactant function by meconium. Am J Obstet Gynecol 164:477–81.
117. Msall MF, Rogers BT Catanzaro N, et al. (1989). Five year neurodevelopmental

outcome of infants less than 28 weeks gestational age enrolled in a surfactant randomized clinical trial. Pediatr Res 25:258A.

118. Revak SD, Merritt TA, Degryse E, et al. (1988). Use of human low molecular weight apoproteins in the reconstitution of surfactant biologic activity. J Clin Invest 81:826–833.
119. Robertson B. (1984) Pathology and pathophysiology of neonatal surfactant deficiency. In: Robertson B, Van Golde LMG, Batenburg JJ, eds. Pulmonary Surfactant. Amsterdam: Elsevier, pp 383–418.
120. Schurch F (1991). Surface Tension Properties of Surfacent Presented at Exosurf Neonatal Treatment IND Investigators Meeting. Nov. 12–14, 1991, Research Triangle Park, NC.
121. Soll RF. Synthetic Surfactant Treatment of RDS. In Chalmers I, ed. Oxford Database of Perinatal trials. January 28, 1990. Updated August 29, 1990, January 29, 1991, July 24, 1991, January 9, 1992.
122. Soll RF. Prophylactic Administration of Synthetic Surfactant. In Chalmers I, ed. Oxford Database of Perinatal trials. January 28, 1990. Updated August 29, 1990, July 24, 1991, February 20, 1992.
123. Soll RF. Prophylactic surfactant vs surfactant treatment of RDS. In Chalmers I, ed. Oxford Database of Perinatal Trials. August 29, 1990, January 29, 1991, July 24, 1991.
124. Strayer DS, Merritt TA, Lwebuga-Mukasa J, et al. (1986). Surfactant-anti-surfactant immune complex in infants with respiratory distress syndrome. Am J Pathol 122:353–362.
125. Strayer DS, Hallman M, Merritt TA. (1991). Immunogenicity of surfactant. I. Human alveolar surfactant. Clin Exp Immunol 83:35–40.
126. Tabor BL, Ikegami M, Jobe AH, et al. (1990). Dose response of thyrotropin-releasing hormone on pulmonary maturation in corticosteroid-treated preterm rabbits. Am Obstet Gynecol 163:669–76.
127. van Houten J, Long W, Mullett M, et al. (1992). Pulmonary hemorrhage in premature infants after treatment with synthetic surfactant: an autopsy evaluation. J Pediatr 120:S40–44.
128. Vidyasagar D, Maeta H, Raju TNK, et al. (1985). Bovine surfactant (Surfactant TA) therapy in immature baboons with hyaline membrane disease. Pediatrics 75:1132–1142.
129. Walter D, McGuinness G, Bose C. (1991). Double blind one year follow-up in 1450 infants randomized to Exosurf, Neonatal or air. Pediatr Res 29:270A.
130. Whitset JA, Hull WM, Luse S. (1991). Failure to detect surfactant protein-specific antibodies in sera of premature infants treated with Surfacta, a modified bovine surfactant. Pediatrics 87:505–510.

20

Strategies for Surfactant Therapy in Established Neonatal Respiratory Distress Syndrome

HENRY L. HALLIDAY
The Queen's University of Belfast
and Royal Maternity Hospital
Belfast, Northern Ireland

CHRISTIAN P. SPEER
University Children's Hospital
Tübingen, Germany

I. Introduction

Studies by Avery and Mead published in 1959 (1) clearly demonstrated that infants dying of respiratory distress syndrome (RDS) had a deficiency of pulmonary surfactant. About 20 years later, Fujiwara and coworkers (2) reported successful treatment of 10 babies with established RDS using a modified bovine surfactant. Since then many trials have used this strategy of "rescue" treatment of babies with established RDS (3–5), although some studies used true prophylaxis of babies during resuscitation (6,7) (see Chapter 19). These randomised controlled trials used both natural (4,6) and synthetic (5,7) surfactant preparations and meta-analysis clearly demonstrates an approximate 40% reduction in the odds of neonatal death after surfactant treatment (3). Pulmonary air leaks are also significantly reduced after surfactant treatment, with the extent of this reduction varying between 70% for natural surfactant preparations and 30% for synthetic surfactants (3,8).

In this chapter, we will concentrate on the use of surfactant to treat established RDS; so-called "rescue" therapy. We will discuss the relative merits of natural versus synthetic surfactant, the timing of surfactant replacement in relation to birth and severity of RDS, the initial dose of phospholipids needed, retreatment criteria, causes of a poor response, the mode of administration, and acute responses to treatment.

II. Types of Surfactants

The first trials of surfactant replacement used aerosolised dipalmitoyl phosphatidylcholine (DPPC) in babies with RDS and were largely unsuccessful (9,10), because the surfactant was ineffective and inadequate amounts would have reached the air-liquid interfaces in the alveoli. Although pulmonary surfactant is predominantly DPPC, it also contains other phospholipids, including phosphatidylglycerol (PG) and phosphatidylinositol (PI). Surfactant also contains neutral lipids and specific proteins (SP-A, SP-B, SP-C, and SP-D) (see Chapter 3). Three of these proteins (SP-A, SP-B, SP-C) enable it to rapidly adsorb, spread, and reform a monolayer during respiration. DPPC alone does not adsorb or spread rapidly enough to function as an effective surfactant. Synthetic surfactants based on DPPC need the addition of compounds to encourage adsorption and spreading; PG, lipoprotein, alcohols, and nonionic surfactants have been used (see below). An alternative strategy is to use natural or modified natural surfactants derived from human amniotic fluid or animal lungs; the so-called natural surfactants. They act rapidly as they contain the proteins SP-B and SP-C (human amniotic fluid surfactant also contains SP-A).

A. Natural Surfactants

At least six different preparations of natural surfactants have been used in clinical trials (Table 1); four derived from bovine lungs and one each from human amniotic fluid and porcine lungs (3,11–14). The dose of phospholipids administered in these trials ranged from 50 to 200 mg/kg in a volume of 1.2–4 ml/kg. In general, up to three or four doses of surfactant have been used for babies who respond poorly or show relapse after an initially good response. Human surfactant, which is derived from amniotic fluid, is the only surfactant preparation to contain SP-A, but it is no longer being used in clinical trials because of the risk of HIV contamination. The other five surfactants listed in Table 1 are produced commercially for use in the United States, Europe, Japan, and other countries.

B. Synthetic Surfactants

Three synthetic surfactant preparations used in clinical trials are listed in Table 2. Artificial lung expanding compound (ALEC) was developed in Cambridge, England, by Morley and Bangham (15). It contains DPPC and PG in a 7:3 weight for weight ratio and is administered in a dose of 100 mg/kg. The

Table 1 Natural Surfactant Preparations: Source, Composition, Dosages, and Volumes Used in Randomized Clinical Trials

Preparation	Source	Dose (phospholipids, mg/kg)	Volume (ml/kg)	No. of doses
Surfactant-TA	Bovine	100	4	4
Survanta	Bovine	100	4	4
Infasurf (CLSE)	Bovine	90–100	3	3
Alveofact	Bovine	50	1.2	4
Amniotic fluid surfactant	Human	60	3	3
Curosurf	Porcine	100–200	1.25–2.5	3

CLSE, calf lung surfactant extract.

Belfast, Northern Ireland, surfactant, Turfsurf, composed of DPPC:HDL (10:1) and given in a dose of only 25 mg/kg, is no longer being used in clinical trials (16) and has not been produced commercially. Exosurf, which contains DPPC, hexadecanol, and tyloxapol is administered in a dose of 67.5 mg/kg and has been used in a number of clinical trials (17–19). It is commercially produced and is licensed for use as prophylaxis or "rescue" therapy when two doses are recommended.

C. Trials Comparing Natural and Synthetic Surfactants

In vitro properties of surfactant preparations are usually assessed by measuring surface adsorption, surface spreading and respreading, film compressibility, and changes in surface tension during cyclic film compression (20). Using the

Table 2 Synthetic Surfactant Preparations Subjected to Randomized Clinical Trials

Preparation	Composition	Dose (phospholipids, mg/kg)	Volume (ml/kg)	No. of doses
ALEC	DPPC, PG	100	1	4
Turfsurf	DPPC, HDL	25	1	1[a]
Exosurf	DPPC, hexadecanol, tyloxapol	67.5	5	2

ALEC, artificial lung expanding compound; DPPC, dipalmitoyl phosphatidylcholine; PG, phosphatidylglycerol; HDL, high-density lipoprotein.
[a]Prophylaxis only.

pulsating-bubble technique (21), Hall and coworkers (22) found that Exosurf at 10 mg/ml had a minimum surface tension of 29 mN/m during 50% surface compression compared with values of <1 and 2 mN/m, respectively, for calf lung surfactant extract (CLSE) and Survanta. In vivo animal studies also demonstrate better oxygenation, pulmonary pressure-volume characteristics, and survival with natural (sheep surfactant) or modified natural surfactants (Infasurf, Survanta) compared with synthetic surfactant (Exosurf) (23) (see also Chapter 12).

Only one clinical trial comparing two surfactant preparations has been published in full (24), but other studies are currently being undertaken. Six hundred and seventeen babies weighing between 501 and 1500 g with RDS who were receiving assisted ventilation with 30% or more oxygen within 6 hr of birth were randomized to receive up to four intratracheal doses of either Exosurf or Survanta. During the 72 hr after the first surfactant dose, the average oxygen requirement and mean airway pressure were lower for the Survanta-treated babies. Death or bronchopulmonary dysplasia (BPD) occurred in 67% of the Exosurf-treated babies compared with 62% of the Survanta-treated infants. This clinically important difference of 5% was not statistically significant with the sample size chosen for this study (24). A trial of 2000 infants would be needed to show statistical significance with these rates of morbidity. Trials currently in progress may be able to clarify whether natural surfactant preparations are indeed superior to synthetic surfactants.

The choice between using a synthetic surfactant (e.g., Exosurf) or a natural surfactant (e.g., Survanta, Surfactant-TA, Infasurf, CLSE, Curosurf, or Alveofact) may be determined by the clinician's opinion of the required speed of response for an individual infant with RDS. Synthetic surfactants with their slower response may be more suitable for prophylaxis or treatment of less severe disease, whereas natural surfactants with their more rapid normalization of blood gases and reduced ventilator pressures may be more suitable for very ill babies at risk of pulmonary barotrauma and air leak. The relative costs of surfactant preparations may also be important determinants of the clinician's choice (25–27).

III. Timing—Early Rather Than Late

There is considerable controversy about the timing of surfactant therapy. From a theoretical viewpoint prophylactic surfactant replacement has potential advantages. In animal experiments, surfactant replacement at birth facilitates initial lung aeration, improves distribution of surfactant at the air-liquid interface, and decreases both barotrauma and alveolar-capillary leakage of inhibitory serum proteins (28). Recent trials with natural surfactants which compared prophylaxis with rescue treatment gave contradictory results. Merritt and coworkers (29) found no differences in outcome between 102 preterm infants who were treated in the delivery room with human surfactant and 101 infants who received surfactant at a mean age of 3.7 hr. In addition, Dunn and colleagues (30) observed a higher incidence of chronic lung disease at 28 days in 62 infants who were treated prophylactically at birth with a bovine surfactant compared with 60 neonates treated at a mean age of 2.9 hr.

In contrast, Kendig and colleagues (31) reported a significant reduction in mortality in 85 very immature infants (<26 weeks' gestational age) treated prophylactically with a bovine surfactant compared with 72 infants treated for respiratory distress syndrome. Similar results have been reported in relatively mature neonates between 29 and 32 weeks of gestation treated with a bovine surfactant (32). Another small trial using a bovine surfactant also favoured the prophylactic strategy (33). A recently completed multicentre trial which compared prophylaxis and rescue treatment with a porcine surfactant enrolled 149 preterm infants of less than 30 weeks' gestation (34). This study favored prophylactic treatment, and a meta-analysis including it with two other similar trials also using Curosurf suggested significant reductions in mortality and severe intraventricular haemorrhage (35).

However, it is important to remember that without knowledge of lung maturity, prophylactic administration of surfactant implies that about 40% of preterm babies will be treated unnecessarily. The possible consequences are unnecessary intubation of a significant number of neonates. unnecessary exposure to possible adverse effects, and increased costs (36). In addition, the prophylactic instillation of relatively large volumes of surfactant in the delivery suite could complicate resuscitation and destabilise the baby during the vulnerable period of postnatal adaptation. Interestingly, follow-up examination of a small group of infants who had received human surfactant has shown an increase in neurodevelopmental delay in babies treated prophylactically compared with those given rescue therapy (37).

Regarding timing of surfactant treatment, a reasonable compromise is to treat infants as soon as clinical signs of respiratory distress syndrome are evident. In fact, recent trails with Curosurf and Exosurf suggest that treatment at an early stage of the disease improves outcome of babies when compared with later treatment (38,39). An Italian multicentre trial clearly indicated that early single dose treatment before severe RDS had developed (oxygen requirement 40–59%) lead to a better survival and reduced the risk of severe intracranial hemorrhage, when compared with late single-dose treatment (≥60% oxygen) (38). The OSIRIS trial (39) provided further evidence that the two strategies—prophylaxis and rescue treatment— are approaching one another. Infants judged to be at risk for respiratory distress syndrome received early surfactant administration at a mean age of about 2 hr; in contrast, delayed selective administration was given a mean age of 3 hr. However, early administration was associated with lower risk of death or oxygen dependency at the expected date of delivery.

There is agreement that early surfactant treatment is highly effective in reducing pulmonary and nonpulmonary complications. Therefore, early treatment should be initiated in all babies less than 31 weeks of gestation as soon as clinical signs develop and mechanical ventilation is needed with >40% oxygen. From a practical viewpoint more mature infants with respiratory distress syndrome could receive later treatment when they require mechanical ventilation with more than 50–60% oxygen (14). Recently, it has been suggested that the cotside application of static respiratory compliance measurement by occlusion can be used to select infants likely to benefit from early surfactant treatment (40). Very immature infants, for example, those of less than 27 weeks' gestation should probably be given surfactant very soon after birth; in the delivery suite if intubation is needed for resuscitation. However, each approach requires careful and continuous clinical assessment over the first hours of life of all infants with or at risk of developing RDS. Moreover, regardless of the time of surfactant administration, the pediatrician and assisting nurse administering surfactant must be experienced in all aspects of neonatal intensive care, including the necessary ventilatory adjustments following rapid changes in gas exchange (see below).

IV. Dosage and Response

The pool size of endogenous alveolar surfactant lipids in healthy neonates is at least 100 mg/kg (41); in preterm infants with RDS, however, it is usually less than 10 mg/kg (42). With the development of RDS, serum-derived protein inhibitors leak into the alveoli and inactivate surfactant (43) so that more exogenous surfactant will be needed to overcome this inhibition.

A. Initial Dose

The initial dose of surfactant used in clinical trials has varied from 25 to 200 mg of phospholipids per kilogram body weight with a corresponding variation in dose volume (1–5 ml/kg; see Tables 1 and 2) (44). Although the optimal dose has not been clearly defined, there is evidence that larger doses are more effective than smaller ones (45,46). Konishi and coworkers (45) clearly demonstrated in a randomized trial with Surfactant-TA that a single dose of 120 mg/kg improved gas exchange and outcome of babies with established RDS when compared with an initial dose of 60 mg/kg. Recently, the effect of two different surfactant doses on pulmonary gas exchange was evaluated in a small randomized trial (46). Infants with severe RDS were treated with either 100 mg/kg or 200 mg/kg of the natural porcine surfactant Curosurf. The dose of 100 mg/kg resulted in a rapid improvement in oxygenation and ventilatory requirement, which was not as striking as that with a 200 mg/kg dose. A similar response of the initial low versus high dose was observed in the largest randomized Curosurf trial which enrolled 2168 babies (47). In this study, although oxygenation was superior in the high-dose group for up to 36 hr, the long-term outcome of death and/or oxygen dependency at expected date of delivery was similar with both doses of surfactant (47). Most investigators recommend at least 100 mg/kg of various surfactant preparations as an initial dose for the treatment of established disease.

B. Retreatment

Preterm infants with RDS who after an initially good response relapse within 48 hr and need continued mechanical ventilation with ≥30% oxygen may benefit from multiple doses of surfactant. It seems likely that repetitive doses of surfactant overcome the functional inactivation of surfactant by serum proteins leaking into the bronchoalveolar system. In several trials, infants were given repeated doses of surfactant; some studies used automatic retreatment schedules (17,18), whereas others allowed retreatment only if there was significant residual lung disease (48,49). However, only two randomized trials have compared single-dose versus multiple-dose treatment in babies with RDS (50,51). In one study which recruited relatively mature infants with RDS, multiple-dose treatment with a bovine surfactant resulted in an improved oxygenation during the first 2 days following surfactant administration (50). In the second multicenter trial, oxygenation, ventilatory requirement, and outcome of babies with severe RDS was further improved by treatment with two additional doses (100 mg/kg) of a porcine surfactant 12 and 24 hr after the initial dose (51). The incidence of pneumothorax was reduced from 18% in the single-dose group to 9% in the multiple-dose group and mortality from 21 to 13%, respectively.

The total cumulative dose of surfactant needed was addressed in the Curosurf 4 trial (47). A total dose of up to 300 mg/kg was as effective as up to 600 mg/kg. In two trials with Exosurf, which is administered in a larger volume (5 ml/kg), different multiple-dose regimens were evaluated. Five hundred and forty-eight neonates with established RDS (birth weight ≥1250 g) were randomized to receive either two or four doses of Exosurf. No significant advantage was found in infants who were treated with four doses (52). These data were confirmed in the larger OSIRIS trial (39) which enrolled almost 7000 babies.

C. Poor Response

Most preterm infants with RDS respond favorably to the initial and subsequent surfactant doses. However, some babies with clinical signs of RDS do not respond adequately or show early relapse. These infants may have other diseases such as lung hypoplasia, structural pulmonary immaturity, pneumonia, or congenital heart disease. In addition, perinatal asphyxia, hypothermia, acidosis, and systemic hypotension may be associated with a poor response to surfactant (53). For an optimal surfactant response anemia, hypotension and acidosis should be corrected by appropriate measures before surfactant treatment. A poor response to surfactant treatment identifies a group of babies at increased risk of dying (54). In a few infants, relapse may be due to the development of pulmonary edema secondary to a patent ductus arteriosus (PDA). Prior to repeat surfactant treatment, PDA should be excluded by clinical examination and echocardiography if necessary. Studies in San Diego and Helsinki have suggested that excessive fluid intake and failure to reduce ventilatory settings after surfactant administration are associated with poorer outcome (55) (see below).

V. Methods of Administration

Surfactants are usually administered through an endotracheal tube in one, two, or more boluses with the infant positioned so that each dependent lung receives surfactant. Before surfactant administration a chest x-ray should be performed in order to confirm the presence of RDS and to estimate its severity, to determine the correct positioning of the endotracheal tube, and to exclude other diagnoses such as pulmonary air leaks. Pneumothorax should be adequately treated before surfactant instillation.

Several protocols have been proposed to obtain reasonably uniform distribution of surfactant to the alveoli, and there are two commonly practised modes of surfactant delivery: the feeding tube technique and the side-port adaptor technique (56). Most procedures imply that the baby is transiently disconnected from the ventilator while the surfactant is delivered into the lower trachea via a premeasured feeding tube attached to a syringe. After instillation, the baby is either manually ventilated for a short time or immediately reconnected to the ventilator. The pressures used for mechanical ventilation push the surfactant rapidly into the lungs. The most extensive administration and positioning maneuvre has been practised with the natural bovine surfactant preparation Survanta; the infant is held in four different positions for administration of each fractional dose (57). In a recent trial, various administration procedures with Survanta were evaluated: two bolus doses with removal of the infant from the ventilator; two bolus doses through a neonatal suction valve without removal of the infant from the ventilator; four bolus doses with the infant's removal from the ventilator. The authors demonstrated that all procedures were equally effective and safe (57). The manufacturers have changed their recommendations for administration of Survanta following the publication of this trial.

The natural porcine preparation Curosurf is usually administered in two aliquots into each dependent bronchus via a feeding tube. After each instillation, the babies are ventilated manually for 1 min. During this period, the insufflation pressure is adjusted to provide adequate chest movements. No suctioning of the airways is performed for about 6 hr unless endotracheal tube obstruction is suspected (51,58).

A different approach to surfactant treatment has been evaluated by a Danish-Swedish group who combined the early use of nasal continuous positive airway pressure (CPAP) and an intratracheal bolus instillation of Curosurf during a brief period of intubation. Seventy-three babies were enrolled in this randomized multicenter trial. A significant reduction in the need for ventilatory treatment was found in babies initially treated with nasal CPAP and Curosurf compared with control infants not treated with surfactant. Surprisingly, this benefit was only seen in boys (59).

In studies with the synthetic preparation, Exosurf, administration has been either rapid (19) or slow (17) through an endotracheal adaptor with a side-port either directly or through a fine catheter inserted through the side-port into the airways. The minimum recommended time for administration of a complete dose is 4 min, although Phibbs and colleagues (19) gave Exosurf rapidly over 5 sec. Each Exosurf dose is instilled in two aliquots of 2.5 ml/kg with the infant initially in midline position, thereafter turned 45 degrees to the right for 30 sec, and with the second aliquot to the left for the same time.

Alternative methods of administration including aerosolization of surfactant are discussed in Chapter 15.

VI. Acute Effects

The acute effects of natural surfactants have only been observed after bolus instillation. In animal experiments, slow infusion of natural surfactant over 45 min leads to nonhomogeneous distribution in the lung and markedly reduced effects on pulmonary gas exchange (60). The rapid changes in oxygenation and effective pulmonary blood flow following bolus administration of natural surfactant have been shown to be associated with a fall in systemic arterial blood pressure (61) and an improvement in cerebral oxygenation (62). However, changes in blood pressure and cerebral blood flow velocity are not inevitable (63,64) and have also been seen with synthetic surfactants (65). In a few babies, transient suppression of the electroencephalogram (EEG) has been observed (66) which is not associated with reduced cerebral blood flow (62,67). To date, there is no evidence that these findings are associated with any adverse long-term effects on the baby (68).

When using an effective natural surfactant preparation, it is important to reduce ventilator settings soon after administration. Inspired oxygen concentrations can be reduced within minutes and other ventilator changes should be geared to preventing overdistension of the lung (44). Functional residual capacity has been shown to increase within one hour of surfactant treatment (69) and is probably due to stabilization of gas exchange units already being ventilated, as well as the recruitment of new units (70). To prevent overdistension of the lung, inspiratory time and positive end-expiratory pressure (PEEP) should be reduced early and peak inspiratory pressure thereafter if improvement in chest wall movement and blood gases persist (44). Lower mean airway pressure and reduced fluid intake have been associated with improved response to human surfactant treatment (55).

Up to 20% of the babies have unilateral surfactant distribution as judged from chest films (71). Apparently, this transient phenomenon is not associated with adverse effects. However, anecdotal unpublished reports indicate that persisting atelectasis can be effectively treated by selective instillation of surfactant into the dependent atelectatic lung.

Synthetic surfactants have a slower onset of action (24,72), so that ventilator settings need to be altered more cautiously after instillation of Exosurf. In a few infants, ventilator settings need to be temporarily increased, and this may be related to the larger volume of fluid that needs to be instilled. Animal studies suggest that synthetic surfactants show sustained responses only if levels of positive end-expiratory pressure (PEEP) are maintained (72). Other problems associated with Exosurf treatment are an increased incidence of apnea of prematurity and pulmonary hemorrhage (73). Apnea has been said to be due to early extubation and pulmonary hemorrhage to the development of a PDA (73). The increased risk of pulmonary hemorrhage after Exosurf treatment appears confined to babies treated prophylactically (74).

VII. Conclusions

Except for very immature babies, early rescue treatment with surfactant is probably the optimal method of managing neonatal RDS (36,44). For babies of <27 weeks' gestation, prophylaxis may be preferable (35). The choice between a natural and a synthetic surfactant will depend on a number of factors, including the previous experience of the clinician, the need to obtain a rapid response, and cost. In general, natural surfactants can be recommended for moderate to severe RDS in immature infants, whereas a synthetic surfactant might be appropriate for the treatment of milder RDS in more mature infants (Table 3). Sufficient phospholipid to replenish the surfactant pool and to overcome inhibitors means that an initial dose of 100–200 mg/kg is appropriate. Repeat doses become necessary if smaller initial doses are used or if relapse occurs. Criteria for retreatment should be flexible and include continued need for ventilation with at least 30% oxygen (Table 3).

Two commonly used methods of administration have been recommended:

Table 3 Recommendations for Surfactant Therapy in Established Neonatal RDS

Items	Recommendations
Type of surfactant	*Natural* for moderate to severe disease and immature babies *Synthetic* for mild to moderate disease and moderately immature babies
Timing	Early rather than late treatment ($Fio_2 \geq 0.40$)
Initial dose	100–200 mg phospholipids/kg
Retreatment	Flexible (about 12 hourly) *Indications*: $Fio_2 \geq 0.30$ and requirement of artificial ventilation
Action according to typical response	*Natural surfactant*: Lower Fio_2 immediately Lower inspiration time and PEEP soon Lower peak inspiratory pressure according to chest wall movements and blood gases *Synthetic surfactant*: Lower Fio_2 cautiously Maintain PEEP Lower peak inspiratory pressure cautiously according to chest wall movement and blood gases Watch for development of PDA and pulmonary hemorrhage!
Some causes of poor response	*Wrong diagnosis*: Lung hypoplasia Pneumonia ARDS Congenital heart disease *Wrong dose*: Inadequate dose to overcome surfactant inhibition *Wrong place*: Surfactant given into one lung or into esophagus *Wrong condition*: Correct hypothermia, acidosis and hypotension before treatment
Causes of early relapse and its management	*Inadequate dose*: Retreat *PDA, diagnosed by Doppler and diastolic blood pressure recordings*: Early resort to indomethacin *Pneumonia, diagnosed by Gram stain and culture of tracheal aspirate*: Early resort to antibiotics *Pulmonary hemorrhage*: Close the ductus Consider retreatment

rapid bolus doses for natural surfactants and slow instillation using an endotracheal tube adaptor for Exosurf. Natural surfactants give rise to a more rapid response allowing inspired oxygen concentration, inspiratory pressure, and PEEP to be lowered within a few minutes of instillation (see Table 3). With synthetic surfactants, the response is slower and it is important to maintain adequate levels of PEEP. PDA, apnea of prematurity, and pulmonary hemorrhage are more likely after surfactant treatment and should be carefully looked for and treated early.

A poor response to surfactant treatment may indicate an inadequate dose, maladministration, failure to stabilize before instillation, or the wrong diagnosis. Failure to respond to surfactant identifies a group of babies with a poorer outcome (54).

Finally, prevention of preterm birth and maternal treatment to enhance fetal lung maturity should not be forgotten as alternative strategies in the fight against RDS (14). Prenatal corticosteroids have clearly been shown to reduce the risk of RDS and neonatal death by 40–50% (75), and there is also convincing evidence that there are synergistic effects when postnatal surfactant treatment is needed later (76,77) (see Chapter 18). Perhaps we should look at the need for postnatal surfactant treatment as a failure to prevent RDS. However, for some babies who need it, surfactant replacement is a rational treatment strategy based on sound physiological principles and thoroughly tested in clinical trials (12). Its introduction has had a major impact in reducing national neonatal mortality rates, with the greatest benefit being seen in infants weighing between 601 and 1300 g at birth (78).

Acknowledgments

We thank Samantha Jameson for typing the manuscript.

References

1. Avery ME, Mead J. Surface properties in relation to atelectasis and hyaline membrane disease. Am J Dis Child 1959; 97:517–523.
2. Fujiwara T, Maeta H, Chida S, et al. Artificial surfactant therapy in hyaline-membrane disease. Lancet 1980; 1:55–59.
3. Soll RF, McQueen MC. Respiratory distress syndrome. In: Sinclair JC, Bracken MB, eds. Effective Care of the Newborn Infant. Oxford, England: Oxford University Press, 1992:325–355.
4. Soll RF. Natural surfactant extract treatment of RDS. In: Chalmers I, ed. Oxford Database of Perinatal Trials. Version 1.3, Disk Issue 7, 1992; Record 5206.
5. Soll RF. Synthetic surfactant treatment of RDS. In: Chalmers I, ed. Oxford Database of Perinatal Trials. Version 1.3, Disk Issue 7, 1992; Record 5252.

6. Soll RF. Prophylactic administration of natural surfactant extract. In: Chalmers I, ed. Oxford Database of Perinatal Trials. Version 1.3, Disk Issue 7, 1992; Record 5207.
7. Soll RF. Prophylactic administration of synthetic surfactant. In: Chalmers I, ed. Oxford Database of Perinatal Trials. Version 1.3, Disk Issue 7, 1992; Record 5253.
8. Halliday HL. Other acute lung disorders. In: Sinclair JC, Bracken MB, eds. Effective Care of the Newborn Infant. Oxford, England: Oxford University Press, 1992:359–384.
9. Robillard E, Alarie Y, Dagenais-Perusse P, et al. Microaerosal administration of synthetic β-γ-dipalmitoyl-L-α-lecithin in the respiratory distress syndrome: A preliminary report. Can Med Assoc J 1964; 90:55–57.
10. Chu J, Clements JA, Cotton EK, et al. Neonatal pulmonary ischemia. Part 1—Clinical and physiological studies. Pediatrics 1967; 40:709–782.
11. Morlcy CJ. Surfactant treatment for premature babies: A review of clinical trials. Arch Dis Child 1991; 66:445–450.
12. Jobe AH. Pulmonary surfactant therapy. N Engl J Med 1993; 328:861–868.
13. Halliday HL. Surfactant replacement. In: Klaus MH, Fanaroff AA, eds. Yearbook of Neonatal/Perinatal Medicine 1991. Chicago: Year Book Medical Publishers, 1991:XIII–XXI.
14. Halliday HL. Current views of the use of surfactant. Contemp Rev Obstet Gynaecol 1993; 5:65–70.
15. Morley CJ, Bangham AD, Miller N, Davis JA. Dry artificial lung surfactant and its effect on very premature babies. Lancet 1981; 1:64–68.
16. Halliday HL, Reid M McC, Meban C, et al. Controlled trial of artificial surfactant to prevent respiratory distress syndrome. Lancet 1984; 1:476–478.
17. Long W, Thompson T, Sundell H, et al. Effects of two rescue doses of a synthetic surfactant on mortality rate and survival without bronchopulmonary dysplasia in 700- to 1350-gram infants with respiratory distress syndrome: The American Exosurf Neonatal Study Group 1. J Pediatr 1991; 118:595–605.
18. Canadian EXOSURF Pediatric Study Group. Effects of two rescue doses of EXOSURF[R] Pediatric in 342 750-1249 gram infants. Pediatric Res 1990; 27:200A.
19. Phibbs RH, Ballard RA, Clements JA, et al. Initial clinical trial of Exosurf, a protein-free synthetic surfactant, for the prophylaxis and early treatment of hyaline membrane disease. Pediatrics 1991; 88:1–9.
20. Keough KMW. Physical chemistry of pulmonary surfactant in the terminal airspaces. In: Robertson B, van Golde LMG, Batenburg JJ, eds. Pulmonary Surfactant: From Molecular Biology to Clinical Practice. Amsterdam: Elsevier, 1992; 109–164.
21. Enhorning G. Pulsating bubble technique for evaluating pulmonary surfactant. J Appl Physiol 1977; 43:198–203.
22. Hall SB, Venkitaraman AR, Whitsett JA, et al. Importance of hydrophobic apoproteins as constituents of clinical exogenous surfactants. Am Rev Respir Dis 1992; 145:24–30.
23. Cummings JJ, Holm BA, Hudak ML, et al. A controlled clinical comparison of four different surfactant preparations in surfactant-deficient preterm lambs. Am Rev Respir Dis 1992; 145:999–1004.

24. Horbar JD, Wright LL, Soll RF, et al. A multicenter randomised trial comparing two surfactants for the treatment of neonatal respiratory distress syndrome. J Pediatr 1993; 123:757–766.
25. Mugford M, Howard S. Cost-effectiveness of surfactant replacement in preterm babies. Pharmaco-Economics 1993; 3:362–373.
26. Egberts J. Estimated costs of different treatments of the respiratory distress syndrome in a large cohort of preterm infants of less than 30 weeks of gestation. Biol Neonate 1992; 61(Suppl 1):59–65.
27. Halliday HL. Introducing new cost effective treatments into the NHS. Surfactant treatment for premature babies: Who cares enough to pay? Qual Health Care 1993; 2:195–197.
28. Enhorning G, Robertson B. Lung expansion in the premature rabbit fetus after tracheal deposition of surfactant. Pediatrics 1972; 50:58–66.
29. Merritt TA, Hallman M, Berry C, et al. Randomized, placebo-controlled trial of human surfactant given at birth versus rescue administration in very low birth weight infants with lung immaturity. J Pediatr 1991; 118:581–594.
30. Dunn MS, Shennan AT, Zayack D, Possmayer F. Bovine surfactant replacement therapy in neonates of less than 30 weeks gestation: a randomized controlled trial of prophylaxis versus treatment. Pediatrics 1991; 87:377–386.
31. Kendig JW, Notter RH, Cox C, et al. A comparison of surfactant as immediate prophylaxis and as rescue therapy in newborns of less than 30 weeks gestation. N Engl J Med 1991; 324:865–871.
32. Kattwinkel J, Bloom BT, Delmore P, et al. Prophylactic administration of calf lung surfactant extract is more effective than early treatment of respiratory distress syndrome in neonates of 29 to 32 weeks gestation. Pediatrics 1993; 92:90–98.
33. Konishi M, Fujiwara T, Chida S, et al. A prospective randomized trial of early versus late administration of a single dose of surfactant-TA. Early Hum Dev 1992; 29:275–282.
34. Egberts J, de Winter JP, Sedin G, et al. Comparison of prophylaxis and rescue treatment with Curosurf in babies less than 30 weeks gestation: A randomized trial. Pediatrics 1993; 92:768–774.
35. Egberts J, Walti H, Bevilacqua G and the Dutch Swedish and Italian Multicenter Collaborators. Meta-analysis of three "prophylaxis versus rescue" trials with Curosurf. 8th International Workshop on Surfactant Replacement, Oslo, May 20–22, 1993.
36. Dunn MS. Surfactant replacement therapy: Prophylaxis or treatment? Pediatrics 1993; 92:148–150.
37. Vaucher YE, Harker L, Merritt TA, et al. Outcome at twelve months of adjusted age in very low birth weight infants with lung immaturity: A randomized, placebo-controlled trial of human surfactant. J Pediatr 1993; 122:126–132.
38. Bevilacqua G, Halliday HL, Parmigiani S, Robertson B on behalf of the Collaborative European Multicentre Study Group. Randomized multicenter trial of treatment with porcine natural surfactant for moderately severe neonatal respiratory distress syndrome. J Perinat Med 1993; 21:3–9.
39. OSIRIS Collaborative Group. Early versus delayed neonatal administration of a synthetic surfactant—The judgment of OSIRIS. Lancet 1992; 340:1363–1369.
40. Wilkie RA, Bryan MH, Tarnow-Mordi WO. Static respiratory compliance in the

newborn. II: Its potential for improving the selection of infants for early surfactant treatment. Arch Dis Child 1994; 70:F16–F18.
41. Jobe AH, Ikegami M, Glatz T, et al. Duration and characteristics of treatment of premature lambs with natural surfactant. J Clin Invest 1981; 67:370–375.
42. Fujiwara T, Robertson B. Pharmacology of exogenous surfactant. In: Robertson B, van Golde LMG, Batenburg JJ, eds. Pulmonary Surfactant: From Molecular Biology to Clinical Practice. Amsterdam: Elsevier, 1992:561–592.
43. Günther A, Grube C, Seeger W. Inhibition of surfactant by plasma proteins. In: Bevilacqua G, Parmigiani S, Robertson B, eds. Surfactant in Clinical Practice. Chur: Harwood Academic Publishers, 1992:87–101.
44. Speer CP, Halliday HL. Surfactant therapy in the newborn. Curr Paediatr 1994; 4:5–9.
45. Konishi M, Fujiwara T, Naito T, et al. Surfactant replacement therapy in neonatal respiratory distress syndrome. A multicentre, randomized clinical trial: comparison of high- versus low-doses of Surfactant TA. Eur J Pediatr 1988; 47:20–25.
46. Herting E, Tubman R, Halliday HL. Einfluβ von 2 unterschiedlichen Dosierungen eines porcinen Surfactants auf den pulmonalen Gasaustausch Frühgeborener mit schwerem Atemnotsyndrom. Monatsschr Kinderheilkd 1993; 141:721–727.
47. Halliday HL, Tarnow-Mordi WO, Corcoran JD, Patterson CC. A multicentre randomised trial comparing high and low dose surfactant regimens for the treatment of respiratory distress syndrome (The Curosurf 4 trial). Arch Dis Child 1993; 69:276–280.
48. Hoekstra RE, Jackson JC, Myers TF, et al. Improved neonatal survival following multiple doses of bovine surfactant in very premature neonates at risk at respiratory distress syndrome. Pediatrics 1991; 88:10–18.
49. Liechty EA, Donovan E, Purohit D, et al. Reduction of neonatal mortality after multiple doses of bovine surfactant in low birth weight neonates with respiratory distress syndrome. Pediatrics 1991; 88:19–28.
50. Dunn MS, Shennan AT, Possmayer F. Single- versus multiple-dose surfactant replacement therapy in neonates of 30 to 36 weeks' gestation with respiratory distress syndrome. Pediatrics 1990; 86:564–571.
51. Speer CP, Robertson B, Curstedt T, et al. Randomized European multicenter trial of surfactant replacement therapy for severe neonatal respiratory distress syndrome: single versus multiple doses of Curosurf. Pediatrics 1992; 89:13–20.
52. Pramanik AK, Dhanireddy R, Walther F, et al. Effect of two compared with up to four doses of synthetic surfactant in a large randomized multicenter trial treating infants with respiratory distress syndrome weighing $\geq$ 1250 grams. Am J Perinatol 1992; 9:507.
53. Collaborative European Multicentre Study Group. Factors influencing the clinical response to surfactant replacement therapy in babies with severe respiratory distress syndrome. Eur J Pediatr 150:433–439, 1991.
54. Hamvas A, Devine T, Cole FS. Surfactant therapy failure identifies infants at risk for pulmonary mortality. Am J Dis Child 1993; 147:665–668.
55. Hallman M, Merritt TA, Bry K, Berry C. Association between neonatal care practices and efficacy of exogenous human surfactant: Results of a multicenter randomized trial. Pediatrics 1993; 91:552–560.

56. Pramanik A, Holtzman RB, Merritt TA. Surfactant replacement therapy for pulmonary diseases. Pediatr Clin North Am 1993; 40:913–936.
57. Zola EM, Gunkel JH, Chan RK, et al. Comparison of three dosing procedures for administration of bovine surfactant to neonates with respiratory distress syndrome. J Pediatr 1993; 122:453–459.
58. Collaborative European Multicenter Study Group. Surfactant replacement therapy in severe neonatal respiratory distress syndrome: An international randomized clinical trial. Pediatrics 1988; 82:683–691.
59. Saugstad OD, Halliday HL, Robertson B, Speer CP. Replacement therapy with porcine natural surfactant—Current status and future challenges. Biol Neonate 1993; 64:269–278.
60. Segerer H, van Gelder W, Angenent FWM, et al. Pulmonary distribution and efficacy of exogenous surfactant in lung-lavaged rabbits are influenced by the instillation technique. Pediatr Res 1993; 34:490–494.
61. Cowan F, Whitelaw A, Wertheim D, Silverman M. Cerebral blood flow velocity changes after rapid administration of surfactant. Arch Dis Child 1991; 66:1105–1109.
62. Skov L, Hellström-Westas L, Jacobsen T, et al. Acute changes in cerebral oxygenation and cerebral blood volume in preterm infants during surfactant treatment. Neuropediatrics 1992; 23:126–130.
63. McCord FB, Halliday HL, McClure G, Reid M McC. Changes in pulmonary and cerebral blood flow after surfactant treatment for severe respiratory syndrome. In: Lachmann B, ed. Surfactant Replacement Therapy in Neonatal and Adult Respiratory Distress Syndrome. Berlin: Springer-Verlag, 1989:195–200.
64. Jorch G, Rabe H, Garbe H, et al. Acute and protracted effects of intratracheal surfactant application on internal carotid blood flow velocity, blood pressure and carbon dioxide tension in very low birth weight infants. Eur J Pediatr 1989; 148:770–773.
65. van de Bor, Ma EJ, Walther FJ. Cerebral blood flow velocity after surfactant instillation in preterm infants. J Pediatr 1991; 118:285–287.
66. Hellström-Westas L, Bell AH, Skov L, et al. Cerebroelectrical depression following surfactant treatment in preterm neonates. Pediatrics 1992; 89:643–647.
67. Edwards AD, McCormick DC, Roth SC, et al. Cerebral hemodynamic effects of treatment with modified natural surfactant investigated by near infrared spectroscopy. Pediatr Res 1992; 32:532–536.
68. Halliday HL. Follow-up data from babies treated with surfactant. In: Bevilacqua G, Parmigiani S, Robertson S, eds. Surfactant in Clinical Practice. Chur: Harwood Academic Publishers, 1992:149–156.
69. Svenningsen NW, Björklund L, Vilstrup C, Werner O. Lung mechanics (FRC and static pressure-volume diagram) after endotracheal surfactant instillation: preliminary observations. Biol Neonate 1992; 6(Suppl 1):44–47.
70. Cotton RB, Olsson T, Law AB, et al. The physiologic effects of surfactant treatment on gas exchange in newborn premature infants with hyaline membrane disease. Pediatr Res 1993; 34:495–501.
71. Schiffmann H, Harms K, Herting E, et al. Radiologische Veränderungen nach Surfactant-Therapie—Ergebnnisse einer randomisierten europäischen Multicenter-

Studie mit porcinem Surfactant (Curosurf[R]). Monatschr Kinderheilkd 1994; 142: 513–519.

72. Rider ED, Jobe AH, Ikegami M, Sun B. Different ventilation strategies alter surfactant responses in preterm rabbits. J Appl Physiol 1992; 73:2089–2096.
73. Dechant KL, Faulds D. Colfosceril palmitate. A review of the therapeutic efficacy and clinical tolerability of a synthetic surfactant preparation (Exosurf[R] Neonatal™) in neonatal respiratory distress syndrome. Drugs 1991; 42:877–894.
74. Raju TNK, Langenberg P. Pulmonary hemorrhage and exogenous surfactant therapy: A meta-analysis. J Pediatr 1993; 123:603–610.
75. Crowley P. Promoting pulmonary maturity. In: Chalmers IM, Keirse MJNC, eds. Effective Care in Pregnancy and Childbirth. Oxford, England: Oxford University Press, 1989:746–764.
76. Farrell EE, Silver RK, Kimberlin CV, et al. Impact of antenatal dexamethasone administration on respiratory distress syndrome in surfactant treated infants. Am J Obstet Gynecol 1989; 161:628–633.
77. Jobe AH, Mitchell BR, Gunkel JH. Beneficial effects of the combined use of prenatal corticosteroids and postnatal surfactant on preterm infants. Am J Obstet Gynecol 1993; 168:508–513.
78. Horbar JD, Wright EC, Onstad L and the members of the National Institute of Child Health and Human Development Neonatal Research Network. Decreasing mortality associated with the introduction of surfactant therapy; an observational study of neonates weighing 601 to 1300 grams at birth. Pediatrics 1993; 92:191–196.

21

Surfactant Therapy for Neonatal Lung Disorders Other than Respiratory Distress Syndrome

FRANS J. WALTHER
Charles R. Drew University
and University of California, Los Angeles
Los Angeles, California

I. Introduction

Recently, surfactant replacement therapy has been used in uncontrolled studies among infants with neonatal lung disorders other than RDS, such as meconium aspiration syndrome (MAS) and congenital pneumonia (1,2), and among pediatric patients and adults with the adult respiratory distress syndrome (ARDS) (4). Searching through our neonatal intensive care database, we found that out of every four newborn infants with respiratory failure, three were premature infants ventilated for RDS and one was a (near)term infant ventilated for congenital pneumonia, MAS, congenital diaphragmatic hernia, or neonatal ARDS (Table 1). These data indicate that newborn infants with lung disorders other than RDS take up a sizeable share of ventilator support in a neonatal intensive care unit and they indicate the need for further research into possible positive effects of surfactant replacement therapy in this group.

II. Meconium Aspiration Syndrome

Meconium aspiration syndrome (MAS) is generally thought to be a consequence of intrauterine hypoxia and acidosis triggering the passage of meconium into the

Table 1 Incidence of Various Types of Respiratory Distress Treated with at Least 24 Hr of Mechanical Ventilation Among 2135 Consecutively Admitted Newborn Infants

Respiratory problem	Incidence	% of admissions
RDS	659	30.9
Congenital pneumonia[a]	118	5.5
Meconium aspiration syndrome[a]	108	5.1
Congenital diaphragmatic hernia	12	0.6
Unspecified, possibly neonatal ARDS	5	0.2

[a]Twenty-three infants out of these groups required ECMO.

amniotic fluid and fetal gasping. MAS affects about 5% of all infants born through meconium. Although DeLee suctioning of the nasopharynx by the obstetrician with the delivery of the infant's head followed by visualization and direct suctioning of the trachea by the pediatrician is highly effective in preventing MAS (4), intrauterine aspiration of large quantities of meconium remains associated with considerable morbidity and mortality. With the onset of respiration, meconium migrates from the central airways to the peripheral airways, leading to mechanical obstruction, hyperinflation, and atelectasis, and, at a later stage, to chemical pneumonitis and interstitial edema. Partial airway obstruction by meconium, producing a ball-valve effect, may predispose to rupture of alveolar spaces and is the cause of the high risk of pneumothorax and pneumomediastinum in these infants. MAS is often accompanied by persistent pulmonary hypertension of the newborn (PPHN) with large right-to-left shunts across the ductus arteriosus and the foramen ovale. PPHN may be caused by intrauterine hypoxia, which can lead to the extension of smooth muscle into the walls of normally nonmuscular intra-acinar arterioles, thereby reducing their luminal diameter and increasing pulmonary vascular resistance, and by active pulmonary vasoconstriction, the result of the severe perinatal hypoxia and acidosis that triggered the passage of meconium. Thirty percent of infants with MAS require mechanical ventilation and about 5% of these infants die (4). Those who do not respond to conventional therapy may require extracorporeal membrane oxygenation (ECMO). At autopsy, infants with MAS have a high incidence of hyaline membrane formation in their lungs (5).

The pathophysiology of MAS is not only related to mechanical obstruction of the airways and chemical injury to the respiratory epithelium, but also to surfactant inactivation by meconium. Instillation of 10% meconium in saline into excised canine lung significantly decreases lung compliance and functional residual capacity (6). Clark et al. (7) demonstrated that meconium and its major free fatty acids increase mean airway pressure and surface tension and decrease static lung compliance and oxygenation when instilled into canine lungs and are able to inactivate alveolar surfactant. Sun et al. (8) mixed fractions of human meconium with the porcine surfactant, Curosurf (Chiesi Farmaceutici, Parma, Italy), and found the chloroform-soluble phase, which contains free fatty acids, triglycerides, and cholesterol, to have the highest specific inhibitory activity in a Pulsating-Bubble Surfactometer or a Wilhelmy balance. In a newborn piglet model (9), an intratracheal bolus of 20% meconium during mechanical ventilation caused an acute decrease in gas exchange, a decrease in dynamic lung compliance, and an increase in neutrophil count, neutrophil chemotactic activity, albumin, and total protein concentrations of tracheal aspirates.

Moses et al. (10) studied serial dilutions of human meconium added to calf lung surfactant extract (CLSE and Infasurf, Forest Laboratories, St. Louis, MO) using a Pulsating-Bubble Surfactometer and demonstrated that even 6500-fold dilutions of meconium are capable of inhibiting the surface tension–lowering properties of pulmonary surfactant. Most interestingly, high doses of surfactant extract reversed the inhibitory effect of meconium. Paranka et al. (11) lavaged the lungs of piglets with MAS twice with 5 ml/kg bovine surfactant (Survanta, Ross Laboratories, Columbus, OH) and detected a significant short-term improvement in oxygenation versus saline lavage and suctioning only. Subsequent experiments showed no differences between surfactant lavage (10 ml/kg) and surfactant only (4 ml/kg) (12). Nearly mature newborn rabbits with MAS respond to treatment with 200 mg/kg Curosurf with a moderate, but significant improvement, in lung compliance (13). However, not all animal studies have shown positive experiences with pulmonary surfactant and MAS. Wiswell et al. (14) recently examined the use of surfactant in a piglet model of MAS using two different surfactants, Exosurf (Burroughs Wellcome, Research Triangle Part, NC) and Survanta, at usual and twice standard doses and randomizing the piglets to either conventional or high-frequency jet ventilation (HFJV). Neither improvement in oxygenation nor in histological alterations in the surfactant-treated animals compared with controls was found, nor were surface tension measurements of airway secretions lower in the majority of surfactant-treated piglets.

In a small uncontrolled clinical study, Auten et al. (1) treated 14 full-term infants with MAS (n = 7) or pneumonia (n = 7), ventilated with a mean airway pressure (MAP) of 13–15 cmH_2O and 100% oxygen, with up to four doses of 90 mg/kg of CLSE. Mean ± SEM arterial/Alveolar (a/A) Po_2 ratios improved from 0.09 ± 0.01 before to 0.22 ± 0.05 at 15 min and 0.24 ± 0.04 at 1 hr after surfactant therapy. MAPs did not change considerably and oxygenation index (OI) values improved from 26 ± 3 before to 11 ± 2 at 15 min and 10 ± 1 at 1 hr after surfactant therapy. Improved oxygenation was maintained for at least 6 hr. Three of the seven infants with MAS received a second dose of surfactant with a similar effect on oxygenation. All infants survived without bronchopulmonary dysplasia (BPD) and none developed tension pneumothorax after surfactant therapy or required ECMO.

Khammash et al. (2) treated 20 term infants with MAS and MAPs ranging from 10 to 26 cmH_2O, with one to six doses of 100 mg/kg Infasurf. Mean a/A Po_2 ratios improved from 0.07 to 0.11 and OI values from 37 to 23 1–3 hr after surfactant therapy, an effect less striking than in the study by Auten et al. (1). Fifteen infants responded with improved oxygenation and one of them died of respiratory failure. Of the five nonresponders, three were treated with ECMO and one infant died after treatment was withdrawn due to severe hypoxic ischemic encephalopathy.

Davis et al. (15) treated 13 term infants with MAS, who had failed conventional mechanical ventilation and CLSE therapy, with HFJV and additional doses of CLSE. The mean $\pm$ SEM a/A Po_2 ratio increased from 0.09 $\pm$ 0.01 to 0.21 $\pm$ 0.04, and the OI decreased from 24 $\pm$ 2 to 14 $\pm$ 2 after surfactant treatment. This improvement in oxygenation did not affect ventilator settings, arterial pH, and $Paco_2$.

We have enrolled 32 term infants on mechanical ventilation for MAS into a randomized trial in which the study group receives up to four doses of 150 mg/kg Survanta, instilled every 6 hr by continuous infusion over 20 min via a side-hole endotracheal tube adapter. Preliminary data show a cumulative improvement in oxygenation after each of the first three doses of surfactant, without a clear beneficial effect of the 4th dose (Fig. 1), and a dramatic absence of air leaks and requirement for ECMO followed surfactant therapy (R. Findlay, personal communication).

The available clinical studies on surfactant replacement therapy for MAS are encouraging, but before widespread clinical use of surfactant for MAS is applied, further clinical trials are indicated.

III. Congenital Pneumonia

Congenital bacterial pneumonia is an important cause of respiratory failure in newborn infants. Pulmonary surfactant has been shown to possess bacteriostatic and opsonic properties (16,17) with surfactant protein A (SP-A) as a major component responsible for enhanced bacterial killing (18). As surfactant plays an important role in the lung's defense against infection, surfactant deficiency may reduce the infant's resistance against pneumonia. Pneumonia and sepsis can affect pulmonary surfactant function in various ways: Damage of the alveolar-capillary barrier floods the alveolar spaces with plasma proteins and blood components that can inhibit surfactant function (19–22), alveolar type II cell injury will compromise surfactant production and secretion, and phospholipases

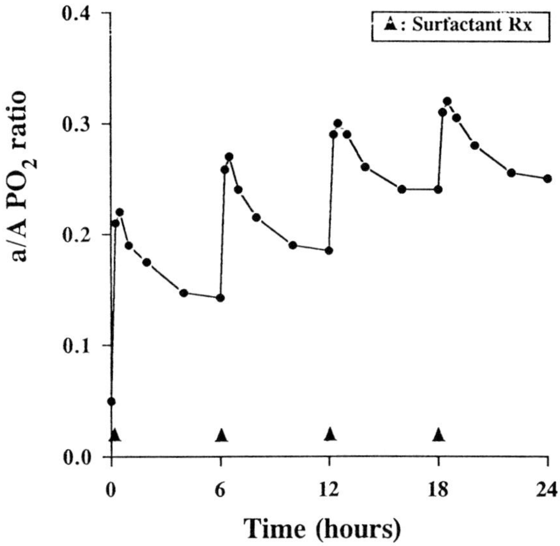

Figure 1 a/A Po_2 ratios in a term infant ventilated for meconium aspiration syndrome and treated with four doses of 150 mg/kg Survanta at 6-hr intervals. Note the cumulative improvement in oxygenation after each of the first three doses of surfactant.

secreted by bacteria are able to inhibit the surface tension–lowering effects of surfactant (23) and mediate injury to the alveolar epithelium (24).

Studies in adults have shown that bacterial pneumonia decreases lung compliance (25), whereas it increases phospholipase activity (25) and reduces dipalmitoyl phosphatidylcholine (DPPC) (26) and SP-A levels (27) in broncho-alveolar lavage. Interestingly, the greatest reduction in SP-A levels is caused by gram-positive organisms, such as *Streptococcus pneumoniae*, *Staphylococcus aureus*, and *Enterococcus* and not by gram-negative organisms, such as *Pseudomonas aeruginosa* and *Haemophilus influenza* (27). A study in nine premature infants with congenital pneumonia, abnormal peripheral white cell counts, and positive cultures from gastric or endotracheal aspirates showed them to have lower endotracheal aspirate phosphatidylcholine (PC) and phosphatidyl-inositol concentrations than matched controls (28). Serial determinations of SP-A/albumin ratios in tracheal aspirates from infants with congenital pneumonia showed low ratios while the infection was evident (29). These data suggest a relation between pneumonia and pulmonary surfactant deficiency.

On theoretical grounds, surfactant replacement therapy may therefore be a worthwhile approach for treatment of respiratory failure caused by pneumonia. In rats with end-stage lethal Sendai virus pneumonia, instillation of 200 mg/kg of a natural bovine surfactant significantly improved their arterial oxygenation within 5 min and this effect lasted for at least 2 hr (30). In mice with end-stage influenza A pneumonia, instillation of an equal amount of surfactant increased thorax-lung compliance and lung volume (31). In rats with severe respiratory failure due to *Pneumocystis carinii* pneumonia, pulmonary function and lung histology improved dramatically after surfactant instillation (32). Although these pneumonia models provide promising effects of surfactant therapy, their implications for newborn infants, whose congenital pneumonia is often of bacterial origin (Group B *Streptococcus*, *Escherichia coli*) is unclear.

Surfactant replacement therapy in newborn infants with congenital pneumonia has been limited to several small, uncontrolled clinical studies. Auten et al. (1) treated seven term infants with pneumonia, who were ventilated with mean ± SEM MAPs of 16.0 ± 1.6 cmH_2O, with up to four doses of 90 mg/kg of CLSE. Oxygenation improved and all infants survived without BPD and none required ECMO. The diagnosis of pneumonia was based on radiographic criteria and all infants had negative blood and tracheal aspirate bacterial cultures, except for one who had urine positive for group B streptococcal antigen. Shinwell et al. (33) treated five infants with pneumonia and severe respiratory failure with multiple doses of Curosurf and also detected a significant improvement in oxygenation. Davis et al. (15) treated two infants with pneumonia, who had failed optimal conventional mechanical ventilation and exogenous surfactant therapy, with HFJV and found that additional doses of CLSE sustained the initial response to HFJV. Anecdotal experience by Khammash et al. (2) in six infants with pneumonia or suspected pneumonia showed only a slight improvement in oxygenation after CLSE treatment.

These studies suggest that surfactant therapy certainly does not harm the pulmonary status in infants with congenital pneumonia, but more extensive, controlled studies are necessary before surfactant therapy can be considered as a treatment modality for this indication.

IV. Congenital Diaphragmatic Hernia and Lung Hypoplasia

Congenital diaphragmatic hernia (CHD) occurs in 1 in 2500–4000 live births. Most infants with this condition are born at term and have a diaphragmatic hernia that passes through the posterolateral foramen of Bochdalek. Long-standing lung compression in utero by bowel and abdominal organs herniated into the chest leads to pulmonary hypoplasia on the ipsilateral side and to a lesser extent on the contralateral side (34). The number of bronchial generations, alveoli per acinus, and arterial vessels are reduced, with an increase in smooth muscle of pulmonary arterioles (34). At birth, when gas fills the bowel, severe respiratory distress occurs. Despite the introduction of new therapeutic approaches, such as high-frequency ventilation, delayed surgery, and ECMO, the mortality for CDH, attributed to the combination of pulmonary hypoplasia and persistent pulmonary hypertension, remains high; about 30–50% in most centers.

Using a fetal lamb CDH model, Glick et al. (35) found that surfactant deficiency may have a significant role in the pathophysiology of CDH. CDH lambs had significantly smaller lungs, decreased total lung capacity and compliance, reduced total lavaged phospholipids, decreased percentage of PC, and higher minimum dynamic surface tension. These findings confirm reports about unusually low lecithin/sphingomyelin ratios and absent phosphatidylglycerol (PG) in amniotic fluid of infants with CDH (36,37) and the presence of low DPPC levels in ipsilateral lung tissue from infants with CDH (34) and indicate that the hypoplastic lung is probably biochemically immature and surfactant deficient.

Management of the infant with CDH remains controversial. Until recently, the standard of care consisted of emergency surgical repair with medical management aimed at treating the combination of lung hypoplasia and pulmonary hypertension. With this approach, most infants do quite well for a few hours and then die of severe reactive pulmonary hypertension complicating their existing lung hypoplasia. When ECMO became available, many programs placed CDH infants on ECMO to treat pre- or postoperative hypoxemia secondary to pulmonary hypertension (38,41).

Bos et al. (40) first reported the use of surfactant replacement therapy in infants with CDH. Four newborn infants with CDH and severe respiratory distress were treated with 150 mg bovine surfactant within 24 hr of birth. Two of them reacted with a transient improvement of oxygenation and survived after surgical correction, whereas the two nonresponders were placed on ECMO, and they died. Glick et al. (41) treated seven newborn infants diagnosed prenatally with CDH with 100 mg/kg of Infasurf prior to the first breath, followed by standard neonatal care and surgical correction. Except for one infant who died because of trisomy 18, all survived and only one had life-threatening pulmonary hypertension. These preliminary findings suggest a potential benefit of prophylactic surfactant therapy and have resulted in an ongoing multicenter study to evaluate the role of surfactant replacement therapy in CDH.

V. Extracorporeal Membrane Oxygenation

ECMO has improved the prognosis for (near)term infants with respiratory failure who do not respond to maximal ventilatory support. Infants over 2000 g with MAS, group B streptococcal sepsis with pneumonia, RDS, PPHN, and CDH have been treated successfully with ECMO. These infants often have diffuse pulmonary atelectasis and poor dynamic lung compliance. Weaning from ECMO support depends on radiographic clearing of their lung fields and improvement in lung compliance, which is quite similar to the clinical course of premature infants with RDS. Studies with tracheal aspirate phospholipids and surfactant proteins in infants receiving ECMO therapy for MAS or pneumonia have shown surfactant insufficiency (42). The cause of the surfactant deficiency is probably multifactorial. Meconium and plasma proteins leaking into the alveoli as a result of damage of the alveolar-capillary barrier by barotrauma, hyperoxia, sepsis, and cardiopulmonary bypass are able to inhibit pulmonary surfactant function. Meconium and inflammation may damage the alveolar type II cells, thereby affecting surfactant production and secretion.

Two recent studies have tested the effects of surfactant therapy on morbidity in infants placed on ECMO. Lotze et al. (43) randomized 56 infants $\geq$34 weeks of gestation, placed on ECMO for severe respiratory failure due to MAS, group B streptococcal sepsis with pneumonia, RDS, or PPHN, to four doses of 100 mg/kg Survanta ($n = 28$) or an equal volume of air ($n = 28$) at ECMO hours 2, 8, 20, and 32. Lung compliance was initially low in both groups but improved faster in the surfactant group, which needed a significantly shorter ECMO treatment period (mean $\pm$ SD: 107 $\pm$ 33 hr versus 139 $\pm$ 54 hr, $p = 0.023$) and had a fewer complications after ECMO (18 versus 46%) than the control group. However, the incidence of intracranial or pulmonary hemorrhage and BPD, time to extubation, duration of oxygen therapy, and duration of hospitalization did not differ between the two groups. Stillerman and Engle (44) instilled up to four doses of either Exosurf or Survanta in 17 infants after placement on ECMO and compared them with 36 infants receiving ECMO but no surfactant therapy. They confirmed the shorter duration of ECMO in the surfactant group (mean $\pm$ SEM: 76 $\pm$ 17 versus 112 $\pm$ 42 hr in the control group, $p = 0.002$) and the absence of other major differences between the two groups during their clinical course. Multicenter clinical trials of Survanta and Exosurf are currently underway to critically evaluate the effectiveness of surfactant in newborn infants referred for ECMO.

VI. Transient Tachypnea of the Newborn

Transient tachypnea of the newborn (TTNB) is characterized by a transient and relatively mild respiratory distress in (near)term infants caused by delayed clearance of fetal lung fluid. TTNB is often seen in infants of diabetic mothers, after delivery by cesarean section, and following heavy maternal sedation. These infants seldom require more than 40% oxygen to maintain adequate oxygenation and they are usually in room air by 24 hr of age. James et al. (28) and Bourbon et al. (45) found reduced PC and PG concentrations in gastric aspirates of infants with TTNB, suggesting that the accumulation of lung fluid in the alveolar spaces and interstitium may be associated with a relative surfactant deficiency.

O'Brodovich and Hannam (46) studied the effect of exogenous surfactant in a TTNB model. In young rabbits ventilated with 100% oxygen, tracheal instillation of 20 ml/kg of warmed saline decreased baseline Pa_{O_2} values to 60 $\pm$ 6.9 (SEM) mmHg. Subsequent administration of 50 mg/kg surfactant increased Pa_{O_2} values to 246 $\pm$ 44 mmHg within 15 min, demonstrating that surfactant replacement therapy improves gas exchange in mature surfactant-replete lungs containing large amounts of saline.

Clinical data on surfactant replacement therapy to (near)term infants with TTNB are anecdotal, probably because of the mildness of the symptomatology and the quick recovery of these infants with conventional therapy.

VII. Neonatal "Adult" Respiratory Distress Syndrome

In pediatric patients and adults, severe hypoxia, shock, sepsis, burns, or drowning can result in a clinical picture resembling RDS (47). This adult respiratory distress syndrome (ARDS) is characterized by damage of the alveolar-capillary membrane, leading to noncardiogenic pulmonary edema and hyaline membrane formation (47,48). Secondary surfactant insufficiency (49) follows intra-alveolar leakage of proteins, albumin, and other surfactant inhibitors (19) and bacterial secretion of phospholipases (23,26) (see Chapter 28). Several reports document successful management of patients with ARDS using large and frequent doses of natural and synthetic surfactant and multicenter randomized clinical studies of Survanta and aerosolized Exosurf in the treatment of ARDS are currently in progress (50). The rationale for use of surfactant replacement therapy in ARDS is founded primarily on the expectation that it improves lung compliance and enhances gas exchange, but in vitro studies have shown that Exosurf inhibits endotoxin-induced cytokine secretion by human alveolar macrophages (51) and that Survanta has similar inhibitory effects on cytokine release from polymorphonuclear neutrophils (52). Modulation of the inflammatory cytokine production in the lung may be a potential additional or alternative mechanism accounting for the apparent clinical benefit of this surfactant preparation in ARDS.

Many of the major predisposing factors for ARDS in children and adults may also occur in newborn infants. Neonatal ARDS was first described in 11 term newborn infants with signs of fetal distress or severe perinatal complications (53). Pfenninger (54) described seven newborn infants with neonatal ARDS. In four infants, the triggering event was group B streptococcal sepsis, two infants presented with severe asphyxia at birth, and the cause was unknown in one infant. All infants had evidence of PPHN and suffered from severe shock, necessitating volume expansion and inotropic support. Despite the use of high-frequency ventilation, four of seven infants died and two survivors had moderate BPD. Surfactant replacement therapy was used by Khammash et al. (2) in a group of 29 term infants with RDS and without evidence for MAS or (suspected) pneumonia. These infants had a mean ± SD a/A Po_2 ratio of 0.1 ± 0.05 and an OI of 27 ± 18 and may fit the diagnosis neonatal ARDS. Twenty-two of the 29 (76%) infants responded with a clinically significant improvement in oxygenation after one to four doses of 100 mg/kg CLSE. Their mean a/A Po_2 ratio improved to 0.3 and their OI to 12 1–3 hr after surfactant replacement therapy.

ARDS is rarely diagnosed in term newborn infants and may be limited to those presenting with respiratory failure after perinatal hypoxia-ischemia injury. The therapeutic effect of surfactant replacement therapy in neonatal ARDS needs to be further delineated.

VIII. Pulmonary Oxygen Toxicity

Prolonged exposure to hyperoxia has been associated with progressive injury to all components of the blood-gas barrier, leading to increased alveolar and pulmonary vascular permeability, pulmonary edema, atelectasis, and eventually death from hypoxia or respiratory failure (53–59). Many of these pathological features are also present in primary (RDS) and secondary (ARDS) deficiency of surfactant. Exposure to hyperoxia can affect both surfactant synthesis and secretion (60), mainly determined by O_2-induced changes in alveolar type II cell biosynthesis and morphology (61,63). Plasma proteins found in increased concentrations in the alveoli of animals exposed to hyperoxia can further compound lung injury by inhibiting the ability of surfactant to absorb and lower surface tension at the alveolar hypophase surface (62).

Rabbits with hyperoxic lung injury develop severe hypoxia and lung edema and have abnormal lung mechanics, decreased alveolar phospholipid, increased alveolar protein, and significantly impaired surface activity in bronchoalveolar lavage (56). In vitro studies have shown that inactivation of lung surfactant by plasma proteins can be abolished by providing sufficient amounts of lung surfactant phospholipid (63). Though the pathophysiology of hyperoxic lung injury is multifactorial and goes beyond surfactant deficiency, Matalon et al. (64) were able to prevent the development of abnormal lung mechanics and alveolar collapse and to reduce the degree of lung edema by intratracheal instillation of 60 mg/kg of CLSE in rabbits exposed to hyperoxia.

Though surfactant replacement therapy may play a probably limited role in the prevention or modification of hyperoxic lung injury, this aspect has received relatively little attention and needs further exploration. A possible combination of surfactant and antioxidant therapy is currently under investigation by several groups (65,66).

IX. Weaning from High-Frequency Ventilation

High-frequency ventilation is increasingly used in infants with respiratory failure who do not respond to conventional mechanical ventilation and would otherwise be candidates for ECMO therapy. Davis et al. (15) described a group of 13 premature infants with RDS and a group of 15 term infants with respiratory failure secondary to group B streptococcal pneumonia (n = 2) and MAS (n = 13), who deteriorated in spite of optimal mechanical ventilation and surfactant therapy with CLSE and were placed on HFJV at a mean age of 2 days. Despite a significant improvement in several respiratory variables after the switch to HFJV, most infants deteriorated subsequently. They were then successfully weaned from HFJV with additional surfactant therapy, with improved oxygenation, but not MAP. Eight-nine percent survived without BPD and none needed ECMO. The effect of surfactant replacement therapy is being evaluated further, both in conjunction with high-frequency jet and oscillatory ventilation in managing patients with RDS and PPHN.

X. Vehicle for Topical Delivery of Other Drugs to the Lung

Although topical drug administration to the lungs by aerosol has many advantages over systemic drug administration, the amount of drug that reaches the subglottic airways is typically less than 10% of the aerosol dose (67). The distribution of aerosolized drugs through the lung is often uneven and dependent on the dimensions of the airways, the particle size of the drug, and distribution of ventilation. Intratracheally instilled surfactant has been shown to distribute rapidly to the alveolar surface and may therefore function as an effective vehicle for delivering drugs to the terminal air spaces, even in a lung that is not surfactant deficient.

Kharasch et al. (68) studied the pulmonary distribution of ^{99m}technetium sulfur colloid mixed with pentamidine in healthy adult hamsters, using either pulmonary surfactant or normal saline as a vehicle. Pentamidine was chosen because of its demonstrated efficacy in the treatment of *Pneumocystis carinii* pneumonia in acquired immunodeficiency syndrome (AIDS). Surfactant increased the fractional area of lung exposed to radioactivity and improved the uniformity of spread of the technetium label in these healthy lungs. The authors raise the crucial question as to how these findings can be applied to drug delivery in pathological states and suggest that the presence of local inflammation would tend to promote protein leaks that in turn increase focal surface tension gradient driving drug convection. As such, drugs in a pulmonary surfactant vehicle might be expected to deposit preferentially in regions where it is most needed.

Our group has focused on surfactant as a tool to deliver antioxidant enzymes to the alveolar epithelium. During the final 10–15% of gestation, both the antioxidant and surfactant systems in the fetal lung show rapid increases in activity (69,70). Prematurity is associated not only with surfactant deficiency, but also with reduced lung antioxidant enzyme activities. Treatment of RDS with oxygen and mechanical ventilation increases the rate of intra- and extracellular production of free oxygen radicals (71), enhancing the susceptibility of premature infants to chronic lung injury (BPD). Pulmonary oxygen toxicity can be reduced by increasing the intracellular antioxidant capacity via the administration of antioxidant enzymes. However, antioxidant enzymes, such as superoxide dismutase (SOD) and catalase, are not able to penetrate across cell membranes because of their large molecular size. SOD and catalase, encapsulated in DPPC:stearylamine:cholesterol liposomes, enter alveolar type II cells, either by fusion with plasma membranes or by endocytosis and render the treated cells more resistant to oxidant challenge (72,73). We found a high uptake by cultured alveolar type II cells of antioxidants encapsulated in liposomes made from surfactant lipids (DPPC: PG:palmitic acid 68:22:9, wt/wt/wt). Antioxidant uptake roughly doubled in the presence of SP-A, which also prevented inhibition of surfactant by encapsulated antioxidants (65). Preliminary data from our laboratory indicate that intratracheally injected antioxidant-surfactant liposomes maintain or boost intracellular antioxidant capacity in 28-day gestational age premature rabbit pups exposed to 24 hr of hyperoxia (74). Liposomes made from pulmonary surfactant can therefore function as a vehicle to target antioxidants toward the alveolar epithelium.

These data indicate that pulmonary surfactant may be a useful vehicle for topical drug administration to the lung. Further studies will be necessary to delineate the clinical applicability of this approach and the presence or absence of interaction between pulmonary surfactant and the drugs to be delivered.

References

1. Auten RL, Notter RH, Kendig JW, et al. Surfactant treatment of full-term newborns with respiratory failure. Pediatrics 1991; 87:101–7.
2. Khammash H, Perlman M, Wojtulewicz J, Dunn M. Surfactant therapy in full-term neonates with severe respiratory failure. Pediatrics 1993; 92:135–139.
3. Lewis JF, Jobe AH. Surfactant and the adult respiratory distress syndrome. Am Rev Respir Dis 1993; 147:218–233.
4. Wiswell TE, Tuggle JM, Turner BS. Meconium aspiration syndrome: Have we made a difference? Pediatrics 1990; 85:715.
5. Seo IS, Gillim SE, Mirkin LD. Hyaline membranes in postmature infants. Pediatr Pathol 1990; 10:539–548.
6. Chen CT, Toung TJK, Rogers MC. Effect of intra-alveolar meconium on pulmonary surface tension properties. Crit Care Med 1985; 13:233–236.
7. Clark DA, Nieman GF, Thompson JE, et al. Surfactant displacement by meconium

free fatty acids: An alternative explanation for atelectasis in meconium aspiration syndrome. J Pediatr 1987; 110:765–70.
8. Sun B, Curstedt T, Robertson B. Surfactant inhibition in experimental meconium aspiration. Acta Paediatr 1993; 82:182–9.
9. Davey AM, Becker JD, Davis JM. Meconium aspiration syndrome: Physiological and inflammatory changes in a newborn piglet model. Pediatr Pulmonol 1993; 16:101–108.
10. Moses D, Holm BA, Spitale P, et al. Inhibition of pulmonary surfactant function by meconium. Am J Obstet Gynecol 1991; 164:477–81.
11. Paranka MS, Walsh WF, Stancombe BB. Surfactant lavage in a piglet model of meconium aspiration syndrome. Pediatr Res 1992; 31:625–8.
12. Walsh W, Paranka M. Treatment of meconium aspiration in piglets with surfactant, and surfactant lavage. Am J Perinatol 1992; 9:506–507.
13. Sun B, Curstedt T, Song G-W, Robertson B. Surfactant improves lung function and morphology in newborn rabbits with meconium aspiration. Biol Neonate 1993; 63:96–104.
14. Wiswell TE, Davis JM, Merritt TA. Surfactant therapy and high frequency jet ventilation in the management of a piglet model of the meconium aspiration syndrome. Pediatr Res 1993; 33:350A.
15. Davis JM, Richter SE, Kendig JW, Notter RH. High-frequency jet ventilation and surfactant treatment of newborns with severe respiratory failure. Pediatr Pulmonol 1992; 13:108–112.
16. LaForce FM. Effect of alveolar lining material on phagocytic and bactericidal activity of lung macrophages against Staphylococcus aureus. J Lab Clin Med 1976; 88:691–699.
17. Coonrod JD, Yoneda K. Detection and partial characterization of antimicrobial factor(s) in alveolar lining material of rats. J Clin Invest 1983; 71:129–141.
18. van Iwaarden F, Welmers B, Verhoef J, et al. Pulmonary surfactant protein A enhances the host-defence mechanisms of rat alveolar macrophages. Am J Respir Cell Mol Biol 1990; 2:91–98.
19. Holm BA, Enhorning G, Notter RH. A biophysical mechanism by which plasma proteins inhibit lung surfactant activity. Chem Phys Lipids 1988; 49:49–55.
20. Amirkhanian JD, Bruni R, Waring AJ, Taeusch HW. Inhibition of mixtures of surfactant lipids and synthetic sequences of surfactant proteins SP-B and SP-C. Biochim Biophys Acta 1991; 1096:355–360.
21. Amirkhanian JD, Taeusch HW. Reversible and irreversible inactivation of preformed pulmonary surfactant surface films by changes in subphase constituents. Biochim Biophys Acta 1993; 1165:321–326.
22. Amirkhanian JD, Bruni R, Waring AJ, et al. Full length synthetic surfactant proteins, SP-B and SP-C, reduce surfactant inactivation by serum. Biochim Biophys Acta 1993; 1168:315–320.
23. Holm BA, Keicher L, Liu M, et al. Inhibition of pulmonary surfactant function by phospholipases. J Appl Physiol 1991; 71:317–321.
24. Wiener-Kronish JP, Sakuma T, Kudoh I, et al. Alveolar epithelial injury and pleural

empyema in acute P. aeruginosa pneumonia in anesthetized rabbits. J Appl Physiol 1993; 75:1661–1669.
25. Sheehan PM, Stokes DC, Yeh Y, Hughes WT. Surfactant phospholipids and lavage phospholipase A2 in experimental pneumocystic carinii pneumonia. Am Rev Respir Dis 1986; 134:526–531.
26. Baughman RP, Stein E, MacGee J, Sahebjami H. Changes in fatty acids in phospholipids of the bronchoalveolar fluid in bacterial pneumonia and in adult respiratory distress syndrome. Clin Chem 1984; 30:521–523.
27. Baughman RP, Sternberg RI, Hull W, et al. Decreased surfactant protein A in patients with bacterial pneumonia. Am Rev Respir Dis 1993; 147:653–7.
28. James DK, Chiswick ML, Harkes A, et al. Non-specificity of surfactant deficiency in neonatal respiratory disorders. Br Med J 1984; 288:1635–1638.
29. Nagai H, Ogawa Y, Eguchi H, et al. Pulmonary surfactant apoprotein-A in neonates with different respiratory disorders. Acta Paediatr Jpn 1992; 34:636–641.
30. Van Daal G-J, So KL, Gommers D, et al. Intratracheal surfactant administration restores gas exchange in experimental adult respiratory distress syndrome associated with viral pneumonia. Anesth Analg 1991; 72:589–595.
31. Van Daal G-J, Bos JAH, Eijking EP, et al. Surfactant replacement therapy improves pulmonary mechanics in end-stage influenza A pneumonia in mice. Am Rev Respir Dis 1992; 145:859–63.
32. Eijking EP, van Daal G-J, Tenbrink R, et al. Effect of surfactant replacement on Pneumocystis carinii pneumonia in rats. Intens Care Med 1991; 17:475–478.
33. Shinwell ES, Zmora E, Karplus M. Surfactant therapy in respiratory failure other than respiratory distress syndrome. Pediatr Res 1992; 31:323A.
34. Nakamura Y, Yamamoto I, Fukuda S, Hashimoto T. Pulmonary acinar development in diaphragmatic hernia. Arch Pathol Lab Med 1991; 115:372–376.
35. Glick PL, Stannard VA, Leach CL, et al. Pathophysiology of congenital diaphragmatic hernia II: the fetal lamb CDH model is surfactant deficient. J Pediatr Surg 1992; 27:382–8.
36. Berk C, Grundy M. 'High-risk' lecithin/sphingomyelin ratios associated with neonatal diaphragmatic hernia. Case reports. Br J Obstet Gynaecol 1982; 89:250–251.
37. Hisanaga S, Shimokawa H, Kashiwabara Y, et al. Unexpectedly low lecithin/sphingomyelin ratio associated with fetal diaphragmatic hernia. Am J Obstet Gynecol 1984; 149:905–906.
38. Nakayama DK, Motoyama EK, Tagge EM. Effect of preoperative stabilization on respiratory system compliance and outcome in newborn infants with congenital diaphragmatic hernia. J Pediatr 1991; 118:793–799.
39. Wilson JM, Lund DP, Lillehei CW, et al. Delayed repair and preoperative ECMO does not improve survival in high-risk congenital diaphragmatic hernia. J Pediatr Surg 1992; 27:368–375.
40. Bos AP, Tibboel D, Hazebroek FWJ, et al. Surfactant replacement therapy in high-risk congenital diaphragmatic hernia. Lancet 1991; 338:1279.
41. Glick PL, Leach CL, Besner GE, et al. Pathophysiology of congenital diaphragmatic hernia III: Exogenous surfactant therapy for the high-risk neonate with CDH. J Pediatr Surg 1992; 27:866–9.
42. Bui KC, Walther FJ, David-Cu R, et al. Phospholipid and surfactant protein A

concentrations in tracheal aspirates from infants requiring extracorporeal membrane oxygenation. J Pediatr 1992; 121:271–4.
43. Lotze A, Knight GR, Martin GR, et al. Improved pulmonary outcome after exogenous surfactant therapy for respiratory failure in term infants requiring extracorporeal membrane oxygenation. J Pediatr 1993; 122:261–8.
44. Stillerman LR, Engle WA. Exogenous surfactant decreases duration of extracorporeal membrane oxygenation with severe respiratory failure. Annual Meeting of the American Academy of Pediatrics, Section on Perinatal Pediatrics, Washington DC, October 30, 1993 (abstract #22).
45. Bourbon JR, Francoual J, Magny JF, et al. Changes in phospholipid composition of tracheal aspirates from newborns with hyaline membrane disease or transient tachypnea. Clin Chim Acta 1990; 189:87–94.
46. O'Brodovich H, Hannam V. Exogenous surfactant rapidly increases PaO2 in mature rabbits with lungs that contain large amounts of saline. Am Rev Respir Dis 1993; 147:1087–1090.
47. Jobe AH. Pulmonary surfactant therapy. N Engl J Med 1993; 328:861–868.
48. Royall JA, Levin DL. Adult respiratory distress syndrome in pediatric patients. I. Clinical aspects, pathophysiology, pathology, and mechanisms of lung injury. J Pediatr 1988; 112:169–180.
49. Gregory TJ, Longmore WJ, Moxley MA, et al. Surfactant chemical composition and biophysical activity in acute respiratory distress syndrome. J Clin Invest 1991; 88:1976–1981.
50. Wiedemann H, Baughman R, deBoisblanc B, et al. A multicenter trial in human sepsis-induced ARDS of an aerosolized synthetic surfactant (Exosurf). Am Rev Respir Dis 1992; 145:A184.
51. Thomassen MJ, Meeker DP, Antal JM, et al. Synthetic surfactant (Exosurf) inhibits endotoxin-stimulated cytokine secretion by human alveolar macrophages. Am J Respir Cell Mol Biol 1992; 7:257–260.
52. Suzuki H, Otake K, Yakuwa N, et al. Effects of artificial surfactant on human peripheral blood polymorphonuclear neutrophil functions. Am Rev Respir Dis 1992; 145:A876.
53. Faix RG, Viscardi RM, DiPietro MA, Nicks JJ. Adult respiratory distress syndrome in full-term newborns. Pediatrics 1989; 83:971–976.
54. Pfenninger J. Adult respiratory distress syndrome in newborn infants. Crit Care Med 1993; 21:S362–363.
55. Clark JM, Lambertsen CJ. Pulmonary oxygen toxicity: A review. Pharmacol Rev 1971; 23:37–133.
56. Holm BA, Notter RH, Siegle J, Matalon S. Pulmonary physiological and surfactant changes during injury and recovery from hyperoxia. J Appl Physiol 1985; 59:1402–1409.
57. Matalon S, Cesar MC. Effects of oxygen breathing on the capillary filtration coefficient in rabbit lungs. Microvasc Res 1985; 29:70–80.
58. Matalon S, Egan EA. Effects of 100% O_2 breathing on permeability of alveolar epithelium to solute. J Appl Physiol 1981; 50:859–863.
59. Matalon S, Egan EA. Interstitial fluid volumes and albumin spaces in pulmonary oxygen toxicity. J Appl Physiol 1984; 57:1767–1772.

60. Ward JA, Roberts RJ. Effect of hyperoxia on phosphatidylcholine synthesis, secretion, uptake and stability in the newborn rabbit lung. Biochim Biophys Acta 1984; 796:42–50.
61. Holm BA, Notter RH, Leary JF, Matalon S. Alveolar epithelial changes in rabbits after a 21-day exposure to 60% O_2. J Appl Physiol 1987; 62:2230–2236.
62. Holm BA, Matalon S, Finkelstein JN, Notter RH. Type II pneumocyte changes during hyperoxic lung injury and recovery. J Appl Physiol 1988; 65:2672–2678.
63. Holm BA, Notter RH, Finkelstein JN. Surface property changes from interactions of albumin with natural lung surfactant and extracted lung lipids. Chem Phys Lipids 1985; 38:287–298.
64. Matalon S, Holm BA, Notter RH. Mitigation of pulmonary hyperoxic injury by the administration of exogenous surfactant. J Appl Physiol 1987; 62:756–761.
65. Walther FJ, David-Cu R, Supnet MC, et al. Uptake of antioxidants in surfactant liposomes by cultured alveolar type II cells is enhanced by SP-A. Am J Physiol 1993; 265:L330–L339.
66. Barnard ML, Baker RR, Matalon S. Mitigation of oxidant injury to lung microvasculature by intratracheal instillation of antioxidant enzymes. Am J Physiol 1993; 265:L340–L345.
67. O'Doherty MJ, Thomas SHL, Page CJ, et al. Delivery of a nebulized aerosol to a lung model during mechanical ventilation. Effect of ventilator setting and nebulizer type, position, and volume of fill. Am Rev Respir Dis 1992; 146:383–388.
68. Kharasch VS, Sweeney TD, Fredberg J, et al. Pulmonary surfactant as a vehicle for intratracheal delivery of technetium sulfur colloid and pentamidine in hamster lungs. Am Rev Respir Dis 1991; 144:909–13.
69. Frank L, Sosenko IRS. Prenatal development of lung antioxidant enzymes in four species. J Pediatr 1987; 110:106–110.
70. Walther FJ, Wade AB, Warburton D, Forman HJ. Ontogeny of antioxidant enzymes in the fetal lamb lung. Exp Lung Res 1991; 17:39–45.
71. Freeman BA, Crapo JD. Biology of disease. Free radicals and tissue injury. Lab Invest 1982; 47:412–426.
72. Buckley BJ, Tanswell AK, Freeman BA. Liposome-mediated augmentation of catalase in alveolar type II cells protects against H_2O_2 injury. J Appl Physiol 1987; 63:359–367.
73. Tanswell AK, Olson DM, Freeman BA. Liposome-mediated augmentation of antioxidant defenses in fetal rat pneumocytes. Am J Physiol 1990; 258:L165–L172.
74. Walther FJ, David-Cu R, Lopez SL. Antioxidant-surfactant liposomes mitigate hyperoxic lung injury in preterm rabbits. FASEB J 1994; 8:A666.

22

Effects of Surfactant Replacement on Lung Mechanics

NILS W. SVENNINGSEN
University Hospital
and Lund University
Lund, Sweden

I. Introduction

Infantile respiratory distress syndrome (RDS) with surfactant deficiency is characterized by changes in pulmonary mechanics with lowered pulmonary compliance, lowered tidal volume, and increased transpulmonary pressure. The function of surfactant is to equalize retractive forces independently of alveolar size. Although surfactant deficiency is a major pathophysiological factor of IRDS (1), both pulmonary atelectasis and increased fluid leakage into the alveoli will also contribute to a decreased lung function as regards elasticity and volume in both animal models and in infants with RDS (2,3).

II. Lung Mechanics Findings in Animal Models

Lung function measurements after endotracheal surfactant instillation at birth in controlled studies in preterm lambs and baboons showed improvement in gas exchange and dynamic compliance occurring immediately after the natural surfactant instillation (4,5). The improved oxygenation was correlated directly to lowering of the alveolar surface tension and increased aeration seen in histological lung preparations. The clinical deterioration gradually occurring in some animals several hours after surfactant instillation could be related to a progressive dilatation of distal airways (6).

In one study comparing natural and synthetic phospholipid endotracheal instillation in preterm lambs, an immediately improved lung function could only be shown with calf lung extract but not with synthetic preparations (7). Oxygenation also improved faster and the response was greater in preterm lambs treated with natural rather than synthetic surfactant in several other studies as well (8,9). Still others have found no difference in the effects with natural versus synthetic protein-free surfactant when pulmonary function was studied later; that is, several hours after surfactant instillation in preterm lambs (10). Pressure-volume curves for preterm rabbits treated with natural sheep surfactant showed lower opening pressure, higher maximal lung volume, and better deflation stability when compared with the effect of bovine (Survanta) or synthetic (Exosurf) surfactant preparations, although the lung physiological effects were still better with these than in the control rabbits (11).

Studies of the modes of administration have shown similar effects on gas exchange and dynamic compliance whether the surfactant was administered as an endotracheal bolus instillation or as a nebulized preparation in preterm lambs (12).

Finally, after natural surfactant replacement in preterm lambs, Clyman et al. (13) found a decreased pulmonary vascular resistance and Vidiyasagar et al. (5) an increased pulmonary blood flow in immature baboons with RDS. These observations from animal studies indicate that not only changes in lung mechanics but also effects on neonatal pulmonary hemodynamics may contribute to the rise in oxygenation after surfactant instillation.

III. Methods Applied in Clinical Research and Practice

The physiological response to endotracheal (ET) surfactant instillation can be evaluated by measurements of degree of aeration and oxygenation before and after instillation as well as evaluations of lung volume, gas exchange, and pulmonary mechanical or kinetic properties. For a review of different techniques for assessing pulmonary function and lung mechanics in newborns, the reader is referred to the overview of McCann et al. (14), Sly et al. (15), and England (16). The complexity of interrelations between pulmonary surfactant action and the viscoelasticity of the lung as related to anatomical dimensions of airways acinar units and fluid-filled alveoli as well as the distribution and types of fibers in lung substructures has been reviewed recently (17) (Table 1).

In comparison with the findings in newborn animal studies, lung function measurements in preterm human infants with RDS have been more difficult to

Table 1 Factors Influencing Surfactant Effects on Pulmonary Function Measurements

Factor
Maturity
age of gestation
birth weight
lung morphology:
size and distribution of inflatable acinar units, alveolar ducts and alveoli as functions of inflation volume
interdependence of lung units
distribution and types of fibers in lung substructures
pulmonary blood flow and shunting
fluid-filling; i.e., lung water content and distribution
Biophysical activity of surfactant
kinetics: turnover, inhibition and alveolar concentration
physicochemical characteristics:
adsorption, distribution, spreading rate, viscosity and bulk effects
apoprotein content—SP-A; SP-B; SP-C
Timing
postnatal age
severity and progression RDS
leakage of proteinaceous fluid into the airways
Mechanical ventilation or spontaneous breathing
rate of ventilation
level of positive inspiratory pressure (PIP)
positive end-expiratory pressure (PEEP)
air and liquid trapping
extra-alveolar air complications

Source: From Ref. 17; with permission.

evaluate for several reasons. First, many practical problems are involved in the clinical management of newborn babies who are often severely ill and therefore difficult to investigate as compared with animal studies. Thus, it is important to avoid any kind of complications related to the method applied per se. Technical methods must be designed to be applicable to the small size of these extremely vulnerable and small infants with birthweights of less than 1500 g and often well below 1000 g. Accurate recordings of airway pressure and flow in general will require muscle relaxation of the baby. For intubated babies, air leakage around the endotracheal tube must be avoided, being especially important in lung function techniques with occlusion and inflation methods (18–20).

The following methods have been applied in clinical studies of neonates before and after surfactant ET administration:

1. Pulmonary x-ray evaluating aeration with degree of clearing of the lung fields within hours after surfactant ET instillation
2. Oxygenation as a/A ratio of the partial pressure of arterial oxygen (PaO_2) to the partial pressure of alveolar oxygen (PAO_2) in millimeters of mercury (mmHg), or kilopascals (kPa), or arterial oxygen saturation with pulse oximetry.
3. Airway pressure (centimeters of water, cmH_2O) and volume (ml/kg body weight) measurements; i.e., P/V curves relating the effect of surfactant treatment to
   a. Opening pressure
   b. Maximal lung volume
   c. Deflation stability
4. Functional residual capacity (FRC) (ml/kg body weight); i.e., the volume of gas remaining in the lungs at the end of the respiratory cycle
5. Compliance (ml/cmH_2O); i.e.,
   (Cdyn) = Dynamic lung compliance measured in spontaneously breathing infants as tidal volume/esophageal pressure, and in ventilator treated infants as tidal volume/ventilator airway pressure swings
   (Crs) = Total respiratory system static compliance measured with airway single breath occlusion technique or by passive flow-volume technique or from volume-pressure measurement during passive, multiple interrupted expiration
6. Total effective pulmonary blood flow measurements with either Doppler flow technique or the fluorocarbon rebreathing method

IV. Clinical Studies of Lung Mechanics During Surfactant Replacement

After endotracheal surfactant replacement in infants with RDS, fragment and often dramatic improvements in oxygenation and gas exchange, lowering of the duration of ventilator therpy, and improved survival rates have been reported in several studies during the 1980s (3,21,22). According to recent studies by Morley et al. (23). Phibbs et al. (24), and Pfenninger et al. (25), differences in oxygenation did not appear until 1–2 hr or more after administration of artificial surfactants (ALEC and Exosurf). In contrast, quite rapid and dramatic improvements in oxygenation and gas exchange, most often within minutes, have been reported in several studies with modified natural surfactants (26–30).

On the other hand, in a 1992 literature review of lung mechanical studies in infants with RDS estimating pulmonary compliance measurements, it was evident that no immediate change occurred until several hours after treatment—

usually after 24 hr or more—and in some studies only after 7 days (31). One study measured lung mechanics in infants with RDS versus the occurrence of persistent ductus arteriosus (PDA) and found higher dynamic compliance in those with spontaneous closure than in those who needed treatment for PDA but still no difference between surfactant treated and controls (32).

Recent studies with both natural and artificial surfactants have confirmed these observations that a rise in dynamic pulmonary compliance is usually delayed for several hours and occur later than expected from the early clinical improvement, with a rapid increase of oxygenation and gas exchange seen in many cases (33,34).

V. Functional Residual Capacity and Compliance Measurements in Infants with RDS

The lung volume at the end of expiration (FRC) is communicating with the airways and tidal breath during respiration. The following gas dilution techniques for FRC measurements have been applied in infants with RDS treated with surfactant:

Nitrogen washout technique (FRC–N_2 washout) (30,35)
Helium dilution technique (FRC–He dilution) (33)
Sulfur hexafluoride washout technique (FRC-SF6 washout) (36–38)

These studies were in 36 infants with RDS treated with endotracheal surfactant instillation—4 with human amniotic fluid extract (35); 10 with synthetic surfactant (Exosurf) and 7 with bovine surfactant (Survanta) (30); 7 with calf lung extract (Infasurf) (33); and 8 with porcine lung extract (Curosurf) (37,38). These investigations all showed an immediate and clear improvement of oxygenation (although sooner and to a greater extent with natural versus synthetic preparations) that was to a certain extent related to an increase in FRC. However, there was no change or a decrease in dynamic compliance in the first hours after surfactant application.

In our studies with porcine surfactant (Curosurf), we also measured pressure-volume (P/V) curves with a computerized interrupter technique during passive expiration. These measurements showed an increase in the slope of the curve soon after surfactant administration (37,38). Kelly et al. (39), measuring both dynamic and static compliance, found no effect on Cdyn directly after a single dose of bovine surfactant. However, they found a significantly increased static Crs, measured with the passive expiratory flow–volume technique (19). Similar observations have been made with an immediate increase in static compliance after surfactant instillation when spontaneous breaths were analyzed (28) and when static Crs was measured—with the single-breath occlusion technique after synthetic surfactant (25) or porcine surfactant instillation (40) or from recording volume and pressure during multiple interrupted passive expiration, as shown in Fig. 1 (37,38).

The lack of improvement or a decrease of Cdyn immediately 1–12 hr after surfactant instillation has been corroborated in other studies (28,30,33,35,41,42). On the other hand, studies have found an improvement in Cdyn at 12–72 hr after surfactant replacement in infants with RDS who improve. This late increase in Cdyn has been observed after bovine surfactant (42), porcine surfactant (38), or synthetic surfactant administration (34). In the study by Kelly et al. (39) using a bovine surfactant replacement, static Crs (measured by the passive flow-volume technique) rose significantly following surfactant instillation, but Cdyn did not differ significantly before and after surfactant therapy (see above). When ventilator peak pressures were reduced rapidly within 2 hr following surfactant treatment (which was administered at a median age of 7 hr), both Crs and Cdyn rose significantly. However, this increase was solely due to a decreased pressure and not recruitment of new lung volume. On the other hand, too rapid reduction of ventilator pressure may cause derecruitment and deterioration with increased shunting and decreased oxygenation. These observations indicate the complexity in the clinical management of surfactant therapy, which may have been overlooked in some studies presented in the literature!

According to Kelly et al. (39), their findings of an immediate change in static compliance measured with the passive flow-volume technique indicate that

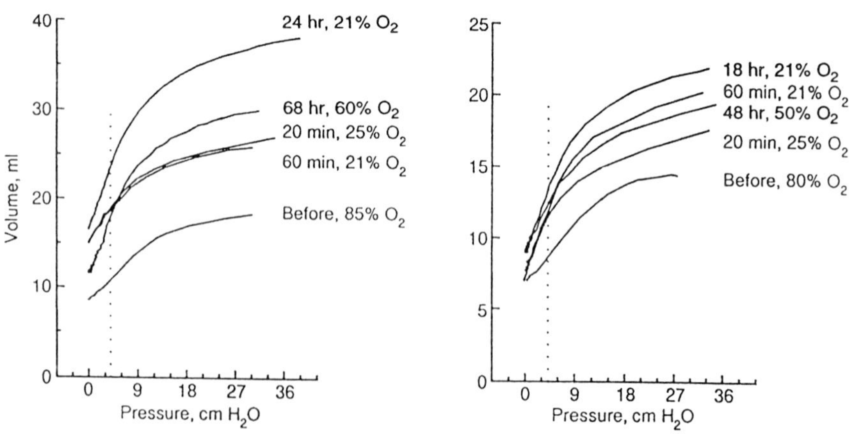

Figure 1 P/V—curves in preterm infants with RDS (left panel, boy, birth weight 1250 g, gestational age 31 weeks; right panel, girl, birth weight 930 g, gestational age 28 weeks) illustrating changes in lung distensibility and decrease in oxygen requirements after a single bolus dose by endotracheal instillation of Curosurf (200 mg/kg). The vertical stippled line indicates the positive end-expiratory pressure (PEEP) kept constant at 4 cmH_2O. The increasing volumes along this line illustrates the rise in FRC after surfactant instillation. (From ref. 37; with permission.)

a substantial volume recruitment occurred in infants with RDS treated on average as early as 7 hr after birth. The mean volume recruited above FRC was 29% in their study, whereas other studies using a direct measure of FRC found increases of 20–153% after surfactant instillation (30,33,35)

It is still unclear whether surfactant administration recruits new gas exchange units or has a stabilizing effect on already open air spaces.

Although only a few infants have been studied with FRC measurements, it is evident that when positive and expiratory pressure (PEEP) is lowered too fast after surfactant instillation, FRC declines with a gradually returning need for increased oxygen (38,39). Nonhomogeneous distribution to open or fluid-filled alveoli in the lungs may occur. One study observed a decrease in compliance after synthetic surfactant before any significant change in FRC, which might be a consequence of the bulk presence of the exogenous liquid surfactant preparation (Exosurf, dose 5 ml per kilogram of body weight) (30). In this particular study, the immediate effects 0–6 hr after treatment with synthetic or natural surfactant were improved oxygenation, accompanied by an increase in FRC, a decrease in compliance, and little or no change in alveolar ventilation. Cotton et al. (30) believed their data were consistent with stabilization of gas exchange units already being ventilated as well as recruitment of new units. The varying duration of the improvement or the lack of improvement in some infants with RDS after surfactant replacement—as well as being dose dependent—may be related to such effects as differences in physicochemical properties, like adsorption and spreading rate, between different surfactant preparations as well as non-homogeneous distribution of both surfactant, open airways, and pulmonary blood flow (43). Besides this, the potential hazard of inactivation of surfactant by proteinacious lung fluid leakage must also be taken into consideration (44).

Contradictory results have been obtained with measurements of effective pulmonary blood flow. Thus, one Doppler flow measurement study showed no increase of total pulmonary blood flow (45), whereas another study showed an acute reduction within 15 min of pulmonary vascular resistance and pulmonary artery pressure (46). This effect was transient and subsided within 12 hr after instillation of surfactant. A similar increase in total pulmonary blood flow of 18% has recently been reported when using a fluorocarbon rebreathing method for evaluation of effective pulmonary blood flow (47). Whether the sometimes dramatic increase in oxygenation after surfactant instillation is the result of a combination of increased aeration with a simultaneous increase in effective pulmonary blood flow is still an open question.

VI. Discussion

A major puzzle in the evaluation of surfactant effects by lung mechanical studies has been the discrepancy between results from animal studies and from human studies.

A major finding in RDS is deficient surfactant function. There is a direct relation between biochemical abnormalities and diminished lung function, at least in the animal models (48,49). It is also evident that if surfactant instillation improves lung function by increased alveolar expansion, increased FRC with decreased shunting would be beneficial (3).

The advantages of surfactant instillation would comprise several factors like

1. Enhancement of oxygenation at lower FiO_2 levels, thereby avoiding toxic levels of oxygen
2. Need of lower end-expiratory pressure with less compromise of circulatory functions
3. Lower ventilator peak inspiratory airway pressures with less barotrauma and a reduced incidence of extra-alveolar air leakage and eventually less risk of severe bronchopulmonary dysplasia

The difficulty in drawing direct comparisons regarding lung mechanical measurements between animal models and the clinical RDS of preterm human infants is related to several confounding factors and circumstances:

1. Some techniques like whole-lung lavage of, for example, rabbits are widely used for testing respirator settings and effects of different surfactants (50) and also present histological changes similar to those seen in RDS (51,52) but applicable only in animal models.
2. In the clinical situation with rescue treatment of infants with progressive RDS, the vascular to alveolar proteinaceous fluid leakage into the alveoli probably plays a major role, as has been shown also in animal studies (2). This may interfere with and delay the effect of surfactant, as has been observed for FRC changes in certain animal studies and postulated for preterm infants with RDS as well (38,53).
3. The degree of parenchymal changes with hyaline membrane formation besides surfactant deficiency as such will also influence the results of the lung mechanical measurements before and after surfactant replacement (54). Thus, Jobe et al. (43) showed that the distribution of surfactant is homogeneous if delivered with the first breaths but very nonhomogeneous when given later after the onset of mechanical ventilation.
4. It is conceivable that the distribution of surfactant is closely related to its effect on lung function. Lung mechanical studies evaluating influence of the instillation technique during surfactant administration have presently been performed only in animal studies showing, for example, in one study that a single bolus of porcine surfactant was preferable to a slow infusion over 45 min via a side channel in the tracheal tube (55). In contrast, another study comparing instilled versus

nebulized surfactant found significant physiological responses to aerosolized surfactant even with low quantities of deposited exogenous surfactant (56).

5. The effects on lung function from combined use of corticosteroids antenatally and postnatal ET surfactant instillation or both administered postnatally have been studied only in animals with lung function measurements (57), although beneficial effects on clinical outcome in preterm infants have been reported (58).

Future lung mechanics functional investigations will be needed to clarify these important but still unsolved questions in order to reach an efficient surfactant therapy with optimal timing and dosage for surfactant application in combination with other therapeutic interventions in the clinical care of newborn infants with various respiratory disorders.

VII. Conclusions

The still fairly limited number of clinical lung mechanic measurements in infants with RDS after treatment with exogenous ET surfactant instillation—both natural and synthetic preparations—indicate the following:

There is an immediate increase of static lung compliance measured with various occlusion techniques but a delay in improvement of dynamic lung compliance seen not until 24–72 hr or more in infants eventually responding with clinical improvement to surfactant.

Direct FRC measurements in some studies have indicated a more rapid change in parallel with improved oxygenation after surfactant instillation, and in general both oxygenation and FRC will improve sooner and to a larger extent with natural as compared with synthetic surfactant.

Heterogeneity in the distribution of open airways versus fluid-filled alveoli may imply a risk of uneven distribution of instilled surfactant with overdistension in some cases—as well as explaining the less impressive or in some cases even lack of effect from the surfactant treatment.

Differences in composition, dispersion, and distribution at instillation of different types of natural versus synthetic preparations probably play an important role.

Since infants treated with surfactant are usually also on ventilator treatment for some time after surfactant instillation, it is important to monitor ventilator settings in relation to clinical and lung mechanical changes, which may be interrelated factors as well.

In the mid 1990s, the era of clinical lung mechanical and functional investigations in newborn infants treated with surfactant is only at its beginning and still awaiting answers to some of the unsolved questions regarding the physiological effects of surfactant on the lung.

Acknowledgment

This work was supported by the Swedish Medical Research Council (grant no. 4732) and Lund University Medical Faculty Grants.

References

1. Avery ME, Mead J. Surface properties in relation to atelectasis and hyaline membrane disease. Am J Dis Child 1959; 97:517–523.
2. Robertson B, Berry D, Curstedt T, et al. Leakage of protein in the immature rabbit lung: Effect of surfactant replacement. Respir Physiol 1985; 61:265–276.
3. Jobe A, Ikegami M. Surfactant for the treatment of respiratory distress syndrome. Am Rev Respir Dis 1990; 142:1137–1142.
4. Sandberg K, Edberg KE, Benton W, et al. Surfactant improves gas mixing and alveolar ventilation in preterm lambs. Pediatr Res 1991; 30:181–189.
5. Vidiyasagar D, Maxta H, Raju TNK, et al. Bovine surfactant (surfactant TA) therapy in immature baboons with hyaline membrane disease. Pediatrics 1985; 75:1132–1136.
6. Jacobs H, Jobe A, Ikegama M, et al. Premature lambs rescued from respiratory failure with natural surfactant. Clinical and biophysical correlates. Pediatr Res 1982; 16:424–439.
7. Egan EA, Notter RH, Kwong MS, et al. Natural and artificial lung surfactant replacement therapy in premature lambs. J Appl Physiol 1983; 55:875–883.
8. Ikegami M, Jobe A, Jacobs H, Jones SJ. Sequential treatment of premature lambs with an artificial surfactant and natural surfactant, J Clin Invest 1981; 68:491–496.
9. Cummings JJ, Holm BA, Hudak BB, et al. A controlled clinical comparison of four different surfactant preparations in surfactant deficient preterm lambs. Am Rev Respir Dis 1992; 145:999–1004.
10. Durand DJ, Clyman RJ, Heymann MA, et al. Effects of protein-free synthetic surfacant on survival and pulmonary function in preterm lambs. J Pediatr 1985; 107:775–780.
11. Rider ED, Jobe A, Ikegami M, Sun B. Different ventilation strategies after surfactant responses in preterm rabbits. J Appl Physiol 1992; 73:2089–2096.
12. Lewis JF, Ikegami M, Jobe A, et al. Aerolized surfactant treatment of preterm lambs. J Appl Physiol 1991; 70:869–876.
13. Clyman RL, Jobe AS, Heymann M, et al. Increased shunt through the patent ductus arteriosus after surfactant replacement. J Pediatr 1982; 100:101–107.
14. McCann EM, Golmann SL, Brady JB. Pulmonary function in the sick newborn infant. Pediatr Res 1987; 21:313–328.
15. Sly PD, Brown KA, Batas JHT, et al. Non-invasive determination of respiratory

mechanics during mechanical ventilation of neonates; a review of current and future techniques. Pediatr Pulmonol 1988; 4:39–47.

16. England SJ. Current techniques for assessing pulmonary function in the newborn and infants: Advantages and limitations. Pediatr Pulmonol 1988; 4:48–53.
17. Goerke J. Surfactant and lung mechanics. In: Robertson B, van Golde LMG, Batenburg JJ, eds. Pulmonary Surfactant: From Molecular Biology to Clinical Practice. Amsterdam: Elsevier Science, 1992:165–192.
18. Fox WW, Schwartz JG, Schaffer TH. Effects of endotracheal tube leaks on functional residual capacity determination in intubated neonates. Pediatr Res 1979; 13:60–64.
19. LeSouef PN, England SJ, Bryan CA. Passive respiratory mechanics in newborns and children. Ann Rev Respir Dis 1984; 129:552–556.
20. Greenough A, Morley CJ. Dynamic compliance in preterm ventilated babies. Arch Dis Child 1984; 59:289–290.
21. Fujiwara T, Maeta H, Chida S, et al. Artificial surfactant therapy in hyaline membrane disease. Lancet 1980; 1:55–59.
22. Collaborative European Multicenter Study Group. Surfactant replacement therapy for severe neonatal respiratory distress syndrome: an international randomized clinical trial. Pediatrics 1988; 82:683–691.
23. Morley CJ, Greenough A. Respiratory compliance in premature babies treated with artificial surfactant (ALEC). Arch Dis Child 1991; 66:467–471.
24. Phibbs RH, Ballard RA, Clements JA, et al. Initial clinical trial of EXOSURF a protein free synthetic surfactant for the prophylaxis and early treatment of hyaline membrane disease. Pediatrics 1991; 88:1–9.
25. Pfenninger J, Aebi B, Bachmann D, Wagner BP. Lung mechanics and gas exchange in ventilated preterm infants during treatment of hyaline membrane disease with multiple doses of artificial surfactant (Exosurf). Pediatr Pulmonol 1992; 14:10–15.
26. Hallman M, Merritt TA, Järvenpää A-L, et al. Exogenous human surfactant for treatment of severe respiratory distress syndrome; a randomized prospective clinical trial. J Pediatr 1985; 106:963–969.
27. Noack G, Berggren P, Curstedt T, et al. Severe neonatal respiratory distress syndrome treated with the isolated phospholipid fraction of natural surfactant. Acta Paediatr Scand 1987; 76:697–705.
28. Davis JM, Veness-Meehan K, Notter R, et al. Changes in pulmonary mechanics after the administration of surfactant to infants with respiratory distress syndrome. N Eng J Med 1988; 319:476–479.
29. Bhat R, Dziedzic K, Bhutani VK, Vidiyasagar D. Effect of a single dose surfactant on pulmonary function. Crit Care Med 1990; 18:590–595.
30. Cotton RB, Olsson T, Law AB, et al. The physiologic effects of surfactant treatment on gas exchange in newborn premature infants with hyaline membrane disease. Pediatr Res 1993; 34:495–501.
31. Svenningsen NW. Pulmonary functional residual capacity and lung mechanics in surfactant-treated infants. A review. Semin Perinatol 1992; 16:181–185.
32. Heldt GP, Pesonen E, Merritt A, et al. Closure of the ductus arteriosus and mechanics of breathing in preterm infants after surfactant replacement therapy. Pediatr Res 1989; 25:305–310.

33. Goldsmith LS, Greenspan JS, Rubenstein SD, et al. Immediate improvement in lung volume after exogenous surfactant: Alveolar recruitment versus increased distention. J Pediatr 1991; 119:424–428.
34. Bhutani VK, Abbasi S, Long WA, et al. Pulmonary mechanics and energetics in preterm infants who had respiratory distress syndrome treated with synthetic surfactant. J Pediatr 1992; 120:S18–S24.
35. Edberg KE, Ekström-Jodal B, Hallman M, et al. Immediate effects on lung function of instilled human surfactant in mechanically ventilated newborn infants with IRDS. Acta Paediatr Scand 1990; 79:750–755.
36. Vilstrup C, Björklund L, Larsson A., et al. Functional residual capacity and ventilation homogeneity in mechanically ventilated small neonates. J Appl Physiol 1992; 73:(1)276–283.
37. Svenningsen NW, Björklund L, Vilstrup C, Werner O. Lung mechanics (FRC and static pressure-volume diagram) after endotracheal surfactant instillation: Preliminary observations. Biol Neonate 1992; 61(Suppl 1):44–47.
38. Björklund L, Vilstrup C, Larsson A, et al. Lung function before and after natural surfactant rescue treatment in neonates with RDS: Roles of early volume recruitment. Am Rev Respir Dis 1995; in press.
39. Kelly E, Bryan H, Possmayer F, et al. Compliance of the respiratory system in newborn infants pre- and post surfactant replacement therapy. Pediatr Pulmonol 1993; 15:225–230.
40. Baraldi E, Pettenazzo A, Filippone M, et al. Rapid improvement of static compliance after surfactant treatment in preterm infants with respiratory distress syndrome. Pediatr Pulmonol 1993; 15:157–162.
41. Tamura M, Kawano T. The effect of reconstituted bovine surfactant on pulmonary mechanics in infants with respiratory distress syndrome Acta Paediatr Jpn (overseas edition) 1989; 31:734–741.
42. Couser RJ, Ferrara TB, Ebert J, et al. Effects of exogenous surfactant therapy on dynamic compliance during mechanical breathing in preterm infants with hyaline membrane disease. J Pediatr 1990; 116:119–124.
43. Jobe A, Ikegami M, Jacobs H, Jones S. Surfactant and pulmonary flow distributions following treatment of premature lambs with natural surfactant. J Clin Invest 1984; 73:848–856.
44. Ikegami M, Jobe A, Berry D. A protein that inhibits surfactant in respiratory distress syndrome. Biol Neonate 1986; 50:120–129.
45. Halliday HL, McCord FB, McClure BG, McReid M. Acute effects on instillation of surfactants in severe respiratory distress syndrome. Arch Dis Child 1989; 64:13–16.
46. Kääpä P, Seppänen M. Kero P, Saraste M. Pulmonary hemodynamics after synthetic surfactant replacement in neonatal respiratory distress syndrome. J Pediatr 1993; 123:115–119.
47. Milner AD. How does exogenous surfactant work (Annotation) Arch Dis Child 1993; 68:253–254.
48. van Golde LMG, Batenburg JJ, Robertson B, et al. The pulmonary surfactant system: biochemical aspects and functional significance. Physiol Rev 1988; 68: 374–405.

49. Jobe AH, Ikegami M, Seidner SR, et al. Surfactant phosphatidylcholine metabolism and surfactant function in preterm ventilated lambs. Am Rev Respir Dis 1989; 139:352–359.
50. Gommers D, Vilstrup C, Bos JAH. Exogenous surfactant therapy increases static compliance and cannot be assessed by dynamic compliance alone. Crit Care Med 1993; 21:567–574.
51. Lachman B, Robertson B, Vogel J. In vivo lung lavage as an experimental model of the respiratory distress syndrome. Acta Anesth Scand 1980; 24:231–236.
52. Kobayashi T, Kataoka H, Ueda T, et al. Effects of surfactant supplement and end-expiratory pressure in lung-lavaged rabbits J Appl Physiol 1984; 57:995–1001.
53. Vilstrup CT, Gommers D, Bos JAH, et al. Natural surfactant instilled in premature lambs increases lung volume and improves ventilation homogeneity within five minutes. Pediatr Res 1992; 32:595–599.
54. Jackson JC, Mackensie AP, Chi EY, et al. Mechanisms for reduced total lung capacity at birth during hyaline membrane disease in premature newborn monkeys. Am Rev Respir Dis 1990; 142:413–419.
55. Segerer H, van Gelder W, Agenent FWM, et al. Pulmonary distribution and efficacy of exogenous surfactant in lung-lavaged rabbits are influenced by the instillation technique. Pediatr Res 1993; 34:490–494.
56. Lewis J, Tabor B, Ikegami M, et al. Lung function and surfactant distribution in saline lavaged sheep given instilled vs. nebulized surfactant. J Appl Physiol 1993; 74:1256–1264.
57. Fiasione J, Jacobs HC, Moya FR, et al. Betametasone increases pulmonary compliance in part by surfactant independent mechanisms in preterm rabbits. Pediatr Res 1987; 22:730–735.
58. Jobe AH, Mitchell BR, Gunkel JH. Beneficial effects of the combined use of prenatal corticosteroids and postnatal surfactant on preterm infants. Am J Obst Gynecol 1993; 168:508–513.

23

Ventilation Strategies in Relation to Surfactant Replacement

ROBERT A. deLEMOS and RANGASAMY RAMANATHAN
LAC + USC Medical Center
Women's and Children's Hospital
Los Angeles, California

JACQUELINE J. COALSON
University of Texas Health Science Center at San Antonio
San Antonio, Texas

I. Introduction

Exogenous surfactant therapy has resulted in improved survival and decreased acute pulmonary morbidity in premature infants with respiratory distress syndrome (RDS) but its effect on the incidence of chronic lung disease has been less dramatic (1). Although in part this may be related to deficiencies in formulation of the presently available surfactants, it is more likely linked to the multifactorial pathogenesis of chronic lung disease and the fact that surfactant deficiency/dysfunction is only one facet of an extremely complex pathophysiology (2).

Recently, there has been increased interest in the interaction between ventilation strategy and the induction of injury in both normal and diseased lungs (3–5). Although in the clinical setting the contribution of mechanical ventilation to disorders of lung mechanics, transcapillary fluid flux, and alterations in lung morphology cannot be separated from perturbations induced by the underlying disease process, data from animal models have clearly pointed to various aspects of mechanical ventilation as major contributing factors to lung injury (2,3,6). Although surfactant therapy has been in clinical use for some time, there has been until recently little objective data on the relationship between ventilation strategy and optimal surfactant effect or on the role of ventilator-induced injury in the pathogenesis of surfactant treatment failure.

II. Ventilator-Induced Lung Injury

Although there has been considerable speculation that the tidal volumes and pressures required to support gas exchange in newborns, children, and adults with respiratory failure might contribute to lung injury, it is only recently that a number of host and ventilator-dependent factors have been definitively identified (5). Several investigators have described the development of pulmonary edema in newborn and adult animals after ventilation with high inspiratory pressures and/or large tidal volumes (3,6,7). Studies in normal rats in which the duration and magnitude of pressure were varied produced a graded lesion affected by both pressure and time (8). Recently, Dreyfuss et al. demonstrated that although both played a role, peak distending volume rather than pressure was the major contributor to the development of pulmonary edema (3,9). Since high alveolar pressures-volumes lead to compression of septal capillaries, pulmonary artery pressure exceeds intra-alveolar pressure to maintain blood flow. With these changes in hydrostatic forces, it is not surprising that increases in pulmonary microvascular pressure, lymph flow, and protein clearance have been observed when comparing lungs of normal animals ventilated at high to those ventilated at lower transpulmonary pressures (10–12). Other investigators have described a relationship between high pulmonary pressures-volumes and increased microvascular premeability. Parker et al. demonstrated increased pulmonary capillary filtration coefficients in dog lungs at high transpulmonary pressures (11). Dreyfuss noted increased transmural flux of albumin after relatively short periods of high-pressure ventilation in rats (3). Finally, morphological studies by Dreyfuss, West, and others have shown both epithelial and endothelial disruption following ventilation with large lung volumes-pressures, even when vascular pressures are controlled (13,14).

From a functional standpoint, alterations in pulmonary mechanics have also been described following mechanical ventilation. Decreased compliance and increased minimum surface tension are found in normal animals ventilated at high but not low pressures (7,8,15,16). As noted previously, lung overdistension can lead to increased microvascular pressure and to increased endothelial and epithelial permeability. The interaction of plasma proteins and the surface layer has been shown to result in either specific or nonspecific inhibition of surfactant function ultimately leading to alveolar edema and atelectasis (17–19).

Although most studies suggest that the end-inspiratory volumes-pressures are likely the major determinant of development of ventilator-associated pulmonary edema, evidence regarding the role of continual distending airway pressure (continuous positive airway pressure [CPAP], positive end-expiratory pressure [PEEP]) in the induction or prevention of such injury is less consistent. Several studies have shown that the use of PEEP prevents or modifies the development of edema (8,9). In a recent study, Dreyfuss et al. reported that although permeability alterations were similar with changes of tidal volume or PEEP, edema was less marked with PEEP, probably due to the induced changes in hemodynamic status (9).

Although there are limited direct data linking these injury mechanisms to the development of chronic lung disease in human premature infants or developmentally relevant animal models, it is highly likely that they do play a role in surfactant treatment failures and in the development of the exudative phase of bronchopulmonary dysplasia (BPD) in premature infants (2,20). There is substantial evidence that lungs from immature animals have a greater propensity to the development of protein leaks than mature lungs after comparable insults (21–23). Adkins et al. reported that the pulmonary capillary coefficient was significantly increased in young as compared with adult rabbits after ventilation at pressures from 15 to 55 cmH_2O for 1 hr (24). Spontaneous or mechanical ventilation for relatively brief periods leads to epithelial necrosis and the development of increased alveolar-capillary permeability and pulmonary edema in surfactant-deficient preterm animals (21,22). This can be prevented by the administration of exogenous surfactant or the use of one of several strategies that minimize lung distention (21,25,26).

Although much of the data on ventilator-associated pulmonary edema was acquired from animal models with normal lungs and presumably uniform overdistension, it is also likely that the same mechanisms are operable in diseased lungs and, particularly, in the presence of focal overdistention. The morphology of lungs from experimental animals and human infants dying from RDS shows markedly nonuniform inflation, with much of the intrapulmonary gas localized in dilated distal conducting airways (27,28) (Fig. 1). Functional studies suggest a two-compartment model with partially expanded relatively compliant acini and noncompliant atelectatic/fluid-filled units. This explains in part why PEEP decreases lung compliance in infants with RDS (29). Overdistension of these areas during spontaneous breathing or mechanical ventilation likely contributes to the progressive protein leak described by Nilsson, Jobe, and others in ventilated preterm animals (21,22). As described elsewhere in this text, the distribution of exogenously administered surfactant is also nonuniform, particularly when administered after the onset of air breathing (Fig. 2). Although lung mechanics and gas exchange improve predictably, the fact that improved compliance occurs in only a portion of the potential air space leads to overdistension of those regions.

These injury mechanisms may also play a role in the development of chronic lung disease. Burnard first suggested that ventilation was markedly nonuniform in immature lung even in the absence of RDS (30). This has been attributed to the

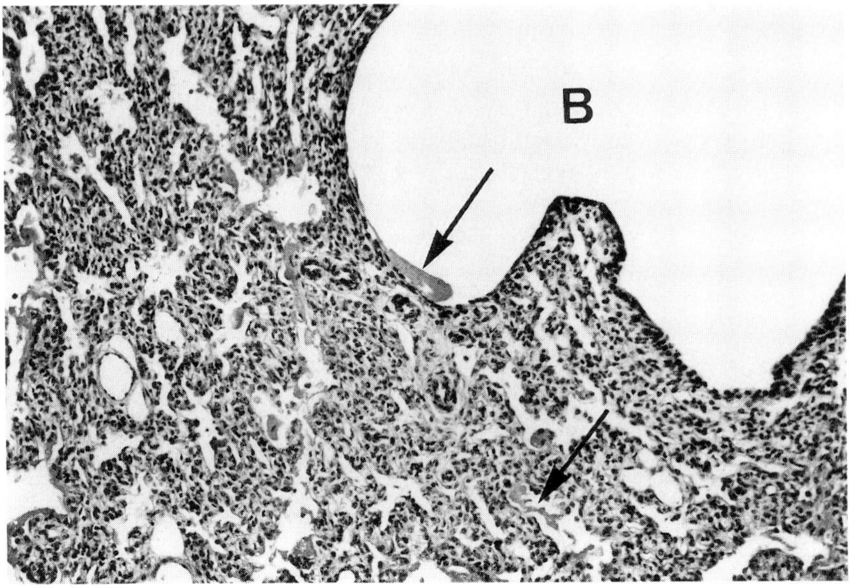

Figure 1 Twenty-four hour specimen. The bronchiole (B) is very dilated. The surrounding saccules are collapsed and hyaline membranes are seen over the surface of the bronchiole and within the saccular walls (arrows). Hematoxylin and eosin; ×140.

extreme distensibility of immature airways and peculiarities of branching geometry of airways. Some investigators have suggested that "choke points" develop during peak flow velocities. Direct measurements in airway segments from premature lambs by Bhutani et al. have confirmed that the conducting airways of immature infants are highly distensible and vulnerable to injury during assisted ventilation (31). The hypothesis that nonuniform ventilatory patterns play a role in the pathogenesis of bronchopulmonary dysplasia (BPD) is also supported by observations in nonhuman primates. In the 140-day gestation premature baboon, the prolonged use of positive-pressure ventilation and hyperoxia results in a pattern of lung injury clinically, radiographically, and morphologically similar to BPD in human premature infants (27,28,32). The unique distribution of the morphological findings with areas of relative underinflation alternating with areas of overinflation and evidence suggesting the relatively underinflated areas are protected from ventilator/oxygen injury strongly suggests that the distributional characteristics of this lesion result from nonuniform ventilation (2) (Fig. 3). Repetitive, prolonged overdistension of the relatively well-aerated segments of the immature lung would lead to increased epithelial and endothelial permeability and the development of alveolar and interstitial edema. This could explain the development of the exudative BPD in immature infants with minimal RDS.

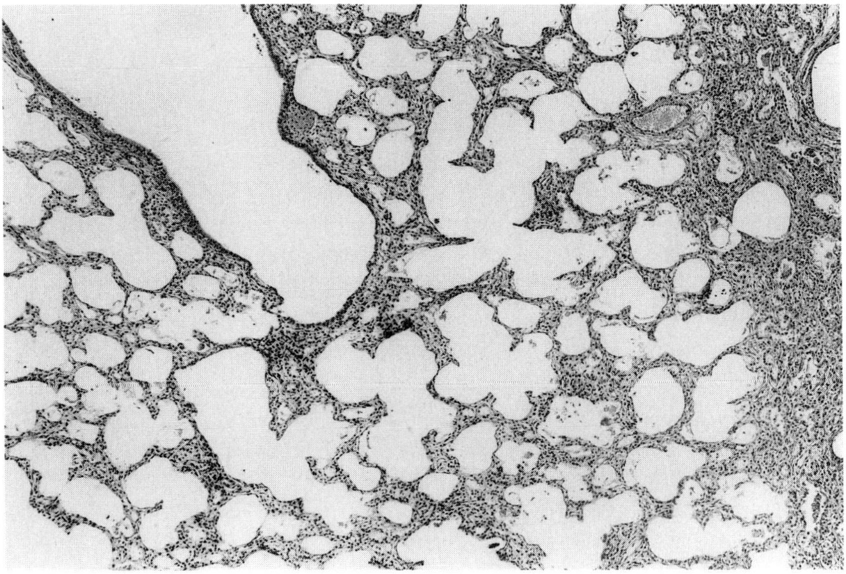

Figure 2 Twenty-four hour specimen. This animal received surfactant and 24 hr of positive-pressure ventilation. There is significant opening especially when compared with the findings in Figure 1, but there is inhomogeneity in inflation. On the right, note the merging of the inflated lung into the collapsed alveolar walls of residual hyaline membrane disease. B, bronchi/bronchioles. Hematoxylin and eosin; ×50.

III. Pulmonary Hemorrhage as a Manifestation of Ventilator-Induced Injury

Pulmonary hemorrhage occurs in association with surfactant-replacement therapy in between 9 and 10% of preterm infants (1). It occurs coincidental with rapid improvement in pulmonary function and gas exchange, is usually associated with relatively low hematocrits in the lung effluent, and is thought to represent hemorrhagic edema secondary to increased pulmonary blood flow through a patent ductus arteriosus or to acute left ventricular failure (33,34).

Another mechanism resulting in pulmonary hemorrhage was described by Bell et al. in the premature baboon (35). In that model of prematurity and RDS, early treatment with exogenous surfactant and/or high-frequency ventilation results in rapid resolution of saccular edema/atelectasis. We described a correlation between rapid clinical and physiological improvement and the presence of focal hemorrhage in the area of the bronchoalveolar (B-A) junctions (35) (Fig. 4). When these treatment modalities resulted in rapid and fairly uniform saccular recruitment, the region of the B-A junction was the most resistant to

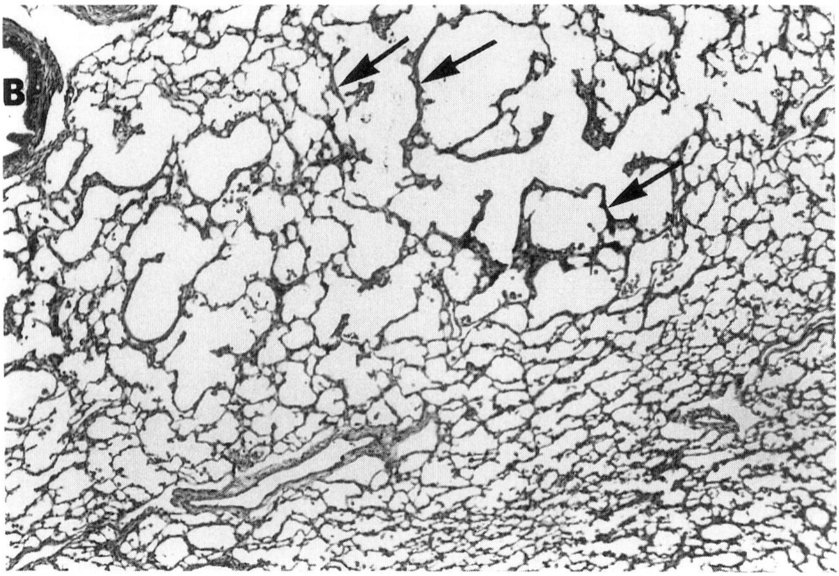

Figure 3 Twenty-one day oxygen-treated specimen. This micrograph depicts the mild to moderate BPD lesion and is characterized by sites of underinflation alternating with those areas of overinflated, fibrosed and remodeled saccular walls (arrows). B, bronchus. Hematoxylin and eosin; ×50.

airway opening. We hypothesize that this results in geometrical distortion, the development of shearing forces, and capillary fracture. Although these B-A hemorrhages were common and usually small in the lungs of premature baboons, coexisting factors such as coagulopathies or pulmonary hypertension could lead to significant intraparenchymal bleeding.

IV. Interaction Between Ventilation Strategy and Surfactant Replacement Therapy

As discussed in another chapter, surfactant replacement therapy changes lung volumes, compliance, gas exchange, and time constants toward those of normal lungs. There was early optimism that this treatment would minimize the need for assisted ventilation, and although the pattern of ventilation was known to affect the surfactant system in both surfactant-sufficient and surfactant-deficient lungs, little research was directed at exploring the interactions between the specific components of ventilation strategy and the outcome with surfactant therapy. In theory, ventilation strategy could impact the efficacy of surfactant

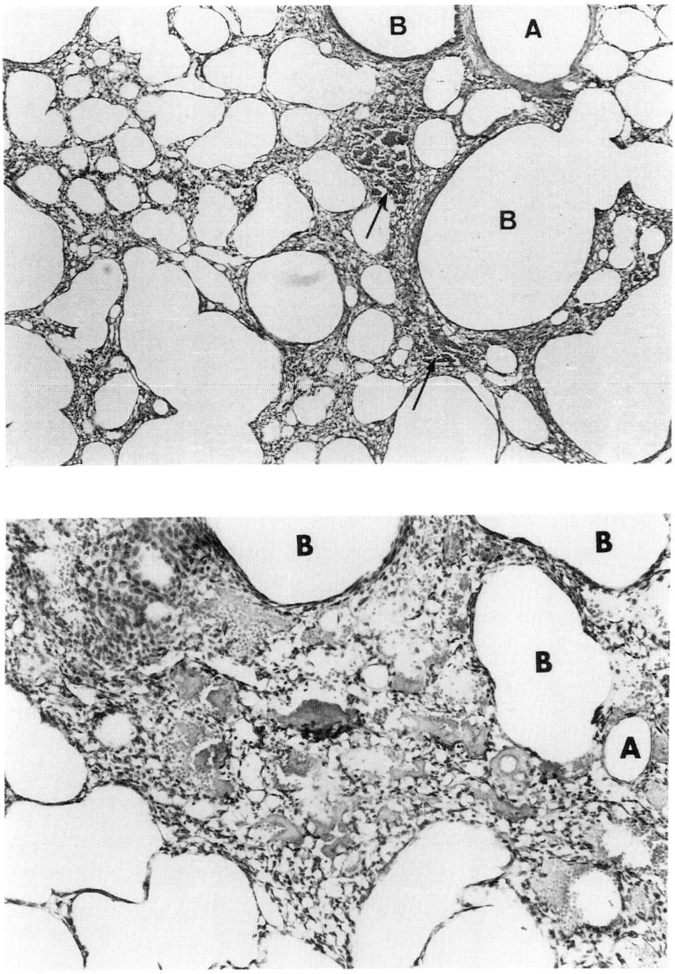

(a)

(b)

Figure 4 Ninety-six hour specimen. (a) The wall of the dilated airway (B) contains accumulations of red blood cells (arrows) that extends into the surrounding saccules with varying degrees of inflation. (b) An intermediate power view of a bronchoalveolar hemorrhage shows the walls of airways and surrounding saccules that contain extravasated RBCs. (Lungs were perfusion fixed.) Pulmonary artery, A. Hematoxylin and eosin; ×50 and ×140, respectively.

therapy by (1) compensating for any limitations in biophysical properties of a particular surfactant, (2) improving distribution, or (3) preventing ventilator-induced lung injury.

Kobayashi et al. noted that lavaged adult rabbits treated with surfactant and ventilated with 4 cmH_2O PEEP had better oxygenation and survival than those managed without PEEP (36). Although looking at only a single variable, these observations supported the hypothesis that specific aspects of ventilatory management might be important in determining outcome with exogenous surfactant therapy. In a comprehensive series of experiments, Rider et al. examined the effect of ventilation strategy on in vivo function of four different surfactants in the preterm rabbit (37). Sheep surfactant resulted in a significant increase in maximal and minimal lung volumes compared with Survanta or Exosurf. The effects of PEEP differed depending on the surfactant used. Air leaks were increased when PEEP was used with sheep surfactant but decreased with Exosurf or Survanta, suggesting that PEEP had a beneficial effect on lung deflation stability when used in combination with less effective surfactants but resulted in gas trapping, overdistension, and saccular rupture with the more efficient therapy. Although sheep surfactant tended to prevent protein leak and the development of pulmonary edema to a greater degree than the other surfactants tested, the use of PEEP resulted in decreased edema in all groups.

The term *high-frequency ventilation* describes a group of ventilatory techniques using specifically designed equipment which are capable of accomplishing adequate oxygenation and ventilation with low tidal volumes and supraphysiological frequencies. When used with the same strategy in experimental animals, high-frequency oscillatory ventilation (HFOV), high-frequency jet ventilation (HFJV), and the high-frequency flow interrupter (HFFI) give similar results (38,39). Froese, Meredith, and others have shown that the use of high-frequency ventilation (HFV) with a strategy designed to achieve alveolar/saccular recruitment and maintain lung volume above closing volume favorably affects lung mechanics, gas exchange and the morphological and biochemical progression of lung injury in lavaged adult rabbits and surfactant-deficient premature nonhuman primates (26,38,40). Surfactant-deficient animals treated with tidal ventilation develop progressive edema/atelectasis and deterioration in lung mechanics, whereas those treated with HFV and maintained at a relatively high mean lung volumes had more uniform inflation, minimal alveolar/saccular edema, and less evidence of inflammation (26,40). These findings suggest that tidal ventilation contributes substantively to the progression of lung injury in surfactant-deficient subjects, presumably by the mechanisms cited earlier in this chapter.

Nilsson et al. reported increased survival of premature rabbits after treatment with HFOV and exogenous surfactant compared with those treated with surfactant alone (25). Dunn noted improved oxygenation at 4 and 6 hr in lavaged adult rabbits and preterm lambs treated with surfactant and HFOV compared with positive-pressure ventilation (PPV), but the levels of PEEP used were probably not optimal (41). Recently, Froese et al. treated lavaged adult rabbits with bovine surfactant and compared outcomes after HFOV or PPV at either high or low end-expiratory volumes (42). They observed outcome to be significantly influenced by both ventilator type and strategy. Animals managed with surfactant and HFOV had lower mean airway pressures, higher blood pressures, and less need for bicarbonate than those managed with tidal ventilation. In terms of lung mechanics and surfactant, rabbits treated with HFOV had larger inflation and deflation volumes at 10 cmH_2O and increased lavage lamellar body phospholipid levels. Deflation stability and lamellar and lavage phospholipid levels were higher after the high end-expiratory volume strategies. These investigators concluded that surfactant therapy was most effective when used with a ventilation strategy that kept end-expiratory volume high enough to prevent atelectasis and simultaneously avoided focal overdistension by using low tidal volumes. This was accomplished with HFOV by initially recruiting atelectatic/fluid-filled alveoli and then maintaining lung volume above closing volume, a strategy which Froese et al. (42) had previously shown to be effective in preventing ventilator-induced injury in the same model.

Based on the experimental evidence cited earlier, the benefit of HFOV in these studies was directly related to the prevention of focal overdistension and intermittent alveolar/saccular collapse, thus minimizing their role in ventilator-induced lung injury. It is not clear whether the use of HFOV also resulted in more uniform distribution of surfactant or had a beneficial effect on utilization or turnover. Harris and others have described nonhomogeneous distribution of exogenous surfactant in injured lungs (43). (see Fig. 2). HFOV has been shown to produce more uniform inflation than tidal ventilation in lung injury models, and although this theoretically might result in better distribution, there are contradictory data with regard to this hypothesis (44).

V. Clinical Implications

There are substantial experimental data that support the hypotheses that (1) mechanical ventilation contributes to lung injury and (2) optimal ventilation strategies can maximize effectiveness of surfactant therapy; yet there are few studies that directly approach these issues in the clinical setting. Nonetheless, despite this caveat, the use of sufficient continual distending presssure to prevent saccular collapse during surfactant administration and in the immediate posttreatment period, with subsequent reduction during recovery to minimize the adverse cardiovascular effects is a wise strategy.

The role of HFV in the routine clinical management of surfactant-treated premature infants is more problematic. When used with a strategy aimed at achieving saccular/alveolar recruitment, avoiding cyclic overdistension, and holding lung volume above closing volume, HFV can prevent lung injury in surfactant-deficient experimental animals and human infants. Nonetheless, some human studies have shown an unacceptably high complication rate (45). This suggests that the appropriate use of the technology requires a high skill level and that the risk/benefit ratio may be small (39).

Even in the absence of surfactant-replacement therapy, HFOV can result in rapid improvement in gas exchange and lung mechanics. Since mean airway pressure (Paw) is independently controlled, failure to lower it coincidental with improved lung compliance will result in increased lung volumes and pleural pressure, decreased venous return, and engorgement of the extrathoracic capacitance vessels. This, coupled with a suboptimal strategy, likely accounted for the lack of benefit and the higher incidence of intraventricular hemorrhage reported in the multicenter HIFI trial (45). Subsequently, Clark et al. reported a decreased incidence of chronic lung disease without increased complications in a single-center controlled trial of HFOV (46). Other investigators have reported similar results, demonstrating that, with experience and close patient monitoring, it is possible to use this technology safely and effectively in preterm infants (47).

Alterations in cerebral blood flow and an increased incidence of intraventricular hemorrhage has been reported in some studies using surfactant replacement therapy and conventional ventilation (48–50). This presumably was due in part to iatrogenic lung overinflation (51,52). Although the combination of HFV and surfactant replacement therapy should result in improved pulmonary outcome, the rapid changes in lung mechanics that result from each technique independently would make the risks of lung overdistension and its resultant complications prohibitive unless careful patient monitoring and appropriate ventilator readjustment are accomplished.

The interaction between use of HFV, ventilation strategy, and cardiovascular function is less clear. Early studies suggested that HFV had less adverse effect on cardiovascular function than conventional positive-pressure ventilation, but the mean airway pressures used in these studies were low (53). Using radiolabled microspheres in the 140-day premature baboon, Kinsella found no difference in cardiac output or blood flow distribution between animals ventilated with PPV or those managed with HFOV and a "high-pressure" strategy (54). In clinical applications, however, several investigators have noted that HFOV and a "high-pressure" strategy are poorly tolerated in infants with hypovolemia or cardiovascular dysfunction (39). We have recently used ECHO-Doppler technology to measure serial changes in cardiovascular function in near-term/term infants with adult RDS (ARDS) and respiratory failure treated with HFOV and high Paw. Although, as previously reported, this approach significantly reduces the need for extracorporeal membrane oxygenation (ECMO) in this patient population (55,56), we have consistently documented decreased preload and increased right ventricular afterload even when lung overdistension is avoided. Whether this is related in part to the relative absence of cyclic changes in lung volumes and pleural pressures and/or the combination of sedation/paralysis is unclear, but the observations are consistent over a large number of infants. To prevent secondary hypotension in this setting, these infants often require volume supplementation that exceeds their estimated blood volume. Although this treatment strategy appears to be safe and effective in the term infant, the premature infant is less tolerant of hypotension and factors that impede venous return and result in an increased requirement for volume resuscitation are thought to contribute to periventricular/intraventricular hemorrhage (57).

Therefore, although there is strong theoretical and experimental evidence to support the combined use of surfactant therapy and HFV in the treatment of lung disease in the immature subject, we feel that additional controlled human trials are necessary before we can accurately determine the overall risk/benefit ratio of this treatment strategy and possibly recommend it for routine use in the premature infant with RDS.

References

1. Horbar JD, Wright LL, Soll, RF, et al. A multicenter randomized trial comparing two surfactants for the treatment of neonatal respiratory distress syndrome. J Peds 1993; 123:757–776.
2. deLemos RA, Coalson JJ. The contribution of experimental models to our understanding of the pathogenesis and treatment of bronchopulmonary dysplasia. Clin Perinatol 1992; 19:521–539.
3. Dreyfuss D, Soler P, Basset G, et al. High inflation pressure pulmonary edema. Respective effects of high airway pressure, high tidal volume, and positive end-expiratory pressure. Amer Rev Respir Dis 1988; 137:1159–1164.
4. Marini JJ, Kelson SG. Re-targeting Ventilatory Objectives in Adult Respiratory Distress Syndrome: New Treatment Prospects—Persistent Questions. Amer Rev Respir Dis 1992; 146:2–3.
5. Parker JC, Hernandez LA, and Peevy KJ. Mechanisms of ventilator-induced injury. Crit Care Med 1993: 21:131–143.
6. Bowton DL, Kong DL. High tidal volume ventilation produces increased lung water in oleic acid-injured rabbit lungs. Crit Care Med 1989; 17:908–911.
7. Kolobow T, Moretti MP, Fumagalli R, et al. Severe impairment in lung function induced by high peak airway pressure during mechanical ventilation. An experimental study. Am Rev Respir Dis 1987; 136:312–315.
8. Webb HH, Tierney DF. Experimental pulmonary edema due to intermittent positive pressure ventilation with high inflation pressures. Protection by positive end-expiratory pressures. Am Rev Respir Dis 1974; 110:556–565.
9. Dreyfuss D, Saumon G. Role of tidal volume, FRC and end-inspiratory volume in

the development of pulmonary edema following mechanical ventilation. Am Rev Respir Dis 1993; 148:1194–1203.
10. Eagan EA. Lung inflation, lung solute permeability, and alveolar edema. J Appl Physiol 1982; 53:121–125.
11. Parker JC, Townsley MI, Rippe B, et al. Increased microvascular permeability in dog lungs due to high peak inflation pressure. J Appl Physiol 1984; 57:1809–1816.
12. Parker JC, Hernandez LA, Longenecker GL, et al. Lung edema due to high peak airway pressures in dogs: Role of increased microvascular filtration pressure and permeability. Am Rev Respir Dis 1990; 142:321–328.
13. Dreyfuss D, Basset G, Soler P, et al. Intermittent positive pressure hyperventilation with high inflation pressures produce pulmonary microvascular injury in rats. Amer Rev Respir Dis 1985; 132:880–884.
14. West JB, Tsukimoto K, Mathieu-Costello O, et al. Stress failure in pulmonary capillaries. J Appl Physiol 1991; 70:1731–1742.
15. Greenfield LJ, Ebert PA, Benson DW. Effect of positive pressure ventilation on surface tension properties of lung extracts. Anesthesiology 1964; 25:312–316.
16. Wyszogrodski I, Abaagye K, Taeusch HW Jr, et al. Surfactant inactivation by hyperventilation: Conservation by end-expiratory pressure. J Appl Physiol 1975; 38:461–466.
17. Berry D, Ikegami M, Jobe A. Respiratory distress and surfactant inhibition following vagotomy in rabbits. J Appl Physiol 1986; 61:1741–1748.
18. Ikegami M, Agata Y, Elkrady T, et al. Comparison of four surfactants: In vitro surface properties and responses of preterm lambs to treatment at birth. Pediatrics 1987; 79:585–592.
19. Holm BA, Enhorning G, Notter RH. A biophysical mechanism by which plasma proteins inhibit lung surfactant activity. Chem Phys Lipids 1988; 49:49–55.
20. Northway WH Jr, Rosan RC, Porter DY. Pulmonary disease following respiratory therapy of hyaline membrane disease. N Engl J Med 1967; 276:357–368.
21. Jobe A, Ikegami M, Jacobs HC, et al. Permeability of premature lamb lungs to protein and the effect of surfactant on that permeability. J Appl Physiol 1983; 55:169–176.
22. Nilsson R, Grossman G, Robertson B. Lung surfactant and the pathogenesis of neonatal bronchiolar lesions induced by artificial ventilation. Pediatr Res 1978; 12:249–255.
23. Jackson JC, MacKenzie AP, Chi EY, et al. Mechanisms for reduced total lung capacity at birth and during hyaline membrane disease in premature newborn monkeys. Am Rev Respir Dis 1990: 142:413–419.
24. Adkins KW, Hernandez LA, Coker PJ, et al. Age affects susceptibility to pulmonary barotrauma in rabbits. Crit Care Med 1991; 19:390–393.
25. Nilsson R, Bergren P, Curstedt T, et al. Surfactant treatment and ventilation by high frequency oscillation in premature newborn rabbits: effect on survival, lung aeration, and bronchiolar epithelial lesions. Pediatr Res 1985; 19:143–147.
26. Meredith KS, deLemos RA, Coalson JJ, et al. Role of lung injury in the pathogenesis of hyaline membrane disease in premature baboons. J Appl Physiol 1989; 66:2150–2158.

27. Coalson JJ, Kuehl TJ, Escobedo MB, et al. A baboon model of bronchopulmonary dysplasia II. Pathologic features. Exp Mol Pathol 1982; 37:335–350.
28. Coalson JJ, Kuehl TJ, Prihoda TJ, et al. Diffuse alveolar damage in the evolution of bronchopulmonary dysplasia in the baboon. Pediatr Res 1988; 24:357–366.
29. Bancalari E, Garcia OL, Jesse MJ. Effects of continuous negative pressure on lung mechanics in idiopathic respiratory distress syndrome. Pediatrics 1973; 51:485–493.
30. Burnard ED, Grattan-Smith P, Picton-Warlow CG, Grauaug A: Pulmonary Insufficiency in Prematurity. Aust Paediatr J 1965; 1:12–38.
31. Bhutani VK, Rubenstein SD, Shaffer TK. Pressure-induced deformation in immature airways. Pediatr Res 1981; 15:829–832.
32. Bonikos DS, Bensch KG, Northway WH Jr, et al. Bronchopulmonary dysplasia: The pulmonary pathologic sequel of necrotizing bronchiolitis and pulmonary fibrosis. Hum Pathol 1976; 7:643–666.
33. Cole VA, Normand CS, Reynolds EOR, and Rivers RPA. Pathogenesis of hemorrhagic pulmonary edema and massive pulmonary hemorrhage in the newborn. Pediatrics 1973; 51:175–185.
34. Trompeter R, Yu VYH, Ansley-Green A, Roberton NRC. Massive pulmonary hemorrhage in the newborn infant. Arch Dis Child 1975; 50:123–127.
35. Bell RE, Kuehl TJ, Coalson JJ, et al. High-frequency ventilation compared to conventional positive-pressure ventilation in the treatment of hyaline membrane disease in primates. Crit Care Med 1984; 12:764–768.
36. Kobayashi TH, Kataoka H, Ueda T, et al. Effects of surfactant supplement and end-expiratory pressure in lung-lavaged rabbits. J Appl Physiol 1984; 57:995–1001.
37. Rider ED, Jobe AH, Ikegami M, Sun B. Different ventilation strategies alter surfactant responses in preterm rabbits. J Appl Physiol 1992; 73(5):2089–2096.
38. Froese AB, Bryan AC. High frequency ventilation. Am Rev Respir Dis 1987; 135:1363–1374.
39. Gerstman DR, deLemos RA, Clark RH. High-frequency ventilation: Issues of strategy. Clin Perinatol 1991; 18:563–578.
40. Hamilton PP, Onayemi A, Smyth JA, et al. Comparison of conventional and high-frequency ventilation: Oxygenation and lung pathology. J Appl Physiol 1983; 55:131–138.
41. Dunn MS, Jefferies AL, Young Tai KF, et al. The role of high frequency oscillation in surfactant replacement. In: Ekelund L, Jonson B, Malm L, eds. Surfactant and the Respiratory Tract. New York: Elsevier 1989:233–242.
42. Froese AB, McCulloch PR, Sugiura M, et al. Optimizing alveolar expansion prolongs the effectiveness of exogenous surfactant therapy in the adult rabbit. Am Rev Respir Dis 1993; 148:569–577.
43. Harris JD, Jackson F, Moxley MA, Longmore WJ. Effect of exogenous surfactant istillation on experimental acute lung injury. J Appl Physiol 1989; 66:1846–1851.
44. Walther FJ, Kuipers IM, Gidding DW, et al. A comparison of high-frequency oscillation superimposed onto backup mechanical ventilation and conventional mechanical ventilation on the distribution of exogenous surfactant in premature lambs. Pediatr Res 1987; 22:725–729.
45. HIFI Study Group. High-frequency oscillatory ventilation compared with conven-

tional mechanical ventilation in the treatment of respiratory failure in preterm infants. N Engl J Med 1989; 320:88–93.
46. Clark RH, Gerstmann DR, Null DM Jr., deLemos RA. Prospective randomized comparison of high frequency oscillatory ventilation and conventional ventilation in respiratory distress syndrome. Pediatrics 1992; 89:5–11.
47. Ogawa Y, Miyasaka K, Kawano T, et al. A multicenter randomized trial of high frequency oscillatory ventilation as compared to conventional mechanical ventilation in preterm infants with respiratory failure. Early Hum Dev 1993; 32:1–10.
48. Cowan F, Whitelaw A, Wertheim D, Silverman M. Cerebral blood flow velocity changes after rapid administration of surfactant. Arch Dis Child 1991; 66:1105–1109.
49. Horbar JD, Soll RF, Schachinger H, et al. A European multicenter randomized controlled tril of single dose surfactant therapy for idiopathic respiratory distress syndrome. Eur J Pediatr 1990; 149:416–423.
50. Gunkel JH, Banks PLC. Surfactant therapy and Intra cranial Hemorrhage: Review of the literature and results of new analysis. Pediatrics 1993; 92:775–786.
51. Jorch G, Rabe H, Garbie M, et al. Acute and protracted effects of intratracheal surfactant application on internal carotid blood flow velocity, blood pressure and carbon dioxide tension in very low birth weight infants. Eur J Pediatr 1989; 148:770–773.
52. Van de Bor M, Ma EJ, Walther FJ. Cerebral blood flow velocity after surfactant instillation in preterm infants. J Pediatr 1991; 118:285–287.
53. Mirro R, Tamura M, Kawano T. Systemic cardiac output and distribution during high-frequency oscillation. Crit Care Med 1985; 13:727–727.
54. Kinsella JP, Gerstmann DR, deLemos RA. Circulatory changes following premature delivery in a baboon model of hyaline membrane disease. Am J Physiol 1991; 261(4):H1148–H1154.
55. Carter JM, Gerstmann DR, Clark RH, et al. High frequency oscillatory ventilation and extracorporeal membrane oxygenation for the treatment of acute neonatal respiratory failure. Pediatrics 1990; 85:159–164.
56. deLemos RA, Yoder B, McCurnin D., et al. The use of high-frequency oscillatory ventilation (HFOV) and extracorporeal membrane oxygenation (ECMO) in the management of the term/near term infant with respiratory failure. Early Human Dev 1992; 29:299–303.
57. deLemos RA, Tomasovic JJ. Effects of positive pressure ventilation on cerebral blood flow in the newborn infant. Clin Perinatol 1978; 5:395–409.

24

Radiographic Evaluation of the Therapeutic Response

DAVID K. EDWARDS III
University of California, San Diego
San Diego, California

I. Introduction

Chest radiography remains the basic and most essential imaging modality in the neonatal intensive care nursery. In recent years, sonography also has become crucial in evaluating the heart, brain, and abdomen in ill infants, but to date no sectional imaging technique exceeds the reliability of plain radiography in assessing the lung parenchyma, airways, bones, and the positions of most catheters. The chest radiograph is unsurpassed in diagnosing the cause of respiratory distress, monitoring the progress of lung diseases, and detecting the various complications of ventilatory support.

In the specific case of preterm infants with respiratory distress syndrome (RDS), the chest radiograph helps establish the initial diagnosis, confirms the placement of endotracheal tubes, and permits surveillance for such complications as air leaks (primarily pulmonary interstitial emphysema and pneumothorax), iatrogenic fluid overload, focal atelectasis, and superimposed pneumonia. The chest radiograph may also suggest the presence of significant left-to-right shunting (usually through the patent ductus arteriosus), although sonography is unquestionably preferable in this regard (1).

With the advent of exogenous surfactant therapy for RDS, the role of chest radiography has expanded to include monitoring those effects of surfactant administration that may be radiographically apparent. These effects are the subject of this chapter. Because it is widely agreed that the radiographic severity of RDS correlates, albeit roughly, with the clinical (2,3) and pathological (4) extent of disease, the radiograph contributes to assessing surfactant effect by demonstrating the extent of clearing and suggesting the potential need for additional surfactant treatment. Probably more importantly, the radiograph functions in its customary way to detect and monitor the numerous secondary cardiopulmonary disturbances that may affect infants with RDS.

II. Radiographic Technique

Chest radiography in the newborn intensive care unit generally employs a mobile ("portable") machine and uses conventional film-screen techniques. At the University of California at San Diego, the initial chest radiograph is treated differently from subsequent chest films. For one thing, a lateral view routinely accompanies the initial anteroposterior (AP) view. This is a cross-table, or horizontal beam, lateral view; overhead, or vertical beam, lateral views distort the lungs (as may be appreciated by examining a decubitus view) and do not provide the advantages of a gravity-dependent examination. A gravity-dependent view permits, for example, the appreciation of air-fluid levels as well as pneumothoraces, with which the free ectopic gas rises superiorly (thus anteriorly) in the chest, facilitating its visualization. The lateral projection also provides the best view of the intrathoracic trachea, the vertebrae, and the sternum. Further, the air bronchogram effect, which is crucial in the radiographic diagnosis of RDS, is often best appreciated in the retrocardiac region on the lateral projection.

The initial lateral view is occasionally omitted, sometimes by accident and sometimes because the infant's condition is too precarious to permit two views. A lateral view is exposed as soon as the patient's condition permits.

The field of view is also wide for the first chest examination (5), with the beam coned from the mouth to the umbilicus. This technique suffers the disadvantage of increased beam scattering, which slightly degrades the image of pulmonary parenchymal detail. This disadvantage, however, is offset by the appreciation the wide field of view offers of the skeleton (permitting, e.g., evaluation of spinal abnormalities and dysplasias), the abdominal viscera (determining, e.g., visceral situs and detecting gastrointestinal atresias), and umbilical arterial and venous catheters.

Radiographs exposed after the initial study are commonly an AP view only, with the beam tightly coned to the infant's chest. In certain circumstances, however, a lateral view accompanying the AP view is helpful (Table 1). Lateral decubitus radiographs are primarily useful in the setting of suspected pneumo-

Table 1 Plain Film Chest Radiography in the Intensive Care Nursery

Initial radiograph: anteroposterior (AP) supine and supine lateral (coned mouth to umbilicus)
Routine surveillance radiographs: AP coned to chest
Lateral projection accompanying AP suggested:
Initial radiograph
Establish AP position of chest tubes
Unexplained clinical deterioration (may reveal, e.g., an occult pneumothorax, esophageal placement of endotracheal tube)
Locate focal intrathoracic masses or other abnormalities
Lateral decubitus radiograph suggested:
Possible pneumothorax (equivocal side up)
Pleural fluid (equivocal side down or, if lungs nearly opaque, up)

thorax. The equivocal side is placed uppermost, with the expectation that free intrapleural gas will rise and the lung fall medially, permitting visualization of the lung edge and confirmation of the pneumothorax. Rarely a lateral decubitus view may be needed to characterize or roughly quantitate a pleural effusion. The affected side is generally placed lowermost. However, when the underlying lung is already radiodense, its compression by the decubitus position may make the lung indistinguishable from the pleural fluid. In this setting, the "wrong" decubitus may be helpful, with the hemithorax in question uppermost; the lung floats peripherally and remains relatively well aerated, permitting visualization of the pleural fluid. Occasionally, a lateral decubitus view may clarify focal infiltrates by moving the mediastinum away from the questionable area (6).

Infants should be radiographed during quiet breathing. Attempts, usually futile, may be made to time the exposure to peak inspiration; however, filming during any phase of respiration is usually fruitful, so long as the infant is not crying. Crying causes large excursions of the diaphragm (7), and filming during crying is a common cause of radiographs that adventitiously suggest hyper- or hypoaeration.

III. The Radiographic Diagnosis of RDS

Most institutions require a chest radiograph as a necessary part of the diagnosis of RDS. The radiograph serves to exclude other causes of respiratory distress and to provide confirmatory evidence that any surfactant deficiency results from RDS and not from some other condition (8). When the radiographic findings of RDS are combined with analysis of surfactant components in lung effluent, the diagnosis of RDS can be made with a high degree of confidence and accuracy (9).

Understanding the radiographic abnormalities in respiratory distress syndrome (RDS) is crucial to appreciating the changes engendered by surfactant therapy. The radiographic findings noted on the initial radiograph in uncomplicated RDS typically consist of a triad of findings: (1) a diffuse "infiltrate" that is typically described as "granular" or resembling ground glass; (2) an air bronchogram; and (3) underaeration (10). Of these, the least reliable is underaeration, largely because commonly the infant is already being treated with mechanically assisted ventilation by the time the first radiograph is exposed, and the degree of aeration is as much a function of ventilator pressure as it is of the extent of underlying atelectasis.

If the radiograph is exposed before assisted ventilation is begun, however, and the infant is not crying, the degree of aeration suggested by the radiograph is at least moderately helpful. The assessment of aeration is best accomplished using the lateral projection. The diaphragm in this view assumes an exaggerated cephalad domed configuration with underaeration (11). The only other condition that typically produces such hypoaeration is pulmonary hypoplasia. Virtually all other parenchymal disorders of newborn infants exhibit normal or hyperaeration. With hyperaeration, which is common with retained fetal lung fluid, neonatal pneumonia, and meconium aspiration syndrome, the diaphragm loses its domed configuration and is situated relatively low; typically, there is flattening of the posterior hemidiaphragms in the lateral projection.

Diffuse granularity of the lungs is seen in conditions other than RDS. With preterm infants without RDS, often because of intrauterine acceleration of the surfactant system, mild granularity may be noted (12). Such patients, however, lack a significant air bronchogram, and often have a small thymic silhouette, reflecting intrauterine stress or maternal steroid therapy. Another common cause of diffusely granular lungs is retained fetal lung fluid in the early hours after delivery, whereas the majority of the excessive fluid is largely alveolar (13,14). The next commonest cause is diffuse neonatal pneumonia. With both of these latter conditions, the lungs tend to be hyperinflated; further, pleural effusion is common, whereas it is uncommon with uncomplicated RDS. Of course, pneumonia and RDS can coexist; in such cases, the presence of pleural effusion should raise a suspicion of concurrent infection (15,16).

An air bronchogram is normally seen in about the central third of a newborn infant's lungs on the AP projection. An abnormal air bronchogram, reflecting airways surrounded by consolidated lung, is seen peripherally, often extending below the hemidiaphragms on the AP view. As noted above, an abnormal air bronchogram may be best appreciated in the lateral projection in the retrocardiac region.

As with diffuse granularity, an air bronchogram is seen in conditions other than RDS, most notably in diffuse pneumonia accompanying sepsis (17,18). A focal air bronchogram, visible only in a lobe or lobes, occurs with pneumonias that are not global; in this setting, it is unlikely that confusion with RDS would arise.

The radiographic differential diagnosis of RDS is presented in Table 2 (12–14,17–20). Of the entities listed, the one that in my experience most commonly causes diagnostic difficulty is the premature infant that does not lack adequate surfactant (the so-called PALM infant, an acronym for *p*remature with *a*ccelerated *l*ung *m*aturity). The PALM infant's small size, and in whom mild granularity commonly occurs, makes an erroneous diagnosis of RDS treacherously easy. This is especially true when an endotracheal tube is in place. In such infants, the lack of an abnormal air bronchogram is helpful, as is the typically small size of the thymic shadow (19).

Occasionally, the initial radiograph in RDS does not reflect the true diagnosis. Instead the radiograph may appear nearly normal (21), or it may suggest retained lung fluid. In such instances, changes suggesting RDS are virtually inevitably appreciable on a second radiograph exposed within 1–2 hr. It may be hypothesized that initially the patient's lungs contain enough

Table 2 Radiographic Differential Diagnosis of RDS

Preterm infant with accelerated lung maturity (12)
Lungs may appear granular, but lack significant air bronchograms
Thymus often small (19)
May exhibit trophic ("growth arrest") lines in bones (20)
(Clinical: little to mild respiratory insufficiency)
Retained fetal lung fluid (13,14)
In first hours of life when excessive fluid is largely alveolar
Pleural fluid not uncommon
Usually term or near-term infant
(Clinical: tachypnea, respiratory distress that is usually mild)
Diffuse pneumonia accompanying sepsis
Group B streptococci and other organisms (17,18)
Usually term or near-term infant
Pleural fluid common
(Clinical: other signs of sepsis)
Severe pulmonary venous congestion
Prototype is total anomalous pulmonary venous connection with obstruction
(Clinical: inability to oxygenate; characteristic sonogram)
Pulmonary hemorrhage
(Clinical: blood from endotracheal tube)

Numbers in parentheses are references.

endogenous surfactant to prevent widespread atelectasis, but this surfactant is expended more rapidly than it is produced, so that the atelectasis and the radiographic findings of RDS ensue. The initial radiograph may also be nondiagnostic when such complications as air leaks or focal abnormalities from endotracheal tube malpositions have predated the radiograph.

IV. Radiographic Progression of RDS

In infants who are not treated with surfactant therapy, sequential radiographs typically reveal a fairly consistent progression of findings (10). The timing of this progression in terms of how rapidly sequential changes occur depends in large part on the severity of the initial RDS, and probably on idiosyncratic factors as well. In patients with RDS that initially is severe, with marked atelectasis and a prominent air bronchogram, resolution is typically slower than it is with infants whose initial radiographs suggest milder disease.

The radiographic abnormalities tend to be most marked on the first 1–2 days of life, followed by clearing over the next several days. Clearing is first notable by an overall decrease in radiopacity, followed by resolution of the abnormal air bronchogram and granularity. The lungs remain abnormally dense for a period of days to 1 or 2 weeks, with a generally hazy appearance (22). This appearance may clear to normal with time, or long-lived abnormalities representing bronchopulmonary dysplasia (BPD) may appear. BPD has its own appearances and radiographic course whose details are beyond the scope of this chapter (23,24).

The "typical" pattern of gradual radiographic clearing, with or without an initial brief worsening, is in fact relatively uncommon. Often other processes supervene, especially in the infants with relatively more severe underlying disease. These processes add their own radiographic characteristics to the sequence of films. Probably the most common of these is left-to-right shunting through a patent ductus arteriosus (PDA). The PDA may result in pulmonary edema that superficially suggests worsening RDS. The diagnosis of PDA is primarily echocardiographic, but may be suggested on the radiograph by noting enlarged central pulmonary arteries and often an increased heart size (25–27). Similar findings may result from iatrogenic fluid overload, although enlarged central arteries are less common in this setting than they are with a PDA. Several causes of increased radiopacity that may cause a "whiteout" effect in infants with RDS are listed in Table 3 (23,28).

Another frequent process that hinders radiographic assessment of RDS is intrathoracic air leak; most commonly pulmonary interstitial emphysema (PIE) and pneumothorax. PIE is usually radiographically obvious, with abnormal lucencies in the affected lobe or lung that may be distinguished from an air bronchogram because they do not branch and smoothly taper peripherally (Fig. 1), and they are usually much larger in the lung periphery than bronchi in this location would be

Table 3 Intrathoracic Radiopacities in Preterm Infants

Diffuse
- Normal
  - Pulmonary vessels
  - Hypoventilatory or underpenetrated examination
- Abnormal (commonly presenting a "whiteout" effect)
  - Granular densities of respiratory distress syndrome
  - Pulmonary edema (left-to-right shunting through patent ductus arteriosus, iatrogenic fluid overload, neurogenic and other causes of edema)
  - "Weaning effect" of decreased ventilator pressure (28)
  - Exudative phase of bronchopulmonary dysplasia (23)
  - Blood (pulmonary hemorrhage)
  - Pus (global infiltrate)
  - Gastric contents (massive aspiration)
  - Extracorporeal membrane oxygenation

Focal
- Normal
  - Thymus
  - Heart and central vessels
  - Superimposed bones (ribs; scapula may be projected over chest, simulating an upper lobe process; sternal ossification centers may be projected over chest with rotated examination, simulating nodules or masses)
- Abnormal
  - Pneumonia
  - Atelectasis
  - Enlarged heart and central vessels
  - Irregular surfactant effect
  - Masses: for example, cystic adenomatoid malformation, sequestration, bronchogenic cyst, pericardial cyst, diaphragmatic hernia

Numbers in parentheses refer to references.

(29). Sometimes, however, the abnormal lucencies may be quite small, requiring close observation to diagnose correctly, producing a "pseudoclearing" of RDS, in which seeming radiographic improvement is accompanied by clinical worsening. The changes of PIE may appear in a single lobe (most commonly an upper lobe, in my experience) or throughout one or both lungs.

A variety of other air leaks are listed in Table 4 (30–44), some of which are relatively uncommon and radiographically confusing. With most of these, the presence of ectopic gas within the thorax acts effectively as a space-occupying mass lesion, diminishing the lung area available for gas exchange and sometimes causing cardiac tamponade ("air block"). In the radiographic assessment of infants with air leaks, probably the most important single factor is the size of

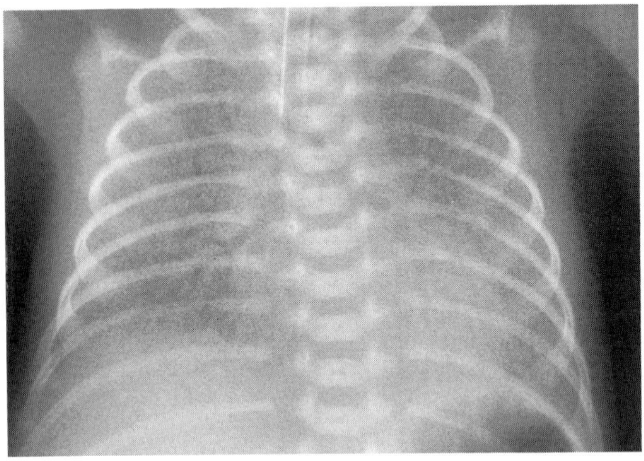

(A)

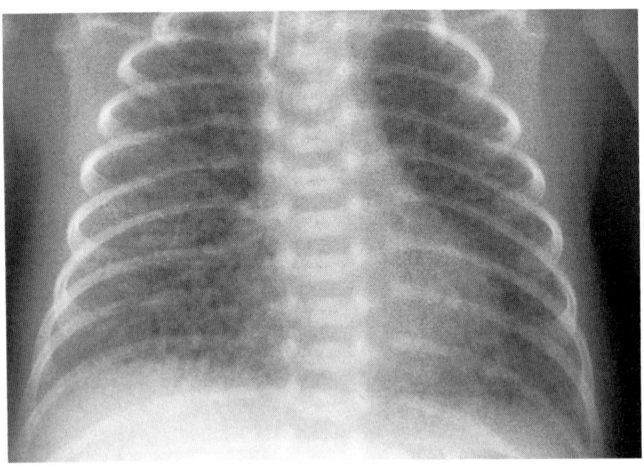

(B)

Figure 1 Pulmonary interstitial emphysema (PIE) developing in two infants after surfactant treatment. In both infants, the initial chest radiographs (A and C, respectively), exposed about 1 hr before treatment, reveal severe respiratory distress syndrome. On films exposed immediately following treatment, both exhibit diffuse bilateral irregular lucencies representing PIE (radiographs B and D, respectively).

the cardiac silhouette as compared with that of prior radiographs or normal standards (45); substantial decrease in heart size suggests tamponade (43) and the need for immediate efforts to drain the ectopic gas.

Other interruptions of the progression of RDS clearing are idiosyncratic and miscellaneous. For example, malpositions of the endotracheal tube may result

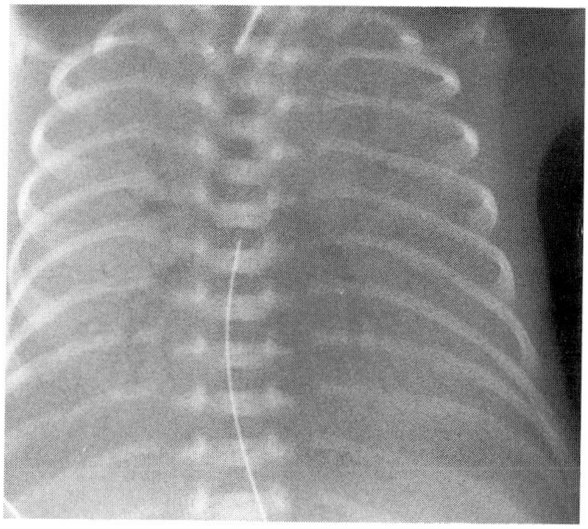

(C)

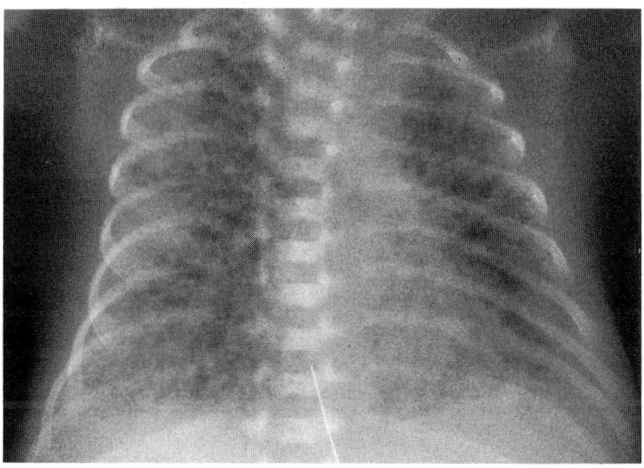

(D)

in asymmetrical aeration. After about the first week of life, foci of atelectasis may appear and disappear, probably the result of mucous plugs. Bacterial, viral, or fungal pneumonia may also occur, although this is more common during chronic care of infants with bronchopulmonary dysplasia.

V. Immediate Radiographic Effects of Exogenous Surfactant Therapy

Typically, surfactant is initially administered to constitute either "rescue" or "prophylactic" therapy. Rescue surfactant therapy is applied after the infant is

Table 4 Air Leaks in Infants with RDS

Pulmonary interstitial emphysema (30)
"Pseudoclearing" of RDS
"Tension": unilateral or bilateral
Subpleural blebs or pseudocysts (31,32)
Blebs can rupture to form pneumothorax (30); rarely can become essentially permanent in lung or lobe (33–35)
Pneumomediastinum
Ordinary: thymic lobes outlined by gas (36)
"Tension": heart forced backward and flattened
Subazygous: gas in azygoesophageal recess (37); may dissect to neck
Inferior pulmonary ligament gas (38)
Periaortic: gas may dissect to peritoneum
Pneumothorax
Ordinary: lung edge outlined by gas; uncommon in supine infants
"Tension": hemidiaphragm depressed, mediastinum shifted, herniated tongue of pleura (39)
Occult on AP view save for unilateral hyperlucency: lung fallen backward (40)
Medial: lucency paralleling the mediastinum (40,41)
Gas below visceral pleura (42)
Usually at lung base
Against a fissure
Pneumopericardium
"Tension" when cardiac silhouette shrinks notably (43)
Gas embolism
Gas in chambers of heart and blood vessels (44)

Numbers in parentheses refer to references.

diagnosed as having RDS, preferably by both biochemical and radiographic criteria (9), and generally after respiratory insufficiency has developed. With prophylactic therapy, the infant is treated with surfactant on the basis of risk factors for RDS, such as small size and considerable prematurity, without waiting for respiratory failure or radiographic confirmation of RDS. The type of therapy employed affects the radiographic evaluation of treated infants.

A. Prophylactic Application

The radiographic effects of surfactant that is administered prophylactally (i.e., immediately after delivery before a radiograph is exposed) obviously cannot be assessed directly; a subsequent film showing no RDS could mean that the surfactant was efficacious or that the infant would not have developed RDS in any case. Neonatologists are familiar with tiny infants who are at risk for RDS but who do not develop it because of accelerated lung maturity (so-called PALM babies; see above), and such infants are to an unknown extent treated needlessly with prophylactic surfactant (46).

In the radiographic assessment of prophylactic treatment, the posttreatment radiographs may be compared with those of untreated controls. When this is done, radiographs of the treated group typically demonstrate a relatively decreased incidence and severity of RDS (47,48). Approximately half of treated infants demonstrate radiographs showing no RDS (49), whereas about three quarters of controls have radiographic RDS (47). An unusual pattern of aeration was noted in 14% of infants treated prophylactically with a bovine surfactant; these infants showed preferentially central clearing, with changes suggesting RDS confined largely to the lung periphery (49). This pattern has not been widely reported, and I have never encountered it.

Prophylactic treatment offers the disadvantage of entailing treatment without prior diagnosis, and it does not appear to offer significant clinical advantages over rescue treatment (50). Although prophylactic treatment may reduce the incidence of BPD compared with that of control infants (51), at least one report suggests that BPD is more common among prophylactically treated than with rescue-treated infants (52).

B. Rescue Application

For the radiologist, at least, the situation in which surfactant is administered only after RDS is diagnosed (rescue treatment) is more satisfactory than is the case with prophylactic therapy. For one thing, an initial radiograph is available to help confirm the diagnosis. Additionally, a second radiograph is typically exposed following surfactant therapy, and this film allows assessment of any changes that are, for the most part, a result of the therapy.

As suggested above, the radiographic findings in untreated RDS remain fairly stable for the first day or two unless complications supervene. The administration of surfactant typically disrupts both this initial stability and the usual radiographic progression of RDS, most typically by ameliorating the parenchymal abnormalities and accelerating clearing and apparent healing of the disease. The radiograph appears to reflect the clinical course of the infants with fair fidelity (53), although it appears that the radiograph may suggest improvement earlier than do clinical and physiological indices of pulmonary mechanics (54,55).

Common radiographic sequelae of surfactant therapy are outlined in Table 5, listed in approximate order of frequency as reflected by the literature and the author's clinical experience (53,56–58). The most common immediate result seems to be global clearing of a slight to moderate degree; marked global clearing (Fig. 2) is also quite common (59). Radiographs of a few infants change little

Table 5 Common Radiographic Sequelae of Surfactant Therapy

Immediate
Global clearing, moderate to slight
Global clearing, marked
Assyemtric clearing (usually but not invariably greatest in the right lung)
No significant change
Central clearing with dense periphery
Appearance of another condition
Left-to-right shunt, usually through a patent ductus arteriosus
Air leak (usually pulmonary interstitial emphysema or pneumothorax)
Short-term (subsequent few hours to days)
Continued clearing
Worsening of findings suggesting RDS ("relapse;" findings may improve after readministration of surfactant)
Appearance of another condition:
Left-to-right shunt, usually through a patent ductus arteriosus
Air leak (usually pulmonary interstitial emphysema or pneumothorax)
Long-term (weeks to months)
Normal
Minimal and nonspecific abnormalities (presumably scars)
Mild, moderate, or severe bronchopulmonary dysplasia

if any (53,60), but radiographic improvement is by far the rule. The type of surfactant used probably makes little difference radiographically; one study comparing human with artificial surfactant under similar radiographic conditions found quite similar radiographic outcomes (58), and similar clinical outcomes have been noted comparing two artificial surfactants (61). It may be noted in passing that among infants treated with surfactant who have underlying diseases other than RDS, radiographic improvement is minimal to nonexistent (62,63).

Asymmetrical clearing (Fig. 3) is another common finding on the immediate postsurfactant radiograph (53,57,60), and it has been described with prophylactic surfactant administration (49) as well as with rescue therapy. Relative clearing is more common in the right lung than the left (53). In a few instances, this has been ascribed to endotracheal tube malposition during surfactant application (57,64), but this is probably not the case in most instances. It may be speculated that the relatively straight angle of the right main bronchus from the trachea could contribute to asymmetrical and predominantly right-sided surfactant deposition, but this explanation is not altogether satisfactory. In a study using a surfactant labeled with radioactive tracer in eight infants, no gross irregularities in deposition were noted as reflected by lung scanning (65). In a lamb model, labeled surfactant given in a prophylactic setting led to homogeneous deposition throughout the

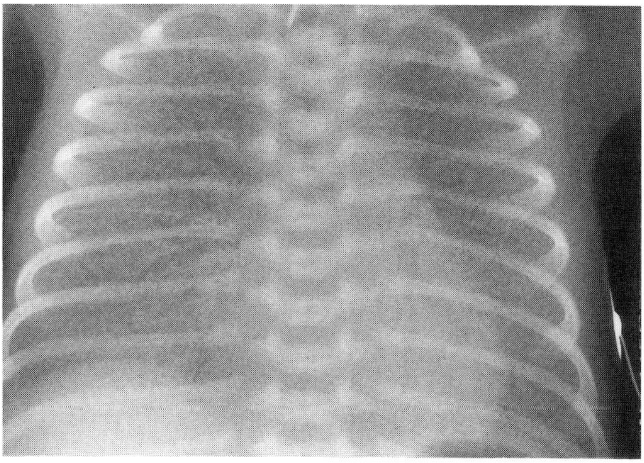

(A)

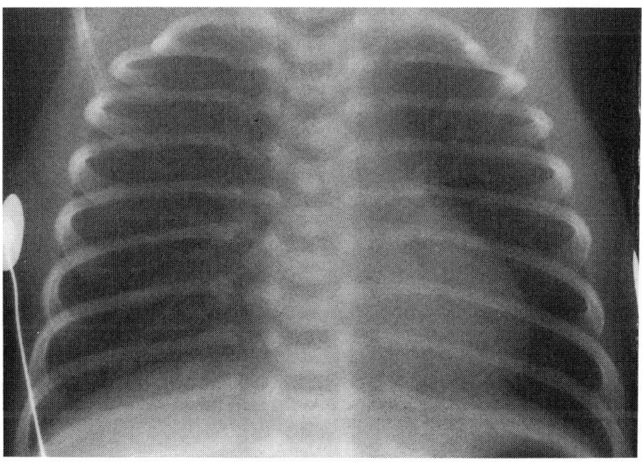

(B)

Figure 2 Effect of surfactant administered in a "rescue" protocol to two infants. A and B, radiographs exposed approximately one hour before and one hour after surfactant administration; A demonstrates severe respiratory distress syndrome, with marked subsequent clearing of both the granularity and the air bronchogram effect (B). C and D, similar radiographs of another infant; postsurfactant radiograph (D) reveals moderate clearing with persistence of some granularity and air bronchogram.

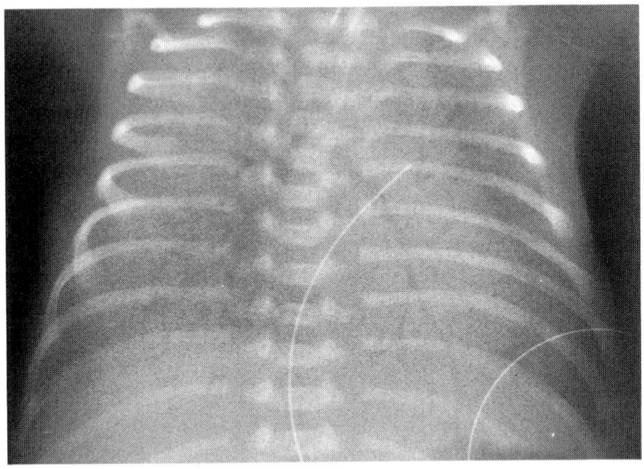

(C)

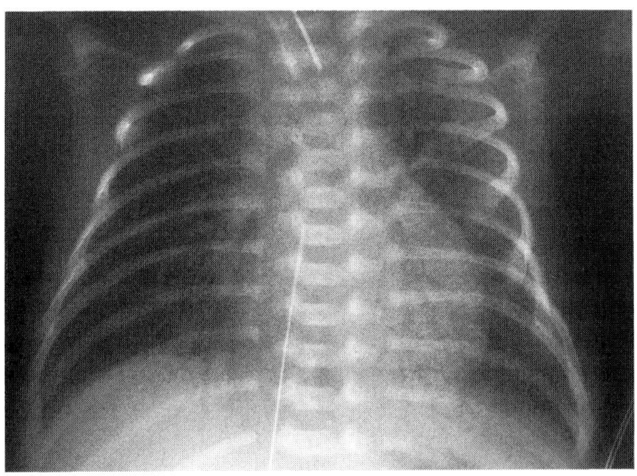

(D)

Figure 2 (*Continued*)

lungs, whereas labeled surfactant administered after mechanical ventilation was markedly inhomogeneously distributed (66). That inhomogeneous radiographic clearing occurs is unequivocal, but its etiology remains uncertain.

C. Radiographic Scoring Systems of RDS

As is quickly demonstrated to anyone who converts photographic radiographs to a digital format, the sheer bulk of information contained on a film of even the smallest infant is prodigious. Nevertheless, it is often desirable to consolidate

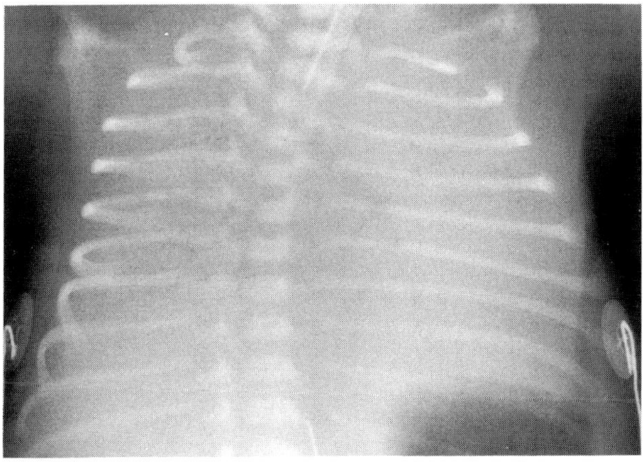

(A)

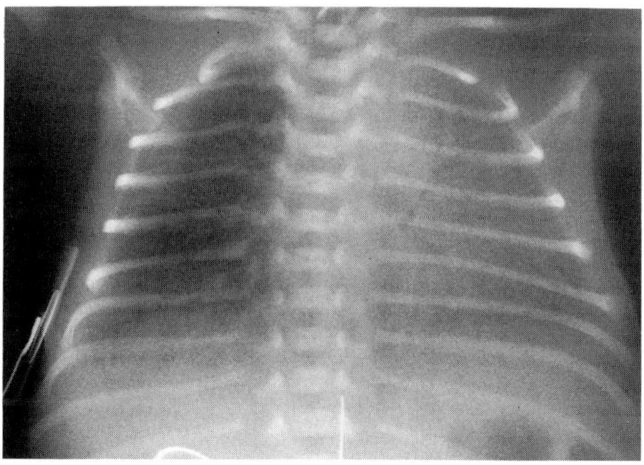

(B)

Figure 3 Asymmetrical clearing following surfactant administration to two infants. A and B are pre- and posttreatment radiographs of an infant who demonstrates primarily right-sided clearing. In the infant whose radiographs are shown in C and D, the clearing is primarily left sided, which is the less common situation.

this information to a single integer that will, it is hoped, summarize the essential information in a form that is easily understood and manipulated. In the case of RDS, which is generally observed radiographically as a diffuse pattern, such an integer might reflect the overall parenchymal density.

To this end, several scoring systems to grade the radiographic severity of RDS have been devised (4,57,67–69). These range from simple categories

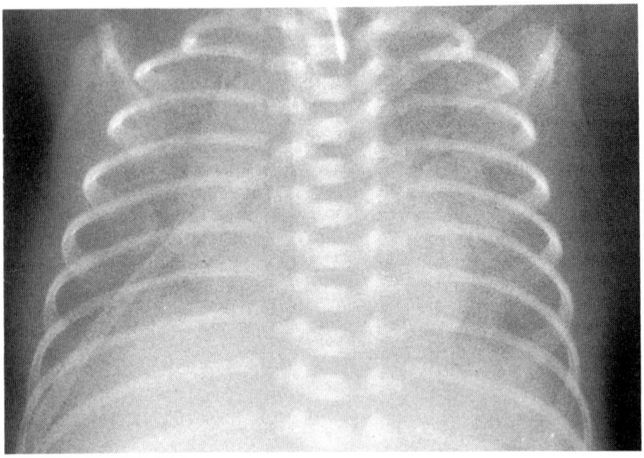

(C)

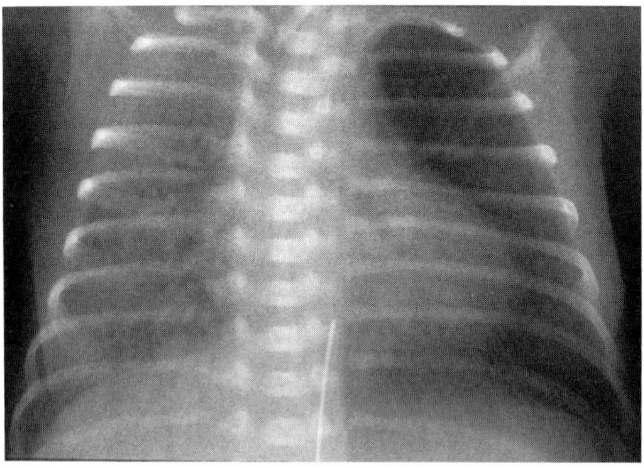

(D)

Figure 3 (*Continued*)

analogous to "mild, moderate, and severe" (48) to more elaborate assessments of specific features that constitute the radiographic findings in RDS (57,68). The more complex scoring systems offer the seeming advantage of presenting a wider numerical range of values, but in fact there is no evidence that these are any more accurate or meaningful than simple categories. In any case, these scoring systems have been widely used in an attempt to quantitate the radiographic changes that occur in infants treated with surfactant; such systems have also been employed with animal models (70).

Typically, radiographic scores are assigned to the pre- and postsurfactant radiographs and possibly to subsequent films as well (57,58). To improve the validity of such scoring, the interpreter is typically blinded to whether or not the infant has received surfactant. Potential reader bias might ideally be diminished by additionally removing identifying marks from all films of all infants, putting these in random order, and scoring them multiple times by a variety of observers, permitting assessment of intra- and interobserver variation. Generally such efforts are not made, and they would perhaps add little if they were.

Probably the most essential feature described by radiographic scores is the overall radiopacity of the pulmonary parenchyma, with worse scores reflecting increased opacity. An immediate "eyeball" assessment of lung density is usually sufficient for categorizing the patient into mild, moderate, or severe RDS. However, it must be recalled that many nonparenchymal densities are also displayed on the radiograph (see Table 3); further, variations in inspiration and filming technique can result in inaccurately ascribing the apparent radiographic parenchymal density to the actual extent of disease. For these reasons, it is probably preferable that scoring of radiographs, as well as general interpretation, be the province of trained and experienced pediatric radiologists.

Most, but not all (60), studies employing radiographic scores show a tendency for improvement from the presurfactant to the postsurfactant radiograph, and relatively favorable scores for prophylactically treated infants compared with control infants. A difficulty with scoring systems arises when there are inhomogeneities within a lung or between one lung and another; this may be dealt with by scoring each lung individually (69) or scoring individual zones within each lung (59).

Considering that lung density is the major feature used to estimate the severity of RDS, it might be appropriate to use optical techniques to evaluate changes in lung density. Indeed, densitometry has been employed with radiographs of rabbits treated with surfactant (71). Densitometry or numerical assessment using digitized radiographs offer promise of reducing observer bias, detecting more subtle changes than are appreciable with the unaided eye, and offering numerical values that are more amenable to statistical manipulation than is a discontinuously distributed set of relatively arbitrary integers.

VI. Short-Term Radiographic Findings After Exogenous Surfactant Therapy

A variety of radiographic findings may occur in the hours to few days following surfactant therapy, the more common of which are listed in Table 5. Probably the most common of these is continued radiographic clearing that follows the usual course of healing RDS, although in a milder form than would have been suggested by the pretreatment radiograph. However, in some patients, radiographic abnormalities suggesting RDS subsequently worsen (57), suggesting that endogenous and exogenous surfactant is being depleted faster than it can replenished ("relapse" of RDS). In this setting, especially if there is decreased respiratory sufficiency, subsequent applications of surfactant may be warranted.

Radiographic findings suggesting left-to-right shunting, most commonly through the PDA, are also commonly encountered (48,53,57) in infants treated with surfactant as well as in untreated infants with RDS. Such findings include enlarged central arteries, pulmonary edema that may be confused with worsening RDS, and variable cardiomegaly (26,27). These observations, none of which is pathognomonic, may be confirmed with sonography to guide medical or surgical closure of the shunt. Surfactant therapy is associated with a more frequent clinically determined need for PDA treatment (72).

Episodes of air leak (intrathoracic ectopic gas) are also commonly seen in infants treated with surfactant (53,57,58,69). The most common of these are pulmonary interstitial emphysema (PIE) and pneumothorax. Of course, as with shunting through a PDA, such air leaks are also common in infants with RDS who are not treated with surfactant. Although early findings suggested that the incidence of PIE might be higher with surfactant therapy (73), most recent studies suggest that surfactant in fact decreases the incidence of air leak (50,51,56,60,74–79). The diagnosis of PIE, which is primarily radiological, is discussed above (see Fig. 1). It should be recalled that once PIE occurs, the affected infant is at increased risk for pneumothorax and various other less common air leaks.

An early radiographic report of surfactant administration described a transient interstitial process that developed 3–4 days following surfactant treatment (57). Such a process has not been described in other reports, although "transient radiologic evidence" of BPD at 14–17 days was noted in one study (56). This phenomenon appears to be rare, and usually a fleeting interstitial prominence represents subtle PIE, iatrogenic fluid overload, or an uncommon manifestion of PDA (80).

Pulmonary hemorrhage has been noted following both rescue (75) and prophylactic (77) administration of an artificial surfactant. Radiographically, the manifestations of this potential complication are a nonspecific increase in global radiopacity (see Table 3); diagnosis is generally presumed when blood is suctioned from the endotracheal tube.

VII. Long-Term Radiographic Findings After Exogenous Surfactant Therapy

Following the crucial first several days of life, survivors of RDS, with or without surfactant therapy, may follow one of several courses (see Table 5). By far the commonest of these in infants who are able to be "weaned" from assisted ventilation is gradual radiographic clearing. During clearing, the granularity and air bronchogram of RDS are replaced by a nonspecific haziness of the pulmonary parenchyma that becomes normal within days to weeks. This progression is often interrupted by transient episodes of parenchymal opacity, usually representing fluid overload, and by focal appearances of atelectasis, which usually reflect mucous plugging. Sometimes bacterial or viral pneumonias supervene. Such episodes may require reestablishment of assisted ventilation, increasing the risk of long-term lung damage.

It is unfortunately apparent that bronchopulmonary dysplasia (BPD) still occurs despite the use of surfactant therapy (47,56,57,68,69,74,78,81). The effect of surfactant therapy on the incidence of BPD is rendered somewhat difficult to analyze by the factor of survival; infants must live long enough to develop the chronic changes of BPD. Still, most studies that have addressed this problem suggest that surfactant therapy decreases the incidence of BPD (51,75, 76) and increases survival without BPD (76,78). It is also apparent, if only from the statistical difficulties in showing a strong effect, that surfactant therapy does not represent a panacea as far as BPD is concerned.

The radiographic course and complications of BPD have been described in detail elsewhere (24). The changes that constitute BPD usually appear in an insidious manner and can be diagnosed with confidence only retrospectively. An important hallmark of these changes is that they are persistent; that is, they do not come and go from film to film. Thus, a period of time must elapse before the lung abnormalities can be appreciated as being chronic. The abnormalities themselves are by no means specific; usually they are a diffuse pattern of interstitial prominence or haziness that may initially be interpreted as fluid excess. These are seldom apparent before 2 weeks of life, and diagnosing BPD radiographically earlier than 2 weeks is fraught with hazard. Generally the changes of BPD appear in the setting of a ventilator-bound infant, with clinical findings of chronic pulmonary insufficiency.

Over subsequent weeks, the radiographic changes may worsen, stay the same, or gradually improve, seemingly depending on whether or not and how rapidly the infant can be extubated and its inspired oxygen level reduced to that of room air. During this period, cystic changes may become apparent, together with emphysema, streaks of abnormal density representing fibrosis, and secondary cardiovascular changes: stage IV BPD (23). More commonly, the radiographic picture evolves to one of diffuse, lint-like opacities with mild to no hyperinflation (Fig. 4A) (82). In some infants, a long-lived appearance of parenchymal radiopacity develops (Fig. 4B), clearing after 3–4 weeks to a more typical picture of BPD (24). The final appearance that evolves in BPD is extremely varied, ranging from nearly normal to a pattern of gross and extensive abnormalities. By and large, the patient's degree of respiratory sufficiency parallels the radiographic appearance.

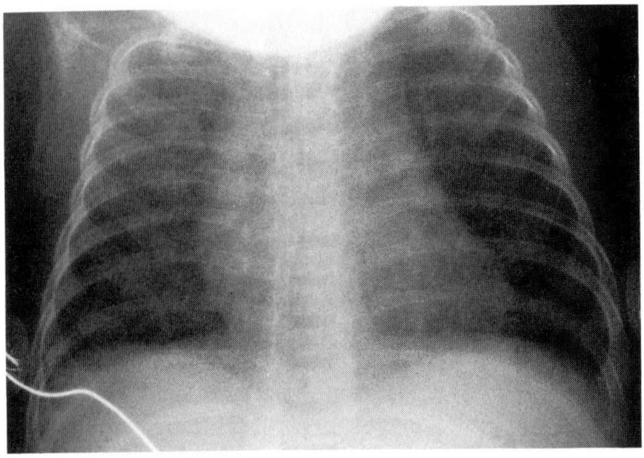

(A)

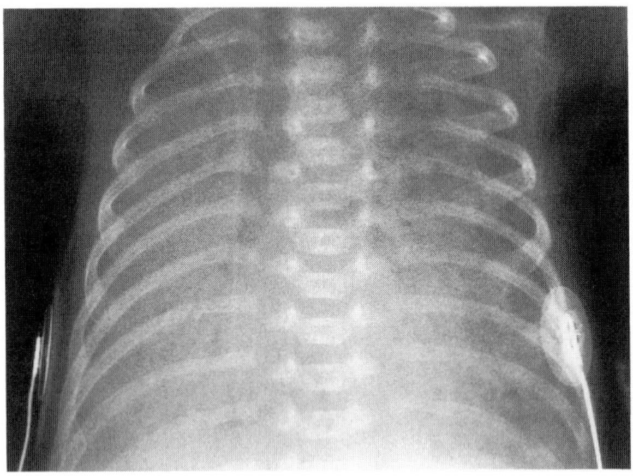

(B)

Figure 4 Bronchopulmonary dysplasia (BPD) in two infants following surfactant therapy. A, 3-month-old infant, with typical changes of mild BPD, with homogeneous, scattered, fluffy abnormal densities throughout both lungs, and mild hyperinflation. B, 1-month-old infant, near the outset of a protracted episode (duration approximately 3 weeks) of pulmonary parenchymal opacity, which ultimately cleared to a more typical appearance of moderately severe BPD.

As with RDS, it is tempting to condense the radiographic findings in BPD into a single numerical score of severity. A scoring system that I devised (83) has been fairly widely used; it provides a scale of 0–10, with 10 reflecting the severest disease. This system has a number of drawbacks beyond those intrinsic to such devices. One defect is that it was primarily based on the model of stage IV BPD as initially described by Northway and Rosan (23) and not on the generally milder variety of BPD more commonly seen today. A probable result of this is that scores among a patient population tend to be quite low or quite high, with but few scores in the middle range. A better scoring system would probably weigh the degree of disturbances of pulmonary architecture revealed on the radiograph.

It should also be noted that this scoring system is intended for infants who have been diagnosed as having BPD by clinical criteria and the presence of chronic radiographic changes. The scoring system was not intended to diagnose BPD and probably should not be so used. In other words, defining radiographic BPD by a score of 3 or more, for example, is probably faulty. Radiographic changes that might produce such a score are seen in many conditions other than BPD.

A few survivors of RDS who do not have clinical BPD demonstrate long-lived, mild, and nonspecific radiographic abnormalities. Although pathological confirmation is lacking, most likely these abnormalities represent trivial degrees of pulmonary or pleural scarring. It is doubtful that such patients should be considered as having BPD in assigning prognosis or assessing outcome of surfactant therapy or other interventions.

VIII. Conclusions

In brief, the application of surfactant usually ameliorates the usual radiographic course and complications of RDS. Surfactant generally causes radiographic clearing that is more rapid than that seen in untreated infants. Further, it tends to reduce the important complications of RDS and its therapy. However, only in rare cases does surfactant therapy seemingly cure RDS altogether, and indeed the best "cure" of RDS remains as it has been for many years: prevention of preterm delivery.

Acknowledgment

I am grateful to Dr. Saskia vW. Hilton for reviewing the manuscript.

References

1. Sahn DJ. Real-time two-dimensional Doppler echocardiographic flow mapping. Circulation 1985; 71:849–853.
2. Kero PO, Mäkinen EO. Comparison between clinical and radiological classifications of infants with respiratory distress syndrome. Eur J Pediatr 1979; 130:271–278.
3. Lischka A, Coradello H, Simbruner G, et al. Comparison of chest radiography and static respiratory compliance in the assessment of the severity of pulmonary diseases in newborns with respiratory distress. Pediatr Radiol 1984; 14:369–372.
4. Tudor J, Young L, Wigglesworth JS, Steiner RE. The value of radiology in the idiopathic respiratory distress syndrome: a radiological and pathological correlation study. Clin Radiol 1976; 27:65–75.
5. Capitanio MA, Kirkpatrick JA Jr. Roentgen examination in the evaluation of the newborn infant with respiratory distress. J Pediatr 1969; 75:896–907.
6. Faerber EN, Darling DB, Leonidas JC. Diagnosis of ill-defined pulmonary infiltrates by lateral decubitus chest radiography. Pediatrics 1983; 71:192–195.
7. Burnard ED, James LS. The cardiac silhouette in newborn infants: a cinematographic study of the normal range. Pediatrics 1961; 27:713–725.
8. Hallman M, Kankaanpaa K. Evidence of surfactant deficiency in persistence of the fetal circulation. Eur J Pediatr 1980; 134:129–134.
9. Harker LC, Merritt TA, Edwards DK III. Improving the prediction of surfactant deficiency in very low-birthweight infants with respiratory distress. J Perinatol 1992; 12:129–133.
10. Weller MH. The roentgenographic course and complications of hyaline membrane disease. Pediatr Clin North Am 1973; 20:381–406.
11. Wesenberg RL. The Newborn Chest. Hagerstown, Maryland: Harper & Row, 1973: pp. 61–68.
12. Edwards DK, Jacob J, Gluck L. The immature lung: radiographic appearance, course, and complications. AJR 1980; 135:659–666.
13. Kuhn JP, Fletcher BD, DeLemos RA. Roentgen findings in transient tachypnea of the newborn. Radiology 1969; 92:751–757.
14. Wesenberg RL, Graven SN, McCabe EB. Radiological findings in wet-lung disease. Radiology 1971; 98:69–74.
15. Jacob J, Edwards D, Gluck L. Early-onset sepsis and pneumonia observed as respiratory distress syndrome. Assessment of lung maturity. Am J Dis Child 1980; 134:766–768.
16. Foote GA, Stewart JH. The coexistence of pneumonia and the idiopathic respiratory distress syndrome in neonates. Br J Radiol 1973; 46:504–511.
17. Vollman JH, Smith WL, Ballard ET, Light IJ. Early onset group B streptococcal disease: clinical, roentgenographic, and pathologic features. J Pediatr 1976; 89:199–203.
18. Weller MH, Katzenstein AA. Radiological findings in group B streptococcal sepsis. Radiology 1976; 118:385–387.
19. Gewolb IH, Lebowitz RL, Taeusch HW Jr. Thymus size and its relationship to the respiratory distress syndrome. J Pediatr 1979; 95:108–111.
20. Edwards DK III. Skeletal growth lines seen on radiographs of newborn infants:

prevalence and possible association with obstetrical abnormalities. AJR 1993; 161:141–145.

21. Feinberg SB, Goldberg ME. Hyaline membrane disease: preclinical roentgen diagnosis. A planned study. Radiology 1957; 68:185–191.
22. Rhodes PG, Hall RT, Leonidas JC. Chronic pulmonary disease in neonates with assisted ventilation. Pediatrics 1975; 55:788–796.
23. Northway WH Jr, Rosan RC. Radiographic features of oxygen toxicity in the newborn: bronchopulmonary dysplasia. Radiology 1968; 91:49–58.
24. Edwards DK III. The radiology of bronchopulmonary dysplasia and its complications. In: Merritt TA, Northway WH, Jr., Boynton BR, eds., *Bronchopulmonary Dysplasia*, Boston, Blackwell Scientific Publications, 1988, pp. 185–234.
25. Higgins CB, Rausch J, Friedman WF, et al. Patent ductus arteriosus in preterm infants with idiopathic respiratory distress syndrome. Radiographic and echocardiographic evaluation. Radiology 1977; 124:189–195.
26. Edwards DK, Higgins CB, Merritt TA, et al. Radiographic and echocardiographic evaluation of newborns treated with indomethacin for patent ductus arteriosus. AJR 1978; 131:1009–1013.
27. Burney B, Smith WL, Franken EA Jr, et al. Chest film diagnosis of patent ductus arteriosus in infants with hyaline membrane disease. AJR 1978; 130:1149–1151.
28. Cleveland RH, Todres ID. Patterns of evolution of x-ray changes in respiratory distress syndrome. Helv Paediatr Acta 1981; 36:43–53.
29. Swischuk LE. Bubbles in hyaline membrane disease. Differentiation of three types. Radiology 1977; 122:417–426.
30. Brewer LL, Moskowitz PS, Carrington CB, Bensch KG. Pneumatosis pulmonalis. Am J Pathol 1979; 95:171–190.
31. Harris H. Pulmonary pseudocysts in the newborn infant. Pediatrics 1977; 59:199–204.
32. Clarke TA, Edwards DK. Pulmonary pseudocysts in newborn infants with respiratory distress syndrome. AJR 1979; 133:417–421.
33. Fletcher BD, Outerbridge EW, Youssef S, Bolande RP. Pulmonary interstitial emphysema in a newborn infant treated by lobectomy. Pediatrics 1974; 54:808–811.
34. Drew JH, Landau LI, Acton CM, et al. Pulmonary interstitial emphysema requiring lobectomy: complication of assisted ventilation. Arch Dis Child 1978; 53:424–426.
35. Stocker JT, Madewell JE. Persistent interstitial pulmonary emphysema: another complication of the respiratory distress syndrome. Pediatrics 1977; 59:847–857.
36. Moseley JE. Loculated pneumomediastinum in the newborn. A thymic "spinnaker sail" sign. Radiology 1960; 75:788–790.
37. Bowen A III, Quattromani FL. Infraazygous pneumomediastinum in the newborn. AJR 1980; 135:1017–1021.
38. Volberg FM Jr, Everett CJ, Brill PW. Radiologic features of inferior pulmonary ligament air collections in neonates with respiratory distress. Radiology 1979; 130:357–360.
39. Fletcher BD. Medial herniation of the parietal pleura: a useful sign of pneumothorax in supine neonates. AJR 1978; 130:469–472.
40. Swischuk LE. Two lesser known but useful signs of neonatal pneumothorax. AJR 1976; 127:523–627.

41. Moskowitz PS, Griscom NT. The medial pneumothorax. Radiology 1976; 120:143–147.
42. Ivey HH, Kattwinkel J, Alford BA. Subvisceral pleural air in neonates with respiratory distress. Am J Dis Child 1981; 135:544–546.
43. Higgins CB, Broderick TW, Edwards DK, Shumaker A. The hemodynamic significance of massive pneumopericardium in preterm infants with respiratory distress syndrome. Clinical and experimental observations. Radiology 1979; 133:363–368.
44. Kogutt M. Systemic air embolism secondary to respiratory therapy in the neonate: six cases including one survivor. AJR 1978; 131:425–429.
45. Edwards DK, Higgins CB, Gilpin EA. The cardiothoracic ratio in newborn infants. AJR 1981; 136:907–913.
46. Tarnow-Mordi W. OSIRIS trial [letter]. Lancet 1993; 341:174.
47. Soll RF, Hoekstra RE, Fangman JJ, et al. Ross Collaborative Surfactant Prevention Study Group. Multicenter trial of single-dose modified bovine surfactant extract (Survanta) for prevention of respiratory distress syndrome. Ross Collaborative Surfactant Prevention Study Group. Pediatrics 1990; 85:1092–1102.
48. Wood BP, Sinkin RA, Kendig JW, et al. Exogenous lung surfactant: effect on radiographic appearance in premature infants. Radiology; 1987; 165:11–13.
49. Clarke EA, Siegle RL, Gong AK. Findings on chest radiographs after prophylactic pulmonary surfactant treatment of premature infants. AJR 1989; 153:799–802.
50. Merritt TA, Hallman M, Berry C, et al. Randomized, placebo-controlled trial of human surfactant given at birth versus rescue administration in very low birth weight infants with lung immaturity. J Pediatr 1991; 118:581–594.
51. Merritt TA, Hallman M, Bloom BT, et al. Prophylactic treatment of very premature infants with human surfactant. N Eng J Med 1986; 315:785–790.
52. Vaucher YE, Harker L, Merritt TA, et al. Outcome at twelve months of adjusted age in very low birth weight infants with lung immaturity: A randomized, placebo-controlled trial of human surfactant. J Pediatr 1993; 122:126–132.
53. Bick U, Müller-Leisse C, Tröger J, et al. Therapeutic use of surfactant in neonatal respiratory distress syndrome. Correlation between pulmonary X-ray changes and clinical data. Pediatr Radiol 1992; 22:169–173.
54. Tamura M, Kawano T. The effect of reconstituted bovine surfactant on pulmonary mechanics in infants with respiratory distress syndrome. Acta Paediatr Jpn 1989; 31:734–741.
55. Couser RJ, Ferrara TB, Ebert J, et al. Effects of exogenous surfactant therapy on dynamic compliance during mechanical breathing in preterm infants with hyaline membrane disease. J Pediatr 1990; 116:119–124.
56. Büky B, Dévai G, Várady E, et al. Treatment of severe hyaline membrane disease with surfactant (Curosurf). A collaborative clinical study. Acta Paediatr Hung 1990; 30:351–365.
57. Edwards DK, Hilton SvW, Merritt TA, et al. Respiratory distress syndrome treated with human surfactant: radiographic findings. Radiology 1985; 157:329–334.
58. Levine D, Edwards DK III, Merritt TA. Synthetic vs. human surfactants in the treatment of respiratory distress syndrome: radiographic findings. AJR 1991; 157:371–374.

59. Namgung R, Lee C, Suh JS, et al. Exogenous surfactant replacement therapy of hyaline membrane disease in premature infants. Yonsei Med J 1989; 30:355–366.
60. Soll RF, Horbar JD, Griscom NT, et al. Radiographic findings associated with surfactant treatment. Am J Perinatol 1991; 8:114–118.
61. Horbar JD, Wright LL, Soll RF, et al. A multicenter randomized trial comparing two surfactants for the treatment of neonatal respiratory distress syndrome. J Pediatr 1993; 123:757–766.
62. Auten RL, Notter RH, Kendig JW, et al. Surfactant treatment of full-term newborns with respiratory failure. Pediatrics 1991; 87:101–107.
63. Lotze A, Knight GR, Martin GR, et al. Improved pulmonary outcome after exogenous surfactant therapy for respiratory failure in term infants requiring extracorporeal membrane oxygenation. J Pediatr 1993; 122:261–268.
64. Svenningsen N, Robertson B, Andreason B, et al. Endotracheal administration of surfactant in very low birth weight infants with respiratory distress syndrome. Crit Care Med 1987; 15:918–922.
65. Charon A, Taeusch HW, Fitzgibbon C, et al. Factors associated with surfactant treatment response in infants with severe respiratory distress syndrome. Pediatrics 1989; 83:348–354.
66. Jobe A, Ikegami M, Jacobs H, Jones S. Surfactant and pulmonary blood flow distributions following treatment of premature lambs with natural surfactant. J Clin Invest 1984; 76:848–856.
67. Giedion A, Haefliger H, Dangel P. Acute pulmonary X-ray changes in hyaline membrane disease treated with artificial ventilation and positive end-expiratory pressure (PEP). Pediatr Radiol 1973; 1:145–152.
68. Kwong MS, Egan EA, Notter RH, Shapiro DL. Double-blind clinical trial of calf lung surfactant extract for the prevention of hyaline membrane disease in extremely premature infants. Pediatrics 1985; 76:585–592.
69. Mortensson W, Noack G, Curstedt T, et al. Radiologic observations in severe neonatal respiratory distress syndrome treated with the isolated phospholipid fraction of natural surfactant. Acta Radiol 1987; 28:389–394.
70. Shimada S, Raju TN, Vidyasagar D, et al. Chest radiographic course after exogenous surfactant therapy in baboons with respiratory distress syndrome. Crit Care Med 1990; 18:969–973.
71. Enhörning G, Robertson B. Densitometric evaluation of lung aeration in chest films. Acta Radiol Diagn 1976; 17:413–416.
72. Heldt GP, Pesonen E, Merritt TA, et al. Closure of the ductus arteriosus and mechanics of breathing in preterm infants after surfactant replacement therapy. Pediatr Res 1989; 25:305–310.
73. Halliday HL, McClure G, Reid MM, et al. Controlled trial of artificial surfactant to prevent respiratory distress syndrome. Lancet 1984; 1(8375):476–478.
74. Speer CP, Harms K, Müller U, et al. Behandlung des schweren Atemnotsyndroms Frühgeborener mit natürlichem Surfactant. [Treatment of severe respiratory distress syndrome in the premature infant with natural surfactant]. Monatsschr Kinderheilkd 1988; 136:65–70.
75. Long W, Corbet A, Cotton R, et al. The American Exosurf Neonatal Study Group I. The Canadian Exosurf Neonatal Study Group. A controlled trial of synthetic

surfactant in infants weighing 1250 g or more with respiratory distress syndrome. N Eng J Med 1991; 325:1696–1703.
76. Bose C, Corbet A, Bose G, et al. Improved outcome at 28 days of age for very low birth weight infants treated with a single dose of a synthetic surfactant. J Pediatr 1990; 117:947–953.
77. Stevenson D, Walther F, Long W, et al. American Exosurf Neonatal Study Group I. Controlled trial of a single dose of synthetic surfactant at birth in premature infants weighing 500 to 699 grams. J Pediatr Supplement 1992; 120(2S):S3–S12.
78. Long W, Thompson T, Sundell H, et al. The American Exosurf Neonatal Study Group I. Effects of two rescue doses of a synthetic surfactant on mortality rate and survival without bronchopulmonary dysplasia in 700- to 1350-gram infants with respiratory distress syndrome. J Pediatr 1991; 118:595–605.
79. Enhorning G, Shennan A, Possmayer F, et al. Prevention of neonatal respiratory distress syndrome by tracheal instillation of surfactant: a randomized clinical trial. Pediatrics 1985; 76:145–153.
80. Wesenberg RL, Wax RE, Zachman RD. Varying roentgenographic patterns of patent ductus arteriosus in the newborn. AJR 1972; 114:340–349.
81. Speer CP, Harms K, Herting E, et al. Surfactant-Substitution beim schweren Atemnotsyndrom Frühgeborener < 1000 g. [Surfactant substitution in severe respiratory distress syndrome in premature infants weighing less than 1,000 g]. Geburtshilfe-Frauenheilkd 1990; 50:359–364.
82. Edwards DK. Radiographic aspects of bronchopulmonary dysplasia. J Pediatr 1979; 95:823–829.
83. Edwards DK. Radiology of hyaline membrane disease, transient tachypnea of the newborn, and bronchopulmonary dysplasia. In: Farrell PM, ed. *Lung Development: Biological and Clinical Perspectives, Vol. II*. New York, Academic Press, 1982, pp. 47–89.

25

Cardiovascular Effects of Surfactant Replacement with Special Reference to the Patent Ductus Arteriosus

GAD ALPAN
Johns Hopkins Bayview Medical Center
and Johns Hopkins University
School of Medicine
Baltimore, Maryland

RONALD I. CLYMAN
University of California, San Francisco
San Francisco, California

I. Introduction

Many studies have been conducted in animals and humans on the pulmonary effects of surfactant administration in sick premature babies. However, little attention has been paid, either in experimental animal work or in human studies, to the cardiovascular effects of surfactant administration. For example, of the 28 randomized trials of surfactant treatment in premature babies reviewed here, none reported data on even as simple a measurement as arterial blood pressure, and in only two trials was the incidence of hypotension published.

Our purpose in this chapter is to review the experimental data on the cardiovascular effects attending surfactant treatment in premature animals and humans. For the purpose of this analysis, surfactants containing animal-derived materials are grouped under "natural surfactants," whereas those not containing chemicals derived from animal products are grouped under "synthetic surfactants."

II. Effects of Surfactant Administration on Cardiac Output and Systemic Circulation

In premature lambs with respiratory distress, treatment with natural (sheep-derived) surfactant did not affect cardiac output in the first few hours following surfactant administration (1). Also, there were no changes in kidney, gastrointestinal, hepatic, or cerebral blood flow following surfactant administration. The findings were similar in premature baboons treated with surfactant and studied over a period of 1 day (2). In another study of premature baboons (3), administration of bovine surfactant (Surfactant-TA) was followed by a transient increase in cardiac output 3 hr following treatment, with a return to pretreatment values 7 hr after surfactant administration. The increase in cardiac output was attributed to the patent ductus arteriosus (PDA).

Mean aortic blood pressure was unaffected by natural surfactant administration to premature lambs studied for 3 hr (1) and 9 hr (4) following treatment, and similar findings were noted in premature baboons studied over 3 days (5). In sick premature human infants, administration of surfactant (Curosurf) caused a small, transient rise in blood pressure, which was neither clinically nor statistically significant; within 30 min there was no difference in blood pressure between surfactant-treated babies and controls (6). After surfactant, the descending aortic pulsatility index rose, but it returned to baseline by 6 hr following surfactant treatment; the rise was attributed to a transient PDA shunt, although there were no clinical signs of a PDA. Similar minor transient (20–30 min) increases in blood pressure were noted in premature babies treated with Exosurf (7) and bovine surfactant (8). In one study, rapid administration of Curosurf was followed by a small decrease in mean arterial blood pressure with a subsequent gradual rise; but at 20 min following surfactant administration, mean blood pressure was still lower (median change of 5 mmHg) than baseline (9). Because the study ended at 20 min, how long it took for the blood pressure to return to baseline values is not known.

In summary: Careful administration of surfactant appears to have little effect on cardiac output, systemic blood flow, or systemic blood pressure (excluding its possible effects on the ductus arteriosus left-to-right shunt, discussed below).

III. Effects of Surfactant on the Pulmonary Circulation

A. Pulmonary Hemorrhage

Concerns about transient, rapid increases in pulmonary blood flow following surfactant administration have existed since the first accounts of pulmonary hemorrhage were reported in 1990 (10). Pulmonary hemorrhage is frequently associated with increased pulmonary blood volume, and it is thought to be due to increased pulmonary blood flow via the ductus arteriosus. Although a recent meta-analysis of the incidence of pulmonary hemorrhage in controlled trials of exogenous surfactant therapy found that the rate of pulmonary hemorrhage was low (<5% of infants with respiratory distress syndrome [RDS]), there was a small but significant increase in this risk when surfactant was used (11). However, this increased risk of pulmonary hemorrhage following surfactant therapy could not be explained solely on the basis of differences in the rate of occurrence of PDA among the trials (11). To really determine whether there was a relationship between PDA and pulmonary hemorrhage, one would need to know the PDA status among those infants with and without pulmonary hemorrhage; unfortunately, such data were not published in the reported trials. It is interesting to note, however, that the group of trials associated with an increased risk of PDA following surfactant (the prophylactic synthetic surfactant trials—see Section IV) was also the group of trials with an increased risk for pulmonary hemorrhage (11). On the other hand, it still is possible that the increased risk of pulmonary hemorrhage following surfactant treatment may be unrelated to pulmonary blood flow and may be due to some cytolytic activity of surfactant; this has recently been demonstrated in vitro (12).

B. Studies of the Pulmonary Circulation

In sick premature lambs that were treated with natural (sheep) surfactant, pulmonary arterial pressure fell transiently (<1 hr) following surfactant administration and then returned to baseline (1). In another study, using younger premature lambs, the untreated control lambs had a progressive increase in pulmonary vascular resistance (compared with systemic resistance) as their pulmonary function deteriorated (13). In the lambs treated with natural sheep surfactant, there was no progressive increase in pulmonary vascular resistance. In this study, the ductus arteriosus was widely patent in both groups of lambs. As a result, surfactant-treated lambs had a greater blood flow to the lungs via the ductus arteriosus when compared with the untreated controls. In premature baboons treated with Surfactant-TA, a significant increase in pulmonary blood flow also was noted 3 hr following treatment (3). Pulmonary blood flow returned to baseline 7 hr following surfactant treatment and did not differ from that of untreated control animals.

In an uncontrolled study in 10 preterm infants with RDS, pulmonary arterial pressure was assessed by Doppler echocardiography immediately before and 45 min after surfactant (Exosurf) instillation (14). Surfactant administration was associated with an average 18.5% decrease in systolic pulmonary arterial pressure (PAP) despite patency of the ductus. In some of these infants, PAP was measured 12 hr after surfactant instillation and was found by then to have returned to baseline values. The same investigators repeated this study with matched controls (15). Again, surfactant administration resulted in a significant decrease (average 20%) in systolic PAP in all infants. These changes persisted for at least 1 hr (the duration of the study) and were significant when compared with baseline pretreatment measurements and to untreated controls who were assessed before and after routine endotracheal suctioning. In six of the surfactant-treated and in four of the untreated control infants there had been right-to-left ductus shunting. Following surfactant treatment, this shunting disappeared in four of the surfactant-treated babies but in no control infants.

In a single small study, effective pulmonary blood flow (i.e., that which perfuses ventilated alveoli) was measured using fluorocarbon inhalation. Treatment of infants with surfactant (Exosurf) was associated with an 18% increase in effective pulmonary blood flow, but owing to the small study size, this failed to achieve statistical significance (16).

In premature infants treated with porcine surfactant, no change in pulmonary blood flow measurements were observed between pre- and postsurfactant treatment or between surfactant-treated babies and untreated controls during a 4-hr observation period (17). However, this study had no information about ductus patency, and pulmonary blood flow was assumed to be proportional to Doppler ultrasound measurements of aortic valve flow velocity. Moreover, the study was small and designed to detect the presence of large (threefold) changes in pulmonary blood flow. It easily could have missed detecting significant, albeit less dramatic, changes in pulmonary blood flow. Similarly, a study using human amniotic surfactant in premature babies found no difference in pulmonary blood flow between infants who had received surfactant and untreated controls (18). Doppler ultrasound studies were performed at 6-hr intervals and could have missed transient changes in pulmonary blood flow.

In summary: Experiments in animals demonstrate that when pulmonary vascular resistance is elevated owing to poor lung expansion, surfactant administration may cause a decrease in this abnormal resistance. As a result, pulmonary blood flow may increase transiently following surfactant treatment. This may be due to the decreased afterload on the right ventricle. If the ductus arteriosus is patent, this also may be due to an increased left-to-right ductus shunt. The limited evidence from clinical studies suggests that these changes in pulmonary vascular resistance may be less dramatic in preterm human infants. This would result in only small changes in pulmonary blood flow.

IV. Effects of a Patent Ductus Arteriosus on the Efficiency of Surfactant Treatment

When the ductus arteriosus is widely patent, the pulmonary vasculature is exposed to systemic blood pressure and increased pulmonary blood flow. The elevated microvascular perfusion pressure that results from a PDA is more likely to increase interstitial and alveolar lung fluid in preterm infants who have RDS because of their low plasma oncotic pressure and increased capillary and epithelial permeability (19). Leakage of plasma proteins into the alveolar space inhibits both endogenous and exogenous surfactant function and increases surface tension in the immature air sacs (20). Experiments performed in preterm lambs with a PDA have shown that patency of the ductus arteriosus is indeed associated with increased fluid and protein movement from the lung vasculature into the interstitium (21). This appears to be due to the increase in pulmonary microvascular filtration pressure associated with an open ductus and not to an increase in surface area or permeability of the vasculature (21). However, the early increase in fluid filtration and protein extravasation appears to be compensated by an increase in lung lymph flow that clears the interstitial fluid and protein. As a result, no net increase in lung water or protein accumulation has been observed when exposure to a PDA has been studied during the first 24 hr after delivery (22,23). As would be expected from these findings, the presence of a large PDA has not been shown to affect the pulmonary mechanics of preterm lambs treated with natural sheep surfactant during the first 24 hr after delivery (23). Similarly, closure of the ductus arteriosus, by either ligation or indomethacin, did not affect pulmonary mechanical function during the first 72 hr after delivery in premature baboons with RDS given Surfactant-TA (5). In another study, using premature baboons with RDS, no association was found between the degree of left-to-right shunting through the PDA and pulmonary response to Survanta (24). The compensatory increase in lung lymph flow, demonstrated in preterm lambs (21), acts as an "edema safety factor," inhibiting fluid accumulation in the lungs. However, if lung lymphatic drainage is impaired, as it may be in the presence of pulmonary interstitial emphysema or fibrosis, the likelihood of edema would increase. Because surfactant therapy is most often limited to the first 24 hr after delivery, which is usually before the onset of impaired lymphatic drainage, the effect of exogenous surfactant on lung mechanics does not appear to be altered by the presence of a large PDA.

Not all of the changes associated with a PDA are necessarily detrimental to the immature infant with respiratory distress syndrome. In fact, following closure of a PDA, decreases in systemic arterial O_2 content have been observed despite no alteration in pulmonary mechanics (23,25). This phenomenon is due to recirculation of arterial blood through partially expanded lungs and suggests that continued ductus patency after birth may serve a temporary but useful function in infants whose lungs are not fully expanded. On the other hand, changes in left-to-right shunt through the ductus due to unrecognized changes in ductal patency (or pulmonary vascular resistance when the ductus arteriosus is patent) may confound the interpretation of arterial Po_2 values, which are commonly, although mistakenly, assumed to reflect only what is happening to the pulmonary air spaces (26). For example, a study aimed at identifying factors that influence the response to treatment with surfactant (Curosurf) found that the group of infants who had a good response measured by the arterial/alveolar oxygen tension ratio (a/A Po_2) 24 hr after treatment also had a higher incidence of PDA compared with the group of infants who responded poorly or to the group of infants whose response was intermediate. This finding was confounded, however, by the fact that those who responded well also had a somewhat higher a/A Po_2 prior to surfactant treatment. Whether this reflected better initial gas exchange or a larger left-to-right ductus shunt was not mentioned in the study. Nevertheless, it appears that the presence of a PDA is *not* associated with a *poor* arterial Po_2 response to surfactant (27).

In summary: Based on a limited number of animal and human studies, there is no evidence that a left-to-right ductus shunt affects the efficiency of surfactant treatment of RDS.

V. Effects of Surfactant on Persistent Patency of the Ductus Arteriosus

The factors regulating ductus patency and closure in the preterm infant have been reviewed previously (28). In 1980, Fujiwara et al. (29) reported that of 10 infants treated with surfactant, 9 developed signs and symptoms of a PDA. Since then considerable concern has persisted as to whether surfactant treatment would be associated with an increased incidence of problematic ductus left-to-right shunts.

Jobe et al. (1) found that in premature lambs (133–136 days' gestation; full term is 145 days), the mean left-to-right ductus shunt was similar before and after instillation of natural sheep surfactant. Clyman et al. (13) studied younger premature lambs (120–124 days' gestation) and found an increased left-to-right ductus shunt when comparing lambs treated with natural surfactant with untreated control lambs. In these very young lambs, the ductus was widely patent in both groups. Surfactant treatment altered the relationship between pulmonary to systemic vascular resistances. In the untreated animals, continued respiratory failure was associated with persistent acidosis and an increased pulmonary vascular resistance relative to systemic resistance. The surfactant-treated animals, however, had no deterioration of the ratio of pulmonary to systemic vascular resistance. In the face of a widely patent ductus arteriosus, the ductus left-to-right shunt is determined by the relationship between pulmonary and systemic vascular resistances; therefore, surfactant-treated animals had a larger left-to-right shunt. Surfactant administration did not affect ductus resistance. Both in vivo and in vitro studies of isolated ductus tissue showed similar ductus contractile behavior and rate of prostaglandin E_2 (PGE_2) synthesis in specimens obtained from both surfactant-treated and control lambs (13).

Administration of Surfactant-TA to premature baboons with RDS was similarly associated with a larger left-to-right ductus shunt 2 hr following surfactant administration (3); ductus shunt was assessed only once during the course of the study. The same investigators conducted another study in premature baboons with RDS treated with Surfactant-TA (5). Surfactant treatment was associated with an earlier, but not necessarily larger, left-to-right PDA shunt. In contrast, the left-to-right PDA shunt in premature baboons treated at birth with natural (baboon) surfactant did not differ from that in untreated control animals when examined at 3, 8, and 23 hr after delivery (2).

In infants treated with human amniotic surfactant, surfactant treatment did not alter the time course of spontaneous or induced closure of PDA with indomethacin (18). The surfactant-treated babies had no greater incidence or larger amounts of a left-to-right shunt than control infants. Surfactant treatment was associated, however, with more frequent overall treatment of PDA; that is, there was a greater perceived need to treat PDA.

In a randomized trial to assess the effects of surfactant (Survanta) on RDS in premature neonates, Reller et al. (30,31) evaluated the effects of surfactant on various manifestations of ductus patency. Diagnosis of PDA was made by Doppler echocardiography, but decisions to treat were made by the neonatal staff, who were unaware of the daily investigational echocardiograms. A similar number of infants from surfactant-treated and control groups received indomethacin in the first 4 days after birth. In those who did not receive indomethacin soon after birth, a similar number of infants from both groups demonstrated spontaneous physiological closure of their PDA. Of those infants who still had a PDA more than 4 days after birth, a similar number from both groups had later spontaneous closure, and requirements for treatments (indomethacin or ligation) were similar. The reduction in ventilatory support with surfactant was present even in the subgroup with persistent ductus patency. Of particular interest was the finding that although surfactant treatment did not affect the incidence of left-to-right PDA shunt, neonates receiving surfactant had a greater tendency to develop audible murmurs.

Although the reduction in pulmonary vascular resistance and pressure following surfactant is thought to increase the left-to-right shunt through the PDA, equally compelling arguments suggest that surfactant may reduce PDA shunts. The improvement in oxygenation may enhance ductus constriction. Furthermore, elevated pulmonary arterial pressure opposes ductus constriction, whereas a drop in pulmonary arterial pressure may facilitate its closure (32).

We therefore carried out a meta-analysis of surfactant trials with the aim of analyzing whether surfactant treatment affects the incidence of PDA. Studies included were those that (1) were in English, (2) were randomized and controlled, (3) included data on incidence of PDA in treated and control groups, (4) had information on diagnostic criteria for PDA, and (5) were independent of each other (i.e., no preliminary reports, for example). Summary odds ratios (estimating relative risks) and their 95% confidence interval (CI) were calculated using the Peto method (33,34). This takes into account variations in sample sizes among the trials. Twenty-eight trials were included in this meta-analysis (a total of 6117 patients). These consisted of 7 trials of prophylaxis with synthetic surfactants (10,35–40), 3 trials of rescue treatment with synthetic surfactant (40–42), 7 trials of prophylaxis with natural surfactants (43–49), and 11 trials of rescue treatment with natural surfactants (50–60).

The meta-analysis of the 28 trials is summarized in Fig. 1. Taken together, all the trials (resuce and prophylaxis, with both synthetic and natural surfactants) did not show an increased risk of PDA in treated versus untreated infants. Similarly, there was no significant difference in PDA occurrence in treated versus control patients in the natural surfactant trials (prophylaxis and rescue) or in the synthetic surfactant trials (prophylaxis and rescue). However, there was a decreased risk of PDA in the combined (natural and synthetic) surfactant rescue trials; as can be seen in Fig. 1, this was due to a substantially reduced risk of PDA in the synthetic surfactant rescue trials. On the other hand, there was an

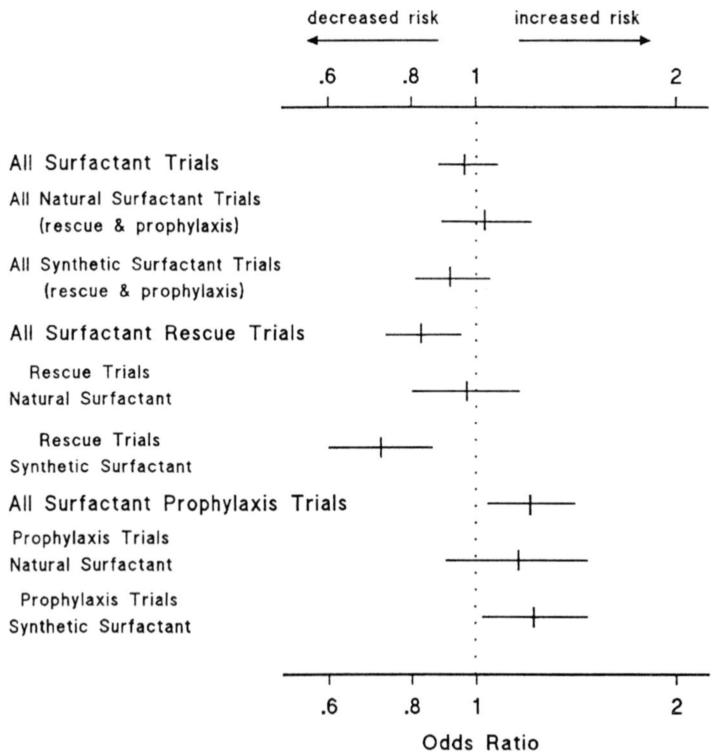

Figure 1 Odds ratio with 95% confidence interval for the incidence of PDA in various surfactant treatment groups. Numbers derived by meta-analysis of 28 randomized controlled studies (references in text).

increased risk of PDA in surfactant-treated infants in the combined (natural and synthetic) surfactant prophylaxis trials; this was due to the increased risk of PDA occurrence in infants treated with synthetic surfactant prophylactically.

The decreased risk of PDA in infants receiving synthetic surfactant as a rescue treatment is attributable to one large study that had this finding (42). This study consisted of 70% of the patients in the synthetic surfactant rescue trials and found an 8% reduction in incidence of PDA with surfactant rescue treatment. A second synthetic surfactant rescue trial found a 9% reduction in incidence of PDA (41), but because of the smaller study size, this was not statistically significant. The smallest of the synthetic surfactant rescue studies (40) reported essentially no difference in PDA incidence between surfactant-treated infants and controls.

In the trials of prophylactic treatment with synthetic surfactants, none of the individual trials found a statistically significant difference in incidence of PDA between treated babies and controls. Surfactant treatment was associated with an average increase of 6.4% in rate of occurrence of PDA (range: 0–19%). The two studies that noted the greatest increase in PDA incidence with surfactant treatment (39,40) (increased incidence of 10 and 19%, respectively) were also the two smallest studies in this group of trials; thus, this finding may have reflected sampling variability.

Of the 28 trials reviewed here, only two individual studies showed a statistically significant difference in incidence of PDA. One was the previously mentioned synthetic surfactant rescue trial (42) in which there was a reduced risk of PDA associated with surfactant treatment. The other was the small study of Surfactant-TA given as a rescue to premature babies with RDS (57). In this study, surfactant treatment was associated with an increased incidence of PDA. However, in this study, improvement in oxygenation occurred early (<24 hr), but the mean age at diagnosis of PDA was 2.9 days. The small size of this study (17 patients treated and 13 controls) also makes it more susceptible to sampling variations.

In all of the surfactant trials reviewed, the diagnosis of PDA was based on physical findings. Occasional confirmation was obtained by echocardiography. The limitations of clinical signs for detecting the presence of a patent ductus arteriosus (61) and of Doppler ultrasound for determining the magnitude of a left-to-right ductus shunt (62) are well known. This is especially so in the very low birth weight infant (63–65), who is at greatest risk for RDS and therefore the likeliest candidate for surfactant treatment. Thus, the incidence of PDA in these trials actually reflects the incidence of certain clinical signs at best. Surfactant treatment may affect the clinical signs of a left-to-right ductus shunt more than it affects the incidence of such a shunt.

In summary: The animal and human studies reviewed above suggest that surfactant treatment is not necessarily associated with an increased incidence of ductus patency; however, it may be associated with an increased incidence of certain clinical signs of a PDA, which may affect the decision of when to treat a PDA in a clinical setting. The magnitude of the left-to-right ductus shunt appears to be determined by factors that influence pulmonary and systemic vascular resistances. These factors and the various ventilatory strategies used may explain some of the variability obtained in the results of the experimental studies. For example, human infants with respiratory distress are usually not allowed to become as acidotic or hypoxemic as are preterm animals. The more abnormal the pretreatment blood gas values have been in the animal studies, the greater the change in pulmonary vascular resistance and the greater the subsequent left-to-right shunt has been following correction of the blood gases with surfactant treatment. Presumably the change in pulmonary vascular resistance and the change in ductus shunting following surfactant treatment in human infants is much less impressive. It is worthwhile to note that the study reporting the greatest increase in symptoms of a left-to-right ductus shunt following surfactant treatment also studied infants with the greatest degree of acidosis and hypoxemia prior to treatment (29). In our opinion, there is little evidence that the incidence of PDA is increased in babies treated with any of the available surfactants; if there is such an effect, it must be very small.

Speculation: A recent review by Konishi et al. (66) of the use of Surfactant-TA during the past decade showed that the incidence of PDA in surfactant-treated babies in 1987–1991 was considerably lower than in surfactant-treated babies treated during 1982–1986. Similarly, the European Multicentre Study of Curosurf recently reviewed its original experience with Curosurf and compared it with its subsequent experience (27,50). In their extended study, the incidence of PDA was 35% (compared with 53% in the original trial; $p < 0.05$). This decrease occurred despite the fact that the later study was carried out at the same centers and with infants with similar entry characteristics as those in the original randomized trial. In our opinion, these figures may well reflect changes in various practices (e.g., fluid balance, colloid administration) that affect the incidence of PDA and attend the initial treatment of the sick premature baby. It may be that these "extrapulmonary" therapies affect the incidence of PDA rather than surfactant administration per se.

Acknowledgments

The authors wish to thank Paul Sagan for his skillful editorial assistance. This work was supported in part by a grant from the U.S. Public Health Service, National Heart, Lung and Blood Institute HL 46691, and by a gift from Perinatal Associates Research Foundation.

References

1. Jobe A, Jacobs H, Ikegami M, Jones S. Cardiovascular effects of surfactant suspensions given by tracheal instillation to premature lambs. Pediatr Res 1983; 17:444–448.
2. Kinsella JP, Gerstmann DR, Gong AK, et al. Ductal shunting and effective systemic blood flow following single dose surfactant treatment in the premature baboon with hyaline membrane disease. Biol Neonate 1991; 60:283–291.
3. Vidyasagar D, Maeta H, Raju TN, et al. Bovine surfactant (surfactant TA) therapy in immature baboons with hyaline membrane disease. Pediatrics 1985; 75:1132–1142.
4. Durand DJ, Clyman RI, Heymann MA, et al. Effects of a protein-free synthetic surfactant on the survival and pulmonary function of preterm lambs. J Pediatr 1985; 107:775–780.
5. Shimada S, Raju TNK, Bhat R, et al. Treatment of patent ductus arteriosus after exogenous surfactant in baboons with hyaline membrane disease. Pediatr Res 1989; 26:565–569.
6. van Bel F, de Winter PJ, Wijnands HB, et al. Cerebral and aortic blood flow velocity patterns in preterm infants receiving prophylactic surfactant treatment. Acta Paediatr 1992; 81:504–510.
7. van de Bor M, Ma EJ, Walther FJ. Cerebral blood flow velocity after surfactant instillation in preterm infants. J Pediatr 1991; 118:285–287.
8. Jorch G, Rabe H, Garbe M, et al. Acute and protracted effects of intratracheal surfactant application on internal carotid blood flow velocity, blood pressure and carbondioxide tension in very low birth weight infants. Eur J Pediatr 1989; 148:770–773.
9. Cowan F, Whitelaw A, Wertheim D, Silverman M. Cerebral blood flow velocity changes after rapid administration of surfactant. Arch Dis Child 1991; 66:1105–1109.
10. Bose C, Corbet A, Bose G, et al. Improved outcome at 28 days of age for very low birth weight infants treated with a single dose of a synthetic surfactant. J Pediatr 1990; 117:947–953.
11. Raju TNK, Langenberg P. Pulmonary hemorrhage and exogenous surfactant therapy—a metaanalysis. J Pediatr 1993; 123:603–610.
12. Findlay RD, Taeusch HW, David-Cu R, Walther FJ. The China syndrome: Cytolysis as a possible mechanism of pulmonary hemorrhage after surfactant treatment. Clin Res 1993; 41:95A.
13. Clyman RI, Jobe A, Heymann MA, et al. Increased shunt through the patent ductus arteriosus after surfactant replacement therapy. J Pediatr 1982; 100:101–107.
14. Kääpä P, Kero P, Saraste M. Synthetic surfactant replacement therapy decreases estimated pulmonary artery pressure in respiratory distress syndrome. Am J Dis Child 1992; 146:961–964.
15. Kääpä P, Seppanen M, Kero P, Saraste M. Pulmonary hemodynamics after synthetic surfactant replacement in neonatal respiratory distress syndrome. J Pediatr 1993; 123:115–119.
16. Milner AD. How does exogenous surfactant work? Arch Dis Child 1993; 68:253–254.

17. Halliday HL, McCord FB, McClure BG, Reid MM. Acute effects of instillation of surfactant in severe respiratory distress syndrome. Arch Dis Chil 1989; 64: 13–16.
18. Heldt GP, Pesonen E, Merritt TA, et al. Closure of the ductus arteriosus and mechanics of breathing in preterm infants after surfactant replacement therapy. Pediatr Res 1989; 25:305–310.
19. Jobe A, Ikegami M, Jacobs H, et al. Permeability of premature lamb lungs to protein and the effect of surfactant on that permeability. J Appl Physiol 1983; 55:169–176.
20. Ikegami M, Jacobs H, Jobe A. Surfactant function in respiratory distress syndrome. J Pediatr 1983; 102:443–447.
21. Alpan G, Scheerer R, Bland R, Clyman R. Patent ductus arteriosus increases lung fluid filtration in preterm lambs. Pediatr Res 1991; 30:616–621.
22. Alpan G, Mauray F, Clyman RI. Effect of patent ductus arteriosus on water accumulation and protein permeability in the premature lungs of mechanically ventilated premature lambs. Pediatr Res 1989; 26:570–575.
23. Pérez Fontán JJ, Clyman RI, Mauray F, et al. Respiratory effects of a patent ductus arteriosus in premature newborn lambs. J Appl Physiol 1987; 63:2315–2324.
24. McCumin D, Seidner S. Effects of surfactant therapy on ductus shunting in premature baboons with hyaline membrane disease. Clin Res 1992; 40:825A.
25. Clyman RI, Mauray F, Heymann MA, Roman C. Cardiovascular effects of a patent ductus arteriosus in preterm lambs with respiratory distress. J Pediatr 1987; 111:579–587.
26. Bratton DL, Mellander M, Krueger ED, et al. Influence of early indomethacin on venous admixture in infants with HMD. Pediatr Res 1984; 18:150A.
27. Collaborative European Multicentre Study Group. Factors influencing the clinical response to surfactant replacement therapy in babies with severe respiratory distress syndrome. Eur J Pediatr 1991; 150:433–439.
28. Clyman RI. Ductus arteriosus. In: Gluckman PD, Heymann MA, eds. Perinatal and Pediatric Pathophysiology: A Clinical Perspective. London: Edward Arnold, 1993:525–528.
29. Fujiwara T, Maeta H, Chida S, et al. Artificial surfactant therapy in hyaline-membrane disease. Lancet 1980; 1:55–59.
30. Reller MD, Buffkin DC, Colasurdo MA, et al. Ductal patency in neonates with respiratory distress syndrome. A randomized surfactant trial. Am J Dis Child 1991; 145:1017–1020.
31. Reller MD, Rice MJ, McDonald RW. Review of studies evaluating ductal patency in the premature infant. J Pediatr 1993; 122:S59–S62.
32. Clyman RI, Mauray F, Heymann MA, Roman C. Influence of increased pulmonary vascular pressures on the closure of the ductus arteriosus in newborn lambs. Pediatr Res 1989; 25:136–142.
33. Yusuf S, Peto R, Lewis J, et al. Beta blockade during and after myocardial infarction: An overview of the randomized trials. Prog Cardiovasc Dis 1985; 27:335–371.
34. Chalmers I, Hetherington J, Elbourne D, et al. Materials and methods used in

synthesizing evidence to evaluate the effects of care during pregnancy and childbirth. In: Enkin M, Keirse MJNC, Chalmers I, eds. Effective Care in Pregnancy and Childbirth. Oxford: Oxford University Press, 1992:39–65.

35. Stevenson D, Walther F, Long W, et al. Controlled trial of a single dose of synthetic surfactant at birth in premature infants weighing 500 to 699 grams. The American Exosurf Neonatal Study Group I. J Pediatr 1992; 120:S3–S12.
36. Corbet A, Bucciarelli R, Goldman S, et al. Decreased mortality rate among small premature infants treated at birth with a single dose of synthetic surfactant: A multicenter controlled trial. American Exosurf Pediatric Study Group 1. J Pediatr 1991; 118:277–284.
37. Morley CJ, Greenough A, Miller NG, et al. Randomized trial of artificial surfactant (ALEC) given at birth to babies from 23 to 34 weeks gestation. Early Hum Dev 1988; 17:41–54.
38. Ten Centre Study Group. Ten centre trial of artificial surfactant (artificial lung expanding compound) in very premature babies. Br Med J Clin Res Ed 1987; 294:991–996.
39. Halliday HL, McClure G, Reid MM, et al. Controlled trial of artificial surfactant to prevent respiratory distress syndrome. Lancet 1984; 1:476–478.
40. Phibbs RH, Ballard RA, Clements JA, et al. Initial clinical trial of EXOSURF, a protein-free synthetic surfactant, for the prophylaxis and early treatment of hyaline membrane disease. Pediatrics 1991; 88:1–9.
41. Long W, Thompson T, Sundell H, et al. Effects of two rescue doses of a synthetic surfactant on mortality rate and survival without bronchopulmonary dysplasia in 700- to 1350-gram infants with respiratory distress syndrome. The American Exosurf Neonatal Study Group I. J Pediatr 1991; 118:595–605.
42. Long W, Corbet A, Cotton R, et al. A controlled trial of synthetic surfactant in infants weighing 1250 g or more with respiratory distress syndrome. The American Exosurf Neonatal Study Group I, and the Canadian Exosurf Neonatal Study Group. N Engl J Med 1991; 325:1696–1703.
43. Hoekstra RE, Jackson JC, Myers TF, et al. Improved neonatal survival following multiple doses of bovine surfactant in very premature neonates at risk for respiratory distress syndrome. Pediatrics 1991; 88:10–18.
44. Enhorning G, Shennan A, Possmayer F, et al. Prevention of neonatal respiratory distress syndrome by tracheal instillation of surfactant: A randomized clinical trial. Pediatrics 1985; 76:145–153.
45. Dunn MS, Shennan AT, Zayack D, Possmayer F. Bovine surfactant replacement therapy in neonates of less than 30 weeks' gestation: A randomized controlled trial of prophylaxis versus treatment. Pediatrics 1991; 87:377–386.
46. Soll RF, Hoekstra RE, Fangman JJ, et al. Multicenter trial of single-dose modified bovine surfactant extract (Survanta) for prevention of respiratory distress syndrome. Ross Collaborative Surfactant Prevention Study Group. Pediatrics 1990; 85:1092–1102.
47. Kendig JW, Notter RH, Cox C, et al. Surfactant replacement therapy at birth: Final analysis of a clinical trial and comparisons with similar trials. Pediatrics 1988; 82:756–762.
48. Kwong MS, Egan EA, Notter RH, Shapiro DL. Double-blind clinical trial of calf

lung surfactant extract for the prevention of hyaline membrane disease in extremely premature infants. Pediatrics 1985; 76:585–592.
49. Merritt TA, Hallman M, Bloom BT, et al. Prophylactic treatment of very premature infants with human surfactant. N Engl J Med 1986; 315:785–790.
50. Collaborative European Multicenter Study Group. Surfactant replacement therapy for severe neonatal respiratory distress syndrome: An international randomized clinical trial. Pediatrics 1988; 82:683–691.
51. Lang MJ, Hall RT, Reddy NS, et al. A controlled trial of human surfactant replacement therapy for severe respiratory distress syndrome in very low birth weight infants. J Pediatr 1990; 116:295–300.
52. Gitlin JD, Soll RF, Parad RB, et al. Randomized controlled trial of exogenous surfactant for the treatment of hyaline membrane disease. Pediatrics 1987; 79:31–37.
53. Fujiwara T, Konishi M, Chida S, et al. Surfactant replacement therapy with a single postventilatory dose of a reconstituted bovine surfactant in preterm neonates with respiratory distress syndrome: Final analysis of a multicenter, double-blind, randomized trial and comparison with similar trials. The Surfactant-TA Study Group. Pediatrics 1990; 86:753–764.
54. Hallman M, Merritt TA, Jarvenpaa A-L, et al. Exogenous human surfactant for treatment of severe respiratory distress syndrome: A randomized prospective clinical trial. J Pediatr 1985; 106:963–969.
55. Horbar JD, Soll RF, Schachinger H, et al. A European multicenter randomized controlled trial of single dose surfactant therapy for idiopathic respiratory distress syndrome. Eur J Pediatr 1990; 149:416–423.
56. Horbar JD, Soll RF, Sutherland JM, et al. A multicenter randomized, placebo-controlled trial of surfactant therapy for respiratory distress syndrome. N Engl J Med 1989; 320:959–965.
57. Raju TN, Vidyasagar D, Bhat R, et al. Double-blind controlled trial of single-dose treatment with bovine surfactant in severe hyaline membrane disease. Lancet 1987; 1:651–656.
58. Gortner L, Bartmann P, Pohlandt F, et al. Early treatment of respiratory distress syndrome with bovine surfactant in very preterm infants: a multicenter controlled clinical trial. Pediatr Pulmonol 1992; 14:4–9.
59. Chen J-Y. Exogenous surfactant for treatment of respiratory distress syndrome in premature infants. J Formosan Med Assoc 1990; 89:110–114.
60. Liechty EA, Donovan E, Purohit D, et al. Reduction of neonatal mortality after multiple doses of bovine surfactant in low birth weight neonates with respiratory distress syndrome. Pediatrics 1991; 88:19–28.
61. Ellison RC, Peckham GJ, Lang P, et al. Evaluation of the preterm infant for patent ductus arteriosus. Pediatrics 1983; 71:364–372.
62. Karsdon J, Clyman RI. A comparison of continuous wave Doppler ultrasonography with microsphere measured left-to-right shunt through the patent ductus arteriosus. Crit Care Med 1983; 11:556–558.
63. Evans N, Moorcraft J. Effect of patency of the ductus arteriosus on blood pressure in very preterm infants. Arch Dis Child 1992; 67:1169–1173.
64. Evans N. Diagnosis of patent ductus arteriosus in the preterm newborn. Arch Dis Child 1993; 68:58–61.

65. Ratner I, Perelmuter B, Toews W, Whitfield J. Association of low systolic and diastolic blood pressure with significant patent ductus arteriosus in the very low birth weight infant. Crit Care Med 1985; 13:497–500.
66. Konishi M, Chida S, Shimada S, et al. Surfactant replacement therapy in premature babies with respiratory distress syndrome: Factors affecting the response to surfactant and comparison of outcome from 1982–86 and 1987–91. Acta Paediatr Jpn 1992; 34:617–630.

26

Effects of Surfactant Replacement on Cerebral Hemodynamics and Oxygenation

E. OSMUND R. REYNOLDS
University College London Medical School
London, England

ANTHONY DAVID EDWARDS
Royal Postgraduate Medical School
Hammersmith Hospital
London, England

DAVID C. McCORMICK
Royal Women's Hospital
Brisbane, Australia

I. Surfactant Deficiency and Perinatal Brain Damage

Brain damage together with respiratory illnesses are the major causes of death in preterm infants, and these infants, particularly the least mature ones, are at considerably increased risk of neurodevelopmental impairments compared with infants born at term. Much of the damage that leads to death or impairment is acquired in the perinatal period and is due to the more severe forms of periventricular hemorrhage (PVH) or to hypoxic-ischemic injury, which causes periventricular leukomalacia (PVL) (1,2).

Abnormalities of cerebral perfusion, often initiated or made worse by respiratory illness, are heavily involved in the pathogenesis of both PVH and PVL. The more severe the respiratory illness, the greater is the risk that a cerebral lesion will occur. For example, in one study carried out on infants born at less than 33 weeks' gestation, only 17% (4/23) of those without a respiratory illness developed PVH, as opposed to 25% (11 of 44) of those with illnesses which did not necessitate mechanical ventilation, 25% (6 of 24) when ventilation was required for conditions other than deficiency of surfactant, 60% (40 of 67) of those ventilated for surfactant deficiency and 87% (13 of 15) of those who acquired pneumothoraces during ventilation (4). A very wide range of obstetrical and perinatal data were collected from these infants, and when it was subjected to analysis of variance only three variables—short gestation (or low birth weight), a diagnosis of surfactant-deficient respiratory distress syndrome (RDS), and pneumothorax emerged as significant predictors of PVH, together accounting for 34% of the variance. The study was done before diagnostic cold lights had been introduced, which is probably why pneumothorax was such a powerful predictor. A number of other factors contributed to the variance, including hypotension, abnormal arterial oxygen (Pao_2) and carbon dioxide ($Paco_2$) tensions and pH, the use of mechanical ventilation, and defective hemostasis. Adverse intrapartum events did not appear to be importantly involved in the pathogenesis of PVH, although there was a trend in that direction. Many other studies have yielded broadly similar results (2,3). Information obtained from studies of animals (5) as well as clinical studies strongly indicates that the cerebral hemodynamic effects of impaired pulmonary gas exchange together with impaired autoregulation, and often acting against a background of hypotension or impaired hemostasis, are the major causal antecedents of PVH. Hypotension, often together with hypoxemia, is also probably the major antecedent of PVL (2,3). Quite frequently, PVH and PVL coexist.

Since surfactant deficiency is so clearly implicated in events which lead up to cerebral damage, it was a reasonable expectation that replacement therapy would lead to a reduction in the incidence of both PVH and PVL. Much information is available relating to PVH, which arises in the first few days of life and can very easily be visualized by ultrasonography, but so far none has appeared relating to PVL, probably because this lesion cannot be diagnosed with certainty until cystic lesions appear several weeks after the initiating insult or insults (6).

II. Surfactant Replacement and PVH

The results of randomized trials of surfactant replacement carried out up to 1991 have been analyzed in detail by Soll and McQueen (3). Meta-analyses of the effects of replacement therapy from a large number of trials show that the effects of prophylactic and rescue therapy by natural and synthetic surfactants yield broadly similar reductions in mortality rates, with typical event rate ratios (ERR) of 0.66–0.74. The pneumothorax rate was also strikingly reduced. However, the incidence of PVH was unchanged, although it was perhaps reassuring that the typical values for ERR were below zero at 0.90–0.94, implying at least that the incidence of PVH was not increased in treated infants. The data from nine trials for infants diagnosed as having "severe" PVH (blood distending the ventricles or in brain parenchyma) is particularly interesting, since these hemorrhages, unlike lesser ones, are very likely to lead to death or serious neurodevelopmental impairments in survivors (7,8). The typical ERR was 0.98.

There are numerous possible explanations why the incidence of PVH has not fallen in infants treated with surfactant. For example, the effects of a reduction in hemodynamic perturbations likely to provoke bleeding may have been balanced by the survival of infants who lived long enough to develop PVH but would otherwise have died beforehand. Or some adverse effect of giving surfactant might have counterbalanced the beneficial effects of doing so.

It is important that these issues are clarified, because the large reduction in mortality rate due to surfactant replacement together with an unchanged severe PVH rate of around 20% in treated infants—some of whom will die and others survive—raises the specter of an increase in the absolute numbers of infants surviving with serious impairments. If so, the numbers are likely to be very small as a proportion of seriously impaired children in general, and far less than the number of children who survive healthy (8).

Although, in general, the incidence of PVH has been found to be the same in surfactant-treated and control infants, the possibility has been raised that under some circumstances PVH might be provoked by treatment. The multicenter study of Horbar et al. (9) raised particular concerns. PVH occurred in 60% (31 of 52) of infants treated for established illness with an enriched extract of bovine lung (Survanta) compared with 27% (14 of 52) of controls. More importantly, hemorrhages graded as severe were found in 39% (20 of 52) of treated versus 15% (8 of 52) of control infants (ERR 2.5). The importance of investigating the cerebral hemodynamic effects of surfactant administration was highlighted by this study in case the procedure or some unexpected mechanical or pharmacological effect was capable of causing serious perturbations which might lead to PVH.

III. Investigations of Cerebral Hemodynamics and Oxygenation

Studies with Doppler velocimetry of cerebral vessels designed to measure the effects of surfactant therapy have given rather variable results probably owing to the employment of different protocols (10–14). For example, van Bel et al. (11) detected fluctuations but no sustained change in mean cerebral blood flow velocity (CBFV) in the internal carotid artery following the administration of Curosurf at 10 mins of age, whereas van de Bor et al. (12) found that mean arterial blood pressure (MABP) and mean CBFV in the pericallosal artery were increased for up to 40 min after giving a synthetic surfactant (Exosurf) at 2–24 hr of age.

Cowan et al. (14) undertook a detailed Doppler study in which continuous rather than intermittent measurements of CBFV were made from the middle cerebral artery before, during, and after administration in two boluses of 200 mg/kg of a porcine natural surfactant (Curosurf). A number of other variables was recorded simultaneously. The 10 infants, who needed an inspired oxygen fraction (Fio_2) of at least 0.60, were briefly disconnected from the ventilator during the procedure. Details of ventilator settings are not given. Within 2 mins of treatment, MABP fell by a median value of 6 mmHg (15%). At the same time, the heart rate (HR) fell by a mean of 35 beats/min. The MABP remained reduced for 20 mins but HR rapidly recovered. CBFV fell sharply during surfactant administration and diastolic velocities were almost completely lost, although recovery usually took place within 20 mins. Subsequently, the expected improvement in Pao_2 was seen. The change in CBFV was thought possible to be due to transiently reduced alveolar ventilation during disconnection from the ventilator, transmission of high airway pressures to the circulation, or a reduction in pulmonary artery pressure allowing left-to-right ductal shunting and a cerebral steal phenomenon. Such an increase in ductal shunt has been demonstrated in laboratory animals (15), and Heldt et al. (16) showed in human infants that left-to-right shunting was more common after surfactant treatment than in controls (see also Chapter 25).

In 1992, two groups of investigators published the results of studies in which near-infrared spectroscopy (NIRS) was used to investigate the acute cerebral effects of surfactant administration as rescue therapy. NIRS is a noninvasive technique in which near-infrared light is shone through the head (17). Characteristic absorption of light by three chromophores in brain tissue, oxyhemoglobin (HbO_2), deoxyhemoglobin (Hb), and oxidized cytochrome oxidase ($cytO_2$), allows changes in the concentrations of these compounds to be measured (18). Methods have been described for measuring cerebral blood flow (CBF), by a modification of the Fick principle which employs a change in $[HbO_2]$ as the tracer (19,20), cerebral oxygen delivery (COD), and cerebral blood volume (CBV) (21): also, the response of CBF and CBV to changes in $Paco_2$ can readily be tested (22). Continuous observations can be made, at the cotside, of changes in cerebral $[HbO_2]$, [Hb], and $[cytO_2]$, together with intermittent, but repeated, measurements of the other variables.

Hellström-Westas et al. (23) and Skov et al. (24), carrying out combined studies in Lund and Copenhagen, investigated the effects of bolus administration, in 1 or 2 aliquots, of 200 mg/kg of Curosurf on cerebral variables measurable by NIRS, as well as those on the electroencephalogram (EEG). Details of ventilator settings are not given. The infants all needed an Fio_2 above 0.60. Surfactant administration was associated with a mean fall in MABP of 9 mmHg, which generally recovered within 5 mins, more quickly than in the studies of Cowan et al. (14). Immediately after the administration, EEG evidence of cerebroelectrical depression was found, as judged by a fall in the burst rate recorded by continuous amplitude-integrated EEG (cerebral function monitor). This depression lasted for up to 10 mins.

Skov et al. (24) compared the effects of endotracheal suctioning, which did not cause EEG depression, with those of surfactant administration. During both procedures, Pao_2 and Sao_2 fell similarly (by about 2 kPa and 8%, respectively), but MABP was shown to fall significantly more (mean value, 8 mmHg) with surfactant than with suctioning (2 mmHg). Little change took place in $Paco_2$. The NIRS studies showed small falls in cerebral [Hbo_2] and reciprocal rises in [Hb] of about 2 mmol/l/cm, lasting for about 2 mins, which were similar with suctioning and surfactant, and implied modest desaturation of intracerebral haemoglobin. CBV increased slightly. Two to 10 mins after surfactant, the expected improvement in lung function led to increasing Pao_2, Sao_2, and cerebral [Hbo_2]. Skov et al. (24) interpreted their findings as indicating that CBV was well maintained during surfactant administration in the face of a considerable fall in MABP and that surfactant treatment was associated with a hyperemic hyperoxic state in the brain, which did not explain the transient EEG depression.

Edwards et al. (25) investigated the effects of administering 200 mg/kg of Curosurf to 20 infants with a median gestation age of 27 weeks and median birth weight of 1 kg. Observations of a range of variables were made, including cerebral variables by NIRS. The infants were quite ill, requiring an Fio_2 of 0.35–1.0 (median 0.72), a mean airway pressure of 18–45 (25) cm H_2O; end-expiratory pressure of 2–5 cmH_2O (3), and respiratory frequency of 30 (20–36) bpm. The surfactant was given as a single bolus during a 2- to 4-sec disconnection from the ventilator (Bourns BP-200 or SLE 150). Subsequent ventilator management was designed to maintain satisfactory movements of the chest wall, and the Fio_2 was simultaneously adjusted to produce an adequate Pao_2 (8–12 kPa). Changes in cerebral [HbO_2], [Hb], and CBV were continuously recorded and CBF, COD and the response of CBV to changes in $PaCo_2$ (CBVR) were measured while the infants were stable shortly before and after surfactant was given. Cerebral [HbO_2] fell transiently after surfactant, giving a median change of –0.21 (range –0.46–0.05) ml/100 g, but quickly recovered so that the median change during the 10 mins after surfactant was 0.01 (–0.46–0.46) ml/100 g (Fig. 1). Multiple linear regression showed that most of the alterations in [HbO_2] depended on concomitant changes in Pao_2. Transient alterations in CBV also took place (see Fig. 1), and although the medain value for the maximum change following surfactant was zero, the range was quite wide—indicating alterations between –12 and 16% of total CBV. Multiple linear regression showed that the changes in CBV were not independently related to surfactant administration per se but were strongly correlated with changes in $Paco_2$ and slightly with changes in Pao_2. They were not related to MABP, which remained almost unchanged. The results of intermittent observations of CBF and COD when the infants were stable before and after surfactant showed considerable scatter and no significant trends (Fig. 2). The major determinant of changes in CBF was found to be $Paco_2$. The conclusions from this study were that surfactant administration, when performed according to the protocol employed, generally

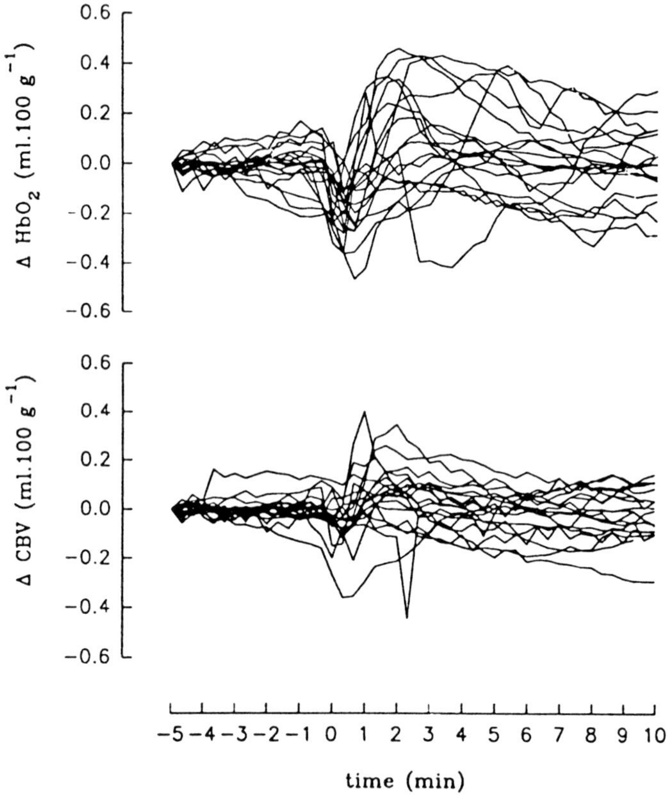

Figure 1 Changes from an arbitrary zero in [HbO_2] and cerebral blood volume (CBV) from 5 mins before to 10 mins after administration of Curosurf. Surfactant was administered at 0 mins. (From ref. 25; used with permission.)

caused only small, transient perturbations in [HbO_2] and CBV and that no important alterations in CBF, COD, or CBVR had been detected. A caveat was included that although on average perturbations in CBV were small, an adverse effect could not be ruled out in individual infants—for example, the maximum increase observed in CBV was 0.40 ml/100 g, or 16% of CBV. Such an acute increase might conceivably provoke bleeding.

IV. Summary and Conclusions

Cerebral hemodynamic perturbations in the first few days of life are heavily implicated in the pathogenesis of PVH and PVL, which are the two most important causes of perinatal brain damage in preterm infants. Respiratory

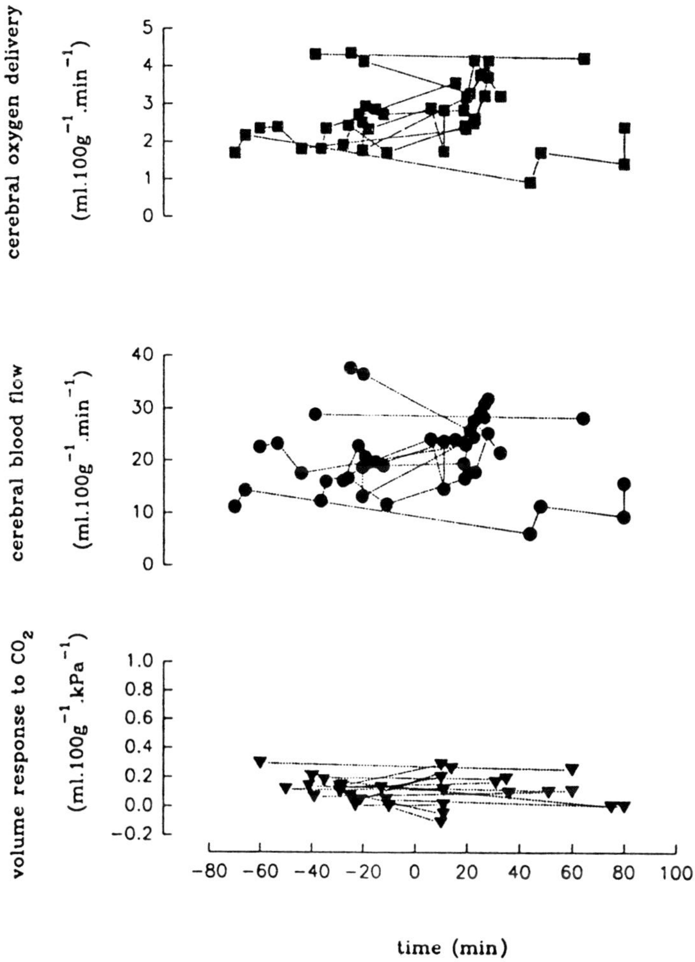

Figure 2 Values for cerebral oxygen delivery (COD, n = 9), cerebral blood flow (n = 9) and the volume response of CBV to changing $Paco_2$ (n = 16). Surfactant was administered at 0 mins. (From ref. 25; used with permission.)

illnesses, particularly RDS due to surfactant deficiency, are potent causes of these perturbations, and there is evidence that stabilization of the cerebral circulation can reduce the incidence of PVH (26). By ameliorating the severity of respiratory illness, it appeared likely that surfactant replacement would also cause a reduction in the likelihood of PVH and perhaps PVL. So far, this has not happened. Meta-analyses show no change in the incidence of PVH, and there is no evidence about the incidence of PVL.

To clarify the effects of surfactant administration on the brain, studies have been performed of cerebral hemodynamics and oxygenation, of electrophysiology, and of systemic variables.

Current evidence is based almost entirely on studies of Curosurf given as rescue therapy. Instillation of this compound has typically been found to lead to a reduction in MABP and HR, which appeared greater than when saline was instilled or endotracheal suction was performed. These falls were associated with a reduction in Pao_2.

Doppler velocimetry has shown that when MABP fell, carotid CBFV was much reduced, with loss of end-diastolic velocities. This effect may be attributed both to transient hypotension and hypoxemia and to increased left-to-right ductal shunting associated with pulmonary vasodilatation.

NIRS has been used to explore the effects of the administration of Curosurf on intracerebral events and also in an attempt to explain the cerebroelectrical depression that has been observed for up to 10 min afterwards. A small transient fall in cerebral [Hbo_2] was found, which was mainly attributable to the fall in Pao_2. The fall in [Hbo_2] appeared insufficient to account for the cerebroelectrical depression. At the same time, minor perturbations of CBV were generally seen, which were largely due to coincident changes in $Paco_2$. In individual infants the change in CBV could, however, be quite large, and conceivably capable of provoking PVH. Within a few minutes of reconnection to the ventilator, [Hbo_2] and CBV were reverting to baseline and remained there while the blood gases normalized as lung function improved. No changes in COD, CBF, and CBVR have been detected, as measured before and after surfactant when the infants were stable.

No satisfactory explanation for cerebroelectric depression was found. Flushing of the skin was reported in association with this depression by Hellström-Westas et al. (23) and was also recorded by another group (14). Edwards et al. (25) did not, however, see any flushing. The phenomenon of cerebroelectric depression needs further study. It has only been described with Curosurf, and the effects of other surfactants have not been investigated. It may have been due to some, possibly variable, fraction in the Curosurf, or perhaps to the washout of a neuroactive substance from the lungs or other tissues in association with pulmonary vasodilatation and improving Pao_2 (27). The depression has not been reported to be associated with physical signs and there is at present no evidence that it is harmful.

The very high incidence of serious PVH in the study of Horbar et al. (9), and to a lesser extent in some other studies, is counterbalanced by a low incidence in others (1). The possibility exists, however, that some aspect of surfactant replacement could provoke bleeding. The occasional acute effect on CBV has been mentioned above. Also, the exact protocol used for instillation could be important. For example, prolonged disconnection from the ventilator is likely to cause more cerebral perturbations than very brief disconnection—and there is a case for administering the surfactant down a sidearm or by aerosol so that there is no disconnection at all. The details of ventilator management could be important, and they are almost never described in publications about surfactant replacement. For example, if a protocol is used where the ventilator is reconnected at the same settings as before, without attention to air entry, the surfactant could clog the airways for a while, causing an acute episode of hypoxemia together with an increase or fall in blood pressure. Alternatively, if the lung rapidly becomes more compliant, it could become overdistended, leading to obstruction of the pulmonary circulation and a situation analogous to a tension pneumothorax, an important antecedent of PVH. This effect would probably be particularly marked at fast (conventional) ventilator rates, because the increasing expiratory time constant of the lung would not allow time for deflation to occur (28).

More studies of the acute cerebral effects of surfactant-replacement both as prophylaxis and rescue therapy, and employing natural and synthetic surfactants, are needed, so that the best way of minimizing potentially damaging effects can be defined. NIRS is probably the method of choice for carrying out these studies. In the meantime, efforts should be made to avoid adverse changes in variables known to affect cerebral hemodynamics and oxygenation, notably Pa_{O_2}, Pa_{CO_2}, and MABP, and to avoid inappropriate ventilator management.

References

1. Volpe JJ. Neurology of the Newborn. 2nd ed. Philadelphia: Saunders, 1987.
2. Reynolds EOR, Wyatt JS. Perinatal brain injury. In: Asbury AK, McKhann GM, McDonald WI, eds. Diseases of the Nervous System. Philadelphia: Saunders, 1992:584–597.
3. Soll RF, McQueen MC. Respiratory distress syndrome. In: Sinclair JC, Bracken MB, eds. Effective Care of the Newborn Infant. Oxford, England: Oxford University Press, 1992:325–358.
4. Hope PL, Thorburn RJ, Stewart AL, et al. Timing and antecedents of periventricular hemorrhage in very preterm infants. In: Second Special Ross Conference on Perinatal Intracranial Hemorrhage. Ohio: Ross Laboratories, 1992:78–101.
5. Goddard-Finegold J. Experimental models of intraventricular hemorrhage. In: Pape KE, Wigglesworth JS, eds. Perinatal Brain Lesions. Oxford, England: Blackwell, 1989:115–134.
6. Hope PL, Gould SJ, Howard S, et al. Precision of ultrasound diagnosis of pathologically verified lesions in the brains of very preterm infants. Dev Med Child Neurol 1988; 30:457–471.
7. Guzzetta F, Shackelford GD, Volpe S, et al. Periventricular intraparenchymal echodensities in the premature newborn: Critical determinant of neurological outcome. Pediatrics 1986; 78:995–1006.

8. Alberman ED. The epidemiology of congenital defects: A pragmatic approach. In: Adinolfi M, Benson P, Gianelli F, et al, eds. Paediatric Research: A Genetic Approach. London: Heinemann, 1982:1–28.
9. Horbar JD, Soll RF, Schachinger H, et al. A European multicentre randomised controlled trial of single dose surfactant therapy for idiopathic respiratory distress syndrome. Eur J Pediatr 1990; 149:416–423.
10. Jorch G, Rabe H, Garbe M, Gortner L. Acute and protracted effects of intratracheal surfactant application on internal carotid blood flow velocity, blood pressure and carbon dioxide tension in very low birthweight infants. Eur J Pediatr 1989; 148:770–773.
11. van Bel F, de Winter PJ, Wijnands HBG, et al. Cerebral and aortic blood flow velocity patterns in preterm infants receiving prophylactic surfactant treatment. Acta Paediatr 1992; 81:504–510.
12. van de Bor M, Ma EJ, Walther FJ. Cerebral blood flow velocity after surfactant instillation in preterm infants. J Pediatr 1991; 118:285–287.
13. McCord FB, Halliday H, McClure G, Reid MMcC. Changes in pulmonary and cerebral blood flow after surfactant treatment for severe respiratory distress syndrome. Arch Dis Child 1989; 64:13–16.
14. Cowan F, Whitelaw A, Wertheim D, Silverman M. Cerebral blood flow velocity changes after rapid administration of surfactant. Arch Dis Child 1991; 66:1105–1109.
15. Clyman RI, Jobe A, Heymann M, et al. Increased shunt through the patent ductus arteriosus after surfactant replacement therapy. J Pediatr 1982; 100:101–107.
16. Heldt GP, Pesonen E, Merritt TA, et al. Closure of the ductus arteriosus and mechanics of breathing in preterm infants after surfactant replacement therapy. Pediatr Res 1989; 25:305–310.
17. Jobsis FF. Non-invasive infrared monitoring of cerebral and myocardial sufficiency and circulatory parameters. Science 1977; 198:1264–1267.
18. Wyatt JS, Cope M, Delpy DT, et al. Quantification of cerebral oxygenation and hemodynamics in sick newborn infants by near infrared spectrophotometry. Lancet 1986; 2:1063–1066.
19. Edwards AD, Wyatt JS, Richardson C, et al. Cotside measurement of cerebral blood flow in ill newborn infants by near infrared spectroscopy. Lancet 1988; 2:770–771.
20. Edwards AD, Richardson C, van der Zee P, et al. Measurement of hemoglobin flow and blood flow by near infrared spectroscopy. J Appl Physiol 1993; 75:1884–1889.
21. Wyatt JS, Cope M, Delpy DT, et al. Quantification of cerebral blood volume in newborn human infants by near infrared spectroscopy. J Appl Physiol 1990; 68:1086–1091.
22. Wyatt JS, Edwards AD, Cope M, et al. Response of cerebral blood volume to changes in arterial carbon dioxide tension in preterm and term infants. Pediatr Res 1991; 29:553–557.
23. Hellström-Westas L, Bell AH, Skov L, et al. Cerebroelectrical depression following surfactant treatment in preterm infants. Pediatrics 1992; 89:643–647.
24. Skov L, Hellström-Westas L, Jacobsen T, et al. Acute changes in cerebral blood volume in preterm infants during surfactant treatment. Neuropediatrics 1992; 23:126–130.

25. Edwards AD, McCormick DC, Roth SC, et al. Cerebral haemodynamic effects of treatment with modified natural surfactant investigated by near infrared spectroscopy. Pediatr Res 1992; 32:532–536.
26. Perlman JM, Goodman S, Kreusser KL, et al. Reduction in intraventricular hemorrhage by elimination of fluctuating cerebral blood flow in preterm infants with respiratory distress syndrome. N Engl J Med 1985; 312:1353–1357.
27. Saugstad OD, Tubman RJ, Gloppestad K, et al. Robertson B. J Perinat Med 1992; 20:379–385.
28. Ramsden CA, Reynolds EOR. Ventilator settings for newborn infants. Arch Dis Child 1987; 62:529–538.

27

Reoxygenation Effects of Surfactant Replacement Therapy

OLA DIDRIK SAUGSTAD
The National Hospital
University of Oslo
Oslo, Norway

I. Introduction

The rapid changes in oxygenation and circulation often seen after instillation of natural surfactant may exert a number of effects on different organs which up to now has poorly been investigated. Does a rapid increase in oxygenation after surfactant instillation influence metabolic rate? There are indications that reoxygenation with 100% oxygen after hypoxia depresses oxygen uptake in the newborn pig brain. Does this occur after surfactant treatment as well?

Hyperoxygenation, if it occurs after surfactant instillation, may also lead to an increased production of oxygen radicals. These reactive substances may have a number of effects on different organs of the preterm baby. Which evidences do we have that oxygen radicals are produced in excess in relation to surfactant therapy?

II. Oxygenation Status Following Surfactant Administration

When Fujiwara and coworkers (1) published the first report on the clinical effects of synthetic surfactant therapy on babies with respiratory distress syndrome, one of their main findings was an improved oxygenation with an increase in Pao_2 from 17–89 to 61–464 mmHg in the course of 20–180 min. Hallman and coworkers (2) could subsequently demonstrate that natural (human) surfactant gave a much more rapid response concerning Po_2 increase compared with synthetic surfactant. They found a $TcPO_2$ increase from in mean 69 mmHg before to 239 mmHg already 5 min after surfactant was instilled (2) (Fig. 1).

The Collaborative European Multicenter Study with porcine surfactant (Curosurf) also showed a rapid increase in oxygenation with a mean peak in Pao_2 of 19.7 kPa 5 min after surfactant instillation (3). This group (4) published data showing that babies with a high Pao_2 response (>30 kPa) during the first 15 min after surfactant instillation had an increased risk of mild intraventricular hemorrhage grade I and II compared with babies with a less clear response (incidence of 21 versus 7%). The incidence of more serious intracranial hemorrhage did not change and the total incidence of intracranial hemorrhage did not differ much between babies with a high Pao_2 response, a moderate (Pao_2 > 15 < 30 kPa) response, or small response (Pao_2 < 15 kPa) (4).

Hyperoxygenation can therefore obviously be seen after surfactant replacement therapy and may have a number of circulatory and biochemical effects both directly and indirectly through for instance the production of oxygen radicals.

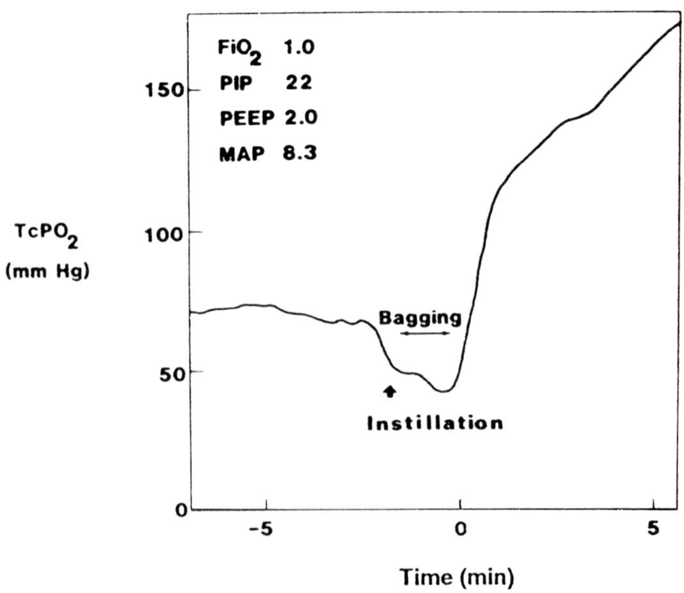

Figure 1 Changes in $TcPO_2$ after administration of human surfactant. (From ref. 2; used with permission.)

III. Effects of Hyperoxygenation on the Lung and Surfactant

The damage after exposure of the lung to hyperoxia is found diffusely throughout the lung parenchyma. Hyperoxia produces pulmonary edema and infiltration of polymorphonuclear leukocytes and alveolar macrophages. In the bronchi and bronchioli, oxidant exposure causes ciliated and nonciliated cells to swell, become necrotic, and slough off during days 2 and 3 of an exposure. In the alveoli, the first sign of damage is swelling of the endothelium; later they undergo cytoplasmic change and fragmentation. The type I cells remain largely intact; the type II cells, however, may start to proliferate (5). Change in cell diameter may also be seen (6). Latcr on fibrosis and a thickened alveolar membrane are observed. Reactive oxygen species activate human neutrophil collagenase (7) and alveolar macrophages have been shown to produce fibroblasts.

Rabbits exposed to 100% oxygen for 64 hr have a decline in phospholipid and increase in protein levels in bronchoalveolar lavage fluid (6). Hyperoxic exposure of rabbits alters gene expression in the lung. A substantial increase in mRNA encoding for the tissue inhibitor of metalloproteinases has been found. This protein plays a key role in regulating connective tissue turnover (8). Rats exposed to 85% oxygen progressively increased the amounts of surfactant proteins SP-A, SP-B, and SP-C in alveolar lavage fluid (9). The increased surfactant protein was associated with increased relative abundance of mRNA encoding each of the proteins in lung tissue.

Type II cells exposed to H_2O_2 or oxygen radicals produced by xanthine-xanthine oxidase demonstrated a decrease in phosphatidylcholine synthesis with only minimal changes in cell viability (10). The activities of choline phosphate cytidyltransferase and choline phosphotransferase, which are specific enzymes in phosphatidylcholine synthesis, did not decrease during exposure (10).

IV. Oxygen Radicals

A. Characteristics

It was Gerschman and coworkers (11) who first pointed out that oxygen may be toxic since oxygen generates oxygen radicals. Today, we know that oxygen radicals are not only toxic but that they also play a role in physiological processes such as regulating the circulation.

A free radical is any atom or molecule with an unpaired electron in the outer electron orbit. There are several reactive oxygen species such as superoxide radical, O_2^-, and the hydroxyl radical, $OH\cdot$. Free radicals are short lived but highly reactive. They may initiate chain reactions and exert a number of effects such as peroxidation of polyunsaturated fatty acids in the cellular membrane, degradation of structural proteins, inactivation of enzymes, and they attack ribonucleic acids (12).

B. Production and Sources

Oxygen radicals are produced in a number of biochemical reactions. In the energy metabolism in the mitochondria, oxygen is reduced to water by accepting four electrons in one step. A small part of the oxygen involved is, however, reduced stepwise, taking up one electron at a time. Reactive oxygen species, such as superoxide radical, hydrogen peroxide, and hydroxyl radical, are formed as intermediates (12). Production of oxygen radicals is therefore part of the normal metabolism.

Activated polymorphonuclear cells produce a burst of oxygen radicals by turning on the NADPH oxidase (13). This is an important part of the defense against invading microorganisms. Surfactant replacement may inhibit this oxygen burst in macrophages (14).

Oxygen radicals can be produced in enzymatic processes as well; for instance, when arachidonic acid is metabolized to prostaglandins or when hypoxanthine (HX) is oxidized to uric acid (UA) in the presence of xanthine oxidase (XO) (15,16):

$$HX + O_2 \xrightarrow{XO} UA + O_2^- \qquad (1)$$

The presence of nonprotein bound iron, when reduced to ferrous ions, enhances the formation of hydroxyl radicals (Haber-Weiss reaction):

$$O_2^- + H_2O_2 \xrightarrow{Fe} OH\cdot . \qquad (2)$$

The hypoxanthine-xanthine oxidase system is of importance, since large amounts of hypoxanthine accumulate in the tissues and body fluids during hypoxia (17–19). We have postulated that during reoxygenation a burst of oxygen radicals is formed which may injure different organs simultanously (20,21). This is the theoretical basis for the so-called “oxygen radical disease in neonatology” (22,23).

There are several other sources of oxygen radicals such as damaged mitochondria with uncoupled oxidative phosphorylation and auto-oxidation of catecholamines.

C. Effects on the Circulation

Oxygen radicals exert effects on the circulation. When generated by the hypoxanthine-xanthine oxidase system, they constrict the pulmonary vessels of isolated rabbit lungs (24) as well as in intact pig lungs (25). The same oxygen radical–generating system dilates isolated ductal rings from fetal sheep (26). The effect of this system on the circulation is inhibited by indomethacin, allopurinol (xanthine oxidase inhibitor and oxygen radical scavenger), and catalase (24–26). The output of prostaglandins, as PGE_2, thromboxane B_2, 6 keto-$PGF_{1\alpha}$ is increased in the presence of hypoxanthine-xanthine oxidase and inhibited by indomethacin, allopurinol, and catalase (26,27). We therefore have suggested that this system may play a role in regulating the perinatal circulation through the initiation of prostaglandin synthesis (28). Free radicals therefore are not only harmful, but they may play an important role in regulating normal physiological processes.

There may as well be a complex relation between oxygen radicals and nitric oxide which is inactivated by oxygen radicals. On the other hand, when NO reacts with superoxide radical, a peroxynitrite is formed which can spontaneously decompose to the toxic hydroxyl radical (29,30). Activated alveolar macrophages secrete both nitric oxide and superoxide in the alveolar lining fluid. These substances combine rapidly to form peroxynitrite, which potently may damage lipids and proteins in biological membranes by oxidation. Peroxynitrite has been shown to inhibit calf lung surfactant extract and damage surfactant proteins (31).

V. Defense Against Oxygen Radicals

The body has a number of defense mechanisms against free radicals such as scavengers and antioxidants, repair agents, and antioxienzymes. Without these we could not exist in an oxygen-rich atmosphere.

Free radical scavengers inactivate free radicals which have already been generated. The action of the scavenging agent is often to replace a highly reactive free radical by a less reactive radical which does not contribute to cascades and which is not harmful. Mannitol, bilirubin, uric acid, and dimethyl sulfoxide are examples of powerful oxygen radical scavengers.

Antioxidants may either inhibit initiation of free radical formation or inactivate preformed free radicals. The last class of antioxidants are the chain-breaking agents, which are good electron donors. Vitamin E is the major lipid-soluble antioxidant and is located in the cell membranes, terminating cascade formation of free radicals derived from polyunsaturated free fatty acids. Vitamin C is a powerful antioxidant and acts also by regenerating vitamin E from vitamin E free radicals. Bilirubin is very powerful in protecting polyunsaturated fatty acids from peroxidation. Maybe it therefore is an advantage for the preterm baby, with its lowered antioxidant defense, to have a higher bilirubin level in plasma and extracellular space than the term baby?

Antioxienzymes are enzymes such as catalase, glutathione peroxidase, and superoxide dismutase. Superoxide dismutases (SOD) catalyse the transformation from superoxide to hydrogen peroxide (12,23).

$$O_2^- + H^+ \xrightarrow{SOD} H_2O_2 \quad (3)$$

Catalase (CAT) converts hydrogen peroxide to molecular oxygen and water:

$$H_2O_2 \xrightarrow{CAT} O_2 + H_2O \quad (4)$$

and glutathione peroxidase (GP) converts hydroperoxides to molecular water and alcohol:

$$ROOH + GSH \xrightarrow{GP} ROH + H_2O + GSSG \quad (5)$$

GSH: reduced gluthathione
GSSG: oxidized glutathione

VI. Perinatal Development of Antioxienzymes

The intracellular defense against free radicals seems to be low during fetal life. Activities of antioxienzymes such as superoxide dismutases, catalase, and glutathione peroxidase increase in the lung and kidney of rats or rabbits during pregnancy (32–34). The maturation of these enzymes seems to occur in parallel with the maturation of the surfactant system (32). In the brain and myocardium, the activities of such enzymes in different species investigated seem, however, to be more stable throughout pregnancy (34,35). In newborn pig intestine mucosa, superoxide dismutase activities have been found to be higher the first day of life compared with 1-month-old piglets; however, glutathione peroxidase was significantly lower and there was no detectable catalase activity, indicating that neonatal piglet intestine has a lower capacity to detoxify hydrogen peroxide than that of older animals (36).

In human preterm babies, the erythrocyte superoxide dismutase activity does not change with gestational age. Further, significant differences have not been observed between preterm babies, term babies, and adults regarding the activities of this enzyme. Erythrocyte catalase and glutathione peroxidase increase, however, during pregnancy (37).

By contrast to the intracellular antioxidant status, the total antioxidant activity of plasma seems to be at about the same level in the preterm and the term baby and in adults (38). The extracellular defense against free radicals, however, is probably less important than the intracellular defense. There is therefore compelling evidence that the defense against oxygen radicals is lower in fetal life than at term. This means that preterm babies may be born with insufficient protection against oxygen free radicals. This is of special significance, since preterm babies often are exposed to a higher load of oxygen radicals than term babies, because they are often treated with high concentrations of oxygen and simultanously have elevated hypoxanthine concentrations in their body fluids (39).

In adult animals exposed to hyperoxia, increased activities of antioxidant enzymes in the lungs have been reported. Hyperoxic antioxidant enzyme induction seems to be an important defense mechanism against hyperoxia. By contrast, premature rabbits exposed to hyperoxia do not seem to respond by an increase in antioxidant enzymes in their lungs (40). The preterm infant therefore has a lowered defense against hyperoxia and a reduced ability to protect itself from hyperoxia by induction of antioxidant enzymes.

VII. Oxygen Radicals and Surfactant Instillation

As mentioned above, the rapid increase in oxygenation often seen after surfactant replacement therapy may increase the production of oxygen radicals in a preterm baby, who may have a reduced capacity to detoxify them.

For this reason, we wanted to investigate whether an important substrate for oxygen radical formation, hypoxanthine, is found in excess concentration in relation to surfactant therapy. We therefore measured plasma hypoxanthine before and immediately after instillation of natural surfactant in human babies with respiratory distress syndrome (RDS).

In our first investigation (41), 12 babies with mean gestational age of 28 weeks and birth weight of 1120 g with severe respiratory distress syndrome (mean Fio_2 of 0.92) were studied before and after treatment with porcine surfactant (Curosurf). Pao_2 increased sharply from a mean of 7.2 kPa, reaching a peak of 25 kPa after 5 min. Fio_2 was then gradually reduced to 0.45 after 1 hr when Pao_2 reached pretreatment values (Fig. 2A). Simultanously plasma hypoxanthine concentration increased from a mean of 5.8 μmol/l to 9.0 μmol/l after 5 min, 9.6 μmol/l after 15 min, and 9.3 μmol/l after 30 min. At 60 min, plasma hypoxanthine concentrations had again reached pretreatment levels (Fig. 2B). Although the peak in plasma hypoxanthine was reached somewhat delayed compared with the peak in Pao_2, it seems that already 5 min after surfactant instillation, a high plasma hypoxanthine concentration coexisted with a high Pao_2. The stage could therefore be set for an augmentation in free radical production the first minutes after surfactant was administered.

We then compared the maximal plasma concentration of hypoxanthine (15 or 30 min after surfactant instillation) between babies who died and babies who survived. Nonsurviving babies had an initial favorable response to surfactant treatment with an adequate increase in Pao_2 and reduction in Fio_2 but could not be stabilized and weaned from the ventilator, and they died during the first week. Judged by birth weight, gestational age, initial Fio_2, and Pao_2, there were no differences between babies who died and those who survived. Table 1. Surviving

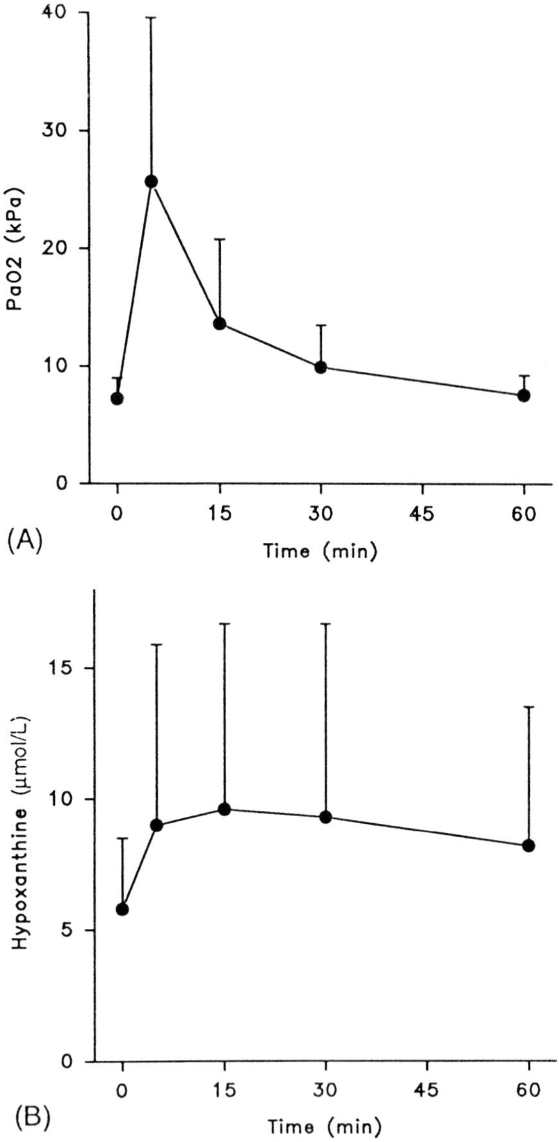

Figure 2 (A) Changes in Pa_{O_2} in babies with RDS the first 60 min after receiving porcine surfactant (Curosurf). (B) Changes in plasma hypoxanthine in the same babies. Mean and SD are given.

Table 1 Clinical Data for Surviving and Nonsurviving Infants

	Survivors	Nonsurvivors
Gestational age (weeks)	28.3 (1.1)	27.5 (2.4)
Birth weight (g)	1196 (162)	1014 (205)
FiO_2[a]	0.93 (0.09)	0.90 (0.09)
PaO_2 (kPa)[a]	7.2 (1.8)	7.1 (1.7)
Plasma hypoxanthine (μmol/l)	5.1 (1.9)	6.8 (3.5)

SD is given in parenthesis. There were no statistically significant differences between surviving and non-surving infants.
[a]Values before surfactant instillation.

babies had a mean maximal plasma hypoxanthine concentration of 1.9 (SD 2.9) μmol/l compared with 9.4 (SD 8.1) μmol/l ($P < 0.05$, Mann-Whitney U-test) in nonsurviving babies (Fig. 3, bottom).

Six out of the 12 babies developed intracranial hemorrhage grades II–IV (32). These babies had a maximal plasma hypoxanthine concentration of 9.6 (SD 7.2) μmol/l compared with 1.1 (SD 0.7) μmol/l in babies who did not develop intracranial hemorrhage ($P < 0.01$, Mann-Whitney U-test) (Fig. 3, top). It therefore seems a raised plasma hypoxanthine level may serve as a prognostic factor in infants treated with natural surfactant.

VIII. Discussion

The rapid increase in oxygenation after replacement therapy with natural surfactant of preterm babies with respiratory distress syndrome described by several investigators has always been a cause of concern to this author. As mentioned above, there are indications that if PaO_2 is elevated too much, an increased risk for intracranial hemorrhage, at least the milder degrees, exists (4). Other adverse consequences of hyperoxygenation in preterm babies due to treatment with natural surfactant is not known in full. We know, however, that only a short period of resuscitation of preterm babies with 80% oxygen induces cerebral vasoconstriction for several hours after the resuscitation period (42). In studies on hypoxic newborn pigs, we have demonstrated that resuscitation with 100% oxygen increases PaO_2 to extremely high levels; that is, up to 50–60 kPa (43). An increased oxygen tension in the dog seems to reduce the oxygen uptake (44). Further, compared with resuscitation with room air, 100% oxygen seems to reduce cerebral oxygen uptake (45). In addition, damage to the immature alveolar wall due to ventilation with a high fraction of oxygen may result in increased leakage of iron-loaded tranferrin into the alveolar spaces. Plasma from

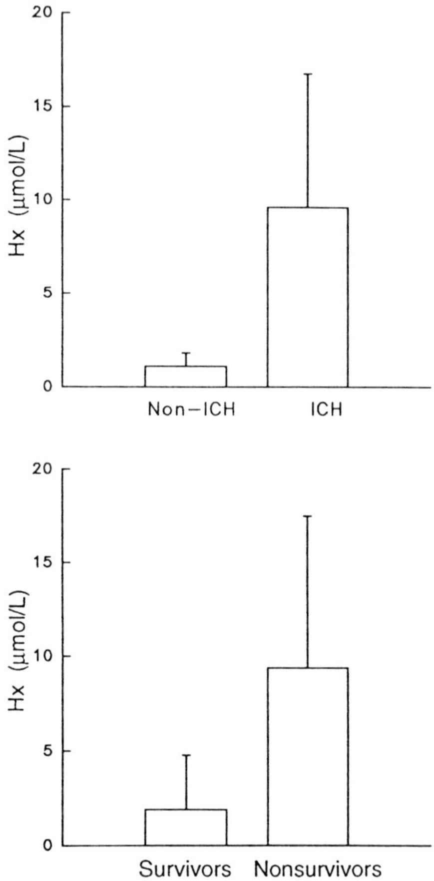

Figure 3 (Bottom) Babies developing intracranial hemorrhage (ICH) (grades II–IV) are compared with the babies who did not develop ICH. Mean and SD are given. Maximal increase in plasma hypoxanthine concentration in surviving and nonsurviving babies with RDS after receiving porcine surfactant (Curosurf). (Top) Plasma hypoxanthine in the same babies.

preterm babies, by contrast to plasma from adults, stimulate iron catalysed peroxidation of pulmonary surfactant liposomes (46). Hyperoxygenation per se may therefore result in inactivation of surfactant owing to leakage of plasma into the alveoli.

Our data showing that plasma hypoxanthine in babies with poor outcome reaches a peak the first minutes after surfactant instillation may give at least partly an explanation for the adverse effects following hyperoxygenation in relation to surfactant therapy. It is known from in vitro studies that the production of oxygen radicals by the hypoxanthine-xanthine oxidase system is dependent both on the degree of oxygenation and the concentration of plasma hypoxanthine (16). Although the distribution of xanthine oxidase is not known in detail in preterm babies, there is now data supporting our hypothesis (21,22) that xanthine oxidase released from liver and intestine in hypoxia and hypovolemia circulates throughout the body generating oxygen radicals which attack several organs simultanously (47,48). In fact, a recent study indicates that xanthine oxidase is released in babies with RDS (48). The significance of elevated plasma hypoxanthine concentration immediately after surfactant therapy therefore becomes more obvious.

The effect of the hypoxanthine-xanthine oxidase system may be due to a direct toxic effect on cells and/or by its action as a vasoactive agent contributing to fluctuations in blood flow in relation to surfactant therapy.

In a recent clinical study (49), we could not find a peak in plasma hypoxanthine after instillation of porcine surfactant. By contrast, the plasma hypoxanthine concentrations decreased from initial high levels to normal levels after surfactant was given. These babies were, however, clinically different from those investigated in our first study, since they had a higher initial plasma hypoxanthine concentration (mean of 11.6 versus 5.8 μmol/l). However, in these babies, as in the first study, a high plasma hypoxanthine concentration indicated poorer prognosis than in babies with nonelevated hypoxanthine concentrations, since babies who died had significantly higher hypoxanthine concentrations before surfactant administration compared with surviving babies (mean 17.0 versus 8.7 μmol/l) (49). Further, it has been shown that preterm babies who develop bronchopulmonary dysplasia have significantly higher plasma hypoxanthine concentration at birth compared with preterm babies who do not develop this condition (50).

We therefore believe it is of importance to study in more detail the factors which may contribute to an elevation of plasma hypoxanthine concentration in relation to surfactant therapy. In animal studies, we are presently investigating whether release of plasma hypoxanthine in relation to surfactant replacement administration is influenced by the clinical status before surfactant is given. We hypothesize that only hypovolemic or hypoxic babies release hypoxanthine to any significant extent into the circulation after treatment with natural surfactant. If this is the case, it clearly indicates how important it is to stabilize the baby before surfactant is given, treating any hypovolemia, hypotension, or hypoxia if possible.

To what extent oxygen free radicals play a role in babies given surfactant is of course not fully known. In this chapter, I have tried to summarize the indications we have that such reactive substances may under certain circumstances be produced in excess immediately after surfactant is given. Since babies with respiratory distress syndrome probably have a lowered defense against free radicals, it must be of importance to reduce their generation of free radicals. The hypoxanthine peak can be reduced by stabilizing the baby and carefully treating any hypovolemia before surfactant is given, and the PO_2 peak should be avoided by quickly reducing Fio_2 after surfactant has been instilled. The oxygenation status of the baby should preferably be followed both by pulse oximetry and transcutaneous PO_2 electrodes in relation to surfactant instillation.

References

1. Fujiwara T, Chida, S, Watabe Y, et al. Artificial surfactant therapy in hyaline-membrane disease. Lancet 1980; 1:55–59.
2. Hallman M, Meritt TA, Schneider H, et al. Isolation of human surfactant from amniotic fluid and a pilot study of its efficacy in respiratory distress syndrome. Pediatrics 1983; 71:473–482.
3. Collaborative European Multicenter Study Group. Surfactant replacement therapy for severe neonatal respiratory distress syndrome: An international randomized clinical trial. Pediatrics 1988; 82:683–691.
4. Collaborative European Multicenter Study Group. Factors influencing the clinical response to surfactant replacement therapy in babies with severe respiratory distress syndrome. Eur J Pediatr 1991; 150:433–439.
5. Finkelstein JN, Horowitz S, Sinkin RA, Ryan RM. Cellular and molecular responses to lung injury in relation to induction of tissue repair and fibrosis. Clin Perinatol 1992; 19:603–620.
6. Holm BA, Matalon S, Finkelstein JN, Notter RH. Type II pneumocyte changes during hyperoxic lung injury and recovery. J Appl Physiol 1988; 65:2672–2678.
7. Saari H, Suomalainen K, Lindy O, et al. Activation of latent human neutrophil collagenase by reactive oxygen species and serine proteases. Biochem Biophys Res Commun 1990; 171:979–987.
8. Horowitz S, Dafni N, Shapiro, DL, et al. Hyperoxic exposure alters gene expression in the lung. Induction of tissue inhibitor of metalloproteinases mRNA and other mRNAs. J Biol Chem 1989; 264:7092–7095.
9. Nogee LM, Wispe JR, Clark JC, et al. Increased expression of pulmonary surfactant proteins in oxygen exposed rats. Am J Respir Cell Mol Biol 1991; 4:102–107.
10. Holm BA, Hudak BB, Keicher L, et al. Mechanisms of H_2O_2-mediated injury to type II cell surfactant metabolism and protection with PEG-catalase. Am J Physiol 1991; 261:C751–757.
11. Gerschman R, Gilbert DL, Nyl SW, et al. Oxygen poisoning and x-ray irradiation: A mechanism in common. Science 1954; 119:624–626.
12. Simic MG, Taylor KA, Ward JF, von Sonntag C. Oxygen Radicals in Biology and Medicine. New York: Plenum Press, 1988.
13. Babior BM, Kipnes RS, Curnutte JT. Biological defense mechanisms. The production by leukocytes of superoxide—A potential bactericidial agent. J Clin Invest 1973; 52:741–744.
14. Sherman MP, D'Ambola JB, Aeberhardt EE, Barett CT. Surfactant therapy of

newborn rabbits impairs lung macrophage bactericidal activity. J Appl Physiol 1988; 65:137–145.
15. McCord JM, Fridovich I. The reduction of cytochrome C by milk xanthine oxidase. J Biol Chem 1968; 243:5753–5760.
16. Fridovich I. Quantitative aspects of the production of superoxide radical by milk xanthine oxidase. J Biol Chem 1969; 244:4053–4057.
17. Saugstad OD. Hypoxanthine as a measurement of hypoxia. Pediatr Res 1975; 9:158–161.
18. Pietz J, Guttenberg N, Gluck L. Hypoxanthine: A marker for asphyxia. Obstet Gynecol 1988; 72:762–766.
19. Thiringer K, Karlsson K, Rosén KG, Kjellmer I. The contribution of heart muscle, liver, skeletal muscle, and placenta to the elevation of hypoxanthine during asphyxia in the acutely exteriorized foetal lamb. Biol Neonate 1984; 45:169–182.
20. Saugstad OD, Aasen AO. Plasma hypoxanthine levels as a prognostic aid of tissue hypoxia. Europ Surg Res 1980; 12:123–129.
21. Saugstad OD. Oxygen radicals and pulmonary damage. Pediatr Pulmonol 1985; 1:167–175.
22. Saugstad OD. Hypoxanthine as an indicator of hypoxia: Its role in health and disease through free radical production. Pediatr Res 1988; 23:143–150.
23. Saugstad OD. Neonatal oxygen radical disease. In: David TJ, ed. Recent Advances in Paediatrics 10. Edinburgh: Churchill Livingstone, 1992:173–187.
24. Tate RM, Morris HG, Schroeder WR, Repine JE. Oxygen metabolites stimulate thromboxane production and vasoconstriction in isolated saline-perfused rabbit lungs. J Clin Invest 1984; 74:608–613.
25. Sanderud J, Norstein J, Saugstad OD. Reactive oxygen metabolites produce pulmonary vasoconstriction in young pigs. Pediatr Res 1991; 29:543–547.
26. Clyman RI, Saugstad OD, Mauray F. Reactive oxygen metabolites relax the lamb ductus arteriosus by stimulating prostaglandin production. Circ Res 1989; 64:1–8.
27. Sanderud J, Bjøro K, Saugstad OD. Oxygen radicals stimulate thromboxane and prostacyclin synthesis and induce vasoconstriction in pig lungs. Scand J Clin Lab Invest 1993; 53:447–455.
28. Saugstad OD, Sanderud J. Circulatory effects of oxygen radicals. Biomed Biochim Acta 1989; 48:20–24.
29. Ignarro LJ. Biological actions and properties of endothelium derived nitric oxide formed and released from artery and vein. Circ Res 1989; 65:1–21.
30. Beckman JS, Beckman TW, Chen J, et al. Apparent hydroxyl radical production by peroxynitrite: Implications for endothelial injury from nitric oxide and superoxide. Proc Natl Acad Sci USA 1990; 87:1620–1624.
31. Haddad IY, Ischiropoulos H, Holm BA, et al. Mechanisms of peroxynitrite-induced injury to pulmonary surfactants. Am J Physiol 1993; 265:L555–564.
32. Frank L, Groseclose EE. Preparation for birth into an O_2-rich environment: the antioxidant enzymes in the developing rabbit lung. Pediatr Res 1984; 18:584–587.
33. Gerdin E, Tydén O, Erikson UJ. The development of antioxidant enzymatic defense in the perinatal rat lung. Activities of superoxide dismutase, glutathione peroxidase and catalase. Pediatr Res 1984; 19:687–691.
34. Hayashibe H, Asayama K, Dobashi K, Kato K. Prenatal development of antioxidant

enzymes in rat lung, kidney, and heart: marked increase in immunreactive superoxide dismutase, glutathione peroxidase, and catalase in the kidney. Pediatr Res 1990; 27:472–475.
35. Mishra OP, Delivoria-Papadopoulos M. Anti-oxidant enzymes in fetal guinea pig brain during development and the effect of maternal hypoxia. Dev Brain Res 1988; 42:173–179.
36. Crissinger KD, Grishma MB, Granger DN. Developmental biology of oxidant-producing enzymes and antioxidants in the pig intestine. Pediatr Res 1989; 25:612–616.
37. Ripalda MJ, Rudolph N, Wong SL. Developmental patterns of antioxidant defense mechanisms in human erythrocytes. Pediatr Res 1989; 26:366–369.
38. Sullivan JL, Newton RB. Serum antioxidant activity in neonates. Arch Dis Child 1988; 63:748–757.
39. Saugstad OD, Rognum TO. High post mortem levels of hypoxanthine in the vitreous humor of premature babies with respiratory distress syndrome. Pediatrics 1988; 81:395–398.
40. Frank L, Sosenko IRS. Failure of premature rabbits to increase antioxidant enzymes during hyperoxic exposure: Increased susceptibility to pulmonary oxygen toxicity compared with term rabbits. Pediatr Res 1991; 29:292–296.
41. Saugstad OD, Tubman TRJ, Gloppestad K, et al. Raised plasma hypoxanthine levels as a prognostic sign in preterm babies with respiratory distress syndrome treated with natural surfactant. J Perinat Med 1992; 20:379–385.
42. Lundstrøm KE, Pryds O, Greisen G. 80% oxygen administered to newborn premature infants causes prolonged cerebral vasoconstriction. Pediatric Res 1993; 35:275 (Abstr).
43. Rootwelt T, Løberg EM, Moen A, et al. Hypoxemia and reoxygenation with 21% or 100% oxygen in newborn pigs: Changes in blood pressure, base deficit, and hypoxanthine and brain morphology. Pediatr Res 1992; 32:107–113.
44. Lodato RF. Decreased O_2 consumption and cardiac output during normobaric hyperoxia in conscious dogs. J Appl Physiol 1989; 67:1551–1559.
45. Rootwelt T, Odden JP, Hall C, et al. Cerebral blood flow and evoked potentials during reoxygenation with 21 or 100% O_2 in newborn pigs. J Appl Physiol 1993; 75:2054–2060.
46. Moison RMW, Palinckx JJS, Roest M, et al. Induction of lipid peroxidation of pulmonary surfactant by plasma of preterm babies. Lancet 1993; 341:79–82.
47. Yokoyama Y, Beckman JS, Beckman TK, et al. Freeman BA, Parks DA. Circulating xanthine oxidase: Potential mediator of ischemic injury. Am J Physiol 1990; 258:G564–G570.
48. Supnet MC, David-Cu R, Walther FJ. Plasma xanthine oxidase activity and lipid hydroperoxide levels in preterm infants. Pediatr Res 1994; 36:283–287.
49. Bell AH, Skov L, Lundstrøm KE, et al. Measurement of global cerebral blood flow in preterm babies after surfactant treatment. Acta Paediatr 1994; 83:910–914.
50. Russell GAB. Antioxidants and neonatal lung disease. Eur J Pediatr 1994; 153(Suppl 2):36–41.

28

Surfactant Therapy for Adult Respiratory Distress Syndrome

FRANCIS X. McCORMACK
University of Cincinnati
Cincinnati, Ohio

ROBERT J. MASON
National Jewish Center for Immunology and Respiratory Medicine
and the University of Colorado School of Medicine
Denver, Colorado

I. Introduction

Surfactant replacement has become the standard of care for neonates with infant respiratory distress syndrome (IRDS). Multiple well-designed trials have demonstrated clear improvements in pulmonary compliance, gas exchange, complications of barotrauma, and mortality in premature infants born with respiratory failure who are treated with synthetic and natural surfactants (1,2). These successes have generated enthusiasm for trials of surfactant replacement therapy in acute lung injury in adult patients. Although surfactant abnormalities have been described in several lung diseases, including pneumonia (3,4), fibrotic lung disease (5,6), atelectasis (7), and radiation injury (8), the adult respiratory distress syndrome (ARDS) is the most logical initial target for surfactant replacement in the adult population. This strategy is based on convincing histopathological and pathophysiological parallels with IRDS, suggesting an important role for abnormalities of surface active material in ARDS. Although trials of surfactant therapy in adults have just begun, preliminary studies support optimism that exogenous surfactant will reduce barotrauma and improve gas exchange in ARDS and that the extent of pulmonary injury and respiratory disability will be attenuated.

The evidence that surfactant plays an important role in the clinical presentation of ARDS is compelling. The characteristic physiological derangements in ARDS, including atelectasis, impaired gas exchange, and decreased compliance, are consistent with the hypothesis that functional inactivation or deficiency of surfactant is important in the pathophysiology of the disease (9,10). Furthermore, surfactant is clearly abnormal in ARDS. The composition of surfactant recovered by bronchoalveolar lavage (BAL) is altered and surface tension–lowering qualities are impaired (11–14). Although definitive conclusions await the results of human trials, studies employing animal models of ARDS demonstrate that surfactant replacement partially restores pulmonary compliance and gas exchange (15–19). The success of surfactant replacement in these models is testament to the importance of surfactant in acute lung injury. Taken together, these data suggest that the impairment of the biophysical qualities of surfactant contributes to the physiological derangements of ARDS. Thus, there is a sound theoretical basis for the use of exogenous surfactant to address the clinical pulmonary dysfunction of ARDS.

Less certain is the role of surfactant in the development and perpetuation of lung injury in ARDS. Although conclusive studies are not available, surfactant abnormalities do not appear to herald the development of ARDS and are present in respiratory failure because of multiple etiologies (14). It is becoming clear that a host of insults which alter the viability, synthetic function, or surfactant metabolism of alveolar type II cells can result in the "characteristic" abnormalities of surfactant phospholipid and protein composition described in patients with ARDS. In support of these findings, Gregory et al. (14) demonstrated that most of the at-risk patients with respiratory failure and ARDS-like surfactant abnormalities never develop ARDS (by standard criteria). Hence, there is no conclusive evidence that primary surfactant abnormalities are necessary or sufficient to develop the syndrome. However, abnormalities of surface activity may play a secondary role in lung injury. Once biophysical qualities of surfactant have been impaired in patients with established alveolar damage, increased surface tension forces may aggravate and perpetuate the pulmonary injury. Atelectasis of alveolar units promotes the apposition and fibrotic fusion of denuded alveolar basement membranes in ARDS (collapse induration) (20). By extrapolation from the infant syndrome, the stretching of surfactant-deficient, poorly compliant alveolar structures results in further epithelial damage and desquamation (21). Thus, it is likely that surfactant derangements play an important, if not etiological, role in the lung injury and subsequent fibrotic scarring in patients with ARDS. On this basis, there is cautious optimism that surfactant therapy will also address the progression of pulmonary injury in ARDS.

II. Clinical Overview of Features of ARDS Relevant to Surfactant Therapy

A. Historical Perspective

The first clinical description of ARDS is attributed to Ashbaugh, et al. (22). They reported 12 patients who developed diffuse pulmonary infiltrates, reduced lung compliance, hypoxemia, and respiratory failure following a variety of traumatic, infectious, and systemic insults. Lung tissue from these patients at autopsy revealed interstitial and alveolar edema, hyaline membrane formation, and widespread atelectasis. These investigators recognized clinical and pathological parallels with the infant respiratory distress syndrome and suggested that pulmonary surfactant was abnormal in ARDS. They further demonstrated that material derived from the minced postmortem lungs of two of the patients had impaired surface tension–lowering characteristics (9,10). The initial recognition and remarkably thorough clinical description of this syndrome has been a lasting achievement. In fact, the only generally accepted modification to the definition of ARDS since that time has been the objective exclusion of cardiogenic pulmonary edema, which was made possible by the development of the Swan-Ganz catheter (Table 1). In addition, the list of pulmonary and systemic insults which have been found to result in ARDS has expanded considerably. Over the past 25 years, however, the advent of critical care, dramatic technological advances, and multicenter trials with steroids (23–25) and prostaglandins (26) have had little impact on mortality in ARDS. Trials with nonsteroidal anti-inflammatory agents, cytokines, various receptor antagonists, and anti-endotoxin antibodies are under discussion or in progress (27). To date, however, no therapeutic intervention or treatment has been reported to interrupt the cycle of biological or mechanical insult and alveolar damage that results in progressive loss of gas exchange units in ARDS. Surfactant treatment in ARDS is a promising therapeutic alternative in a disease that has frustrated clinicians for nearly three decades.

Table 1 Criteria for the Diagnosis of ARDS

1. Appropriate risk factor
2. Severe arterial hypoxemia
3. Increased intrapulmonary shunt fraction
4. Decreased lung volumes (functional residual capacity, total lung capacity)
5. Decreased lung compliance
6. Diffuse infiltrates on chest x-ray
7. Exclusion of cardiogenic cause for pulmonary edema

Source: From ref. 114; with permission.

B. Clinical-Pathological Correlations and Pathogenesis

The uniformity of the pathological lesion in ARDS irrespective of the inciting insult suggests that pulmonary injury is either due to a common mediator or that the lung has a limited repertoire of response to injury. Despite intensive research, no unifying mechanism implicating a single mediator has emerged (28). The general scheme below is assembled from animal data and human observations (29) but is not representative of ARDS from all etiologies. The histopathological evolution of the disease is arbitrarily divided into the exudative (or injury) phase, the repair (or proliferative) phase, and the healed phase. A variety of pulmonary or systemic insults, such as prolonged hypotension, pneumonia, or sepsis, leads to platelet and neutrophil accumulation in the pulmonary microvasculature (30). There is substantial evidence that neutrophils are important in the pathogenesis of ARDS, although the syndrome also occurs in neutropenic patients (28). Activated leukocytes trapped in pulmonary capillaries release or secrete toxic products resulting in alveolar damage. The mediators of injury may include but are not limited to cytokines (31), arachidonic acid intermediates (32), phospholipases (33), reactive oxygen species (34), lysosomal enzymes and proteases (35), and complement proteins (36) (Table 2). Clinically, respiratory distress usually develops between 12 and 48 hr after the initial insult and more than 90% of cases are apparent by 80 hr (37). This latency period represents a window of opportunity for therapeutic intervention, especially after high-risk events (e.g., gastric aspiration).

The *exudative phase* begins within hours of the precipitating injury. The interstitium of the lung becomes edematous and the air spaces become filled with proteinaceous exudate and red blood cells. Destruction of alveolar type I cells and endothelial injury are the proximate causes of the alveolar edema (38). The flooding of the alveoli with serum proteins and other factors inactivates surfactant

Table 2 Potential Mediators of Lung Injury in ARDS

Complement
Oxygen radicals
Proteases
Endotoxin
Eicosanoids
Platelet-activating factor
Cytokines (TNF, interleukins, endothelin)
Growth factors
Kallikreins (kinins)
Fragment D

Source: From ref. 28; with permission.

and results in atelectasis. Protein, cellular debris, and fibrin condense to form hyaline membranes which marginate along the air space lumens (39,40). The alveolar septa and air spaces become infiltrated with polymorphonuclear leukocytes, and bronchoalveolar lavage at this stage usually demonstrates neutrophilia. These diverse histopathological changes which develop soon after lung injury are termed diffuse alveolar damage (DAD).

The *repair phase* usually occurs in the interval from 7 to 28 days after onset, although there is significant variability. During this period, the alveolar exudate must be cleared and the epithelial barrier restored. The proliferation of hypertrophic type II cells over denuded alveolar basement membranes and subsequent terminal differentiation into type I cells repopulates the alveolar epithelium. Fibroblasts infiltrate the pulmonary parenchyma and may predominate either in the interstitium or in the air spaces (40,41). In an unfortunate subset of patients, collagen is deposited resulting in fibrotic distortion of the alveolar architecture. Patients with exuberant fibroproliferation on open lung biopsy from 1 to 3 weeks following the initial insult may be especially responsive to treatment with prednisone (42,43). Even in the absence of treatment, post-ARDS pulmonary fibrosis may spontaneously reverse with the return of normal or near-normal pulmonary function. This phenomenon involves the elimination of fibroblasts, collagen and other connective tissue matrices, and capillaries followed by repopulation of the alveolar spaces with type I cells. The role of apoptosis in the elimination of the cellular infiltrate during tissue remodeling is under investigation (44). The effectiveness of this remodeling process contrasts with many forms of pulmonary fibrosis which typically result in permanent and progressive scarring (45).

The *healed phase* of ARDS may be associated with a broad range of histopathological changes. The post-ARDS lung tissue may be normal or may show increased alveolar macrophages, nonspecific interstitial scarring, or mural scarring in the small airways. In some patients, particularly those exposed to high airway pressures or high oxygen tensions for prolonged periods, residual scarring is more severe, and it may resemble usual interstitial pneumonia. These patients may suffer irreversible pulmonary disability owing to restrictive lung disease. In most survivors of ARDS, however, pulmonary function improves over the first 6–12 months, and estimates of chronic pulmonary disability should not be made in the sixth month of recovery (46).

III. Abnormalities of Surfactant in ARDS

A. Quantitative Compositional and Biophysical Abnormalities of Surfactant in ARDS

There have been several studies describing the biochemical and biophysical qualities of surfactant isolated from patients with ARDS (Table 3) (see Chapter

Table 3 Surfactant Abnormalities in Patients with ARDS

First author	Year	n	PL	PC	DPPC	PG	Min surf tension	SP-A	SP-B
Ashbaugh (22)	1967	2					I		
Petty (9)	1977	1	NC				NC		
Petty (10)	1979	6					NC		
Hallman (13)	1982	26	NC	D		D	I		
Pison (11)	1989	17	D	D		D	NC		
Pison (12)	1990	30	D	D		D			
Gregory (14)	1991	66	D	D	D	D	I	D	D
Pison (48)	1992	19	D	D		D		D	

D, decreased; I, increased; NC, no change.
Source: Modified from ref. 55; with permission.

9). Early reports examined the characteristics of surface-active material derived from ex vivo lungs of patients who died of ARDS (9,22). Lavage phospholipid recovery was reduced and the surface activity of the BAL surfactant was low but confounding postmortem changes in the lung could not be excluded. In a subsequent report, Petty and coworkers described a lighter buoyant density and an increased compressability of surfactant recovered from patients with ARDS shortly after death (10). Hallman et al. (13) subsequently reported the phospholipid composition and biophysical characteristics of surfactant isolated by bronchoalveolar lavage from 26 patients with ARDS compared with 12 normal controls. They found that the phosphatidylcholine to sphingomyelin ratio, disaturated phosphatidylcholine and phosphatidylglycerol were reduced, whereas sphingomyelin and phosphatidylserine were elevated. The lipid-protein complexes isolated on sucrose density centrifugation from patients with ARDS demonstrated increased minimum surface tension compared with normal controls. The importance of the epithelial layer as a barrier to contaminating serum proteins was underscored by Holter et al. (47). These authors described the molecular mass distribution of proteins recovered by bronchoalveolar lavage from patients with ARDS compared with normal controls and patients with cardiac edema. Large proteins were recovered in much greater abundance from patients with ARDS than in the patients with pulmonary edema due to elevated left ventricular pressures. They concluded that the normal size selectivity of the epithelial barrier was preserved in cardiac edema but lost in ARDS. Protein inactivation of surfactant is now thought to be a major determinant of the early pulmonary manifestations of ARDS (see below and Chapter 13). Pison examined surfactant characteristics and the time course of surfactant changes of 17 patients with posttraumatic pulmonary dysfunction (11). These patients were stratified into a high and low ARDS severity groups using a multifarious clinical scoring system. Serial lavages were performed daily for 2 weeks and the surfactant composition and surface tension–lowering qualities were measured. Total phospholipid content was unchanged but there was a progressive decrease in the phosphatidylcholine and phosphatidylglycerol content of lavage over time. Abnormalities in the surface activity of the surfactant pellet paralleled these changes. The decrease in phosphatidylcholine and the magnitude of derangement in surface activity were more pronounced in patients with a higher ARDS score than in those with less severe pulmonary dysfunction. Protein leakage into the alveolar space was also greater in patients with more severe respiratory failure. A subsequent study examined the time course of surfactant protein A (SP-A) abnormalities in pulmonary parenchymal injury associated with polytrauma (48). SP-A is the most abundant surfactant-associated protein in the alveolar space and is synthesized primarily by alveolar type II cells. SP-A in lavage was reduced and the magnitude of reduction correlated with the severity of the lung injury. In patients with mild to moderate pulmonary injury, the SP-A levels normalized, whereas in patients with severe injury SP-A remained low over the time period examined. A multicenter study of surfactant abnormalities in 66 patients with ARDS was recently completed (14). Gregory et al. found that total surfactant phospholipid recovered by lavage was decreased in ARDS. In addition, phosphatidylcholine and phosphatidylglycerol were depleted, whereas disaturated phosphatidylcholine was unchanged and phosphatidylinositol was elevated. Surfactant proteins A and B were significantly reduced in ARDS relative to normal controls by factors of 4 and 2, respectively (Fig. 1). Total protein in the surfactant pellet was reduced despite the flooding of the air spaces with protein-rich edema fluid, a finding perhaps due to the purification procedure employed. The minimum surface tension of the surfactant pellet was also increased in ARDS patients. Surprisingly, very similar (but less severe) surfactant abnormalities were found in the group of 20 at-risk patients who had developed respiratory failure, only one of whom ultimately met the criteria for ARDS. The impairment of the biophysical activity of surfactant was intermediate between normals and patients with ARDS (Fig. 2). This result suggests that changes in surfactant composition and biophysical characteristics may be a nonspecific response to lung injury and serves to highlight the importance of surfactant inhibitors in the development of ARDS. At the current time, however, it is not possible to determine if surfactant abnormalities are the cause or the result of lung dysfunction in ARDS.

Thus, the abnormalities in surfactant composition which have been described in ARDS include a reduction in total phospholipid, total phosphatidylcholine (PC), dipalmitoyl phosphatidylcholine (DPPC), phosphatidyl-

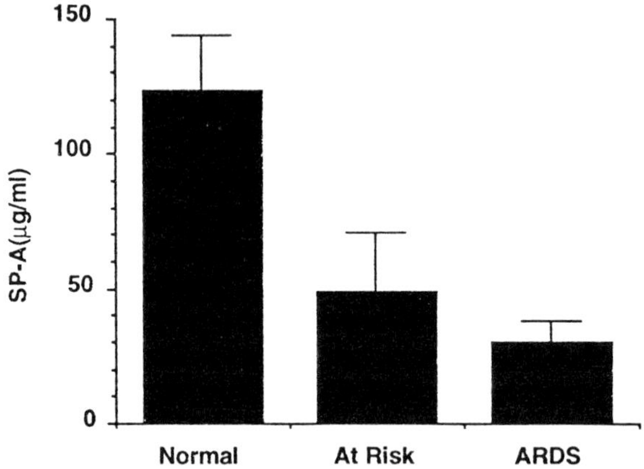

Figure 1 Surfactant protein A in normal subjects and at-risk and patients with ARDS. (Redrawn from ref. 14; with permission.)

glycerol (PG), SP-A and SP-B, and an increase in phosphatidylinositol, phosphatidylethanolamine, and phosphatidylserine (49). Surfactant recovered by BAL in ARDS has altered surface tension–lowering characteristics, but the extent to which quantitative and compositional surfactant abnormalities directly contribute to the atelectasis, gas exchange abnormalities, and decreased compliance in ARDS is not known. Several investigators have suggested that inhibitors or inactivators of surfactant function are responsible for most of the surfactant dysfunction of ARDS (50).

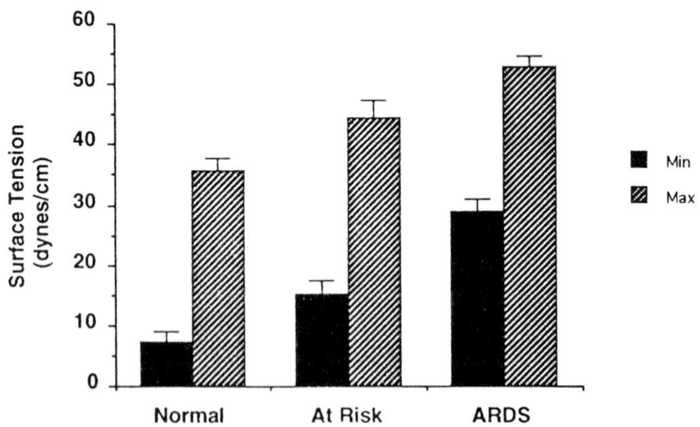

Figure 2 Biophysical activity of the crude surfactant pellet in normal subjects and at-risk and patients with ARDS. (Redrawn from ref. 14; with permission.)

B. Surfactant Inactivation in ARDS

Surfactant inactivation may occur through several mechanisms (Table 4) (see Chapter 13). Surfactant may be diluted with pulmonary edema fluid or depleted by foaming (51,52). In addition, the well-described abnormalities of surfactant composition may be responsible for the altered biophysical characteristics of surfactant in ARDS. It is more likely, however, that depletion of surfactant or abnormal surfactant composition renders the alveolar lining layer more susceptible to potent inhibition by protein-rich pulmonary edema (Fig. 3) (53,54). This notion is supported by data from animal models in which subtotal surfactant depletion produced by limited bronchoalveolar lavage enhances the physiological dysfunction induced by intratracheal instillation of plasma proteins (54). In several animal injury models, normal surface tension–lowering characteristics of surfactant are restored when foreign proteins are separated from the phospholipid components of BAL fluid (15). This finding has also been confirmed in patients with ARDS (55).

There is clinical and experimental evidence to suggest that serum proteins are capable of producing profound surfactant inhibition. Flooding of the alveolar spaces with serum-derived proteins through the injured epithelial barrier is common to ARDS of all etiologies (54). Proteins enter the alveolar space in rough proportion to their concentration in serum (47). The rank order of potency for surfactant inhibition is fibrin monomer > fibrin > immunoglobulin G > albumin. Protein contamination of surfactant decreases both the rate of adsorption of surfactant to the air-liquid interface and the ability of surfactant to reduce surface tension to low values on dynamic compression (56). The mechanism of surfactant inhibition by serum-derived proteins is not fully understood but several theories have been advanced. Serum proteins may directly interfere with phospholipid physiochemical properties in the bulk phase or in the monolayer. Alternatively, foreign proteins may compete with surface-active phospholipids for occupancy of sites in the monolayer (57). Inhibition of surfactant by foreign proteins is dose dependent and can be stoichiometrically overcome by increasing

Table 4 Substances Capable of Inhibiting Surfactant Function

Whole serum	Phospholipases
Albumin	Lysophospholipids
Fibrinogen	Oxygen radicals
Fibrin monomer	Proteases
IgG	Membrane lipids
Hemoglobin	

Source: From ref. 114; with permission.

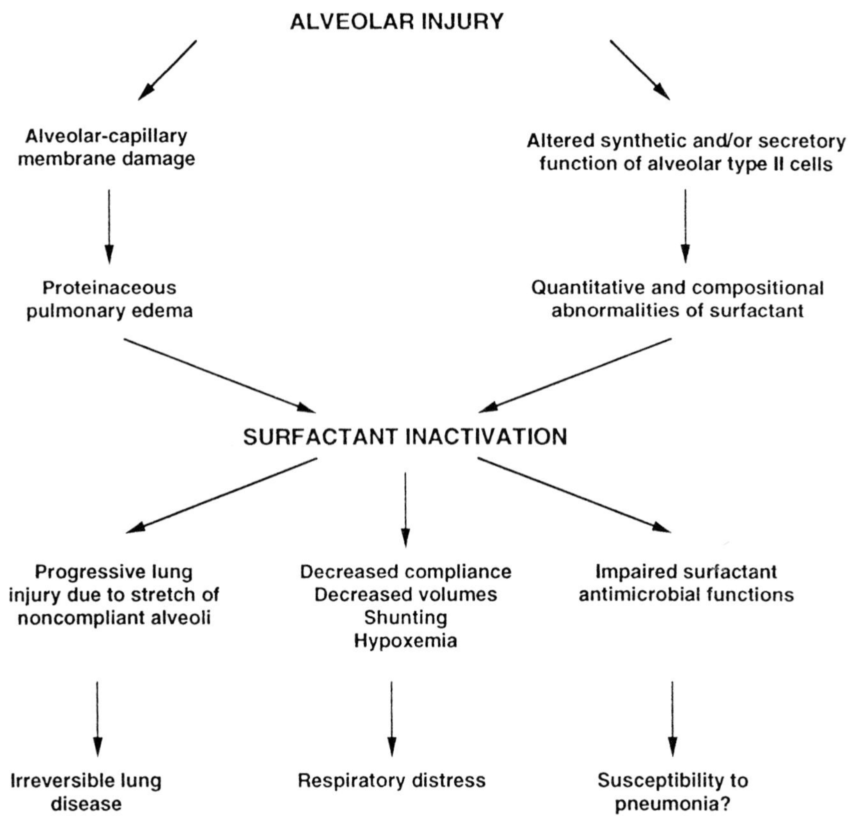

Figure 3 Role of surfactant in the adult respiratory distress syndrome.

the ratio of lipid to protein (58,59). In the whole organism, this can be accomplished either by administering exogenous surfactant or by presurfactant therapeutic bronchoalveolar lavage to reduce the burden of alveolar protein (18,19). The finding that synthetic surfactants are more susceptible to protein inhibition than natural surfactants suggests that an endogenous component or characteristic of surfactant reduces surfactant inactivation (60). Recently, the surfactant proteins SP-B and SP-C (61) and to a lesser extent SP-A (49,62) have been shown to increase the resistance of surfactant preparations to contaminating serum protein inhibition. These discoveries have important implications for the design of optimal surfactants for the treatment of ARDS.

Surfactant can also be inactivated in ARDS by reactive oxygen species, proteases, and phospholipases. Exposure to hyperoxic conditions has multiple deleterious effects on the surfactant system. The alveolar epithelium is damaged, surfactant synthesis is depressed (63), and surfactant function is impaired (64). Reactive oxygen species inactivate surfactant through the formation of free radicals and reactive intermediates which oxidize and modify protein and lipid species (65). Unsaturated lipid species, surfactant protein A, and α_1-antitrypsin have each been shown to be vulnerable to oxidative attack (55). Oxidation of surfactant apoproteins may in turn enhance susceptibility to attack by proteases (66–69). Finally, oxidative inactivation of antiproteases in the alveolus may render the lung more susceptible to injury by neutrophil elastase and other proteases (35).

Phospholipases hydrolyze acyl side chains from phospholipids resulting in the formation of lysophospholipids and free fatty acids. Thus, these enzymes simultaneously decrease the concentration of phospholipid in the alveolar space and generate lipid species which are disruptive to monolayers and surfactant aggregates (70). Phospholipase A_2 (PLA_2) has profound effects of the surface activity of surfactant lipids in vitro (70). In addition, subtoxic concentrations of phospholipases which are below the threshold for surfactant inactivation greatly potentiate the inhibitory potency of exogenous proteins (70). Patients with respiratory failure on the basis of pancreatitis have reduced levels of phosphatidylcholine and increased levels of phospholipase A_2 in bronchoalveolar lavage (33). The phospholipase activity of bronchoalveolar lavage fluid is also increased in patients with ARDS of other etiologies (70). Surfactant inhibition by phospholipases may not be easily overcome by exogenous surfactant, since phospholipases act on the added substrate to generate more lysophospholipid and fatty acid species (54). Phospholipases other than PLA_2 have also been shown to inactivate surfactant (70).

C. Impaired Antimicrobial Defenses of Surfactant

Several studies have suggested that whole surfactant (71,72), surfactant phospholipids and the surfactant proteins A (73,74) and D (75) have antimicrobial qualities. Patients with ARDS are at increased risk for the development of pneumonia. Although no data are available, it is possible that abnormalities of surfactant in ARDS (both phospholipids and surfactant proteins) may contribute to altered host defenses. (See Chapter 4)

IV. Comparison of ARDS and IRDS with Regard to Surfactant Replacement

It is useful to explore the clinical-pathological-physiological parallels and differences between ARDS and IRDS (Tables 5 and 6). Comparison topics relevant to surfactant replacement which are discussed include the roles of (1)

Table 5 Adult Respiratory Distress Syndrome and Infant Respiratory Distress Syndrome

Similarities	ARDS	IRDS
Surfactant deficiency	Probably	Yes
Abnormality in composition	Yes	Yes
Microatelectasis/overdistention	Yes	Yes
Importance of barotrauma	Yes	Yes
Dissimilarities	**ARDS**	**IRDS**
Mechanism	Alveolar injury	Immaturity
Alveolar damage	Early, 1 degree	Late, 2 degrees
Population	Heterogeneous	Homogeneous
Onset predictable	Generally not	Yes
Critical role of inflammation	Yes	No
Clinical course	Highly variable	Less variable
Multi-organ failure	Yes	No
Mortality	50%	15%
Surfactant deficiency	Late	Early
Surfactant inactivation	Early	Late
Improved PaO_2 after surfactant Rx	Incomplete(?)	Often Dramatic

Table 6 Rationale for Surfactant Replacement in ARDS

Pathogenetic	
reduce protein and fluid leak	Yes
attenuate inflammation	Maybe
limit lung injury	Maybe
Physiological	
improve gas exchange	Yes
reduce intrapulmonary shunt	Yes
improve compliance	Probably
reduce barotrauma	Yes
Sequelae	
reduce pulmonary infections	Maybe
reduce nonpulmonary infections	No
limit pulmonary fibrosis	Maybe
reduce panendothelial permeability	No
prevent multi-organ failure	No
reduce mortality	Maybe

alveolar injury, (2) surfactant deficiency, (3) surfactant inhibitors in the two syndromes.

The data for the study of lung pathology in IRDS are derived from the autopsy material of infants who do not survive (76). In very premature infants (<500 gs), the lungs are atelectatic or filled with a low-protein fluid, but there is no obvious cell death or hyaline membrane formation. The lungs are normal in weight and pink (77). Infants who survive for 4 hr to 5 days develop hyaline membranes comprised of plasma proteins, nucleic acids, and lipids in the alveolar spaces (78). Hyaline membranes first appear in the central air spaces and terminal airways which are preferentially ventilated in the noncompliant lung. The periphery of the lobules are relatively spared. Overdistention in conjunction with atelectasis is associated with vacuolization of capillary endothelium, sloughing of the alveolar epithelium, and alveolar permeability (21). The process of repair may begin as early as the second day. Hypertrophic alveolar epithelial cells line the alveolus producing an almost glandular appearance. Pathological data beyond this stage is scarce. Of three infants who suffered crib death 6–8 weeks following RDS, two had histologically normal lungs and one had extensive goblet cell hyperplasia (76).

Thus, like ARDS, the lungs of patients with IRDS demonstrate a pattern of alveolar damage, alveolar membrane permeability resulting in protein leak, amorphous exudative debris in the alveolar space, and hyaline membrane formation. However, along with features of lung immaturity, deficiency of surfactant is the primary abnormality in IRDS and alveolar damage and permeability are secondary to overdistension of airways and air spaces. In contrast, in ARDS, a primary alveolar insult results in a promiscuous permeability defect and vicious cycle of surfactant inactivation, atelectasis, and worsening gas exchange. The observation that surfactant deficiency in IRDS results in alveolar injury may have relevance to ARDS. It suggests that progressive lung injury following the inciting insult in ARDS may be related, in part, to the absence of a functional alveolar lining layer (14,13). Although an absolute deficiency of surfactant has not been conclusively demonstrated in ARDS, there is ample evidence that the biophysical qualities of surfactant are severely compromised. It is possible that progression of lung injury following the initial insult may be thwarted by surfactant supplementation. Inactivation of surfactant is the proposed mechanism whereby one-third of patients with IRDS fail to respond to surfactant supplementation. Because of routinely elevated alveolar protein concentrations, the threat of inactivation of exogenous surfactant is greater in ARDS than in IRDS. Additional consideration must be given to replacement strategies which limit inactivation. This may involve lavage to remove debris before the instillation of surfactant, greater doses of surfactant than used in infants to stoichiometrically overcome inactivation or additives which resist inactivation. In particular, surfactant proteins A, B, and/or C may be beneficial in surfactant preparations to protect the surface activity of administered surfactant.

Finally, surfactant replacement in ARDS differs in concept from its infant counterpart, at least in its early stages, in that the lung is injured and parenchymal architecture is distorted by cellular infiltrates and increased connective tissue. Thus, the decreased lung compliance in ARDS is the result of both surfactant dysfunction and abnormal elastic recoil of lung tissue. Exogenous surfactant does not affect the tissue compliance of the lung and incomplete responses should be anticipated. In addition, patients with ARDS represent a more heterogeneous population than infants with IRDS and the outcome may be less predictable. The duration of the illness, the diversity of etiological insults, and concomitant illness and organ failure all complicate the treatment of patients with ARDS. Despite the differences between IRDS and ARDS in the early stages, it is also probable that infants with severe IRDS pass through stages similar to ARDS as their disease progresses to bronchopulmonary dysplasia.

V. Surfactant Replacement in Experimental Models of ARDS

Several animal models have been developed to reproduce the alveolar damage, protein-rich pulmonary edema, hyaline membrane formation, impaired gas exchange, atelectasis, and decreased compliance of ARDS. (See also Chapter 12.) Comparisons with the human syndrome must be made cautiously, since the pathology and physiology of many lung injury models can mimic that of ARDS without necessarily directly reflecting the mechanisms involved in the development of ARDS. The models which have been developed include detergent aerosol, smoke inhalation, in vivo lung lavage, antilung serum, bilateral cervical vagatomy, oxygen toxicity, viral infection (79,80), and N-nitroso-N-methyl-urea infusion. A few of the best characterized models which have included studies of surfactant replacement are discussed (see Chapter 12).

In vivo lung lavage depletes the intra-alveolar pool of surfactant with a limited immediate effect on the cellular compartments (16,17). This procedure produces respiratory failure due to reduced lung compliance and impaired gas exchange, similarly to ARDS (81,82). Histological examination of animals killed 5 min after the last lavage shows atelectasis and mild cellular changes. Animals who are mechanically ventilated after lavage develop lung injury characterized by hemorrhagic pulmonary edema, necrosis and desquamation of bronchiolar and alveolar epithelium, and hyaline membrane formation. There is dramatic improvement in oxygenation (Po_2 95–300 mmHg) and ventilation ($Paco_2$ 95–55 mmHg) in animals treated with exogenous surfactant composed of DPPC, unsaturated PC, PG, and 6% other surfactant lipids (Curosurf). Administration of exogenous surfactant 15 and 45 min after the lavage procedure prevents intra-alveolar edema and damage to the airway epithelium (83). Thus, alveolar permeability is increased by the lavage procedure alone, but alveolar damage is the result of ventilation of poorly compliant air spaces. However, this model is of limited utility in the study of ARDS, since there is limited primary alveolar epithelial injury. Nonetheless, it is suitable for testing the feasibility of surfactant replacement in the surfactant-depleted lung.

Exposure of animals to 100% oxygen produces severe lung injury resulting in increased alveolar permeability, decreased compliance, and atelectasis (63,84–87). Histological lung sections from animals exposed to hyperoxic conditions for 2–3 days shows hemorrhagic intra-alveolar edema, alveolar accumulation of neutrophils, necrosis of alveolar and bronchiolar epithelium, and migration of histiocytes and fibroblasts into the interstitium (88). Pressure volume curve studies of saline filled lungs demonstrate that the most of the observed decrease in lung compliance is the result of surfactant inactivation rather than lung tissue changes. The surfactant abnormalities described in the hyperoxic injury model mimic those of ARDS. Total phospholipid, phosphatidylcholine, dipalmitoyl phosphatidylcholine, and phosphatidylglycerol are decreased in BAL fluid, whereas phosphatidylinositol is increased. There is a marked increase in the total protein in bronchoalveolar lavage, and the surface tension–lowering qualities of surfactant are impaired. Surfactant replacement improves mortality, reduces protein leak into the alveolar space, and partially restores surface tension–lowering qualities of the surfactant isolated by BAL (89,90).

The compound N-nitroso-N-methyl urea (NNNMU) produces a syndrome very similar to human ARDS within a few days of infusion into animals (91–93). NNNMU injection results in alveolar type II cell injury, edema, atelectasis, neutrophilic infiltration, decreased lung compliance, and increased intrapulmonary shunt. Furthermore, surfactant abnormalities are similar to those of ARDS, with a reduction in surfactant phospholipids, decreased phosphatidylglycerol, and increased phosphatidylinositol (91). Surfactant protein A is also reduced. In animals with lung injury due to NNNMU, treatment with a modified bovine lung surfactant (Survanta) normalized the phospholipid composition of the surfactant recovered by lavage. Gas exchange and surface activity of recovered surfactant was also significantly improved. The survival of Survanta-treated animals was significantly increased at 24 hr over air or saline controls (60% vs 13 or 20%, respectively) (94).

Intratracheal hydrochloric acid instillation results in damage to the alveolar-capillary membrane, flooding of the alveolar spaces with protein-rich pulmonary edema, and surfactant inhibition (95–97). The physiological changes produced by this procedure are similar to ARDS and include diminished compliance, atelectasis, intrapulmonary shunting, and hypoxemia. Surfactant replacement has generally demonstrated only a limited or partial response on the pulmonary mechanics and gas exchange in this model. This has been attributed to inhibition of the function of exogenous surfactant by abundant serum-derived inhibitors in the air spaces. A recent study (19) demonstrated that rats given intratracheal HCl developed profound hypoxemia that was not reversed with surfactant replacement (freeze dried, natural, bovine surfactant). Only those acid-treated animals who were lavaged with saline prior to surfactant replacement or who were lavaged with diluted surface active material had a significant improvement in Pa_{O_2}. This finding is consistent with the notion that surfactant inhibition by serum-derived proteins or other factors must be stoichiometrically overcome either by increasing the amount of exogenous phospholipid or reducing the amount of endogenous inhibitor. In a subsequent study (18) these investigators also demonstrated that exogenous surfactant given immediately (1 or 10 min) after intratracheal HCl prevented the development of respiratory failure. The total protein accumulation in the alveolar space was not different in the surfactant- versus saline-treated animals, suggesting that the instilled surfactant did not directly protect the alveolar-capillary membrane. This study suggests that respiratory failure from acid aspiration can be prevented by surfactant replacement but only if it is given before gas exchange deteriorates.

VI. Practical Clinical Considerations for Surfactant Replacement in Adults

The logistical questions which must be answered for the optimal delivery of surfactant therapy include (1) what delivery method?, (2) how much surfactant?, (3) who gets it?, (4) when?, (5) how often?, (6) how long?, (7) what criteria should be used to withdraw therapy?, (8) what cost is reasonable?

The dose and method of administration of surfactant in patients with ARDS is controversial (see Chapter 30). There is limited data available on the dose response of exogenous surfactant on the physiological abnormalities of ARDS. In newborn infants, surfactant treatments are generally given in one to four doses at 60–200 mg/kg over the first 24–48 hr of life. In adults, the surfactant alveolar pool size is estimated to be about 10 mg/kg, although the optimal treatment dose is likely to be much higher because of inefficient distribution, surfactant inhibitors, and altered metabolism. The most promising trial to date employed doses of phospholipid up to 400 mg/kg ideal body weight. Equally uncertain in adults is the number of doses and/or duration of treatment. At its earliest and simplest stage, IRDS has a clearly defined endpoint; that is, competence of the patient to synthesize pulmonary surfactant. In adults, the initial targets are likely to be improvement in defined physiological parameters and gas exchange. The objectives of limitation of barometric injury, liberation from the ventilator, and improvements in mortality are the initial goals which will justify the use of this expensive therapy.

The options for administration include slow or bolus administration through the endotracheal tube or bronchoscope, aerosol administration via in-line nebulizer, and presurfactant saline followed by surfactant administration or dilute surfactant lavage. Bolus administration through the endotracheal tube or bronchoscope is rapid, extrapulmonary losses are negligible, and safety has been demonstrated in preliminary trials (98–100). Although routinely used in IRDS, the bolus method may not be optimal for ARDS because of the volume required to treat the immense surface area of the adult lung (250–300 ml for 70-kg adult at 100 mg/kg) and inefficient distribution and cost considerations (as high as $35,000/patient). Slow intratracheal infusion of surfactant to lavaged rabbits through an indwelling endotracheal catheter resulted in an inhomogeneous distribution of surfactant and no changes in gas exchange, whereas bolus administration led to a prompt and sustained increase in Pa_{O_2} (101). No trials of slow intratracheal infusion are available in humans. Nebulized surfactant therapy has been shown to be safe and effective in preliminary human trials (102,103) (see Chapter 30). Nebulization therapy has the potential to reduce the dosage requirements by 20- to 50-fold (104) and the pattern of distribution is more homogeneous than bolus administration in animals with uniform lung injury (105). In nonuniform lung injury models, however, aerosolized surfactant is preferentially deposited in the less affected areas of the lung that receive the greatest share of ventilation (106). This diversion of surfactant away from the severely damaged areas of the lung to less severely damaged areas attenuates the beneficial physiological effects of surfactant therapy (106). In addition, aerosolized therapy is complicated by lengthy delivery times, losses from deposition of surfactant droplets along the ventilator circuit, and the clogging of filters and exhalation valves. Nebulization strategies are being developed which optimize the dose of surfactant, duration of aerosolization, particle size, and ventilator hardware. These parameters can only be adequately addressed empirically through carefully designed trials. The optimal method of delivery of surfactant in ARDS may ultimately be a combination of instilled and aerosolized therapy.

The timing of surfactant therapy can be divided into four periods: prophylactic; postinsult, pre-ARDS; acute ARDS; and established ARDS. Prophylactic therapy in humans is a useful concept for discussion but is obviously not practical. Animal studies provide evidence that prophylactic surfactant treatment can be protective against a variety of insults, including oxygen toxicity and acid aspiration (18,19). Perhaps the most exciting prospect for surfactant therapy in humans will be during the latency period from precipitating insult to the development pulmonary infiltrates. Intervention during this postinsult, pre-ARDS phase has the potential to interrupt the cycle of flooding of the alveolar space with serum proteins, surfactant inactivation, and respiratory failure. Unfortunately, identification of the subset of patients who are likely to benefit from early postinsult surfactant treatment is problematic. At present, there is no single clinical parameter which is predictive of the development of ARDS following the initial insult. Multiple defined risk factors for ARDS in a given individual enhance the likelihood of the development of ARDS. In a prospective study of 993 patients at risk for ARDS, the syndrome developed in 7% of patients with one risk factor and 24% in patients with two or more risk factors (107). The risk factor which had the highest incidence of ARDS was witnessed aspiration of gastric contents (35%). Thus, it may be possible to identify subsets of patients who have a 1:3 to 1:4 chance of developing ARDS. Even this degree of accuracy in predicting the development of ARDS may not be adequate to justify costly early postinsult treatment.

Surfactant treatment during the acute phase of ARDS is also promising. During this phase, many patients experience rising Fio_2 and positive end-expiratory pressure (PEEP) requirements related to progressive pulmonary injury from inflammation or surfactant inactivation. Surfactant replacement has the potential to overcome atelectasis and mechanical injury to the lung by restoring alveolar surface activity. The subset of patients who may be least likely to respond are those with established ARDS. These patients may have substantial remodeling of their pulmonary parenchyma and a significant tissue component to their decreased lung compliance. They are less likely to be liberated from the respirator by surfactant treatment. It is entirely possible that this subgroup of patients may derive benefit from surfactant therapy, and the cost-benefit analysis should be periodically reviewed as surfactant therapies become less expensive.

The candidacy criteria for surfactant replacement therapy have not been determined. Physicians must take into account the cause of the ARDS, the predicted duration of ventilatory support, and the stage and prognosis of the illness. Patients should be stratified by their precipitating injury, at least initially, so that differential responsiveness to surfactant therapy can be determined. The expanded definition of ARDS proposed by Murray et al. (108) classifies the syndrome into acute or chronic; mild, moderate, or severe; and by specific cause. The ARDS due to contrast dye is more likely to be self-limited than ARDS related to unrelenting sepsis. The ARDS due to pancreatitis may prove to be more refractory to surfactant therapy than ARDS due to drowning. In the coming era of limited resources, these considerations may be important. If the expense of surfactant treatment remains at current levels, only treatments which limit or obviate the need for mechanical ventilation are likely to be considered cost effective. Patients with established ARDS who have been ventilated for weeks are less likely to be weaned from the ventilator as a result of surfactant therapy than patients in the acute phase. The prognosis for meaningful recovery should be assessed. It is clear that optimization of pulmonary mechanics and oxygenation alone do not assure survival. Realistic expectations for surfactant replacement therapy include the limitation of barotrauma and optimization of gas exchange. There is cautious optimism that surfactant therapy may even limit progressive lung injury and retard the development of fibrosis and pneumonia. It is not likely, however, that surfactant replacement will affect the development of multiorgan failure and persistent sepsis which are the terminal events in most nonsurvivors of ARDS.

VII. Clinical Observations and Preliminary Results of Trials of Surfactant Replacement in ARDS

Although a monolayer of DPPC harbors almost all of the surface tension–lowering activity of pulmonary surfactant, aerosolized DPPC alone is an ineffective therapy for the treatment of IRDS (109). One explanation for this apparent paradox was not forthcoming until the discovery of the surfactant proteins in 1972 (110). It is now clear that the rapid adsorption and spreading of DPPC at the air-liquid interface is dependent on the presence of the hydrophobic surfactant proteins SP-B and SP-C and to a lesser extent SP-A (111). Successful surfactant therapies require synthetic or natural components to enhance the adsorption and spreading of surface-active material at the air-liquid interface. The ideal surfactant replacement reagent in ARDS adsorbs rapidly to the air-liquid interface, lowers surface tension to near zero, and is resistant to inactivation by protein inhibitors (56). At least three preparations of surfactant have been used in pilot studies of surfactant replacement in ARDS. These include Survanta, Curosurf, and Exosurf (see Chapter 11).

The safety, feasibility, and acute effects of a single dose of porcine surfactant (Curosurf) were studied in six patients with ARDS (112) due to sepsis, aspiration, trauma, or pancreatitis. The patients were studied within 2 days of the onset of lung injury. A total dose of 4 g (50–60 mg/kg lean body weight [LBW]) of surfactant was administered in divided doses into each of the five pulmonary lobes by instillation through the bronchoscope. This treatment resulted in an average 49 ± 16 mmHg improvement in Po_2, peaking 5–120 min posttreatment. This improvement was sustained for up to 2 hr in five of the six patients. In one patient, improvement in gas exchange persisted for 24 hr. There were no significant changes in the chest radiograph or in pulmonary compliance. The composition of BAL fluid 3 hr after the instillation of surfactant revealed no change in cell count, albumin, or α_1-proteinase inhibitor specific activity. BAL lavage phospholipid concentrations were elevated 3 hr after surfactant administration relative to preadministration levels and fell by 24 hr. Two patients demonstrated reduced levels of surfactant inhibition in BAL after surfactant replacement. Although this study was hampered by the relatively small doses of surfactant employed, the investigators demonstrated that exogenous surfactant can be safely administered through the bronchoscope to patients with ARDS with a modest improvement in gas exchange.

Several preliminary studies of surfactant replacement with Exosurf in patients with ARDS have been reported. A randomized, double-blind, multicenter dose comparison pilot study of aerosolized Exosurf in 52 ventilated patients with sepsis-induced ARDS was performed (102). Patients received either 12 or

24 h/day of Exosurf via in line nebulizer on the ventilator for up to 5 days. The total daily dose administered was 6 or 12 mg/kg of dipalmitoyl phosphatidylcholine in the two groups. Control groups received nebulized 0.1*N* saline. Mortality, percentage shunt, and static respiratory compliance were compared over the first 72 hr. Trends toward improvements in mortality, shunt, and compliance were demonstrated in the patients receiving Exosurf relative to saline-treated controls. In a follow-up study, patients were treated in a similar manner, but the concentration and consequently the total dose of surfactant administered was three- and sixfold higher (103). In patients treated with a minimum of 5 days of surfactant therapy, there was a modest but significant improvement in $P(A\text{-}a)O_2$. A similar trend in improvement in mortality was demonstrated in treated versus control groups (25–35% vs 45%).

Although these early studies of Exosurf therapy in patients with ARDS appeared promising, the results of the most recent multicenter trial have been disappointing (115). This study was designed as international, placebo-controlled randomized comparison of aerosolized Exosurf versus aerosolized saline given for up to 5 days to patients with sepsis-induced ARDS. The patients were stratified by APACHE III score. Data were available for 294 patients who received Exosurf and 294 patients who received placebo. Although the therapy was shown to be safe and well tolerated, there were no significant differences in physiological measurements or mortality at 30 days. For the present, it is our understanding that the study of Exosurf replacement in ARDS has been terminated. The successes of Exosurf in infants with IRDS and the apparent lack of benefit in patients with ARDS may be related to difference in the pathophysiology of these two diseases. One hypothesis is that Exosurf is susceptible to surfactant inactivation by protein-rich pulmonary edema in ARDS because of the absence of the hydrophobic surfactant proteins or other components which preserve surface activity.

In a preliminary report from a multicenter trial, Survanta was given to subjects with ARDS due to trauma, multiple blood transfusions, sepsis syndrome, or aspiration of gastric contents (113). When compared with patients who received standard supportive therapy, subjects who received a maximum of 400 mg phospholipid/kg lean body weight in four divided doses demonstrated improved FiO_2 requirements (–35% vs –14%, $P < 0.05$) and decreased mortality (44% vs 18%, $P < 0.05$) at 120 hr. Patients who received a maximum of 800 mg/kg LBW in eight doses also showed a trend toward decreased mortality (44% vs 21%, $P < 0.053$). The investigators concluded that Survanta supplementation may be an effective therapy in ARDS.

VIII. Conclusions

In summary, the surfactant replacement in infant respiratory distress syndrome has been a towering achievement. There is a sound scientific basis to believe that surfactant replacement will also be a useful therapeutic alternative in a subset of patients with ARDS. The optimal surfactant replacement strategy in this population may be different from those successfully used to treat to IRDS, given the differences in the pathogenesis of these two processes. The surfactant used for ARDS may need to be more concentrated, more resistant to protein inhibition, and may need to be optimized for nebulization. Patient selection and decisions regarding allocation of resources will be more difficult than with the infant syndrome. In addition, the responses to surfactant treatment are not likely to be as dramatic as they have been in infants. Nonetheless, preliminary reports are promising and the outcomes of carefully designed prospective trials will be forthcoming soon. At the least, the refinement of the science of surfactant replacement in pulmonary disease is a model of partnership between basic scientists, clinical researchers, and clinicians. At best, surfactant therapy may give new hope to the patients who develop ARDS each year and their families.

References

1. Mercier CE, Soll RF. Clinical trials of natural surfactant extract in respiratory distress syndrome. In: Long WA, Ed: Clinics in Perinatology. Philadelphia: Saunders, 1993:711.
2. Corbet A. Clinical trials of synthetic surfactant in respiratory distress syndrome of premature infants. In: Long WA, Ed: Clinics in Perinatology. Philadelphia, Saunders, 1993, p. 737.
3. Baughman RP, Sternberg R, Hull W, et al. Decreased surfactant protein A in patients with bacterial pneumonia. Am Rev Respir Dis 1987; 147:653.
4. Baughman RP, Stein E, MacGee J, et al. Changes in fatty acids in phospholipids of the bronchoalveolar fluid in bacterial pneumonia and in adult respiratory distress syndrome. Clin Chem 1984; 30:521.
5. McCormack FX, King TE Jr, Voelker DR, et al. Idiopathic pulmonary fibrosis. Abnormalities in the bronchoalveolar lavage content of surfactant protein A. Am Rev Respir Dis 1991; 144:160.
6. Robinson PC, Watters LC, King TE, Mason RJ. Idiopathic pulmonary fibrosis. Abnormalities in bronchoalveolar lavage fluid phospholipids. Am Rev Respir Dis 1988; 137:585.
7. Oyarzun MJ, Stevens P, Clements JA. Effect of lung collapse on alveolar surfactant in rabbits subjected to unilateral pneumothorax. Exp Lung Res 1989; 15:909.
8. Hallman M, Maasilta P, Kivisaari L, Mattson K. Changes in surfactant in bronchoalveolar lavage fluid after hemithorax irradiation in patients with mesothelioma. Am Rev Respir Dis 1990; 141:998.
9. Petty TL, Reiss OK, Paul GK, et al. Characteristics of pulmonary surfactant in adult respiratory distress syndrome associated with trauma and shock. Am Rev Respir Dis 1977; 115:531.
10. Petty TL, Silvers GW, Paul GW, Stanford RE. Abnormalities in elastic properties and surfactant function in adult respiratory distress syndrome. Chest 1979; 75:571.

11. Pison U, Seeger W, Buckhorn R, et al. Surfactant abnormalities in patients with respiratory failure after multiple trauma. Am Rev Respir Dis 1989; 140:1033.
12. Pison U, Obertacke U, Brand M, et al. Altered pulmonary surfactant in uncomplicated and septicemia-complicated courses of acute respiratory failure. J. Trauma 1990; 30:19.
13. Hallman M, Spragg R, Harrell JH, et al. Evidence of lung surfactant abnormality in respiratory failure. J Clin Invest 1983; 70:673.
14. Gregory TJ, Longmore WJ, Moxeley, MA, et al. Surfactant chemical composition and biophysical activity in acute respiratory distress syndrome. J Clin Invest 1991; 88:1976.
15. Berry D, Ikegami M, Jobe A. Respiratory distress syndrome and surfactant inhibition following vagatomy in rabbits. J Appl Physiol 1986; 61:1741.
16. Lachmann B, Robertson B, Vogel, J. In vivo lung lavage as an experimental model of the respiratory distress syndrome. Acta Anaesth Scand 1980; 24:231.
17. Lachmann B. Surfactant therapy. Resuscitation 1989; 18:S37.
18. Eijking EP, Gommers D, So KL, et al. Surfactant treatment induced by hydrochloric acid aspiration in rats. Anesthesiology 1993; 78:1145.
19. Eijking, EP, Gommers D, So, KL, et al. Prevention of respiratory failure after hydrochloric acid aspiration by intratracheal surfactant instillation in rats. Crit Care Trauma 1933; 76:472.
20. Burkhardt A. Alveolitis and collapse in the pathogenesis of pulmonary fibrosis. Am Rev Respir Dis 1989; 140:513.
21. Gandy G, Jacobson W, Gairdner D. Hyaline membrane disease. I. Cellular changes. Arch Dis Child 1970; 45:289.
22. Ashbaugh DG, Bigelow CB, Petty TL, Levine BE. Acute respiratory distress in adults. Lancet 1967; 2:319.
23. Bone RC, Fisher CJJ, Clemmer TP, et al. Early methylprednisolone treatment for septic syndrome and the adult respiratory distress syndrome. Chest 1987; 92: 1032.
24. Bernard GR, Luce JM, Sprung CL, et al. High dose corticosteroids in patients with the adult respiratory distress syndrome. N Engl J Med 1987; 317:1565.
25. Luce JM, Montgomery AB, Marks JD, et al. Ineffectiveness of high dose methylprednisolone in preventing parenchymal lung injury and improving mortality in patients with septic shock. Am Rev Respir Dis 1988; 138:62.
26. Bone RC, Slotman G, Maunder R, et al. Randomized double blind, multicenter trial of prostaglandin E1 in patients with the adult respiratory distress syndrome. Chest 1989; 96:114.
27. Petty TL, Bone RC, Gee MH, et al. Contemporary clinical trials in acute respiratory distress syndrome. Chest 1992; 101:550.
28. Repine JE. Scientific perspectives on adult respiratory distress syndrome. Lancet 1992; 339:466.
29. Fraser RG, Paré JAP, Paré PD, et al. Pulmonary hypertension and edema. In: Diagnosis of Disease of the Chest. Philadelphia: Saunders, 1990:1823.
30. Connell RS, Swank RL, Webb MC. The development of pulmonary ultrastructural lesions during hemorrhage shock. J Trauma, 1975; 15:116.
31. Turner CR, Lackey MN, Quinlan MF, et al. Therapeutic intervention in a rat model

of adult respiratory distress syndrome. III. Cyclooxygenase pathway inhibition. Circ-Shock 1991; 34:270.

32. Matthay MA, Eschenbacher WL, Goetzl EJ. Elevated concentrations of leukotriene D4 in pulmonary edema fluid of patients with adult respiratory distress syndrome. J Clin Immunol 1984; 4:479.
33. Passi RB, Possmayer F. Surfactant metabolism in acute pancreatitis. Prog Respir Res 1981; 15:136.
34. Cochrane CG, Spragg R, Revak SD. Pathogenesis of the adult respiratory distress syndrome. Evidence of oxidant activity in bronchoalveolar lavage fluid. J Clin Invest 1983; 71:754.
35. Baird BR, Cheronis JC, Sandhaus RA, et al. Scientific perspectives on adult respiratory distress syndrome. Lancet 1992; 339:466.
36. Hammerschmidt DE, Weaver LJ, Hudson LD, et al. Association of complement activation and elevated plasma C5a with adult respiratory distress syndrome. Pathophysiologic relevance and possible prognostic value. Lancet 1980; 1:947.
37. Petty TL. The acute respiratory distress syndrome: historic perspective. Chest 1994; 105:44.
38. Weibel ER. Looking into the lung: what can it tell us? Am J Roentgenol 1979; 133:1021.
39. Nash G, Langlinais PC. Pulmonary interstitial edema and hyaline membranes in adult burn patients. Electron microscopic observations. Hum Pathol 1974; 5:149.
40. Fukuda Y, Ishizaki M, Masuda Y, et al. The role of intraalveolar fibrosis in the process of pulmonary structural remodeling in patients with diffuse alveolar damage. Am J Pathol 1987; 126:171.
41. Fukuda Y, Ferrans VJ, Schoenberger CI, et al. Patterns of pulmonary structural remodeling after experimental paraquat toxicity. Am J Pathol 1985; 118:452.
42. Hooper RG, Kearl RA. Established ARDS treated with a sustained course of adrenocortical steroids. Chest 1990; 97:138.
43. Meduri GU, Belenchia JM, Estes RJ, et al. Fibroproliferative phase of ARDS. Clinical findings and effects of corticosteroids. Chest 1991; 100:943.
44. Polunovsky V, Chen B, Henke C, et al. Role of mesenchymal cell death in lung remodeling after injury. J Clin Invest 1993; 92:388.
45. Schwarz MI. Clinical overview of interstitial lung disease. In: Schwarz MI, King TE Jr, Eds: Interstitial Lung Disease. St. Louis: Mosby, 1993:1.
46. Hudson LD. What happens to survivors of the adult respiratory distress syndrome? Chest 1994; 105:123.
47. Holter JF, Welland JE, Pacht ER, et al. Protein permeability in the adult respiratory distress syndrome. J Clin Invest 1986; 78:1513.
48. Pison U, Obertacke U, Seeger W, Hawgood S. Surfactant protein A is decreased in acute parenchymal lung injury associated with polytrauma. Eur J Clin Invest 1992; 22:712.
49. Venkitaraman AR, Hall SB, Whitsett JA, Notter RH. Enhancement of biophysical activity of lung surfactant extracts and phospholipid-apoprotein mixtures by surfactant protein A. Chem Phys Lipids 1990; 56:185.
50. Brown DL, Pattishal EN. Other uses of surfactant. In: Long WA, Ed: Clinics in Perinatology. Philadelphia: Saunders, 1993:761.

51. Harlan WR Jr, Said SI, Banerjee CM. Metabolism of pulmonary phospholipids in normal lung and during acute pulmonary edema. Am Rev Respir Dis 1966; 94:938.
52. Said SI, Avery ME, Davis RK, et al. Pulmonary surface activity in induced pulmonary edema. J Clin Invest 1965; 44:458.
53. Seeger W, Storh G, Wolfe HRD, Neuhof H. Alteration of surfactant function due to protein leakage: special interaction with fibrin monomer. J Appl Physiol 1985; 58:326.
54. Holm BA, Notter RH. Effects of hemoglobin and red blood cell membrane lipids on the biophysical and physiological activity of pulmonary surfactant. J Appl Physiol 1987; 63:1434.
55. Spragg RG, Gilliard N, Richman P, et al. The adult respiratory distress syndrome: Clinical aspects relevant to surfactant supplementation. In: Robertson B, van Golde LMG, Batenburg JJ, Eds: Pulmonary Surfactant from Molecular Biology to Clinical Practice. Amsterdam: Elsevier, 1992:753.
56. Keough KMW. Physical chemistry of surfactant in the terminal airspaces. In: Pulmonary Surfactant from Molecular Biology to Clinical Practice. Amsterdam: Elsevier 1992:109.
57. Holm BA, Enhorning G, Notter RH. A biophysical mechanism by which plasma proteins inhibit lung surfactant activity. Chem Phys Lipids 1988; 49:49.
58. Holm BA, Notter RH, Finklestein JN. Surface property changes from interactions of albumin with natural lung surfactants and extracted lipids. Chem Phys Lipids 1985; 38:287.
59. Fuchimukai T, Fujiwara T, Takahashi A, Enhorning G. Artificial pulmonary surfactant inhibited by proteins. J Appl Physiol 1987; 62:429.
60. Cummings JJ, Holm BA, Hudak ML, et al. A controlled clinical comparison of four different surfactant preparations in surfactant deficient preterm lambs. Am Rev Respir Dis 1992; 145:999.
61. Amirkhanian JD, Bruni R, Waring AJ, et al. Full length synthetic surfactant proteins, SP-B and SP-C, reduce surfactant inactivation by serum. Biochim. Biophys Acta 1993; 1168:315.
62. Cockshutt A, Weitz J, Possmayer F. The effects of surfactant-associated protein A on surface tension reduction and blood protein inhibition in two surfactant preparations. FASEB 1990; 4:A2147.
63. Holm BA, Matalon S, Finkelstein JN, Notter RH. Type II pneumocyte changes during hyperoxic lung injury and recovery, J Appl Physiol 1988; 65:2672.
64. Seeger W, Lepper H, Hellmut RD, Neuhof H. Alteration of alveolar surfactant function after exposure to oxidative stress and to oxygenated and native arachadonic acid in vitro. Biochim Biophys Acta 1985; 835:58.
65. Gilliard N, Heldt G, Merritt TA, et al. Functional consequences of porcine lung surfactant oxidation. Am Rev Respir Dis 1990; 141:A635.
66. Davies KJ, Goldberg AL. Oxygen radicals stimulate intracellular proteolysis and lipid peroxidation by independent mechanisms in erythrocytes. J Biol Chem 1987; 262:8220.
67. Haagsman HP, Hawgood S, Sargeant T, et al. The major lung surfactant apoprotein, SP-28-36, is a calcium-dependent carbohydrate binding protein. J Biol Chem 1987; 262:13877.

68. Pison U, Tam EK, Caughey GH, Hawgood S. Proteolytic inactivation of dog lung surfactant-associated proteins by neutrophil elastase. Biochim Biophys Acta 1989; 1989:251.
69. Ryan S, Ghassibi Y, Liau, D. Effects of neutrophils on surfactant. Chest, 1989; 95:30.
70. Holm BA, Keicher L, Liu M, et al. Inhibition of surfactant function by phospholipases. J Appl Physiol 1991; 71:1.
71. La Force FM, Kelly WJ, Huber GL. Inactivation of staphylococci by alveolar macrophages with preliminary observations on the importance of alveolar lining material. Am Rev Respir Dis 1973; 108:784.
72. Coonrod JD, Lester RL, Hsu LC. Characterization of the extracellular bactericidal factors of rat alveolar lining material. J Clin Invest 1984; 74:1269.
73. van Iwaarden F, Welmers B, Verhoef J, et al. Pulmonary surfactant protein A enhances the host-defense mechanism of rat alveolar macrophages. Am J Respir Cell Mol Biol 1990; 2:91.
74. van Iwaarden JF, Strijp JAG, Ebskamp MJM, et al. Surfactant protein A is opsonin in phagocytosis of herpes simplex virus type 1 by rat alveolar macrophages. Am J Physiol 1991; 261:L204.
75. Kuan S, Rust K, Crouch E. Interactions of surfactant protein D with bacterial lipopolysaccharides. J Clin Invest 1992; 90:97.
76. Tomashefski JF Jr, Vawter GF, Reid LM. Pathological observations on infants who do not survive the respiratory distress syndrome. In: Pulmonary Development. New York: Marcel Dekker, 1985:526.
77. Chu J, Clements JA, Cotton MH, et al. The pulmonary hypoperfusion syndrome. Pediatrics 1965; 35:733.
78. Buckingham S, Sommers SS. Pulmonary hyaline membranes. Am J Dis Child 1960; 99:216.
79. van Daal GJ, Eijking EP, So KL, et al. Acute respiratory failure during pneumonia induced by Sendai virus. Adv Exp Med Biol 1991; 316:319.
80. van Daal GJ, So KL, Gommers D, et al. Intratracheal surfactant administration restores gas exchange in experimental adult respiratory distress syndrome associated with viral pneumonia. Anesth Analg 1991; 72:589.
81. Brendenberg CE, Paskanik AM, Nieman GF. High surface tension pulmonary edema. J Surg Res 1983; 34:515.
82. Nieman GF, Brendenberg CE. High surface tension pulmonary edema induced by detergent aerosol. J Appl Physiol 1985; 58:129.
83. Berggren P, Lachmann B, Curstedt T, et al. Gas exchange and lung morphology after surfactant replacement in experimental respiratory distress syndrome. Acta Anaesthesiol Scand 1986; 30:321.
84. Holm BA, Notter RH, Siegle J, Matalon S. Pulmonary physiological and surfactant changes during injury and recovery from hyperoxia. J Appl Physiol 1985; 59:1402.
85. Holm BA, Notter RH, Leary JF, Matalon S. Alveolar epithelial changes in rabbits after a 21 day exposure to 60% O_2. J Appl Physiol 1987; 62:2230.
86. King RJ, Coalson JJ, Seidenfeld JJ, et al. O_2 and pneumonia induced lung injury. II. Properties of pulmonary surfactant. J Appl Physiol 1989; 67:357.
87. Loewen GM, Holm BA, Milanowski L, et al. Alveolar hyperoxic injury in rabbits receiving exogenous surfactant. J Appl Physiol 1989; 66:1087.

88. Ennema JJ, Kobayashi T, Robertson B, Curstedt T. Inactivation of exogenous surfactant in experimental respiratory failure induced by hyperoxia. Acta Anaesthesiol Scand 1988; 32:665.
89. Matalon S, Holm BA, Notter, RH. Mitigation of pulmonary hyperoxic injury by administration of exogenous surfactant. J Appl Physiol 1987; 62:756.
90. Piantadosi CA, Young SL, Fracica PJ, Crapo JD. Artificial surfactant diminishes pathologic injury in hyperoxia in primates. Am Rev Respir Dis 1992; 145: A609.
91. Harris JD, Jackson FJ, Moxley MA, Longmore WJ. Effect of exogenous surfactant instillation on experimental acute lung injury. J Appl Physiol 1989; 66:1846.
92. Liau DF, Barrett CR, Bell AL, Ryan SF. Functional abnormalities of lung surfactant in experimental acute alveolar injury in the dog. Am Rev Respir Dis 1987; 136:395.
93. Ryan SF, Liau DF, Bell ALL, et al. Correlation of lung compliance and quantities of surfactant phospholipids after acute alveolar injury from N-nitroso-N-methylurethane in the dog. Am Rev Respir Dis 1981; 123:200.
94. Anderson BM, Jackson FJ, Moxley MA, Longmore WJ. Effects on experimental acute lung injury 24 hours after exogenous surfactant instillation. Exp Lung Res 1991; 18:191.
95. Strohmaier W, Redl H, Schlag G. Studies of a semisynthetic surfactant preparation in an experimental aspiration trauma in rats. Exp Lung Res 1990; 16:101.
96. Lamm WJ, Albert RK. Surfactant replacement improves lung recoil in rabbit lungs after acid aspiration. Am Rev Respir Dis 1990; 142:1279.
97. Kobayashi T, Ganzuka M, Taniguchi J, et al. Lung lavage and surfactant replacement for hydrochloric acid aspiration in rabbits. Acta Anaesthesiol Scand 1990; 34:216.
98. Nosaka S, Sakai T, Yonekura M, Yoshikawa K. Surfactant for adults with respiratory failure. Lancet 1990; 336:947.
99. Richman PS, Spragg RG, Robertson B, et al. The adult respiratory distress syndrome: First clinical trials with surfactant replacement, Eur Respir J 1989; 2(suppl 3):109.
100. Lachmann B. The role of pulmonary surfactant in the pathogenesis and therapy of ARDS. In: Vincent JL, ed: Update in Critical Care and Emergency Medicine. New York: Springer Verlag, 1987:123.
101. Segerer H, van Gelder W, Angenent FWM, et al. Pulmonary distribution and efficacy of exogenous surfactant in lung-lavaged rabbits are influenced by the instillation technique. Pediatr Res 1993; 34:490.
102. Weg J, Reines H, Balk R, et al. Safety and efficacy of an aerosolized surfactant (Exosurf) in human sepsis induced ARDS. Chest 1991; 100:137.
103. Weidemann H, Baughman R, deBoisblanc B, et al. A multicenter trial in human sepsis-induced ARDS of an aerosolized synthetic surfactant (EXOSURF). Am Rev Respir Dis 1992; 145:A184.
104. Lewis J, Ikegami M, Higuchi R, et al. Nebulized vs. instilled exogenous surfactant in an adult lung injury model. J Appl Physiol 1991; 71:1270.
105. Lewis JF, Tabor B, Ikegami M, et al. Lung function and surfactant distribution in saline lavaged sheep given instilled vs. nebulized surfactant. J Appl Physiol 1993; 1991:1256.

106. Lewis JF, McCaig L. Aerosolized vs. instilled exogenous surfactant in a nonuniform pattern of lung injury. Am Rev Respir 1993; Dis, 148:1187.
107. Fowler AA, Hamman RF, Good JT, et al. Adult respiratory distress syndrome: Risk with common predisposition. Ann Intern Med 1983; 98:593.
108. Murray JF, Mattham MA, Luce JM, Flick MR. An expanded definition of the adult respiratory distress syndrome. Am Rev Respir Dis 1988; 138:720.
109. Chu JTY, Clements JA, Cotton MH, et al. Neonatal pulmonary ischemia Part 1. Clinical and physiologic study. Pediatrics 1967; 65:709.
110. King RJ, Clements JA. Surface active materials from dog: 1. Method of isolation. Am J Physiol 1972; 223:707.
111. Hawgood S, Benson BJ, Schilling J, et al. Nucleotide and amino acid sequences of pulmonary surfactant protein SP 18 and evidence for cooperation between SP 18 and SP 28-36 in surfactant lipid adsorption, Proc Natl Acad Sci USA 1987; 84:66.
112. Spragg RG, Gilliard N, Richman P, et al. Acute effects of a single dose of porcine surfactant on patients with the adult respiratory distress syndrome. Chest 1994; 105:195.
113. Gregory TJ, Gadek JE, Weiland JE, et al. Survanta supplementation in patients with acute respiratory distress syndrome, Am Rev Respir Dis, 1994; 149:A567.
114. Holm, BA, Surfactant inactivation in the adult respiratory distress syndrome. In: Robertson B, van Golde LMG, Batenburg JJ, Eds: Pulmonary Surfactant: From Molecular Biology to Clinical Practice. Elsevier: Amsterdam, 1993: 665–684.
115. Anzueto A; Baughman R, Guntopalli R, et al. An international, randomized, placebo controlled trial evaluating the safety and efficacy of aerosolized surfactant in patients with sepsis induced ARDS. Am J Respir Crit Care Med 1995; 149:A567.

29

Outcomes of Surfactant-Treated Infants

Analysis of Developmental Outcome and the Economic Impact of Surfactant Therapy

T. ALLEN MERRITT and TERRY TURNER
University of California, Davis
Medical Center
Sacramento, California

YVONNE VAUCHER
University of California, San Diego
San Diego, California

MIKKO HALLMAN
University of California, Irvine
School of Medicine
Irvine, California

MARY JESSE WILSON
California Children's Services
Department of Health Services
Sacramento, California

I. Introduction

The "bench-to-bedside" translation of biomedical research on pulmonary surfactant into lifesaving therapy in the neonatal intensive care unit has heralded a new era in the care of the premature infants with RDS (1,2). During the years of the randomized trials using human surfactant, calf lung surfactant extract, Exosurf, Curosurf Neonatal® and Survanta®, and the years 1989–1990 during Treatment Investigation New Drug (TIND) protocols for Exosurf Neonatal® and Survanta®, the US infant mortality rate declined faster (infant mortality 1989–1990 dropped from 9.7 to 9.1:1,000 births and deaths due to RDS dropped from 86.6 to 59.1:100,000) than during any previous year during the last two decades (3,4,5). Much of this improvement in infant survival was believed to be due to a substantial reduction of deaths due to RDS and related to surfactant treatment (6). Former Secretary of Health and Human Services, Louis Sullivan, MD, and the Centers for Disease Control have credited the reduced infant mortality, which translated to the survival of an additional 1200 neonates in 1990 alone in the US, to the widespread investigational use of exogenous surfactant. Now that surfactant is universally used, this impact must be even greater.

Horbar and colleagues (7) (Figure 1) demonstrated that birth weight specific mortality among infants 601–1300 grams declined significantly in several neonatal centers in the months immediately after participation in surfactant trials when compared to the months immediately preceding participation in the TIND trials for both Survanta® and Exosurf Neonatal®. Although the absolute change in mortality varies by birth weight, a consistent trend of improvement was noted. This change was attributed to use of surfactant since there appeared to be no other major changes in any other neonatal practice or nursing care at these centers over the time of study. Exogenous surfactant given soon after birth (among infants <28 weeks gestation) or after the clinical recognition of RDS is now "the standard of care."

Thus, surfactant therapy for RDS must be viewed as a single powerful intervention that has immediate effects of reducing the severity of RDS; yet many morbidities of prematurity resulting in functional impairment, limitations, and disabilities in later childhood (8) have etiologies that have not been positively influenced by surfactant therapy. The enthusiasm for the clinical advances offered by surfactant for RDS treatment or prevention and for newer uses including meconium aspiration pneumonitis, with pulmonary hypertension, bacterial and viral pneumonia, persistent pulmonary hypertension, and after the initiation of ECMO (9) and the childhood form of adult respiratory distress syndromes needs to be tempered by the significant neonatal and post neonatal problems experienced in the very low birth weight infant, especially including the social environment into which they are born and to which they return after surviving the hazards of premature birth (10,11). Therefore, discussion of the neurodevelopmental outcome and risk for functional limitations and disabilities of infants must be considered along with the economic impact of providing this exogenous surfactant since more infants survive but are also at subsequent developmental risk. While many advances in medicine occur with a shift from mortality to some added morbidity, this shift can only be detected by extensive analysis of cohorts in randomized, placebo-controlled trials, as well as in studies reflecting extensive clinical experiences at many centers. Rosenblatt has suggested that "these advances come at a price that can be measured in subsequent infant disability, family disruption, ethical quagmires for physicians, government intervention and, or course, dollars" (12).

Fortunately this "perinatal paradox" appears to have been overcome to a large extent as exogenous surfactant is the "standard of care" for premature infants either at significant risk for or after the development of RDS. This chapter will review the available data to determine the critical question of whether the use of exogenous surfactant has resulted in increased survival of some infants only to have them develop significant neurodevelopmental delays placing additional burdens on their parents, the health care system and society, or whether the advent of surfactant therapy is an unalloyed boon.

Unlike many other therapies introduced for newborn infants, surfactant therapy was systematically studied in over 35 randomized clinical trials (13) affording researchers the opportunity to evaluate the developmental course of infants randomized to placebo or surfactant therapy. At the time of this writing, school age performance of children treated with surfactant as infants is being reported; so, analyses of these outcome measures remain tentative.

II. Neurodevelopmental Outcome

McCormick (14) has emphasized that "the efficacy of neonatal intensive care, either in terms of selected single interventions (such as surfactant) or as a combination of interventions to improve survival is no longer in doubt." From a meta-analysis of 111 studies including 26,099 births (12,064 from the USA), Escobar and coworkers (15) have suggested that, even though there has been a substantial reduction of mortality of very low birth weight (VLBW) infants (<1500g), survivors are at higher risk for neurodevelopmental problems. These authors estimate a median 25% incidence of disabilities among VLBW, with an approximate 8% incidence of cerebral palsy. McCormick has emphasized that "this neurodevelopmental disability may reflect the fact that VLBW infants in the United States are disproportionately from disadvantaged families . . .", suggesting that socioeconomic and educational factors contributing to LBW births in the first place may also strongly influence their subsequent post-neonatal outcome, regardless of the efficacy of neonatal intensive care (16,17). VLBW infants consistently have an increased risk for re-hospitalizations, learning disabilities and hyperactivity when compared to age-matched controls; however, it remains unclear what morbidities or factors contribute to the decrease in cognitive function of these VLBW infants. Furthermore, analysis of the neurodevelopmental outcomes of surfactant recipients must take into account not only the effect on RDS survival, and early neurodevelopmental outcome (1 to 2 years), but also the power of additional influences (socioeconomic, parental education, environmental factors such as passive tobacco smoke exposure or other environmental toxins) on later developmental outcome and measures of school age performance. Although early assessments at one to two years using Bayley Scales of Infant Development may be reassuring if normal, they may not necessarily predict cognitive function assessment later in early childhood. Saigal and coworkers (18) and Collin et al (19) have stressed the need for longitudinal evaluation of infants since a single time assessment minimizes cortical and motor dysfunctions that may be evident in later years, but are not evident in early assessments. Nonetheless, the survival of more infants at risk for developmental problems secondary to premature birth may complicate interpretation of the efficacy of surfactant. Although large randomized trials included various outcome measures to determine the frequency of developmental and health problems at one–two years of age, these follow-up studies used strict criteria for entry, were aimed at specific gestational or birth weight categories, and had specific exclusions (e.g., chorioamnioitis, some malformations, lack of parental consent, or age or weight limitations after birth) that are presently not used as exclusion criteria for surfactant treatment. Currently, most neonatologists offer surfactant therapy to categories of infants for whom the efficacy of surfactant on survival was not statistically significant (e.g., infants <700 g birth weight). Thus, outcomes reported from the randomized controlled trials must be viewed as incomplete evidence in predicting outcomes now that surfactant therapy has become routine.

Analysis and direct comparison of neurodevelopmental follow-up of surfactant treated infants is problematic because of differences in surfactant preparations, total dose, timing of administration and total number of doses. Entry criteria for many studies were based on gestational age estimates of <30 weeks gestation while other studies were based on birth weight. Most of the developmental reports have combined prophylactic and rescue infants for analysis; duration of follow-up, rate of return rate for follow-up for examination, instruments used to evaluate neurodevelopmental performance (Bayley Scales of Infant Development, Griffith Scales, Gesell-Knobloch, and others), and estimates of health status have varied between investigators. Numbers of subjects enrolled in follow-up studies vary between a handful of infants in smaller studies at single centers to over 1400 infant studies evaluated longitudinally in pharmaceutical company supported randomized trials. While some reports have been peer reviewed, some of the larger (and more recent) are available only in abstracted form or from non-peer reviewed publications derived from data generated by studies supported and analyzed by the manufacturers of therapeutic surfactants.

Table 1 summarizes reports of neurodevelopmental follow-up that have appeared both as peer reviewed (A) and as non-reviewed (B) articles or abstracts (C). Each report cited in the table indicates type of trial, prophylactic or treatment usage, type of surfactant, number of patients, percent of total survivors, and the outcomes. Since duration of follow-up varies in some trials, the age(s) at evaluation and the test instruments are summarized. In all trials to date, there have been no differences in neurodevelopmental outcome suggesting that surfactant treated infants have mental or psychomotor performances equivalent or slightly improved compared to placebo treated infants. Indeed, some studies have shown a significant reduction in cerebral palsy among surfactant treated infants.

A possible bias in follow-up studies exists when a greater percentage of sicker infants are evaluated, or disproportionately those in whom parents are concerned about development return for examination (20). Analysis of follow-up studies in aggregate suggests that survivors treated with one or more doses of the various surfactants fare at least as well as placebo treated infants. Specifically,

Table 1 Summary of Reports of Neurodevelopmental Follow-up

Study peer review	Surfactant	Trial	Types of infants	Treatment	No. of doses	Dosage	N	Birth weight	GA
Halliday 1986	DPPC:HDLP	RCT	<34 wks	Prophylactic	Single	20 mg/kg	49	1569 ± 389	30.6 ± 1.9
	Control						51	1672 ± 40.3	31.3 ± 1.6
Vaucher 1988	Human surfactant	RCT	<30 wks	Prophylactic/ Treatment	1–4	70 mg/kg/dose	28	957 ± 57	27.4 ± 0.3
	Control						18	1010 ± 46	27.2 ± 0.4
Ware 1990	Survanta®	RCT	700–1750 g	Treatment	1–4		15	1271 ± 38	29.5 ± 0.5
	Control						17	1229 ± 37	29.5 ± 0.4
Morley 1990	ALEC	RCT	25–29 wks	Given at birth	Single		121		
	Control						114		
Robertson 1992	Curosurf	RCT	700–2000 g	Rescue/ Treatment	Single	200 mg/kg	45	1305 ± 312	29.9 ± 1.9
	Control						31	1227 ± 350	28.7 ± 2.5
Vaucher 1993	Human Prophyl	RCT	<30 wks	Prophylactic/ Treatment	1–4	80 mg/kg/dose	34	1051 ± 251	27.5 ± 1.7
	Human Treat						29	1038 ± 213	27.4 ± 1.7
	Placebo						17	1117 ± 116	28.0 ± 1.6
Ferrara 1994	Survanta®	Compare	23–26 wks	Prophylactic	1–4	100 mg/dose	100	613–863	23–26
	No treatment						100	559–830	23–26
Gunkel 1994	Survanta®	RCT	600–1250 g	Prophylactic/ Treatment	1–4	100 mg/dose	295		
	Placebo						266		

Study peer review	Surfactant	1-year follow-up rate	CLD ($\%O_2$ at > 28 days)	1-year growth			1-year developmental			
Halliday 1986	DPPC:HDLP									
	Control									
							None (%)	Mild (%)	Mod (%)	Severe (%)
Vaucher 1988	Human surfactant	28/33 (84.8%)		No difference			55	23	4	18
	Control	18/33 (54.5%)					35	41	6	18
Ware 1990	Survanta®									
	Control									
Morley 1990	ALEC									
	Control									
				Wt (kg)	Length (cm)	OFC (cm)				
Robertson 1992	Curosurf	45/49 (92%)		8.4 ± 1.4	72.4 ± 3.8	46.1 ± 2.2				
	Control	31/33 (97%)		8.4 ± 1.1	72.2 ± 3.2	45.2 ± 2.0				
				Wt %ile	Length %ile	OFC %ile				
Vaucher 1993	Human Prophyl	25/34 (73.5%)		26 ± 31	33 ± 29	29 ± 27				
	Human Treat	25/29 (86.2%)		23 ± 26	31 ± 30	35 ± 27				
	Placebo	11/17 (68.5%)		30 ± 25	35 ± 25	33 ± 29				
Ferrara 1994	Survanta®									
	No treatment									
Gunkel 1994	Survanta®									
	Placebo									

Study peer review	Surfactant	1-year neuro-logical						1-year sensory			1-year pulmonary function	18-month follow-up rate
Halliday 1986	DPPC:HDLP											
	Control											
				None (%)	Quest (%)	Abnormal (%)	CP (%)				Recurrent Lung Disease (%)	
Vaucher 1988	Human surfactant			59	19	22	14				23	
	Control			53	24	23	28				57	
Ware 1990	Survanta®											
	Control											
Morley 1990	ALEC											212/231
	Control											combined
				CP	DQ	Major Disability (%)	Minor Disability (%)		Visual (%)	Auditory (%)		
Robertson 1992	Curosurf			7%	94.8 (10.2)	9	9		0	4		
	Control			0%	90.8 (9.3)	10	10		0	3		
		MDI	PDI		Handicap—Normal (%)	Handicap—Major (%)	Handicap—Minor (%)	ROP3 or 4 (%)	Blind (%)	Hearing (%)		
Vaucher 1993	Human Prophyl	78 ± 25	73 ± 20		28	48	24	16	7	2		
	Human Treat	96 ± 16	87 ± 22	48	20	32	16	2	3			
	Placebo	93 ± 17	83 ± 19	64	27	9	4	0	0			
Ferrara 1994	Survanta®											
	No treatment											
Gunkel 1994	Survanta®											
	Placebo											

Study peer review	Surfactant	18-months develop-ment				18-month sensory			18-month rehospital-ization (%)	18-month recurrent infection (%)	2-year follow-up rate	2-year growth
Halliday 1986	DPPC:HDLP										39/49 (79%)	
	Control										41/51 (80%)	
Vaucher 1988	Human surfactant											
	Control											
												Wt (kg)
Ware 1990	Survanta®										32/32	11.7 ± 0.5
	Control										29/31	11.6 ± 0.4
		<30 wks MDI	<30 wks PDI	>30 wks MDI	>30 wks PDI	Visual	Hearing (%)	CP (%)				
Morley 1990	ALEC	95 ± 19	90 ± 15	103 ± 17	95 ± 14	NA	4	14.70	46	54		
	Control	97 ± 20	88 ± 19	107 ± 20	95 ± 14	NA	8	9.80	44	47		
Robertson 1992	Curosurf											
	Control											
Vaucher 1993	Human Prophyl											
	Human Treat											
	Placebo											
Ferrara 1994	Survanta®										96/100 (96%)	
	No treatment										71/100 (71%)	
Gunkel 1994	Survanta®										295/470 (63%)	
	Placebo										266/426 (62%)	

Study peer review	Surfactant	2-year development					2-year mild CP (%)	2-year severe CP (%)	2-year sensory		2-year rehospitalization (%)	2-year lung disease (%)	2-year allergy (%)
				DQ									
Halliday 1986	DPPC:HDLP			100 (75–120)			10	1			31	28	
	Control			95 (13–110)			2	10			51	34	
Vaucher 1988	Human Surfactant												
	Control												
		Length (cm)	OFC (cm)	MDI	PDI				Visual (%)	Auditory (%)			
Ware 1990	Survanta®	85.1 ± 1.0	48.2 ± 0.8	94.8 ± 5.4	92.7 ± 4.6				0	7.60	21.40	21.40	14.20
	Control	85.9 ± 0.9	48.9 ± 0.6	106.1 ± 7.1	88.4 ± 4.0				6.30	0	26.70	26.60	12.50
Morley 1990	ALEC												
	Control												
						CP (%)	Minor Disability (%)	Major Disability (%)	Visual (%)	Auditory (%)			
Robertson 1992	Curosurf					7	9	11	0	0			
	Control					0	21	3	4.50	6.80			
Vaucher 1993	Human Prophyl												
	Human Treat												
	Placebo												
Ferrara 1994	Survanta®						21	14	4				
	No treatment						16	13	1				
				MDI	PDI	CP (%)							
Gunkel 1994	Survanta®			47.1	85.4	8.99			14.30				
	Placebo			96.4	88.4	14.30			16.70				

growth at 1–2 years (adjusted for prematurity) are equivalent between groups. While instruments to assess development have varied, there is no evidence that surfactant treatment has increased the proportion of infants with disabilities at 1–2 years. Indeed, the largest of trials using Exosurf Neonatal® suggests an increase in survival and an overall decrease in morbidity among the surfactant group with mean and median developmental scores within the "normal" range (21,22).

Among infants treated with Curosurf® for the European Multicenter Trial, the relative number of survivors without significant disability was significantly higher in the surfactant treated group (56%) compared to the placebo control group (35%; $p = 0.02$) (23). Rates of rehospitalization and frequency of recurrent respiratory illness were decreased among surfactant treated infants, suggesting that the severity of chronic lung disease over the first year of life may be diminished with surfactant therapy. Clinically, most neonatologists are witnessing "milder" forms of bronchopulmonary dysplasia in the surfactant era (as measured by total days on mechanical ventilation, duration of supplemental oxygen, radiographic scores, or numbers of discharged infants on oxygen). Credence for these impressions comes from a recent report by Long (24), who evaluated radiographic severity of BPD using Edward's criteria among infants treated with two doses of Exosurf Neonatal®. Among surviving infants 700–1350g at birth, radiographic BPD at 28 days was consistently lower ($p = 0.057$); similarly, surviving infants > 1250 g at birth had significantly lower Edward's scores at 28 days ($p = 0.049$). While the proportion of infants with identifiable auditory or visual impairment was low, none of the reports indicated differences.

No difference in prevalence of cerebral palsy was identified in these studies. O'Shea and coworkers (25) found a significant reduction in the rate of cerebral palsy when comparing its occurrence in a 17 county area of North Carolina in the pre and post surfactant eras (16% vs 2%; $p < 0.01$). These changes were evident after controlling for birth weight, gestational age, gender, race, and cranial ultrasonographic diagnosis. As McCormick stressed (15), "although such trial analyses are useful, the focus on a single treatment modality (e.g. surfactant therapy, *author's words*) may mask considerably heterogeneity in other nursery practices that might influence morbidity and, thus, must be interpreted with caution."

Retinopathy of prematurity (ROP) occurs most frequently among infants <1000 g birth weight. Surfactant therapy does not appear to increase either the incidence or severity of this disorder. Dunn and coworkers (26) reported a non-significant difference in the incidence of acute ROP (stages 2, 3 and 4) from 8% (5/60) among placebo control infants to 3% (2/62) among surfactant treated infants. A similar trend was reported by Rankin et al (27) who studied effects of Curosurf®; however, the study was uncontrolled. Repka and coworkers (28) reported ROP (of any stage) was reduced by calf lung surfactant extract, with the greatest effect observed for 500–1000 g infants. Using this surfactant as prophylaxis and treatment and Survanta® given only as prophylaxis, the combined data from two intensive care nurseries reported a non significant increase in the rate or severity of ROP (pre-threshold ROP surfactant 21% versus control 14%; or threshold ROP, surfactant 7% versus 5% controls, P = NS) among surfactant treated infants compared to placebo treated infants (29). These authors acknowledge that the small size of their study groups may not have sufficient power to detect actual differences (Type II error), and they speculated that there would be an absolute increase in the prevalence of threshold ROP requiring cryotherapy because of the increased survival of VLBW infants. In a direct comparison of delivery room prophylaxis in 55 infants <30 weeks gestation to rescue treatment of RDS at 2–4 hr after birth in 50 infants, Merritt et al (30) found significantly more ROP> Stage 1 (13/55 prophylaxis versus 3/50 rescue; $p < .01$) (but no more frequent stage III, IV or plus disease) among infants treated prophylactically with human surfactant than among those treated after development of RDS.

Extremely low birthweight infants of 23–26 weeks or those <750g birthweight have not generally been included in randomized, placebo-controlled trials of surfactant efficacy. Stevenson et al (31) found among infants with birthweights 500–699g who were treated with Exosurf-Neonatal®, there was no improvement in overall survival, although there was a decrease in deaths attributable to RDS and an increase in pulmonary hemorrhage. Among infants 23–25 weeks treated by Allen et al with Infasurf® at birth, only 2% of infants born at 23 weeks gestation survived without severe abnormalities on cranial ultrasonography, as compared to 21% at 24 weeks and 69% at 24 weeks. These infants required 2–3 months of supplemental oxygen and retinopathy of prematurity occurred in 83% of those at 23 weeks versus 53% and 32% at 23 and 25 weeks gestation, respectively. Ferrara and coworkers (33) evaluated neurologic outcome of infants treated with Survanta® and a comparison group of untreated infants. Approximately 25% of infants 23–26 weeks gestation treated with Survanta® were developmentally normal at a mean adjusted age of 23 months. Among these extremely low birthweight infants, surfactant treatment appears to improve survival in some studies, but there is no evidence of improved neurodevelopmental outcome.

Two studies have reported serial lung function measurements performed in the neonatal period following surfactant replacement therapy (34,35). Both demonstrated that the use of surfactant was associated with improvement in pulmonary mechanics early in the neonatal period; however, by 28 days of age, there was no significant difference between surfactant or control infants. Among infants 26–29 gestation treated with Exosurf Neonatal® within 2 hours of birth, Yuksel and coworkers (36) found on evaluation at 6–12 months no differences in functional residual capacity or thoracic gas volume, but airway resistance and conductance were significantly improved among surfactant treated infants. These outcomes also were reported by Abbasi et al (37) in 47 infants treated with Exosurf Neonatal®. Among infants with mean birthweights near 1900g, follow-up pulmonary function testing at 3 to 6 months found no differences between clinical correlates of chronic lung disease. Similar to other reports, total pulmonary resistance was lower among surfactant treated infants. Resistive work of breathing was also lower for surfactant treated infants. Forced expiratory flow measurements demonstrated significant improvement in expiratory reserves and reduced evidence of airflow obstruction. These data, like those of Yuksel et al suggest that surfactant treatment for RDS is associated with beneficial effects on airflow resistive properties of premature infants at 9–12 months of age. Couser et al (38) evaluated 30/44 (68%) survivors treated with Survanta® and 17/35 (49%) of survivors in the placebo control group. Respiratory illnesses by questionnaire showed the Survanta® treated infants to have similar respiratory symptoms to control infants, although wheezing was more frequent in the control group ($p < 0.1$). Bronchitis was also less frequent in the Survanta® treated babies, but bronchopulmonary dysplasia was similar in both groups. There was no difference in pulmonary function tests at 2.5 years between the groups, suggesting that Survanta® neither improves pulmonary outcomes nor produces any long term adverse effects on the developing respiratory system.

A. Economics of Neonatal Intensive Care

Technological advances, including the use of novel and expensive pharmaceutical agents, have contributed to the dramatic rise in the cost of health care and have been blamed for the growing percentage of the gross national product spent on medical care (39). Concern over the cost of neonatal intensive care has raised questions concerning its cost-effectiveness; (40–42). The immediate cost for surfactant therapy is approximately $1000–2000 per treatment course. This is a small price to pay for an individual premature infant surviving from RDS; however, the costs to the parents, the medical insurer, and ultimately society are now being questioned in an era of prospective payment and "rationing" of health care (43). Surfactant therapy reduces individual infants' hospital charges from 5–25% in England, (44) and Maniscalco and coworkers (45) reported a mean reduction in hospital costs of approximately $13,500 per survivor (not including the cost of surfactant). This reduction primarily related to decreased ancillary charges ($p < 0.05$) for radiology, drugs, laboratory tests, although room charges were higher (~ $5,000), presumably reflective of the resultant longer average hospital stay among surfactant treated infants. These findings were supported by Sittington et al, (46) who reported that the introduction of surfactant increased the consumption of hospital resources (e.g. respiratory days, incubator use, parental nutrition days). Among infants <30 weeks gestation receiving a single dose of calf lung surfactant extract, Shennan et al (47) found a reduction of 27% ($p < 0.04$) in neonatal intensive care costs, along with a significant reduction of supplemental oxygen treatment ($p < 0.02$) and reduced mean NICU stay ($p < 0.014$). In Belfast, Tubman and Halliday (48) calculated that the cost for achieving an additional survivor with surfactant was £13,294 per survivor with cost per Quality Adjusted Life Year (QALY) per surviving surfactant treated infant of £690. These costs were generally similar to the cost of £10,000–15,000 for producing a surviving very low birth weight infant in other cities in the England area prior to the introduction of surfactant), therefore they concluded that surfactant use was cost neutral. These authors further argue that, when compared to the costs per infant QALY, surfactant is inexpensive compared to the costs of other medical interventions such as renal transplantation (£1400), single vessel coronary artery bypass grafting (£6000), or hemodialysis (£9000) (based on the 1990 £). This conclusion is in agreement with Mammel et al (49) who found that among 700–1350 g infants the mean cost for each extra survivor treated with surfactant was approximately $38,042. Given a life expectancy of 70 years, Mammel estimated that the true cost of surfactant therapy per QALY was $543/year. Among infants > 1350 gm birth weight, the savings per extra survivor was approximately $375,000 yielding a cost savings of over $5,000/ QALY (50). Furthermore, daily charges were significantly reduced in the surfactant treated group compared to controls. In a more recent analysis, Mugford et al (51) confirms the suspicion that the therapeutic success of surfactant will lead to a total increase in the cost of neonatal care because of costs of care for very low birth weight survivors and increased expenses for care for infants who still die but previously would have died sooner. While the cost per survivor would decrease the total cost of care in a cohort of infants <31 weeks gestation, surfactant treatment will increase the total cost of neonatal care (survivors + nonsurvivors) by 18 to 32% depending on drug costs. Soll and coworkers (52) reported among 210 infants randomized to prophylactic Survanta® or placebo that there was no significant difference in length of hospital stay or room charges during the first 28 days; however, cost per survivor was decreased by $3,404 using selective rescue treatment of infants with RDS. However, because of an 18% increase in survival, total costs (by day 28) were increased $4,442. Mugford and Howard (53) have reviewed costs expressed as total cost per 100 infants, cost per survivors, and additional costs or savings per additional survivor for studies using prophylaxis or rescue treatment. While preliminary data from Shennan et al suggested a cost savings with the prophylactic approach, most other groups have reported a cost of between £7000–9600 per additional survivor. For example, among infants >30 weeks gestation, prophylaxis was significantly more costly ($34,729/case) versus early rescue treatment ($27,367) (54). Mugford and Howard, however, found that for infants between 700–1500 g at birth the cost per additional survivor could range from a net savings of £6000 to a cost of £37,700.

Phibbs et al (55) examined the costs of care from independent randomized clinical trials evaluating Exosurf-Neonatal® using either prophylaxis or rescue therapy. Cost models were developed using multiple regression analysis to examine the effect of Exosurf-Neonatal® on total hospital costs (charges), cost per day, duration of stay, and mortality rate while controlling for the possible independent effects of birth weight, gestational age, sex, multiple birth, type of delivery maternal glucocorticoid therapy, and discharge to another hospital for recovery care.

Cost effectiveness analysis used regression models to assess the effects on cost and mortality rate for both prophylactic and rescue surfactant Exosurf-Neonatal therapy, and wholesale cost of drug was added to obtain net savings or net added costs. The cost and mortality effects of Exosurf-Neonatal therapy were estimated by calculating the predicted values from the regression models for the control cases as though they had received surfactant therapy. These predicted values were compared with the actual costs and mortality rates of the control groups to obtain the estimated effects of treatment. The estimated cost and mortality effects were compared to obtain a cost per life saved, where costs per life year saved was defined as the estimated change in treatment costs divided by the change in the number of survivors. They found that while prophylaxis increased costs by $8,000/case, rescue treatment saved $15,700. Costs per life saved over the first were reduced by $74,4000 in the rescue group but increased in the prophylactic infants and QALY analysis suggested a $1,200 savings/year for early treatment versus an additional cost of $1,200 for prophylaxis.

An analysis of resource use in Neonatal Intensive Care prior to surfactant use in 3922 infants was compared to costs of care in 1707 after surfactant had been approved (56). Infants in both groups had similar birthweight distributions although there was a 16% increase in the numbers of publicly funded patients in the surfactant era. Among infants <1250 grams birthweight, the odds of dying were reduced 30–40% with surfactant use and lethal bronchopulmonary dysplasia was reduced by 40%. Among survivors only the incidence of necrotizing enterocolitis and intraventricular hemorrhage increased, with the preponderance (70%) of bronchopulmonary dysplasia confined to male infants with an overall rate of 25% among survivors (increased by 3% over the pre-surfactant era).

Hospital costs were reduced by 8% among survivors, and by 31% among infants who died. Ancillary charges were reduced by 53% although length of stay was not altered. Schwartz and co-workers concluded on the basis of their analysis that the use of surfactant was associated with a national savings of approximately $90 million per annum, and that these cost savings more than offset the increased costs incurred by the increase in the number of low birth weight infants who now survive who would have otherwise died without surfactant.

Therefore costs/survivor are reduced by the use of surfactant and that overall costs per day in hospital may be reduced by infants being less dependent on expensive mechanical ventilation, associated respiratory care costs, and certain drugs. Cost savings are more pronounced in larger infants because the severity of the respiratory course is lessened. Clearly costs or savings from the initial hospitalization are simplistic because the long term costs of rehabilitation for handicapped children are not accounted for in these calculations. Furthermore, the majority of handicapped infants result from term birth.

As summarized above, more infants will survive with surfactant, and while the percentage of handicap or neurodevelopmental delay is not increased by surfactant, more surviving infants may well mean that overall costs, even when adjusted for the life span of all infants saved, may increase. Most parents and neonatologists, when given a choice about whether to opt for the benefit offered by surfactant, despite the possible risks for handicap among increased numbers of survivors, have welcomed surfactant's role in the NICU. Nonetheless, parents must be informed that surviving premature infants, even in the surfactant era, have significant rates of morbidity, handicap, and school-age dysfunction and that there are limits to our technological success. The ethical limitation of all possible therapy for these infants has been thoughtfully articulated by Silverman (57). The extremely high risk of impairment requiring extended health care is evident among infants 23–24 weeks gestation (20–28% have developmental quotients <70 at two years adjusted age and 14% have severe cerebral palsy) (58). Until data regarding the neurodevelopmental outcome at school age from infants 500–750 g at birth are known, as well as the economic reality confronting the health care and educational systems for such infants, extrapolation of the overall encouraging results in larger and more mature infants is not warranted. This increase in total cost for the care of very low birth weight infants would, therefore, be expected to offset any anticipated savings resulting from the decreased mortality and morbidity from larger weight infants resulting from surfactant. Eidelman (59) has estimated that the total additional cost to the US. health care system from the introduction of surfactant is between $280–350 million dollars, rather than the $90 million saved as reported by Schwartz et al. His estimate may be correct if one adds the total costs for public and mandated programs for the severely disabled. Supplemental Security Income provides approximately $477 per month (equivalent to $103,000 by age 18 using 1990 dollars) as mandated by the U.S. Supreme Court Zebley decision (60). Other special education programs coordinated through programs for all infants and children with special needs (not just premature infants) approach $500,000,000 annually (61), using rates of handicap from low birth weight infants treated prior to the introduction of exogenous surfactant (62).

The strategy of maternal administration of glucocorticoids before preterm delivery also effectively reduces the incidence of RDS (63–65). Egbert (66) found that a policy of combined glucocorticoid and prophylactic surfactant reduced costs by $19,500 per survivor contrasted to prophylactic surfactant alone and saved $14,000 contrasted to glucocorticoids alone. Surfactant treatment administered following maternal treatment with glucocorticoids was less costly than surfactant alone suggesting that the most cost effective approach requires perinatal and neonatal collaboration. If antenatal steroids were used in all women whose infants were likely to benefit and surfactant treatment alone was given to the remaining infants, Mugford et al (51) estimate that for gestations <35 weeks RDS cases and deaths would be reduced 36%. Costs of care for surfactant treatment and/or steroid pre treatment reduces cost by 1–10% for infants 31–35 weeks, but reduces costs up to 16% per survivor even if the cost of surfactant equals $950 per dose; however, with these cost savings in mind, the combined use of prenatal corticosteroids, as discussed by Jobe et al (67), decreases not only overall deaths, but deaths from RDS, air leaks, etc. improves infant outcome and saves money.

III. Summary

It is clear that surfactant treatment has reduced neonatal mortality in infants >700 g birth weight in multiple studies conducted throughout the world. Data are less clear regarding infants 500–699 g birth weight at gestational ages 23–25 weeks gestation, in whom mortality remains approximately 40–50% but in whom death is less frequently directly related to RDS. Surfactant treated babies fare at least as well, and with considerable cost saving both during initial hospitalization and thereafter when compared with control infants. No decisive data suggest that reduced mortality has been converted to either increased or decreased rates of handicap or developmental delay in infancy. Several trials suggest that the prevalence of cerebral palsy may be less in the surfactant treated groups; however, this claim must be viewed as preliminary. It is encouraging that there is no systematic trend towards greater incidence of surviving infants having abnormal neurodevelopmental outcome, lower Bayley or Griffiths scores, or increased rates of visual or auditory impairments because of surfactant treatment. It is noteworthy that Vaucher et al (68) found lower Bayley Scales Scores among infants treated in the delivery room, while others suggest that prophylactically treated infants develop less cerebral palsy.

The economic considerations of surfactant use are favorable compared to other medical interventions in adults. Analysis of costs reveals a savings based on cost/survivor from the placebo controlled trials because the denominator for the surfactant treated infants is larger. These savings are approximately $10,000 per survivor, not counting the costs of surfactant, reflecting lower costs for ancillary services such as radiology, laboratory, and other pharmaceuticals. Nonetheless, the costs for caring for the increased number of survivors still at risk for neurodevelopmental delay adds to overall health care costs. Societal costs for advances in medical care continue to be targeted for political criticism and public debate. However, parents and physicians continue to advocate for these tiny citizens, (69), and QALY costs for surfactant treatment of premature infants are among the most favorable of many medical or surgical interventions for adults. Data are missing for the long term cognitive function and school age performance especially for the tiniest infants presently saved as a result of contemporary neonatal intensive care, of which surfactant therapy is but a part. Continued assessment and surveillance of infants entered into the randomized, placebo controlled trials, the treatment IND phase, and newer uses of surfactant pre and post ECMO for conditions other than RDS continue to demand our attention.

References

1. Jobe AH. Pulmonary surfactant therapy. N Engl J Med 1993; 328:861–868.
2. Merritt TA, Hallman M, Vaucher Y, et al. Impact of surfactant treatment on cost of neonatal intensive care: A cost-benefit analysis. J Perinatol 1990; 10XX:416–419.
3. Zola EM, Overbach AM, Gunkel JH, et al. Treatment investigational new drug experience with Survanta (beractant). Pediatrics 1993; 92:546–531.
4. Wegman ME. Annual summary of vital statistics—1990. Pediatrics 1991; 88:1081–1092.
5. Wegman ME. Annual summary of vital statistics—1991. Pediatrics 1992; 90:835–845.
6. Pear R. US reports rise in low-weight births. New York Times; April 22, 1992, A12.
7. Horbar JD, Wright EC, Onstad L, et al. Decreasing mortality associated with the introduction of surfactant therapy: An observational study of neonates weighing 601–1300 grams at birth. Pediatrics 1993; 92:191–196.
8. Pope AM, Tarlow AR, eds. Disability in America. Toward a National Agenda for Prevention. Washington, DC: National Academy Press, 1991.
9. Lotze A, Knight R, Martin G, et al. Improved pulmonary outcome after exogenous surfactant therapy for respiratory failure in term infants requiring oxygenation extracorporal membrane oxygenation. J Pediatr 1993; 122:261–268.
10. Kliegman RM. Perpetual poverty: Childhood and the underclass. Pediatrics 1992; 89:710–713.
11. Fuchs VR, Reklis DM. America's children: Economic perspectives and policy options. Science 1992; 255:1–46.
12. Rosenblatt RA. The perinatal paradox: Doing more and accomplishing less. Health Affairs 1989; 8:153–168.
13. Lucey JF. The surfactant era: starting off right. Pediatrics 1991; 88:168.
14. McCormick MC. Has the prevalence of handicapped infants increased with improved survival of the very low birth weight infant? Clin Perinatol 1993; 20:263–77.

15. Eschobar GJ, Littenberg B, Petitti DB. Outcome among surviving very low birth weight infants: A met-analysis. Arch Dis Child 1991; 66:204–211.
16. McCormick MC, Brooks-Gunn J, Workman-Daniels K, et al. The health and developmental status of very low-birth-weight children at school age. JAMA 1992; 267:2204–2208.
17. McCormick M, Workman-Daniels K, Brooks-Gunn J, Peckham GJ. Hospitalization of very low birth weight children at school age. J. Pediatr 1992; 122:360–365.
18. Saigal S, Szatmari P, Rosenbaum P, et al. Intellectual and functional status at school entry of children who weighed 1000 grams or less at birth. A regional perspective of births in the 1980's. J Pediatr 1990; 116:409–416.
19. Collin M, Halsey C, Craig A. Emerging developmental sequelae in the "normal" extremely low birth weight infant. Pediatrics 1991; 88:115–120.
20. McCormick MC, Baker J, Brooks-Gunn J, et al. Cohort reconstruction: Which infants can be re-studied at school age? Paediatr Perinat Epidemiol 1991; 5:410–422.
21. Sauve R: Developmental outcome at one year of infants treated with Exosurf Neonatal. Long W, Tilson H, eds. Proceedings of the Exosurf Neonatal Investigators' Meeting, Langhorne, PA; Adis International, 1992.
22. Walter D, McGuinness G, Bose C, et al. The American Exosurf Neonatal Study Group I, and the Canadian Exosurf Neonatal Study Group: Double blind one-year follow up in 1,450 infants randomized to Exosurf Neonatal or air. Pediatr Res 1991; 29:270A.
23. Robertson G. The dilemmas of surfactant replacement. J Perinat Med 1991; 19: (Suppl 1):183–188.
24. Long, W. Synthetic surfactant. Semin Perinatol 1993; 17:275–284.
25. O'Shea M, Klinepeter K, deRegnier R-A, et al. Decreased risk of cerebral palsy (CP) with increasing use of surfactant therapy. Pediatr Res 1993; 33:269.
26. Dunn MS, Shennan AT, Hoskins EM, et al. Two year follow-up of infants enrolled in a randomized trial of surfactant replacement for prevention of neonatal respiratory distress syndrome. Pediatrics 1988; 82:543–547.
27. Rankin STA, Tubman TRAJ, Halliday HL. Surfactant and ROP incidence. Ophthalmology 1991; 98:1148–1149.
28. Repka MX, Hudak ML, Parsa CF, Tielsch JM. Calf lung surfactant extract prophylaxis and retinopathy of prematurity. Ophthalmology 1992; 99:531–536.
29. Repka MX, Hardy RJ, Phelps DL, Summers CG. Surfactant prophylaxis and retinopathy of prematurity. Arch Ophthalmol 1993; 111:618–620.
30. Merritt TA, Hallman M, Berry C, et al. Randomized, placebo-controlled trial of human surfactant given at birth versus rescue administration in very low birth-weight infants with lung immaturity. J Pediatr 1991; 118:581–594.
31. Stevenson D, Walther F, Long W. controlled trial of a single dose of synthetic surfactant at birth in premature infants weighing 500–699 g. J Pediatr 1992; 120–153 (Erratum 1992; 120:762).
32. Allen MC, Donohue PK, Dusman AE. The limits of viability—Neonatal outcome of infants born at 22–25 weeks' gestation. N Engl J Med 1993; 329:1597–1601.
33. Ferrara TB, Hoekstra RE, Couser RJ, Gaziano EP. Survival and follow up of infants born at 23–26 weeks of gestational age: Effects of surfactant therapy. J Pediatr 1994; 124:119–124.

34. Bhutani VK, Abbasi S, Long W, Gerdes J. Pulmonary mechanics and energetics in preterm infants who had respiratory distress syndrome treated with synthetic surfactant. J Pediatr 1992; 20:518–523.
35. Goldman SL, Bosque E, McCann E, Lewis K. Pulmonary mechanics one month after treatment with synthetic surfactant. J Pediatr 1992; 120:525–528.
36. Yuksel B, Greenough A, Gamsu HR. Respiratory function at follow-up after neonatal surfactant replacement therapy. Respir Med 1993; 87:217–221.
37. Abbasi S, Bhutani VK, Gerdes JS. Long-term pulmonary consequences of respiratory distress syndrome in preterm infants treated with exogenous surfactant. J Pediatr 1993; 122:446–452.
38. Couser RJ, Ferrara TB, Wheeler W, McNamara J, et al. Pulmonary follow-up 2.5 years after a randomized, controlled, multiple dose bovine surfactant study of preterm newborn infants. Pediatr Pulmonol 1993; 15:163–167.
39. Ellwood PM. Shattuck Lecture—Outcomes management: A technology of patient experience. N Engl J Med 1988; 318:1549–1556.
40. Boyle MH, Torrance GW, Sinclair JC, Horwood SP. Economic evaluation of neonatal intensive care of very-low-birth-weight infants. N Engl J Med 1983; 308:(92)1330–1337.
41. Hernandez JA, Offutt J, Butterfield J. The cost of care of the less than 1000 gram infant. Clin Perinatol 1986; 13:461–466.
42. Walker D-JB, Feldman A, Vohr BR, Oh W. Cost-benefit analysis of neonatal intensive care for infants weighing less than 1000 grams at birth. Pediatrics 1984; 71:20–26.
43. Steinbrook R, Lo B. The Oregon Medicaid Demonstration Project: Will it provide adequate medical care? N. Engl J Med 1992; 326:300–303.
44. Mugford M, Piercy J, Chalmers I. Cost implications of different approaches to the prevention of respiratory distress syndrome. Arch Dis Child. 1991; 66:757–764.
45. Maniscalco WM, Kendig JW, Shapiro DL. Surfactant replacement therapy: Impact on hospital charges for premature infants with respiratory distress syndrome. Pediatrics 1989; 83:1–6.
46. Sittington N, Tubman TRJ, Normand E. Cost of surfactant treatment in Belfast. Proceedings of the less than 30 weeks gestation. Pediatr Res 1989; 25:231A.
47. Shennan A, Dunn M, Possmayer F. Cost-effectiveness of single dose surfactant prophylaxis in infants of less than 30 weeks gestation. Pediatr Res 1989; 25:231A.
48. Tubman TRJ, Halliday, HL, Normand C. Cost of surfactant replacement treatment for severe neonatal respiratory distress syndrome: A randomized controlled trial. Br Med J 1990; 301:842–845.
49. Mammel M, Mullett M, Derleth DL, et al. Economic impact of two rescue doses of Exosurf® in 700–1350 gram infants. Pediatr Res 1991; 29:260A.
50. Schumacher R, Burchfield D, Vaughan R, et al. Economic impact two doses of Exosurf® neonatal in > 1350 gram infants. Pediatr Res 1991; 29:269A.
51. Mugford M, Piercy J, Chalmers I. Cost implications of different approaches to the prevention of respiratory distress syndrome. Arch Dis Child 1991; 87:587–597.
52. Soll RF, Jacobs J, Pashko S, Thomas R. Cost-Effectiveness of Beractant (Survanta®) in the prevention of respiratory distress syndrome. 1993. In press.

53. Mugford M, Howard S. Cost effectiveness of surfactant replacement in preterm babies. PharmacoEconomics 1993; 3:362–373.
54. Bloom BT, Delmore P, Katwinkel J. Surfactant prophylaxis increases costs >30 weeks. Pediatr Res 1994; 35:217A.
55. Phibbs C, Phibbs R, Wakeley A. cost effects of surfactant therapy for neonatal respiratory distress syndrome. J Pediatr 1993; 123:953–962.
56. Schwartz RM, Luby A, Scanlon J, Kellogg RJ. Effect of surfactant on morbidity, mortality and resource use in newborn infants weighing 500 to 1500 grams. N Engl J Med 1994; 330:1476–1480.
57. Silverman WA. Overtreatment of neonates? A personal retrospective. Pediatrics 1992; 90:971–976.
58. Whyte HE, Fitzhardinge PM, Shennan AT, et al. Extreme immaturity: Outcome of 568 pregnancies of 23–26 week's gestation. Obstet Gyn 1993; 82:1–7.
59. Eidelman AI. Economic consequences of surfactant therapy. J Perinatology 1993; 13:137–139.
60. Sullivan v Zebley, 88-1377 (US Supreme Court, 20 Feb 1990).
61. Perrin JM, Stein REK. Reinterpreting disability: Changes in supplemental security income for children. Pediatrics 1991; 88:1047–1051.
62. Hack M, Horbar SD, Malloy MH. Very low birth weight outcomes of the national institute of child health and human development neonatal network. Pediatrics 1991; 87:587–597.
63. Crowley P, Chalmers I, Keirse MJNC. The effect of corticosteroid administration before preterm delivery: An overview of the evidence from controlled trials. Br J Obstet Gynaecol 1990; 97:11–15.
64. Avery ME. The argument of prenatal administration of dexamethasone to prevent respiratory distress syndrome. J Pediatr 1984; 104:240.
65. Soll RF (ed). Overview 5206, 5207, 5252, 5253 Oxford. Oxford Database of Perinatal Trials, 1991.
66. Egberts J. Estimated costs of different treatments of the respiratory distress syndrome in a large cohort of preterm infants of less than 30 weeks gestation. Biol Neonate 1992; 61 (Suppl 1): 59–65.
67. Jobe AH, Mitchell BR, Gunkel JH. Beneficial effects of the combined use of prenatal corticosteroids and postnatal surfactant on preterm infants. Am J Obstet Gyncol 1993; 168:508–513.
68. Vaucher YE, Harker L, Merritt TA, et al. Outcome at twelve months of adjusted age in very low birth weight infants with lung immaturity: A randomized, placebo-controlled trial of human surfactant. J Pediatr 1993: 122;126–132.
69. Lee SK, Penner PIL, Cox M. Comparison of the attitudes of health care professionals and parents towards active treatment of very low birth weight infants. Pediatrics 1991; 88:110–114.

30

Postscript: Perspectives for the Future

BENGT ROBERTSON
Karolinska Institute
Stockholm, Sweden

H. WILLIAM TAEUSCH
University of California, San Francisco
and San Francisco General Hospital
San Francisco, California

I. Introduction

The principal aim of this volume has been to discuss state-of-the-art aspects of a novel approach to treatment of lung disease, which we believe will be of increasing importance in the future. However, the making of a book of this format is a comparatively slow process, at least in relation to the rapid development in the field. During the writing, editing, and printing of the 29 preceding chapters, new data have been accumulating continuously, new ideas generated, new possible targets for surfactant therapy identified, and new combinations of surfactant therapy and other clinical interventions explored. In this brief postscript, we would like to indicate areas where the perspective is changing most rapidly and where significant expansion of knowledge can be expected in the next few years.

II. Function of Surfactant Proteins and Development of New Artifical Surfactants

Modified natural surfactants, isolated from animal lung tissue or bronchoalveolar lavage fluid by extraction with organic solvents, are highly effective for clinical use, especially for treatment of babies with respiratory distress syndrome (RDS) (reviewed in Chapters 19 and 20). These surfactants contain only lipids and the hydrophobic proteins SP-B and SP-C (see Chapter 11), in proportions depending on the methods used for isolation of the product. As a logical extension of experimental and clinical studies documenting efficacy of such modified natural surfactants, several attemps have been made to develop entirely synthetic surfactant substitutes, based on dipalmitoylphosphatidylcholine (DPPC; either alone or in combination with other lipid constituents of natural surfactant) and synthetic homopolymeric or composite polypeptides mimicking the native hydrophobic proteins (1–7). One such peptide, KL_4, is made from repeated sequences of one lysine and four leucine residues (altogether 21 residues), simulating the hydrophobic and hydrophilic domains of the native SP-B molecule. An artificial surfactant based on this peptide is physiologically active in ventilated immature newborn rabbits (8) and rhesus monkeys (9) and has been tested in premature babies with RDS, with promising preliminary results (10). Interestingly, KL_4 surfactant is more resistant to inactivation by reactive oxygen species than are surfactants containing the native hydrophobic proteins (11).

Another amphipathic model peptide, made from 10 residues forming an α-helix, has recently been developed by McLean et al. (12); this artificial decapeptide seems to be physiologically active when mixed with DPPC but so far no clinical studies have been reported. SP-C and analogs of SP-C, produced by biotechnology or direct protein synthesis, respectively, have also been used for making artificial surfactant. Data from recent experiments indicate that the physiological activity of the peptides depends on their α-helical configuration (13), which seems to be a prerequisite for the interaction between the peptide and lipid membrane systems such as those present in native surfactant.

Recent work has focused on how the hydrophobic proteins enhance movement of phospholipids to the surface of alveoli. Hydrophobic peptides immediately associated with the monolayer apparently have the capacity of attracting phospholipids from the hypophase to the air-liquid interface, thereby increasing the surface pressure (14). Data from in vitro studies recently published by Taneva and Keough (15,16) furthermore indicate that although both SP-B and SP-C enhance movement of phospholipids to an air-water interface, SP-B may leave the lipid monolayer during compression (expiration) and aid recruitment of lipids into the surface during expansion (inspiration). However, the precise molecular interactions during these processes remain obscure. As explained elsewhere in this volume (Chapter 1), the adsorption of modified natural surfactants containing only polar lipids and hydrophobic proteins is extremely rapid and probably implies the simultaneous insertion of large numbers of surfactant lipid molecules (preferentially DPPC) into the monolayer (17).

Although many fundamental problems concerning the secondary structure of the natural and artificial hydrophobic polypeptides in their interaction with surfactant lipids remain to be solved, and methods used for "recombining" lipids with synthetic peptides in an artificial surfactant may need to be improved, we believe there will be a rapid development of new artificial surfactants based on synthetic analogs of SP-B or SP-C or on α-helical model amphipathic peptides. This development will probably be fueled by commercial interests and may soon result in a new generation of surfactant substitutes for clinical use.

These new artificial surfactants will have to be subjected to the same rigorous experimental evaluation and clinical trials as were employed during the development of currently used modified natural surfactants. Particular attention will have to be paid to the metabolic fate and clearance of artificial peptides or other nonnatural components of synthetic surfactants. Various constituents of modified natural surfactants are catabolized by different pathways and clearance rates (for review, see Ref. 18). For example, studies in adult rabbits indicate that clearance of DPPC is slow compared with that of SP-A, with half-life values in total lung of 12 and 6.5 hr, respectively (19). Only a few clearance studies in babies have been reported; Hallman et al. (20) found an apparent half-life of exogenous phosphatidylglycerol ranging from 20 to 36 hr independent of the dose of surfactant, suggesting no overloading of the clearance pathways. The half-life for SP-A in exogenous human surfactant administered to babies with RDS is about 9 hr (21).

The catabolism of hexadecanol and tyloxapol, the two nonnatural components of Exosurf, has been studied in animal experiments. Hexadecanol is apparently rapidly oxidized in the lungs to palmitic acid and then enters the pathways of intermediary lipid metabolism. Tyloxapol, on the other hand, is retained in the lungs for several days after tracheal instillation; it is released to the systemic circulation with a half-life of 5–6 days to be eliminated via fecal and urinary excretion (22). The metabolic fate of KL_4 and other model peptides in the lungs deserves to be investigated.

III. New Methods for Surfactant Delivery

Rapid instillation of exogenous surfactant as a bolus in the central airways, followed by a brief period of manual ventilation or direct reconnection of the tracheal tube to the ventilator system, results in a fairly uniform distribution of material in the lungs and seems to be the most effective mode of administration, judged from both animal experiments (23) and clinical experience (see Chapters 15 and 20). Nevertheless there is room for development of alternative methods for surfactant delivery, such as aerosolization, especially for neonatologists who want to treat babies during the early stage of RDS without a potentially painful intubation procedure. With the methods currently employed, large amounts of the aerosolized material are lost in the delivery system (see Chapter 15). On the other hand, it seems that the aerosolized material that actually enters the lungs is relatively more "active" than is the same amount administered conventionally, as a bolus. The "economy" of surfactant aerosolization can probably be improved by refining the systems for aerosol generation and conduction of the aerosol to the patient. Clinical trials of aerosolized surfactant for treatment of spontaneously breathing babies with RDS are expected in the near future.

Intra-amniotic administration of surfactant for prevention of RDS has been evaluated experimentally in animal models. A slight improvement of static pressure-volume properties was demonstrated in preterm fetal rabbits receiving Exosurf by this route (24), and after injection of Survanta into the amniotic cavity of immature fetal baboons, there was a modest improvement of oxygenation during a 24-hr period of mechanical ventilation beginning soon after birth (25). These effects were obtained with very large doses of surfactant (25 and 40 times larger than the recommended clinical dose, respectively), suggesting that for simple economical reasons this is not a rational approach to clinical prophylaxis of RDS.

IV. New Targets and Strategies for Surfactant Therapy

Exogenous surfactant is now part of the routine clinical management of babies with RDS requiring mechanical ventilation. As reviewed in Chapter 21 and indicated elsewhere in this volume, other potential targets for surfactant therapy include meconium aspiration syndrome, pneumonia, lung hypoplasia especially in babies with congenital diaphragmatic hernia, bronchiolitis, weaning from extracorporeal membrane oxygenation, adult respiratory distress syndrome (ARDS), and ARDS-like conditions in infants and children.

Despite initial positive results in small pilot studies (e.g., Ref. 26), surfactant treatment in ARDS is not as clearly effective as surfactant treatment of RDS in premature infants—presumably because ARDS is a disease wherein surfactant inactivation is more important than surfactant deficiency. Surfactant treatment of ARDS may become more effective when surfactants are produced specifically to overcome inactivation, perhaps by the addition of epitopes of SP-A (27). Weg and co-workers (28) recently published the first full report of a randomized trial of surfactant treatment for ARDS. A total of 51 patients with sepsis-induced ARDS were randomized to receive 12 or 24 hr of aerosolized Exosurf per day or saline. Ventilatory data and arterial blood gases were measured during 5 days of treatment and mortality was also assessed. There was a dose-dependent trend in reduction of mortality from 47% in the combined placebo groups to 41% and 35% in the groups treated with 12 and 24 hr of surfactant per day, respectively, but no statistically significant differences in physiological parameters between the groups. Data from ongoing randomized clinical trials of modified natural surfactant for treatment of ARDS are not yet available.

It has also been proposed that exogenous surfactant might prevent airway occlusion in patients with bronchiolar constriction associated with hypersecretion and thus have a therapeutic effect during acute asthma attacks. This new concept is supported by in vitro model experiments (29), observations in antigen-exposed immunized guinea pigs (30), and data from a clinical pilot study (31).

The advent of nitric oxide (NO) therapy for conditions wherein high pulmonary vascular resistance plays a role in neonatal lung disease (32) raises a number of questions regarding the interplay of NO and surfactant. Synergistic effects need to be further evaluated in animal models, and possible toxic effects of NO on various lipid and protein components of the alveolar surfactant film should be investigated before NO becomes part of the arsenal for routine clinical management of RDS, meconium aspiration syndrome, and other forms of lung disease.

Yet another new strategy for the treatment of neonatal lung disease is partial liquid ventilation using perfluorocarbon. The safety and efficacy of this approach have been documented in a recent clinical pilot study on newborn infants who did not repond well to surfactant therapy (33).

Most likely, the targets and strategies listed above will be actively explored in coming years, and we believe that surfactant replacement will eventually be used on indications wider than those applied today.

V. Neonatal Lung Pathology and Surfactant Replacement

Only a few reports have been published on lung pathology of infants with RDS treated with surfactant (34–36). These studies indicate no significant differences between surfactant-treated babies and controls except for a lower incidence of interstitial emphysema in treated babies (34), confirming clinical observations. We suggest that the lungs of babies and other patients who die after surfactant therapy should be carefully examined with standardized protocols to clarify the cause of treatment failure. Immunostaining with antibodies to surfactant proteins may be used to identify surfactant-producing cells in the lungs and to visualize distribution of exogenous surfactant. In addition, the localization of mRNAs for surfactant proteins can be studied by in situ hybridization. Fixation of the lungs under controlled distending pressure allows meaningful quantification of lung expansion in the histological sections and, hence, an evaluation of alveolar stability as influenced by surfactant treatment (37).

VI. Concluding Remarks

Despite the breadth of knowledge about surfactant function and the spectacular success in newborn infants with this therapy, understanding both of the molecular mechanisms explaining surfactant function and of the full clinical utility of this new therapy is limited. We anticipate that discoveries in the clinical areas will continue to foment discoveries in basic mechanisms of surfactant and vice versa. The most recent example is the finding of congenital SP-B deficiency (38–41) (see also Chapter 5) and the elucidation not only of the spectrum of resulting clinical disease, but also definition of the genetic processes responsible. Better understanding of basic mechanisms may result in an expanded understanding of lipid-protein interactions in cell membranes, of which surfactant may be viewed as a more liquid adaptation.

Initial investigations on the use of surfactant liposomes for delivery of additional therapeutic agents to the lung (42) have not yet reached clinical testing. The possibility of introducing plasmids for gene transfer to somatic cells is particularly attractive with regard to the lung because the distribution of the material in the air spaces can be enhanced using the dispersive properties of surfactant. Using surfactant with cationic liposomes to disperse DNA to animal lungs has been found to double transfection rates of a plasmid encoding full-length cDNA regulated by a cytomegalovirus promoter (43). The fullest expression of clinical utility may thus come from the use of surfactant, not only as therapy in its own right, but as a delivery means for an array of therapies directed at the lung.

References

1. Waring A, Taeusch W, Bruni R, et al. Synthetic amphipathic sequences of surfactant protein-B mimic several physicochemical and in vivo properties of native pulmonary surfactant proteins. Peptide Res 1989; 2:308–313.
2. Venkitaraman AR, Hall SB, Notter RH. Hydrophobic homopolymeric peptides enhance the biophysical activity of synthetic lung phospholipids. Chem Phys Lipids 1990; 53:157–164.
3. Baatz JE, Sarin V, Absolom DR, Baxter C, Whitsett JA. Effects of surfactant-associated protein SP-B synthetic analogs on the structure and surface activity of model membrane bilayers. Chem Phys Lipids 1991; 60:163–178.
4. Bruni R, Taeusch HW, Waring AJ. Surfactant protein B: lipid interactions of synthetic peptides representing the amino-terminal amphipatic domain. Proc Natl Acad Sci USA 1991; 88:7451–7455.
5. Revak SD, Merritt TA, Hallman M, et al. The use of synthetic peptides in the formation of biophysically and biologically active pulmonary surfactants. Pediatr Res 1991; 29:460–465.
6. Vincent JS, Revak SD, Cochrane CD, Levin IW. Interactions of model human pulmonary surfactants with a mixed phospholipid bilayer assembly: Raman spectroscopic studies. Biochemistry 1993; 32:8228–8238.
7. McLean LR, Lewis JE. Biomimetic pulmonary surfactants. Life Sci 1995; 56:363–378.
8. Cochrane CG, Revak SD. Pulmonary surfactant protein B (SP-B): structure-function relationships. Science 1991; 254:566–568.

9. Cochrane CG, Revak SD. Protein-phospholipid interactions in pulmonary surfactant. Chest 1994; 105(Suppl 3):57S–62S.
10. Cochrane CG, Revak SD, Cunningham D, et al. Efficacy of KL_4-surfactant in premature infants with RDS. Pediatr Res (abstract). In press.
11. Merritt TA, Amirkhanian JD, Helbock H, Halliwell B, Cross CE. Reduction of the surface-tension-lowering ability of surfactant after exposure to hypochlorous acid. Biochem J 1993; 295:19–22.
12. McLean LR, Lewis JE, Krstenansky JL, et al: An amphipathic α-helical decapeptide in phosphatidylcholine is an effective synthetic lung surfactant. Am Rev Respir Dis 1993; 147:462–465.
13. Johansson J, Nilsson G, Strömberg R, Robertson B, Jörnvall H, Curstedt T. Secondary structure and biophysical activity of synthetic analogues of the pulmonary surfactant polypeptide SP-C. Biochem J 1995; 307:535–541.
14. Oosterlaken MA, Haagsman HP, van Golde LMG, Demel RA. Characterization of lipid insertion into monomolecular layers mediated by lung surfactant proteins SP-B and SP-C. Biochemistry 1991; 30:10965–10971.
15. Taneva SG, Keough KM. Dynamic surface properties of pulmonary surfactant proteins SP-B and SP-C and their mixtures with dipalmitoylphosphatidylcholine. Biochemistry 1994; 33:14660–14670.
16. Taneva SG, Keough KM. Pulmonary surfactant proteins SP-B and SP-C in spread monolayers at the air-water interface. I. Monolayers of pulmonary surfactant protein SP-B and phospholipids. Biophys J 1994; 66:1137–1148.
17. Schürch S, Schürch D, Curstedt T, Robertson B. Surface activity of lipid extract surfactant in relation to film area compression and collapse. J Appl Physiol 1994; 77:974–986.
18. Jobe AH, Rider ED. Catabolism and recycling of surfactant. In: Robertson B, van Golde LMG, Batenburg JJ, eds. Pulmonary Surfactant. Amsterdam: Elsevier, 1992:313–337.
19. Ueda T, Ikegami M, Jobe AH. Clearance of surfactant protein A from rabbit lungs. Am J Respir Cell Mol Biol 1995; 12:89–94.
20. Hallman M, Merritt A, Pohjavurori M, Gluck L. Effect of surfactant substitution on lung effluent phospholipids in respiratory distress syndrome: evaluation of surfactant phospholipid turnover, pool size, and the relationship to severity of respiratory failure. Pediatr Res 1986; 20:1228–1235.
21. Hallman M, Merritt TA, Bry K. The fate of exogenous surfactant in neonates with respiratory distress syndrome. Clin Pharmacokinet 1994; 26:215–232.
22. DeAngelis RL, Findlay JWA. Metabolism of synthetic surfactants. Clin Perinatol 1993; 20:697–710.
23. Segerer H, van Gelder W, Angenent FWM, et al. Pulmonary distribution and efficacy of exogenous surfactant in lung-lavaged rabbits is influenced by the instillation technique. Pediatr Res 1993; 34:490–494.
24. Galan HL, Kuehl TJ. Effect of intra-amniotic administration of Exosurf in preterm rabbit fetuses. Obstet Gynecol 1992; 80:604–608.
25. Galan HL, Cipriani C, Coalson JJ, Bean JD, Collier G, Kuehl TJ. Surfactant replacement therapy in utero for prevention of hyaline membrane disease in the preterm baboon. Am J Obstet Gynecol 1993; 169:817–824.

26. Spragg RG, Gilliard N, Richman P. et al. Acute effects of a single dose of porcine surfactant on patients with the adult respiratory distress syndrome. Chest 1994; 105:195–202.
27. Yukitake K, Brown CL, Schlueter MA, Clements JA, Hawgood S. Surfactant apoprotein A modifies the inhibitory effect of plasma proteins on surfactant activity in vivo. Pediatr Res 1995; 37:21–25.
28. Weg JG, Balk RA, Tharratt RS, et al. Safety and potential efficacy of an aerosolized surfactant in human sepsis-induced adult respiratory distress syndrome. JAMA 1994; 272:1433–1438.
29. Enhorning G, Holm BA. Disruption of pulmonary surfactant's ability to maintain openness of a narrow tube. J Appl Physiol 1993; 74:2922–2927.
30. Kurashima K. Experimental and clinical study on surfactant inhalation therapy in bronchial asthma. J Juzen Med Soc 1991; 100:772–787 (in Japanese).
31. Kurashima K, Ogawa H, Ohka T, Fujimura M, Matsuda T, Kobayashi T. A pilot study of surfactant inhalation for the treatment of asthmatic attack. Jpn J Allergol 1991; 40:160–163.
32. Roberts J, Polander DM, Lang P, Zapol WM. Inhaled nitric oxide in persistent pulmonary hypertension of the newborn. Lancet 1992; 340:818–819.
33. Leach CI, Greenspan JS, Rubenstein SD, et al. Partial liquid ventilation with perfluorocarbon (LiquiVent): a pilot safety and efficacy study in premature newborns with severe RDS who have failed conventional therapy and exogenous surfactant. J Perinatol. In press.
34. Collaborative European Multicenter Study Group. A two year follow-up of babies enrolled in a European multicenter trial of porcine surfactant replacement for severe neonatal respiratory distress syndrome. Eur J Pediatr 1992; 151:372–376.
35. Pinar H, Makarova N, Rubin LP, Singer DB. Pathology of the lung in surfactant-treated neonates. Pediatr Pathol 1994; 14:627–636.
36. Thornton CM, Halliday HL, O'Hara MD. Surfactant replacement therapy in preterm neonates: a comparison of postmortem pulmonary histology in treated and untreated infants. Pediatr Pathol 1994; 14:945–953.
37. Robertson B. Surfactant replacement and neonatal lung pathology. In: Askin FB, Langston C, Rosenberg HS, Bernstein J, eds. Pulmonary Disease. Perspect Pediatr Pathol. Basel: Karger, 1995; 18:5–31.
38. Nogee LM, deMello DE, Dehner LP, Colten HR. Deficiency of pulmonary surfactant protein B in congenital alveolar proteinosis. N Engl J Med 1993; 328:406–410.
39. deMello DE, Nogee LM, Heyman S, et al. Molecular and phenotypic variability in the congenital alveolar proteinosis syndrome associated with inherited surfactant protein B deficiency. J Pediatr 1994; 125:43–50.
40. deMello DE, Heyman S, Phelps DS, et al. Ultrastructure of lung in surfactant protein B deficiency. Am J Respir Cell Mol Biol 1994; 11:230–239.
41. Hamvas A, Cole FS, deMello DE, et al. Surfactant protein B deficiency: antenatal diagnosis and prospective treatment with surfactant replacement. J Pediatr 1994; 125:356–361.
42. Kharasch VS, Sweeney TD, Fredberg J, et al. Pulmonary surfactant as a vehicle

for intratracheal delivery of technetium sulfur colloid and pentamidine in hamster lungs. Am Rev Respir Dis 1991; 144:909–913.

43. Kaser MR, Boncuk P, Taeusch HW. Enhanced expression of a human pulmonary surfactant apoprotein A cDNA plasmid in the adult rat lung using cationic liposomes mixed with Exosurf. Pediatr Res (abstract). In press.

AUTHOR INDEX

Italic numbers give the page on which the complete reference is listed.

B

C

D

E

F

G

H

I

J

K

N

O

Q

R

S

U

V

W

X

Y

Z

SUBJECT INDEX

D

I

K

L

M

Q

R

S

T

V

W

X